MEDICAL RADIOLOGY
Diagnostic Imaging

Editors:
A. L. Baert, Leuven
K. Sartor, Heidelberg

R. Lencioni
D. Cioni · C. Bartolozzi (Eds.)

Focal Liver Lesions

Detection, Characterization, Ablation

With Contributions by

A. Adam · T. Albrecht · V. Apell · R. S. Arellano · C. Bartolozzi · R Basilico · E. Batini
M. Bazzocchi · C. D. Becker · L. Bolondi · M. P. Bondioni · G. Brancatelli · L. Bonomo
F. Caseiro-Alves · M. Celestre · D. Cioni · M. Colombo · A. Conti · D. O. Cosgrove
L. Crocetti · C. Del Frate · C. Della Pina · A. D'Errico · F. Di Fabio · K. Eichler · J. Fasel
M. P. Federle · A. Ferreira · A. Filippone · D. A. Gervais · A. R. Gillams · J. A. Goode
L. Grazioli · R. M. Hammerstingl · T. K. Helmberger · M. Holtappels · K. M. Josten
C. Kuhnna · R. Lagalla · A. Laghi · T. Lehnert · R. Lencioni · S. Leoni · J. Lera · K. H. Link
P. Loubeyre · M. Mack · P. Majno · D. Mathieu · G. Mentha · M. Midiri · M. Mörschel
S. Montagnani · P. Morel · K. Mortelè · P. R. Mueller · P. Paolantonio · R. Passariello
F. Piscaglia · R. Pozzi-Mucelli · E. Rocchi · G. Ronchi · T. Sabharwal · T. A. Sagban
I. Sansoni · W. Schima · W. V. Schwarz · L. Staib · R. Straub · S. Terraz · R. Thimm
K. Tischbirek · A. Venturi · V. Vilgrain · T. J. Vogl · T. F. Weigel · K. Zayed · C. Zuiani

Foreword by

A. L. Baert

With 268 Figures in 727 Separate Illustrations, 83 in Color and 39 Tables

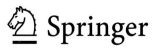
Springer

Riccardo Lencioni, MD
Dania Cioni, MD
Carlo Bartolozzi, MD
Division of Diagnostic and Interventional Radiology
Department of Oncology, Transplants, and Advanced Technologies in Medicine
University of Pisa
Via Roma 67
56126 Pisa
Italy

Medical Radiology · Diagnostic Imaging and Radiation Oncology
Series Editors: A. L. Baert · L. W. Brady · H.-P. Heilmann · M. Molls · K. Sartor

Continuation of Handbuch der medizinischen Radiologie
Encyclopedia of Medical Radiology

Library of Congress Control Number: 2004110091

ISBN 3-540-64464-4 Springer Berlin Heidelberg New York

Springer is a part of Springer Science+Business Media

http//www.springeronline.com
© Springer-Verlag Berlin Heidelberg 2005
Printed in Germany

Medical Editor: Dr. Ute Heilmann, Heidelberg
Desk Editor: Ursula N. Davis, Heidelberg
Production Editor: Kurt Teichmann, Mauer
Cover-Design and Typesetting: Verlagsservice Teichmann, Mauer

Printed on acid-free paper   21/3150xq – 5 4 3 2 1 0

Foreword

The radiological diagnosis and management of focal liver lesions is a common problem confronting many radiologists in their daily clinical activity.

Moreover, during recent years numerous new developments have taken place in the non-invasive diagnosis of focal liver lesions due to the rapid progress in the cross-sectional modalities: ultrasonography, computed tomography and magnetic resonance imaging.Parallel to these important diagnostic advances, several innovative techniques for the percutaneous radiological management of malignant focal liver lesions have been introduced in clinical practice.

This volume comprehensively covers all these new and fascinating radiological techniques both in the diagnostic and the therapeutic field and represents an excellent up-to-date review of our current knowledge on the radiological approach to focal liver lesions. The eminently readable text is complemented by numerous superb illustrations.

The editors are world-renowned experts in the field with a longstanding dedication to imaging of the liver and percutaneous treatment of malignant liver lesions, as proven by their highly praised previous scientific work, including handbooks, book chapters and numerous articles on liver radiology .The department of diagnostic and interventional radiology of the University of Pisa is internationally known for its fundamental and innovative research activities in liver imaging and ablation techniques.

The authors of the individual chapters were invited to participate because of their outstanding experience and major contributions to the radiological literature on the topic.

I would like to thank the editors and the authors and congratulate them most sincerely for their superb efforts which have resulted in this excellent volume, a much-needed comprehensive update of our knowledge of focal liver lesions .This book will be of great interest not only for general and gastrointestinal radiologists but also for abdominal surgeons and gastroenterologists. I am confident that it will meet the same success with the readers as the previous volumes published in this series.

Leuven   ALBERT L. BAERT

Preface

Few fields of medicine have witnessed such impressive progress as the diagnosis and treatment of liver tumors. Advances in imaging technology, the development of novel contrast agents, and the introduction of optimized scanning protocols have greatly facilitated the non-invasive detection and characterization of focal liver lesions. Furthermore, image-guided techniques for percutaneous tumor ablation have become an accepted alternative treatment for patients with inoperable liver cancer.

This book provides a comprehensive and up-to-date overview of the role of diagnostic and interventional radiology in respect of liver tumors. The volume moves from background sections on methodology and segmental liver anatomy to the main sections on the diagnosis of benign and malignant liver lesions. An integrated approach, focused on the correlation of ultrasound, CT, and MR imaging findings, is presented. Finally, an exhaustive section describes the principles, methods, and results of percutaneous tumor ablation techniques.

The volume is the expression of the efforts of many distinguished experts from throughout the world. We are greatly indebted to them for their enthusiastic commitment and support. Also, we would like to thank most sincerely the Medical Radiology series editor, Professor Albert Baert, for his confidence and advice. We sincerely hope that the book fulfills the expectations of our colleagues – radiologists, clinicians, and surgeons – who are interested in this important and rapidly evolving field.

Pisa

RICCARDO LENCIONI
DANIA CIONI
CARLO BARTOLOZZI

Contents

Technique and Methodology
in Liver Imaging

1 Ultrasound and Contrast Ultrasound

David O. Cosgrove

CONTENTS

1.1
Introduction

Ultrasound is a tomographic imaging technique that can provide anatomical and functional images with high resolution and great flexibility at low cost (KREMKAU 1997; McDICKEN 1991). Structural detail down to around a millimetre is available without the need for contrast agents (Fig. 1.1). The high intrinsic contrast is produced by the tissues' structure at a submillimetre level and is chiefly attributable to the differences in rigidity and density between fluids, watery tissue, connective tissue and fat. The tomograms are formed very rapidly, allowing real time imaging so that studies are quick and interactive. Immediate viewing of tissue motion is intrinsic to ultrasound imaging; examples include the effects of respiration or palpation and the direct visualisation of the position of a biopsy needle (PEDERSON et al. 1993). The tomograms can be taken in any plane, allowing optimal display of critical anatomy and pathology. Small, self-contained scanners can be made and these can be taken to the patient's bedside (MACHI and SIGEL 1996). No or minimal preparation is required so that

D. O. COSGROVE, MD
Department of Imaging Sciences, Imperial College School of Medicine, Hammersmith Hospital, 150, Du Cane Road, London W12 0HS, UK

the procedure is well tolerated, the only practical problem for the liver being abdominal tenderness that may make probe contact painful. The hazards of ionising radiation do not exist and the acoustic powers used in diagnosis appear to be completely safe, though there are emerging concerns over the possibility that its interaction with the microbubbles used as contrast agents may produce free radicals that could be injurious.

The flexibility of ultrasound technique has led to several specialised applications. Small transducers can be mounted on an endoscope with the advantage that higher quality images are obtained because higher frequency ultrasound can be used (BEZZI et al. 1998). Endoscopic ultrasound is, of course, somewhat invasive and only tissues with a few centimetres of the gut wall are accessible. The same is true of intravascular ultrasound. Small transducers suitable for use in the operating theatre offer the benefit of higher resolution as well as of guiding needle placement for biopsies or cannulation of small portal vein branches while the development of transducers small enough to fit into standard laparoscopic instruments extends these advantages to minimally invasive surgery (HERMAN 1996; BARBOT et al. 1997; KLOTTER et al. 1986).

Doppler has extended the role of ultrasound in the diagnosis and management of vascular pathology of the liver and is now an indispensable component of hepatic imaging (GRANT 1992). It is particularly helpful in liver transplants, both pre-operatively [to establish portal vein (PV) and caval patency] and post-operatively (for the PV and hepatic artery) and in the Budd Chiari syndrome. In cirrhosis Doppler can establish the patency of the PV and of many types of shunts. For spectral (pulsed) Doppler, a sensitive gate is positioned over a vessel and the temporal pattern of flow analysed to display its velocity spectrum; volume flow can also be estimated, though with less precision (Fig. 1.2). In colour Doppler, a vascular map is presented as an overlay on the grey scale scan to provide a form of angiogram that gives a non-invasive picture of vascular anatomy (Fig. 1.3)

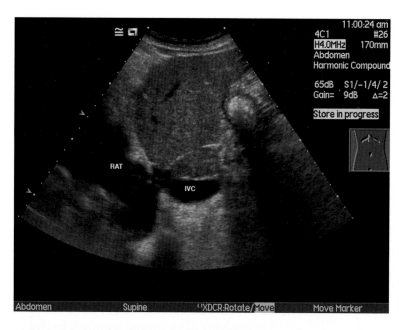

Fig. 1.1. In a sagittal section through the left liver, the caudate lobe (segment 1) can be seen posterior to segments 2 and 3. Note the fine stippled texture of the liver's parenchyma. *IVC*, inferior vena cava; *RAT*, right atrium

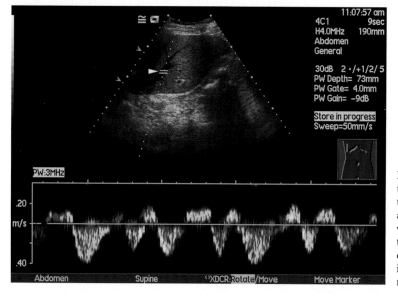

Fig. 1.2. In this spectral Doppler tracing the sensitive gate has been placed over the middle hepatic vein (*arrowhead*) and the trace shows the normal pattern where the predominant flow towards the heart (shown below the line to indicate flow away from the transducer) is interrupted by reverse flow as blood is returned to the liver in cardiac systole

(FOLEY and LAWSON 1992). Though the haemodynamic information is limited (only mean velocity or, in power Doppler, the number of moving red cells, is presented) the anatomical information gained is an extremely valuable addition to imaging. Colour and spectral Doppler are complementary, the former providing images, the latter functional information on blood flow.

However, this description omits some important limitations to the uses of ultrasound. Image quality is affected by body habitus, slim patients giving the best images because resolution deteriorates with depth as

inevitable result of the greater attenuation of higher frequencies; for this reason ultrasound is particularly valuable in paediatrics. This problem has been reduced by the development of non-linear (tissue harmonic) imaging and by the increasing bandwidth of newer transducers so that the most appropriate frequency can be selected electronically (KONO et al. 1997). Bone and gas are impenetrable; in practical terms this is only an occasional problem for the liver because the intercostal spaces allow adequate access in almost all patients if the subcostal route is difficult to use.

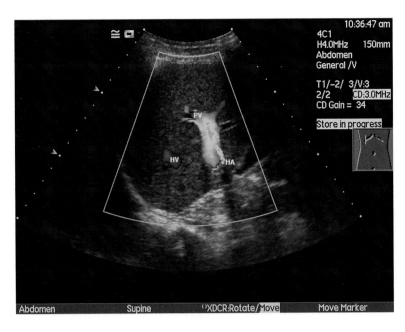

Fig. 1.3. In colour Doppler, flow towards the transducer is coded in reddish tints so that both the portal vein and the hepatic artery have similar colours. Hepatic vein branches are seen in blue. *HA*, hepatic artery; *HV*, hepatic vein; *PV*, portal vein

The small field of view of a real time ultrasound image makes the scan difficult to review and can also lead to difficulty in repeating the same tomogram for follow-up. It makes explanation to referring physicians and surgeons difficult; understandably, they find the more complete tomographic images of CT or MR more believable. Extended field of view displays have been introduced to minimise this limitation. Another interesting approach is to superimpose the real time ultrasound images on the appropriate slice derived from a previous 3D CT scan of the patient using. This virtual image co-registration is very promising for interventional applications such as tumour ablation because it combines the anatomical display of the CT with the interactiveness of ultrasound (BRYANT et al. 2004).

The interactive nature of ultrasound renders it very operator dependent: a skilled and motivated operator can produce consistently good results but lack of experience and working without essential clinical information can severely devalue a study.

Recent technological developments have reduced some of these limitations. Tissue harmonic imaging, by selecting returning echoes at double the transmitted signals (these are generated as the ultrasound pulse propagates through the tissue, rather like the breaking of a wave as it approaches the shore), reduces the artefacts from heavily built patients and gives cleaner images. Intravascular contrast agents in the form of microbubbles not only rescues Doppler studies that would otherwise have been failures but also opens out important new diagnostic possibilities. Application of sophisticated transducer technologies and of powerful computer systems has resulted in better image and particularly Doppler quality.

Thus ultrasound is continuing to develop rapidly and its progress shows no sign of slowing down.

1.2
Technology

Ultrasound is a high frequency, mechanical vibration consisting of alternate waves of compression and rarefaction (KREMKAU 1997; McDICKEN 1991). The waves are generated by piezo-electric crystals shaped into a transducer which focuses the ultrasound waves into a beam. Commonly used frequencies for the liver are 5.0 or 3.5 MHz corresponding to wavelengths in tissue of 0.3 and 0.5 mm respectively, and this is the theoretical best spatial resolution that can be achieved.

The small proportion of the ultrasound that is absorbed by the tissue disappears as heat. The remainder is reflected as the beam crosses between tissues of different acoustic properties, known as acoustic impedance, a complex of tissue density and rigidity. Both these components are familiar in that they are palpable; however, the ultrasound pulse responds to tissue structure in the sub-millimetre range. The smallest structure that can be resolved in practice depends on the contrast in reflectivity: well-defined structures such as ducts can be traced down to a millimetre or so in calibre but low contrast lesions such as liver metastases must be much larger, perhaps 5–10 mm in diameter before they can be detected confidently.

The portion of the reflected sound beam that returns to the transducer is used to form the image. The depth (range) of a reflecting interface is calculated from the delay between the sending of the pulse and the detection of the returning echo, and its direction from the angle at which the transducer faces; this is the same "pulse-echo" method used in Radar and Sonar. The velocity of ultrasound in different tissues is not quite constant but varies so little that the minor errors in calculating the depth of reflecting surfaces can be ignored.

The strength of the echoes is proportional to the change in acoustic impedance at the interface. At risk of oversimplifying a complex phenomenon, the acoustic impedance correlates with tissue rigidity. In the body this ranges from gases at the one extreme, through fluids and soft tissue, to bone and calcified tissue at the other. For soft tissues, the collagen content is usually the main contributor and this is found in a condensed form in fascia and in a diffuse form as the micro-skeleton of the parenchyma that surrounds blood vessels. It is probably the characteristic vascular pattern as reflected in the ultrasound image that lends tissue-specific textures to sonograms. Fatty tissue is strongly echogenic because of the abundant lipid/watery interfaces at cellular or lobular level.

Real time scanners rapidly sweep the beam through the volume of tissue to be examined: the scan is repeated 10–30 times a second to give a moving image. The sweep may be angled from a point on the skin to form a triangular image in sector scanning. This method provides good access through small windows and so is particularly useful for intercostal scans of the liver. However, the triangular field of view does not display superficial structures well and linear arrays are more convenient in this respect. Here the ultrasound beam is swept electronically along a block of piezo-electric material some 2 cm wide and 5–10 cm long. Curved linear arrays combine some of the advantages of the two geometries and is used for all the ultrasound images shown in this chapter.

For Doppler a different type of signal processing is used to assess the movement of blood. By comparing the signals from a series of perhaps ten pulses sent along the same direction, changes caused by a moving structure (typically red blood cells) can be extracted. The slower the flow the more pulses must be transmitted and this, as well as the fact that solid tissues also move, sets a limit to the sensitivity of Doppler. The display shows motion along the line of the beam and so a correction for flow in oblique directions needs to be applied for flow velocity measurements. The spectrum from a pulsed Doppler scanner is displayed as a chart of (blood) velocity against time, in which flow towards the transducer is shown above the zero line. The amount of blood flowing at any particular point is indicated by the degree of whitening of the trace. Simultaneous imaging and Doppler (known as "duplex scanning", from their operation in two modes) allows the Doppler sensitive gate to be positioned precisely over the vessel of interest (Fig. 1.2).

In colour Doppler, similar processing is applied across the image. The colour Doppler signals are shown as an overlay conventionally coded in shades of red for flow towards, and blue for flow away from the transducer (Fig. 1.3). Another way to display flow information depicts only the Doppler signal intensity as a power Doppler scan. It has higher sensitivity than frequency-based colour Doppler but lacks directional information and so is more useful for the small vessels, for example, in tumours, than for the portal vein where flow direction is important.

Ultrasound guided biopsies make use of the real-time interactiveness of ultrasound (CHUAH 2000). It may be used to plan the biopsy by marking the appropriate skin site for puncture; this is useful for simple procedures such as paracentesis where the main value of ultrasound is to check that loops of bowel in the ascites will not be punctured. For biopsy guidance two general approaches are the freehand and needle-guided methods. The former is simpler in that any transducer can be used. The needle site and path are chosen and the needle (or its tip) is monitored continuously as it is advanced into the lesion. Keeping the needle path in view requires a high degree of hand/eye co-ordination and is not feasible for small or deep lesions where the needle guide approach is more reliable. For this, an attachment to the probe with a needle channel constrains the needle along a path that runs diagonally across the scan area; its line is indicated on screen and, once this has been positioned over the lesion, the needle should pass in the correct direction.

To make a scan the transducer is contacted to the skin using a coupling gel, and the examination consists of moving the probe gently across the surface of the abdomen. For the liver, subcostal views in transverse and longitudinal directions are convenient and access may be improved if the patient holds a deep breath. No preparation is needed for liver scans but the gallbladder is easier to assess when distended in the fasting state.

For Doppler the main constraint is the fact that the signals are angle dependant, being maximal when flow is in the direction of the ultrasound beam and falling off with a cosine function to zero when the flow is at right angles to the beam. Thus, choice of the scanning angle is critical to obtaining good Doppler signals and avoiding misdiagnosis of absence of flow (PARVEY et al. 1989). For quantitative velocity and volume flow measurements the beam-to-vessel angle must be measured; scanners are equipped with appropriate calculation packages to transform the Doppler shift into true linear velocity and to calculate the mean velocity from the spectrum of the velocities in the Doppler gate.

1.3
Microbubble Contrast Agents

Microbubbles represent a new class of contrast agent whose effects depend on the compressibility of gasses which is markedly different from the near-incompressibility of tissue (GOLDBERG 1997; STRIDE and SAFFARI 2003; DAWSON et al. 1999). This difference can be exploited using multipulse sequences that cancel tissue signals and emphasise those from the microbubbles. As well as displaying major vessels, microbubbles within the microvasculature can be detected because these methods do not depend on microbubble flow but merely on their presence. In practice these specific modes have found major clinical application in the liver for detecting and characterising focal lesions.

Microbubbles are also ideal tracers because of the small injected volumes and this has been exploited in the liver to identify conditions characterised by arteriovenous shunting such as cirrhosis and metastases: an early hepatic vein transit time indicates a haemodynamic abnormality (BLOMLEY et al. 1998). The dynamics of the wash-in and wash-out phases following a bolus injection can be calculated and used to form functional images which are truly quantitative (ECKERSLEY et al. 1998).

1.3.1
Principles

The microbubbles used as ultrasound contrast agents are designed to be smaller than 7 µm in diameter so that they can cross capillary beds. These agents flood the blood pool after iv injection and are confined to the vascular compartment (unless there is ongoing bleeding). Both the gas they contain (usually air or a perfluoro compound) and the stabilising shell (denatured albumin, surfactants or phospholipids) are critical to their effectiveness as contrast agents and to rendering them sufficiently stable that they survive for several minutes after injection. The first widely used agent, Levovist (Schering, Berlin), is made of galactose microcrystals whose surfaces provide nidation sites on which air bubbles form when they are suspended in water; these microbubbles are then stabilised by a trace of the surfactant palmitic acid. A widely used albumen coated agent, Optison (GE-Amersham, UK), is filled with perfluoropropane, while a family of perfluoro gas-containing agents such as SonoVue (Bracco, Milan) and perflutren (Definity, Bristol, Meyers, Squibb, Billerica, NJ) that use phospholipids as the membrane are becoming important in clinical practice.

1.3.2
Interactions of Microbubbles with Ultrasound Waves

The change in density at the surface of a bubble in plasma forms a major impedance mismatch and the strong echoes this produces is exploited in the uses of microbubbles to improve Doppler studies, so-called Doppler rescue.

However, more specific responses of microbubbles to ultrasound arise because microbubbles undergo pulsatile contraction and expansion in the pressure changes of the ultrasound field (MINE 1998). All oscillating systems have a resonance frequency at which they vibrate most readily. For clinical microbubbles this turns out to correspond to the frequencies typically used in diagnostic ultrasound (2–10 MHz) and this is why they are so intensely reflective. These oscillations are symmetrical (i.e. their behaviour is "linear") at low ultrasound powers so that the frequency of the scattered signals is the same as the transmitted pulse. However, microbubbles resist compression more strongly than expansion so that, as the acoustic power is increased, the expansion and contraction phases become unequal and in this "non-linear" mode the returning signals contain multiples of the transmitted frequency (harmonics). At still higher powers (though within accepted limits for diagnostic imaging), highly non-linear behaviour occurs and the microbubbles may be disrupted and disappear from the sound field.

These harmonics can be detected by tuning the scanner's receiver circuitry to the second harmonic at double the transmitted frequency so that the harmonics can be separated from the fundamental signals. However, tissues also produce harmonics, especially when higher acoustic powers are used, and distinguishing between them is challenging; in practice in many of the simple contrast modes available, the two signals are inextricably mixed together.

Separating tissue from microbubble harmonics completely has been achieved in two ways. The high MI approach was the first to be discovered (Burns et al. 1995). The microbubbles are deliberately disrupted and visualised using colour Doppler or variations of it. The sudden disappearance of a signal from its previous location (loss of correlation between sequential echoes) is detected as a major Doppler shift and is registered as colour signals. Known as stimulated acoustic emission (SAE), it is particularly useful with contrast agents that show liver tropism in the late phase a few minutes after injection such as Levovist. Because it highlights the normal liver and spleen, lesions that do not contain functioning tissue, such as malignancies, are shown as colour voids. It is a very sensitive method and shows the microbubble signature exclusively in the colour layer overlain over the conventional grey scale image. However, the contrast agent is destroyed rapidly so real time scanning cannot be used, and a rather clumsy sweep-and-review approach has had to be been developed.

The alternative approach relies on the property of newer microbubbles, particularly those with phospholipid shells, to produce harmonics at much lower acoustic powers than are necessary to generate tissue harmonics (Burns 1996; Burns et al. 2000). Thus, when very low acoustic powers are used, the harmonics derive exclusively from microbubbles so that they can be separated from all tissue signals.

The phase inversion mode (PIM) was the first of these modes and was developed to avoid frequency filtering with which the narrower bandwidth degrades spatial resolution. In the PIM, a pair of pulses is sent along each scan line, the second being inverted in phase from the first. The returning echoes from the pair are summed so that the linear echoes cancel because they are out of phase, leaving only the nonlinear components, mainly the second harmonic. PIM gives excellent quality images in both vascular and late phases. In its initial implementation, the PIM used a high MI and therefore tissue harmonics contaminated the microbubble signals. At the low powers needed to avoid tissue harmonics the image tends

to become noisy and methods to minimise this have been developed. One approach is to send a stream of pulses with alternating phase and use colour Doppler circuitry to pick out the harmonics; essentially this method (known as power pulse inversion, PPI, and implemented on the Philips HDI 5000) exploits the high sensitivity of Doppler to overcome the signal-to-noise limitation. It has the advantage of displaying the microbubble image in the colour plane with the tissue image as a grey scale underlayer, in the same way as colour Doppler and allows either image to be viewed separately.

Another approach also uses a series of pulses, typically three per line, but here the amplitude of the pulses is changed as well as the phase; this preserves more of the non-linear content of the received signals and thus improves sensitivity. Implemented as contrast pulse sequences (CPS, Siemens Sequoia), the harmonics are displayed in a colour tint over the B-mode picture or as a split screen so that both can be viewed as required. In another approach the direction of flow in larger vessels is detected with low MI Doppler, while slow moving and stationary microbubbles are detected with a phase inversion sequence and depicted in green. This combined mode, known as 'vascular recognition imaging' (Toshiba Aplio), also allows the microbubble signature to be displayed separately from or combined with the B-mode and provides additional information on the flow direction in larger vessels.

All of these modes allow simultaneous display of the microbubble and tissue images. They operate at very low transmit powers and, as well as avoiding excitation of tissue harmonics, this has the important advantage that bubble destruction is minimised so that scanning can be in real time which makes contrast studies much easier to perform since no special scanning techniques are required.

1.3.3
Safety of Microbubbles

The safety of ultrasound contrast agents must be considered under two categories, the agents themselves and the effects of their interaction with the ultrasound beam (ter Haar 1999). The constituents of microbubble contrast agents have been carefully chosen to be inert with biocompatible membranes and gases that are either metabolised (oxygen in air-filled microbubbles) or breathed out (nitrogen, perfluorocarbons and sulphur hexafluoride) and are non-toxic. No toxic effects have been attributed to their components. However, they are a form of particle and there is the possibility that they embolize, blocking microvessels though any blockage is likely to be transient since they dissolve within a few minutes of injection. Nevertheless, the product characteristics summary usually recommends caution in patients with severe heart failure or pulmonary hypertension. A well recognised though uncommon adverse event after injection of many microbubble agents is low backache; it has been suggested that this arises from microbubble emboli, either in the kidneys or in bone marrow. Some are hypertonic when reconstituted and this can cause pain at the site of injection.

Much more important is the possibility of harm arising from the interactions of ultrasound with the microbubbles. This may be mechanical or chemical. Microbubbles can expand to twice their resting diameter during the low pressure phase of the ultrasound wave and this has been shown to rupture capillaries in animal microscopy studies. While capillary rupture is a normal event (coughing and running usually rupture lung and foot capillaries), the possibility that this might cause permanent damage in some tissues such as the brain cannot be excluded. During the rebound from their expansion, microbubbles may collapse and fragment and in this phase very high temperatures can be reached. Though the heating is extremely short lived, surrounding molecules can be altered to release highly active free radicals such as atomic oxygen and ozone. These reactive species can damage macromolecules such as RNA and DNA. Free radicals are produced naturally by chemical and nuclear processes such as cosmic rays and cells are equipped with mechanisms that rapidly neutralise them. It is not clear whether free radical formation from microbubbles is actually harmful or not.

Sensible precautions suggest that the lowest dose and the lowest transmit powers consistent with the need to make a diagnosis – the "as low as reasonably attainable" (ALARA) principle – should be used.

1.4
Normal Appearance

The uniform stippled liver texture is interrupted by vessels which help define its segmental anatomy (Fig. 1.1) (COUINAUD 1957). The hepatic veins, with their thin walls, appear as branching, tubular "defects" converging to the upper IVC. The portal tracts have strongly reflective walls from the associated vessels and fibrous tissue(WACHSBERG et al. 1997). The left portal vein curves anteriorly from the main portal vein to supply the more anteriorly situated left liver. The liver vessels are clearly displayed by colour Doppler using conventional colour coding, normal hepatopetal flow is shown in red (Fig. 1.3). The accompanying artery is seen as a narrow red line lying anteriorly (LAFORTUNE and PATRIQUIN 1999). On spectral Doppler the portal vein has continuous flow with a peak velocity of some 15 cm/s while fasting; this can increase greatly in the postabsorptive state. The hepatic veins appear as blue bands on colour Doppler because their flow is away from the transducer. On spectral Doppler their flow pattern is complex being predominantly towards the IVC but reversed at each atrial systole (Fig. 1.2). This is because the IVC communicates directly with the right atrium, so that in systole blood is pumped retrogradely into the cava and hepatic veins.

1.5
Focal Lesions

A wide variety of focal liver lesions can be diagnosed by ultrasound, notably cysts, for which it is the most specific and sensitive test (GAINES and SAMPSON 1989). They are seen as echo-free spherical spaces with thin, smooth walls and a characteristic band of brighter liver distally, caused by the lower attenuation of ultrasound by their fluid compared to the liver (Fig. 1.4) (BRYANT et al. 2004). The same appearance characterises the individual cysts of dominant polycystic disease except that they may be very numerous (KUNI et al. 1978). The lesions themselves and the heterogeneous liver texture that results from the numerous bands of increased sound transmission make the detection of co-existent liver disease difficult or impossible. Similarly, haemorrhage into a cyst or superinfection are not usually detectable with ultrasound.

Hydatid cysts have a variety of appearances depending on the condition of their contents, but consistently have a prominent capsule that is lacking around simple cysts (HADDAD et al. 2001). In endemic countries, ultrasound guided aspiration (perhaps with injection of a sclerosant) is widely used for symptomatic control with good safety (FILICE and BRUNETTI 1997). Abscesses are typically seen as shaggy-walled cavities that are often multiple (MOAZAM and NAZIR 1998; N'GBESSO and KEITA 1997; DEWBURY et al. 1980). On Doppler the hyper-

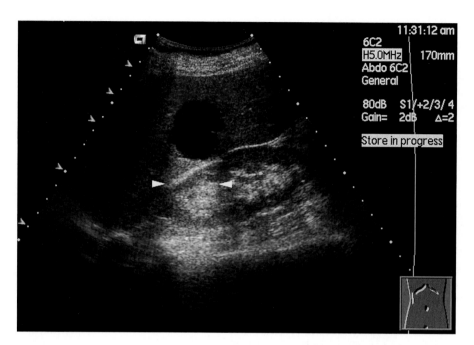

Fig. 1.4. Liver cyst. The typical features of a simple cyst, an echo-free space with smooth walls and increased sound transmission (*arrowheads*), permit a confident diagnosis and normally no further investigation is needed

aemia of the surrounding tissue is often obvious (Fig. 1.5). However, in the initial stages of abscess formation, before pus has collected, a solid mass is found and the lesions can be very subtle (DEWBURY et al. 1980). The microabscesses of fungal septicaemia often have a characteristic appearance of a cavity containing a central echogenic dot which is believed to be the artery in which the hyphae have embolized (PASTAKIA et al. 1988). However, the abscesses may be too small to detect with normal transducers used for liver imaging but may be resolved if a high frequency (small parts) transducer is used. Though these only allow the superficial 4 or 5 cm of liver to be imaged, the wide dissemination of these microabscesses usually allows a firm diagnosis to be made.

Haemangiomas are the commonest benign liver tumour and typically appear as uniformly echogenic masses (KIM et al. 2000). On Doppler they are hypovascular, only occasionally showing weak venous signals.

Focal nodular hyperplasia contains normal liver elements in an abnormal arrangement (CASARELLA et al. 1978; DI STASI et al. 1996; WANG et al. 1997). Some have a vascularized central scar which is seen as an echo-poor streak with Doppler signals that typically radiate outwards in a spoke-wheel fashion and these arterial features are elegantly dem-

onstrated after contrast enhancement (WANG et al. 1997).

Trauma may be very difficult to detect on unenhanced ultrasound unless there is a haematoma which is seen as an echo-poor cavity (SINGH et al. 1997). However, there are interesting reports of the value of contrast agents here. Infarcts in the liver are uncommon except in the HELPP syndrome and following major liver surgery involving vascular reconstruction, such as liver transplantation (CHRISTENSEN et al. 1997). They may be subtle on B-mode imaging but on colour Doppler are seen as non-perfused segments. Again, microbubble enhancement seems to improve the detection rate.

While fatty deposition in the liver is usually diffuse, producing a uniform increase in reflectivity, sometimes it is patchy. Focal fatty change produces echogenic regions, most often close to the gall bladder, that typically have a geometric shape (presumably reflecting the vascular territory that seems to underlie their formation) (Fig. 1.6). The reverse, focal fatty sparing, produces echo-poor patches. These changes can be confusing and may mimic metastases. Contrast enhancement is helpful because the lesion has normal haemodynamics and disappears as both it and the surrounding liver fill in the sinusoidal phase at around 2 min post injection.

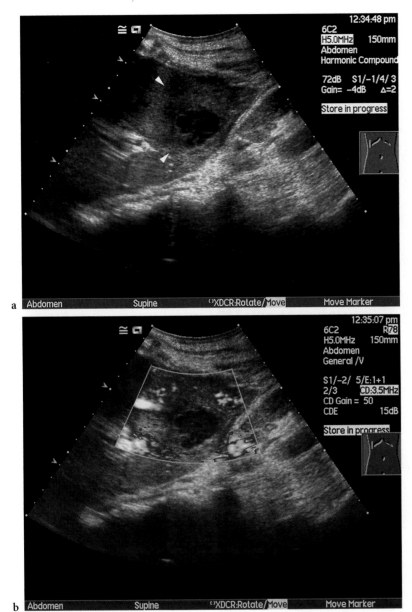

Fig. 1.5. a This liver abscess formed by extension from an aggressive chole-cystitis is seen as a region of slightly reduced reflectivity (*arrowheads*) with a small central cavity that is multiloculated. b The inflamed tissue is markedly hyperaemic on colour Doppler

The variety of appearances of metastases on ultrasound is bewildering and remains largely unexplained (Fig. 1.7) (Middleton et al. 1997; Pain et al. 1984). Though there are trends, for example, echogenic metastases are typically of gastro-intestinal or urogenital tract origin and echo-poor lesions are usual in carcinoma of the breast and bronchus, it has not been possible to relate particular patterns with the primary site. The success of ultrasound in liver staging has been exaggerated in the past, quoted accuracies around 80% being calculated on a per patient basis rather than for individual lesions (Carter et al. 1996). Contrast enhancement offers a significant improvement.

Hepatocellular carcinomas can be detected as masses of varying echogenicity and often a heterogeneous texture (Itoh and Akamatsu 1998). Their typical hypervascularity can be depicted with colour Doppler (Fig. 1.8). However, HCCs are often multicentric and highly invasive so that they may not have well defined borders and this, together with the fact that they often arise in cirrhotic livers with an irregular texture, can make them difficult to detect and size. They may also be confused with regenerating nodules.

Cholangiocarcinomas are also often difficult to detect, probably again because they are infiltrative. For both these primary liver malignancies, microbubble contrast agents have proved useful.

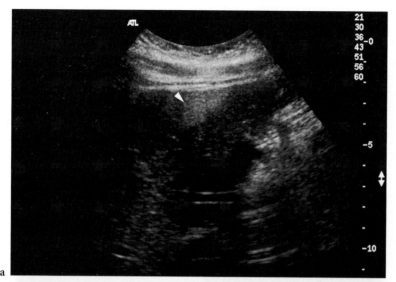

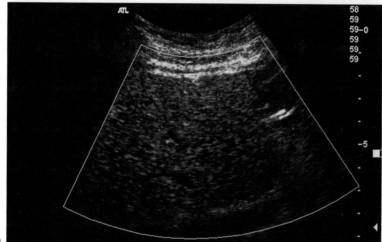

Fig. 1.6. a An echogenic wedge-shaped region (*arrowhead*) of the liver was found in this patient being staged for a colorectal cancer. Its geometric shape projecting onto the liver's surface suggested the diagnosis of focal fatty change. b In view of the importance of establishing the diagnosis with certainty, a microbubble contrast agent (SonoVue, Bracco, Milan) was administered. The microbubble-specific mode Power Pulse Inversion (Philips-ATL, Bothel, Wa.) was used to demonstrate that the *lesion* vanished in the sinusoidal phase at 3 min. In this mode the distribution of the microbubbles is shown as a *red coloured overlay* on the grey-scale scan

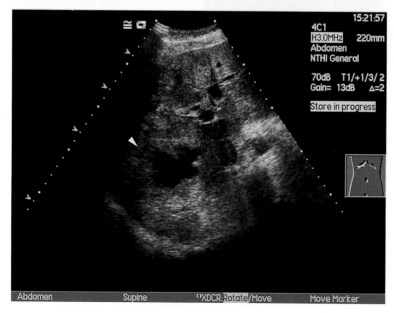

Fig. 1.7. Large heterogeneous masses occupy much of the right liver in this patient being staged for a colorectal carcinoma. One of the lesions has an echo free irregular central region (*arrowhead*) indicating haemorrhage or necrosis

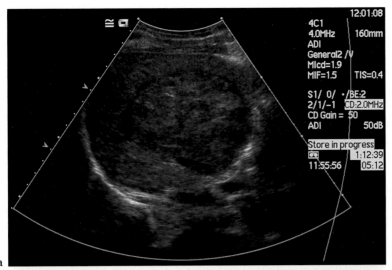

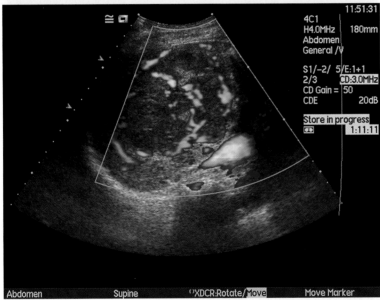

Fig. 1.8. a The heterogeneous texture of large hepatocellular carcinomas is shown in this example which is typically hypervascular on colour Doppler. **b** The complex, chaotic pattern of the malignant neovasculature is well demonstrated

1.5.1
Contrast Enhanced Ultrasound

After injection of one of the newer contrast agents, the enhancement first appears in the hepatic artery and then some 20 s later in the portal vein (WILSON and BURNS 2001). Gradually thereafter the liver parenchyma returns increasingly stronger signals until there is a near-complete parenchymal filling at around 1 min, the exact times depending on cardiac output as well as on the dose of microbubble administered; this late or sinusoidal phase is believed to represent pooling in the sinusoids or attachment to Kupffer cells. Contrast appears in the hepatic veins normally around 40 s after injection and 12 or more seconds after the artery lights up. Overall, the duration of useful liver enhancement is 4–5 min when a bubble-preserving low MI mode is used.

Microbubbles can also be used as tracers; in the liver the time taken for them to cross into the hepatic veins (normally 30 s or more, owing to the slow flow in the liver sinusoids) is shortened when there is arteriovenous shunting, as occurs in metastases and cirrhosis (ALBRECHT et al. 1999; BLOMLEY 1997). This simple test seems to be able to detect occult metastases, for example in colorectal cancer, and might prove useful in selecting patients for adjuvant chemotherapy.

Since the parenchymal (late) phase depends on an intact functioning microcirculation, lesions that lack this appear as dark defects; this applies to cysts and ischaemic regions such as trauma, scars and the rare infarcts and, importantly, to metastases which are detected with greatly improved sensitivity (Fig. 1.9) (WILSON and BURNS 2001; BLOMLEY et al. 1999). Even sub-centimetre metastases are readily detected against the enhanced background of normal liver tissue. Cholangiocarcinomas have the same appearance and this lesion, considered "difficult" for imaging in general, is well delineated with this technique.

Lesions that contain haemodynamically normal liver fill in the same way as the normal surrounding tissue and so tend to disappear in this late phase. Examples include focal fatty sparing/change, regenerating nodules in cirrhosis and focal nodular hyperplasia in which the central scar is often seen as a stellate defect at this stage (Fig. 1.6). The arterial phase is useful for characterising lesions based on their blood supply; hypervascular lesions such as hepatocellular carcinomas and vascular metastases (i.e. those from renal and neuroendocrine carcinomas) have one or more supply arteries that enter the lesion's periphery and fill rapidly in a centripetal fashion (TANAKA et al. 2001). FNH typically shows a different pattern with a single supply artery that feeds the mass from its centre in a centrifugal spoke-wheel fashion. Haemangiomas often have a pathognomonic haemodynamic pattern with arterial filling of the lesion's margin to form peripheral clumps from which the contrast slowly percolates towards the centre of the lesion. It may eventually fill completely and disappear in the sinusoidal phase but sometimes, especially with larger lesions, there are irregular non-filling regions which presumably represent thrombus or fibrosis. This centripetal slow filling also occurs in haemangiomas that are atypical on B-mode scans. Not all haemangiomas behave in this typical fashion on contrast ultrasound but when they do, no further investigation is needed.

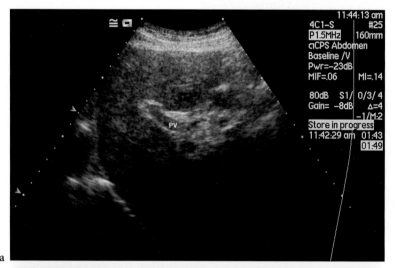

a

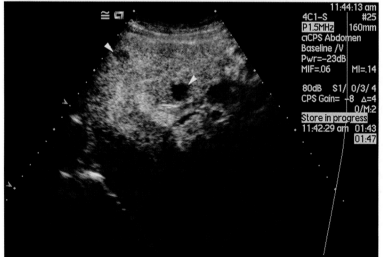

b

Fig. 1.9. a The staging liver ultrasound in this patient with a gastric carcinoma revealed a slightly irregular texture but no definite focal lesion. **b** In the sinusoidal (late) phase, almost 2 min after injection of 2.4 ml of the microbubble contrast agent SonoVue, several signal-free foci representing metastases were detected (*arrowheads*). The mode used was Contrast Pulse Sequences (CPS) which detects the presence of microbubbles whether stationary, as in the liver sinusoids shown here, or moving, as in the portal vein (*PV*). It operates at low transmit powers – an MI of 0.2 was used in this study – so that microbubble destruction is minimised

Metastases may be unimpressive in the arterial phase but sometimes have a peripheral artery that forms a halo; this must be distinguished from the nodular peripheral contrast around a haemangioma (WILSON and BURNS 2001). Metastases that are hypervascular fill rapidly and often heterogeneously from their supply artery. The contrast washes out more rapidly than from the normal liver (a manifestation of their small vascular volume) so that metastases become prominent as enhancement defects in the sinusoidal (late) phase (Fig. 1.9).

Hepatocellular carcinomas have complex patterns that do not always allow a diagnosis on a contrast study (KIM et al. 2002). They are usually hypervascular and show rapid and sometimes spectacular increase in signal a few seconds after the injection, though some are hypovascular. Their late phase appearance is variable, presumably because of the spectrum of differentiation they show on histology. Many behave in the same way as metastases and become prominent as defects from around 45 s after injection and this finding is clinically useful. Unfortunately some (perhaps 25%) retain contrast to a greater or lesser extent in this phase and thus simulate benign lesions. This obviously limits the value of contrast studies in evaluating cirrhotic patients for HCC.

A particularly useful application of contrast agents is in evaluating the completeness of ultrasound-guided interstitial therapy: when all tumour appears to have been destroyed, microbubbles often reveal residual portions of perfused tumour that can be ablated immediately so that the patient does not have to be moved to CT (LENCIONI et al. 1997; SOLBIATI et al. 1999).

1.6
Conclusions

Ultrasound technology has continued its rapid progress and many of the innovations have quickly become accepted as routine tools. Examples include tissue harmonic imaging and extended field of view scans. An important invention is the development of microbubble contrast agents that allow a contrast-enabled scanner to depict both the macro and microcirculation. In the liver they have proved to be especially valuable for detecting and characterising focal lesions and their use as tracers can reveal the arteriovenous shunting that is part of the metastatic process, even when the deposits are undetectable on conventional staging.

References

Albrecht TA, Blomley MJK, Cosgrove D, et al (1999) Non-invasive diagnosis of hepatic cirrhosis by transit time analysis of an ultrasound contrast agent. Lancet 353:1579–1583

Barbot DJ, Marks JH, Feld RI, et al (1997) Improved staging of liver tumors using laparoscopic intraoperative ultrasound. J Surg Oncol 64:63–67

Bezzi M, Silecchia G, De Leo A, et al (1998) Laparoscopic and intraoperative ultrasound. Eur J Radiol 27:S207–214

Blomley M (1997) Functional techniques with microbubbles. In: Nanda N, Schleif R, Goldberg B (eds) Advances in echo-contrast. Kluwer, Dordrecht

Blomley MJ, Albrecht T, Cosgrove D et al (1998) Liver vascular transit time analyzed with dynamic hepatic venography with bolus injections of an US contrast agent: early experience in seven patients with metastases. Radiology 209:862–866

Blomley MJ, Albrecht T, Cosgrove D, et al (1999) Improved imaging of liver metastases with stimulated acoustic emission in the late phase of enhancement with the US contrast agent SH U 508A: early experience. Radiology 210:409–416

Bryant TH, Albrecht T, Sidhu P, et al (2004) Liver phase uptake of a liver specific microbubble improves characterization of liver lesions: a prospective multi-center study. Radiology (in press)

Burns P (1996) Harmonic imaging with ultrasound contrast agents. Clin Radiol 51 [Suppl 1]:50–55

Burns P, Fritsch T, Weitschies W (1995) Pseudo Doppler shifts from stationary tissue due to the stimulated emission of ultrasound from a new microsphere contrast agent. Radiology P197

Burns P, Wilson SR, Simpson DH (2000) Pulse inversion imaging of liver blood flow: improved method for characterizing focal masses with microbubble contrast. Invest Radiol 35:58–71

Carter R, Hemingway D, Cooke TG, et al (1996) A prospective study of six methods for detection of hepatic colorectal metastases. Ann R Coll Surg Engl 78:27–30

Casarella W, Knowles D, Wolff M, et al (1978) Focal nodular hyperplasia and liver cell adenoma. AJR Am J Roentgenol 131:393–402

Christensen S, Herold N, Ravn P (1997) Ultrasound examination of the liver in HELLP syndrome. Radiologe 37:170–172

Chuah SY (2000) Liver biopsy under ultrasound control: implications for training. Gut 46:583–584

Couinaud C (1957) Le Foie. Etude anatomiques et chirurgicales. Masson, Paris

Dawson P, Cosgrove D, Grainger R (1999) Textbook of Contrast Media. Isis Medical, Oxford

Dewbury K, Joseph A, Sadler G, et al (1980) Ultrasound in the diagnosis of early liver abscess. Br J Radiol 53:1160–1167

Di Stasi M, Caturelli E, De Sio I, et al (1996) Natural history of focal nodular hyperplasia of the liver: an ultrasound study. J Clin Ultrasound 24:345–350

Eckersley R, Cosgrove D, Blomley M, et al (1998) Functional imaging of tissue response to bolus injection of an ultrasound contrast agent. Proc. IEEE Ultrasonics Symposium 2:1779–1782

Filice C, Brunetti E (1997) Use of PAIR in human cystic echinococcosis. Acta Tropica 64:95–107

Foley W, Lawson T (1992) Abdomen. In: Foley W (ed) Color Doppler flow imaging. Andover Medical, Boston

Gaines PA, Sampson MA (1989) The prevalence and characterization of simple hepatic cysts by ultrasound examination. Br J Radiol 62:335–337

Goldberg B (1997) Ultrasound contrast agents. Martin Dunitz, London

Grant E (1992) Doppler imaging of the liver. Ultrasound Quarterly 10:117–154

Haddad MC, Al-Awar G, Huwaijah SH, et al (2001) Echinococcal cysts of the liver: a retrospective analysis of clinico-radiological findings and different therapeutic modalities. Clin Imaging 25:403–408

Herman K (1996) Intraoperative ultrasound in gastrointestinal cancer. An analysis of 272 operated patients. Hepato-gastroenterology 43:565–570

Itoh Y, Akamatsu K (1998) Relationships between echo level and histologic characteristics in small hepatocellular carcinomas. J Clin Ultrasound 26:295–301

Kim KW, Kim TK, Han JK, et al (2000) Hepatic hemangiomas: spectrum of US appearances on gray-scale, power Doppler, and contrast-enhanced US. Korean J Radiol 1:191–197

Kim TK, Kim AY, Choi BI (2002) Hepatocellular carcinoma: harmonic ultrasound and contrast agent. Abdom Imaging 27:129–138

Klotter H, Ruckert K, Mentges B, et al (1986) Intraoperative ultrasound study in surgery. Ultraschall Med 7:224–230

Kono Y, Moriyasu F, Nada T, et al (1997) Gray scale second harmonic imaging of the liver: a preliminary animal study. Ultrasound Med Biol 23:719–726

Kremkau F (1997) Diagnostic ultrasound: principles and instruments. WB Saunders, Philadelphia

Kuni CC, Johnson NL, Holmes JH (1978) Polycystic liver disease. J Clin Ultrasound 6:332–334

Lafortune M, Patriquin H (1999) The hepatic artery: studies using Doppler sonography. Ultrasound Quarterly 15:9–26

Lencioni R, Bartolozzi C, Ricci P, et al (1997) Hepatocellular carcinoma: use of contrast enhanced color Doppler US to evaluate response to treatment with percutaneous ethanol injection. Eur Radiol 7:792–794

Machi J, Sigel B (1996) Operative ultrasound in general surgery. Am J Surg 172:15–20

McDicken W (1991) Diagnostic ultrasound, physical principles and use of instruments, 3rd edn. Churchill Livingstone, Edinburgh

Middleton WD, Hiskes SK, Teefey SA, et al (1997) Small (1.5 cm or less) liver metastases: US-guided biopsy. Radiology 205:729–732

Mine Y (1998) Harmonic imaging. Nippon Rinsho 56:881–885

Moazam F, Nazir Z (1998) Amebic liver abscess: spare the knife but save the child. J Pediatr Surg 33:119–122

N'Gbesso RD, Keita AK (1997) Ultrasonography of amebic liver abscesses. Proposal of a new classification. J Radiol 78:569–576

Pain JA, Bailey ME, Bloomberg TJ (1984) Liver metastases: the role of preoperative ultrasound. J R Coll Surg Edinb 29:85–87

Parvey HR, Eisenberg RL, Giyanani V, et al (1989) Duplex sonography of the portal venous system: pitfalls and limitations. AJR Am J Roentgenol 52:765–770

Pastakia B, Shawker TH, Thaler M (1988) Hepatosplenic candidiasis: wheels within wheels. Radiology 166:417–421

Pederson J, Pederson ST, Karstrup S (1993) Ultrasound guided biopsies. In: Cosgrove D, Meire HB, Dewbury K (eds) Clinical ultrasound. Churchill Livingstone, London

Singh G, Arya N, Safaya R, et al (1997) Role of ultrasonography in blunt abdominal trauma. Injury 28:667–670

Solbiati L, Goldberg S, Ierace T, et al (1999) Radio-frequency ablation of hepatic metastases: postprocedural assessment with a US microbubble contrast agent. Radiology 211:643–649

Stride E, Saffari N (2003) Microbubble ultrasound contrast agents: a review. Proc Inst Mech Eng [H] 217:429–447

Tanaka S, Ioka T, Oshikawa O, et al (2001) Dynamic sonography of hepatic tumors. AJR Am J Roentgenol 177:799–805

ter Haar G (1999) Interactions between the ultrasound beam and microbubbles. In: Dawson P, Cosgrove D, Allison D, Grainger R (eds) Contrast agents in radiology. Isis Medical, Oxford

Wachsberg RH, Angyal EA, Klein KM, et al (1997) Echogenicity of hepatic versus portal vein walls revisited with histologic correlation. J Ultrasound Med 16:807–810

Wang LY, Wang JH, Lin ZY, et al (1997) Hepatic focal nodular hyperplasia: findings on color Doppler ultrasound. Abdom Imaging 22:178–181

Wilson SR, Burns PN (2001) Liver mass evaluation with ultrasound: the impact of microbubble contrast agents and pulse inversion imaging. Semin Liver Dis 21:147–159

2 Computed Tomography

Andrea Laghi, Ilaria Sansoni, Michela Celestre, Pasquale Paolantonio, and Roberto Passariello

CONTENTS

2.1
Introduction

Following its introduction in a clinical setting in 1974, computed tomography (CT) underwent an extraordinary technical revolution in terms of both scanning time and spatial resolution. Nevertheless, CT remained a cross-sectional technique with sequential acquisition of axial slices until the introduction of spiral (helical) CT at the end of 1980s. Spiral technology, made possible by improvements in tube technology and electronic computing, has transformed CT from a two-dimensional into a true volumetric imaging modality (Kalender et al. 1990). Faster image acquisition, more rational use of contrast agent administration as well as use of image reformation on multiple planes offered incredible advances in terms of lesion identification, characterization and staging and opened up new indications for CT study (i.e. CT angiography for arterial vascular assessment and replacement of catheter angiography; CT colonography for evaluation of colonic disorders).

A second revolution occurred when multi-slice (multidetector-row) CT (MDCT) was introduced (Klingenbeck-Regn et al. 1999). Although the first MDCT was a "dual-slice" scanner, presented already in 1992 and consisting of two parallel detector rows that allowed the simultaneous acquisition of two interwoven helices, the real impact of multi-slice technology was observed at the end of 1998, when the first four-slice CT equipment was introduced in a clinical setting (Berland and Smith 1998; Liang and Kruger 1996). MDCT, based on a four-row configuration of detectors, together with the development of sub-second gantry rotation time, offered the opportunity to overcome common limitations of single-slice CT scanners, especially in terms of scanning time and limited z-axis resolution (Hu et al. 2000). Technical evolution was followed by the development of 8- and 16-slice scanners, which became available between 2001 and 2002, and will continue with the 64-slice equipment expected by the end of this year (Prokop 2003a; Flohr et al. 2002).

Technological development was followed by a change in liver imaging protocols. The real advance in liver imaging was due to multiplanar and multiphasic capabilities of MDCT. Multiplanarity, due to the acquisition of 3D data sets with isotropic or near-isotropic voxels, resulted in the ability to analyse CT images on multiple planes (i.e. sagittal, coronal and oblique) making diagnosis of lesions in critical anatomic localization easier; isotropic volume also made the use of 3D rendering algorithms available, which is especially useful in the case of vascular reconstructions and virtual endoscopic views (Prokop 2003b). The multiphasic approach, made possible by fast scanning time, makes it possible to scan the liver parenchyma during pure vascular phases, offering a real arterial, portal and delayed phase (Brink 2003; Fleischmann 2003b). Optimization of vascular enhancement together with improved spatial resolution along the z-axis are expected to improve diagnostic accuracy in liver imaging (Kang et al. 2003).

A. Laghi, MD; I. Sansoni, MD; M. Celestre, MD;
P. Paolantonio, MD; R. Passariello, MD
Department of Radiological Sciences, University of Rome "La Sapienza", Policlinico Umberto I, Viale Regina Elena 324, 00161 Rome, Italy

2.2
Technique

MDCT has transformed CT from a transaxial cross-sectional technique into a 3D imaging modality. Whereas single-slice CT took at least 5 years to gain general acceptance, MDCT has been more rapidly accepted in the radiological community, with exponential growth in the use of these scanners in clinical practice. Major improvements (z-axis coverage speed and longitudinal resolution) translated into rapid hepatic imaging and the use of new imaging protocols, not possible with single-slice spiral CT. Thin sections, that can now be routinely used within a single breath-hold, resulted in improved lesion detection and nearly isotropic image acquisition providing high-resolution datasets available for multiplanar reformations (HONDA et al. 2002; KAMEL et al. 2003). Moreover, the possibility to scan through the entire liver in 10 s or less allowed MDCT to demonstrate three clear separate and distinct hepatic circulatory phases of iodine contrast distribution, i.e. pure arterial, arterioportal, venous and equilibrium phases (FOLEY et al. 2000). MDCT with the improvements in morphological and functional information compared with single-slice CT enables a comprehensive approach to hepatic imaging within a single examination. MDCT brings new challenges, concerning contrast injections protocols (including optimal timing and rate of contrast injection, total volume of contrast agent and ideal iodine concentration of contrast medium) and patients' dose exposure (FLEISCHMANN 2003b; PROKOP 2003a).

2.2.1
Detector Configuration

The reason for a brief discussion about detector configuration, which might be beyond the aims of this chapter, lies in the differences among detector arrays of different CT constructors, especially when considering four-slice scanners; in fact, detector arrays of 16-slice machines are more homogeneous. The major consequence of a different design is the choice of scan parameters, which cannot be simply transferred from scanner to scanner, as with single-slice CT. This means that scanning parameters need to be optimized as a function of the available equipment according to only a few general rules.

At present, MDCT scanners may acquire 2, 4, 6, 8, 10 or 16 simultaneous sections. In all MDCT scanners, the number of slices that can be acquired is usually smaller than the number of detector rows (N), in order to obtain more than one collimation setting by adding together the signals of neighbouring detector rows.

The arrangement of detectors along the z-axis and widths of available slices vary among different systems. In particular three different detector array designs are currently available: "matrix", "adaptive" and "hybrid" detector arrays. "Matrix" detectors consist of parallel rows of equal thickness; "adaptive" detectors use detector rows with varying thickness. In the former type, the width of detector elements determines the thinnest possible section thickness and thicker sections are obtained by adding the signal from neighbouring detector rows; in contrast, in the latter type, various section thicknesses can be gained using partial collimation and addition of signal of adjacent rows. Finally, "hybrid" detectors use smaller detector rows in the centre and larger ones towards the periphery of the array. This design has been adopted mostly for 16-row scanners from all companies (PROKOP 2003a; KOPP et al. 2002).

2.2.2
Scan Parameters

In single-slice CT, the most important scan parameters can be provided in the form of a triplet including slice collimation (SC, in mm), table feed/rotation (TF, in mm) and reconstruction increment (RI, in mm). Depending on clinical indications, a compromise has to be reached between z-axis resolution and required scan length. The effective slice thickness or slice width (SW) can be calculated from slice collimation and pitch, P (=TF/SC). The suggested scan parameters for single-slice spiral CT of the liver are 5/8/4 (SC/TF/RI) and the SW is 6.2 (UGGOWITZER 2003).

In four-slice spiral CT the same acquired raw data set can be used to reconstruct two or more data sets of varying thickness. For this reason, it is important to distinguish between acquisition parameters, given as (NxSC/TF), and reconstruction parameters, expressed as (SW/RI) (CADEMARTIRI et al. 2003). With multislice scanners, two definitions of pitch factor are used, depending on whether a section (P*=TF/SC) or total collimation of the detector array (P=TF/NxSC) is chosen as the reference (PROKOP 2003c).

The image quality of any given four-slice CT system depends on collimation, pitch, reconstruction interval. Collimation should be tailored to the purpose of the study, because a decreased collimator width (thus, an increase in pitch) results in a narrow reconstructed section thickness and improved spatial resolution, but in increased image noise and decreased length of coverage. However, maximization of pitch may also result in a decrease in contrast resolution (WANG and VANNIER 1999). Thus, the most appropriate choice of scanning parameters depends also on clinical indication to CT study. In fact, for example, for CT angiography where imaging is devoted to structures with very high attenuation, loss of contrast resolution caused by maximization of pitch can be disregarded. This is not the case with liver imaging where both good spatial and contrast resolutions are required; a practical approach for liver imaging is to use relatively thin collimation, increasing the pitch as needed to cover the entire liver. A small reconstruction interval with overlapping sections is advantageous both for multiplanar reconstructions and for detection of small lesions, because the smaller the reconstruction interval, the greater the longitudinal (z-axis) resolution; one major drawback is the loss of z-axis coverage (JI et al. 2001).

The choice of scan parameters with a four-slice CT scanner can follow two different approaches: "fast spiral acquisition", with the use of 5-mm slice thickness, similar to single-slice spiral CT, but with the advantage of much shorter scanning time; "volumetric imaging" using a high-resolution protocol consisting of thin collimation and lower pitch, necessary to acquire an almost isotropic volume that can be further post-processed using multiplanar reformations, maximum intensity projection and volume-rendering algorithms (SAINI and DSOUZA 2003). For liver imaging a compromise between fast scanning, necessary to obtain pure vascular phases, and high-resolution scanning, necessary to reformat the datasets, has to be performed.

This obligatory choice between scanning time and spatial resolution is not necessary any more with 16-slice spiral CT systems, as they combine the ability to acquire very thin slice images (narrow collimation) with a very fast scanning time.

2.2.3
Strategy of Dataset Acquisition

The major impact of spiral CT technology on liver imaging is represented in the short scanning time, allowing the evaluation of the entire liver parenchyma during a single breath-hold. Fast scanning opened the era of multiphasic protocols, consisting of multiple passes through liver parenchyma during different vascular phases. Using a single detector spiral CT the examination usually consists of a biphasic scan

with images acquired during arterial dominant phase followed by a portal venous phase (VALLS et al. 2004). The rationale of this imaging protocol is based on the differences of blood supply between normal parenchyma and liver tumours, as hepatic vascularization comes predominantly from the portal vein, whereas each kind of liver tumour receives blood mainly from the hepatic artery; exceptions to this rule are often represented by regenerating nodules and early well-differentiated hepatocellular carcinomas (ALTMANN 1978; FERRUCCI 1991; BERNARDINO and GALAMBOS 1989; LANIADO and KOPP 1997; HOLLETT et al. 1995). Therefore, if the arterial dominant phase is acquired as part of the imaging protocol, diagnosis of hypervascular benign and malignant tumours (focal nodular hyperplasia, hepatic adenomas, hepatocellular carcinomas, islet cell tumour and carcinoid) is improved compared with analysis of delayed phase of enhancement alone (FERRUCCI 1991; BARON et al. 1996; OLIVER et al. 1997). On the contrary, hypovascular liver tumours (such as metastases), show low attenuation compared with normal parenchyma during both arterial and subsequent portal venous phases (FERRUCCI 1991).

However, the scanning time of a single-slice spiral CT scanner is too slow to obtain a pure arterial phase; the result is a hybrid phase, with mixed arterial and portal venous enhancement (usually slices acquired first in the volume have a pure arterial enhancement whereas subsequent slices show portal dominant enhancement).

Only with the advent of MDCT could the entire upper abdomen be scanned within 10 s or less (JI and ROS 2001). Fast acquisition offers the possibility to scan the liver during multiple phases of vascular enhancement. A complex multiphasic imaging protocol was optimized soon after the introduction of four-slice scanners (Fig. 2.1) (FOLEY et al. 2000). It consists of four separate passes through liver parenchyma following i.v. injection of contrast medium (Fig. 2.2). The first two passes performed respectively in craniocaudal and caudocranial direction following the arrival of bolus of contrast medium are acquired within a single breath-hold of approximately 24 s; the delay time for scanning is calculated with a preliminary bolus test or is automatically defined using a bolus tracking technique. The first pass, the so-called early arterial phase (EAP) acquires images where only arterial vessels are enhanced; the second pass, the so-called late arterial phase (LAP) obtains images during arterioportal enhancement. The first breath-bold is followed by a second 10-s scan during the portal enhancement (portal venous phase,

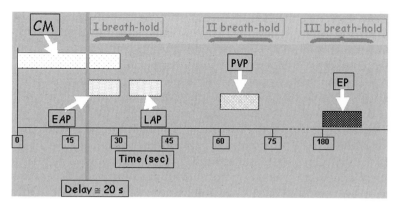

Fig. 2.1. Diagram of multiphasic vascular enhancement of the liver. Around 20 s (representing the average delay time usually calculated on the basis of bolus test) following the beginning of contrast medium injection first breath-hold acquisition of two consecutive scans is obtained. At around 60 s the second breath-hold scan is acquired followed by the equilibrium phase. *CM*, contrast medium; *EAP*, early arterial phase; *LAP*, late arterial phase; *PVP*, portal venous phase; *EP*, equilibrium phase

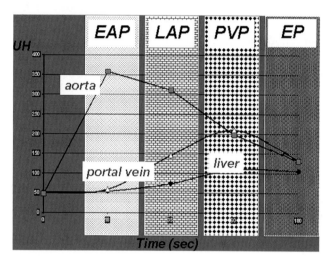

Fig. 2.2. Time-density curves representing enhancement of aorta, portal vein and liver parenchyma during each scan. Please note clear separation of different vascular phases with early arterial phase demonstrating exclusive enhancement of arterial vessels with absolutely no venous contamination. *EAP*, early arterial phase; *LAP*, late arterial phase; *PVP*, portal venous phase; *EP*, equilibrium phase

PVP) beginning 60 s after the injection of contrast medium. Finally, a 3-min delayed scan (equilibrium phase, EP) is acquired. The rationale for performing multiphasic examination is to maximize detection of hypervascular liver neoplasms, particularly in cirrhotic patients.

At this time, no consensus has been reached about the use of a so-called double arterial phase. Some authors reported that double arterial phase imaging of the liver with MDCT is effective for improving detectability of hypervascular hepatocellular carcinoma and for reducing the number of false-positive diagnoses (due to arteriovenous shunts); in particular sensitivity and positive predictive value for hypervascular HCC were 54% and 85% for EAP, 78% and 83% for LAP, and 86% and 92% for double arterial phase, respectively (Fig. 2.3) (Murakami et al. 2001). However, radiologists should recognize that the application of double arterial phase imaging to the liver may have crucial disadvantages for patients in terms of radiation exposure, as well as workload for personnel due to the huge number of acquired images, gen-

erating problems of filming, image interpretation and storage ("image pollution") (Ichikawa et al. 2002). On the other hand, other studies demonstrated that hypervascular neoplasms are best seen during LAP, with no contribution from EAP in terms of sensitivity (Foley et al. 2000; Ichikawa et al. 2002; Laghi et al. 2003). In our personal experience sensitivity and positive predictive value of respectively 48.5% and 96.4% in the EAP, 87.1% and 94% in the LAP were obtained, with no tumours detected in the EAP which were not visible in the LAP (Fig. 2.4) (Laghi et al. 2003). In another study, similar results were reported, with sensitivity of 88% with LAP and 90% combining EAP and LAP; both the values were statistically significant higher than 67% obtained with EAP alone (Fig. 2.5) (Ichikawa et al. 2002). The role of an EAP is the acquisition of pure arterial vascular datasets, where only arterial vessels are opacified. If the acquired volume is obtained with thin collimation and a reconstruction interval it can be used to generate high-quality vascular maps (CT angiography); these vascular maps may have an important role in pre-op-

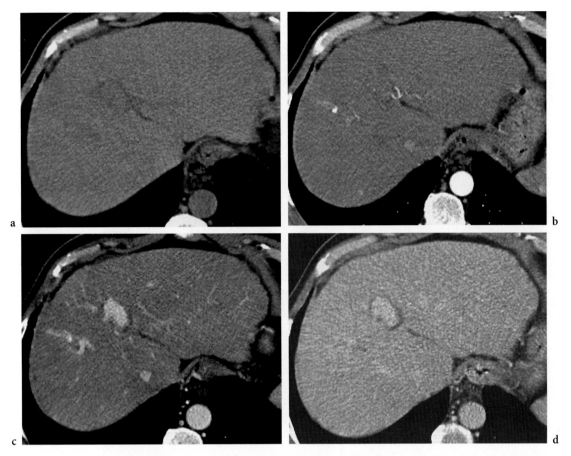

Fig. 2.3a–d. Arterioportal shunt. **a** On basal scan no lesion is detected. **b** On early arterial phase, intense enhancement of a pseudo-lesion is clearly depicted. **c** The enhanced pseudo-lesion follows vascular enhancement, with density similar to portal vein. **d** Delayed scan shows enhancement similar to surrounding parenchyma

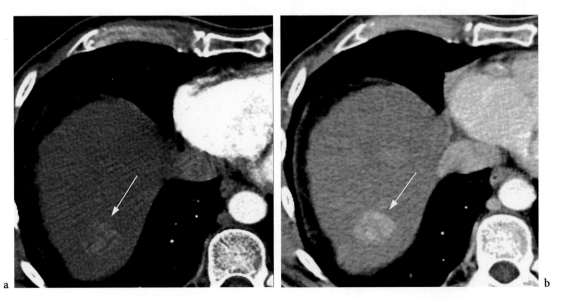

Fig. 2.4a,b. Hepatocellular carcinoma. **a** On early arterial phase hypervascular nodule is fairly seen (*arrow*). **b** Best conspicuity in lesion detection is obtained during late arterial phase (*arrow*)

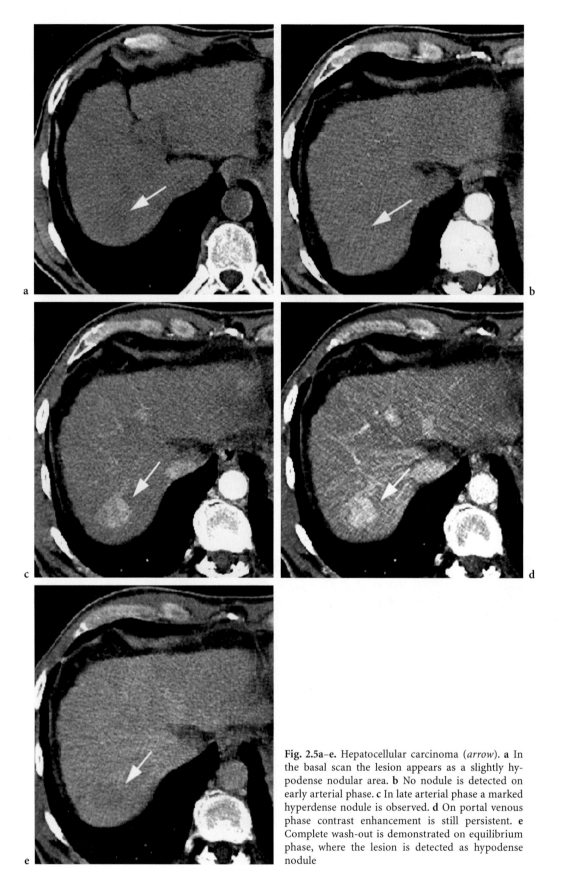

Fig. 2.5a–e. Hepatocellular carcinoma (*arrow*). **a** In the basal scan the lesion appears as a slightly hypodense nodular area. **b** No nodule is detected on early arterial phase. **c** In late arterial phase a marked hyperdense nodule is observed. **d** On portal venous phase contrast enhancement is still persistent. **e** Complete wash-out is demonstrated on equilibrium phase, where the lesion is detected as hypodense nodule

erative assessment of surgical candidates (liver resection or transplantation) or candidates for interventional procedures (catheter angiography) (Fig. 2.6) (LAGHI et al. 2003).

The third imaging pass, the so-called portal venous phase (PVP), enables evaluation of isoattenuation or hypoattenuation of hypervascular lesions. In addition, in some patients, relatively hypovascular hepatocellular carcinomas and metastases from islet cell or carcinoid tumours may be detected only during this later acquisition scan (FOLEY et al. 2000). As is well known, the portal venous phase not only has the advantage of depicting hypovascular lesions but also is useful in demonstrating portal venous thrombosis, differentiating neoplasms from vessels, and identifying varices and shunts (LAGHI et al. 2003).

Within the past decade, some investigators have advocated the use of delayed phase imaging for its potential added value in dynamic spiral CT imaging of the liver. Lesion detection and conspicuity has been reported to be higher in the delayed phase than in the portal venous phase, resulting in an improved detection rate of well-differentiated hypovascular hepatocellular carcinomas, depicted as low-attenuating lesions and sometimes missed when only arterial and portal venous phase scans are obtained (HWANG et al. 1997; LIM et al. 2002). Furthermore, delayed phase imaging has additional value in characterization of hepatic lesions because it offers better visualization of capsule and mosaic patterns seen in some hepatocellular carcinomas, delayed peripheral enhancement of cholangiocarcinoma and "filling-in" patterns of haemangioma (Figs. 2.7, 2.8) (LIM et al.

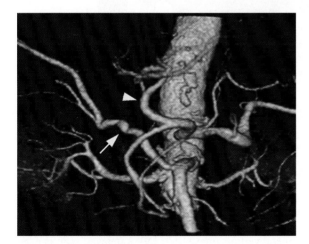

Fig. 2.6. Volume-rendered 3D reconstruction of celiac trunk and superior mesenteric artery. Anomalous origin of right hepatic artery from superior mesenteric artery is demonstrated (*arrow*). Left hepatic artery has a normal origin from common hepatic artery (*arrowhead*)

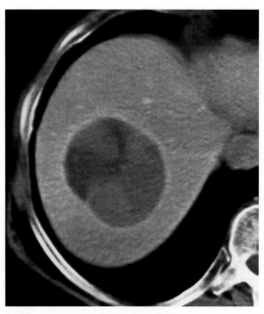

Fig. 2.7. On delayed scan better visualisation of capsule and mosaic pattern of hepatocellular carcinoma is demonstrated

2002). In contrast, other authors demonstrated that the portal venous phase showed no significant differences in lesion detection compared with delayed phase imaging, or better still when combined, spiral CT of the arterial and the delayed phases revealed 91% of lesions, whereas a combination of the arterial and portal venous phases or the combination of all three phases revealed 92% of lesions; therefore, the combination of the arterial and portal venous phases is equal to the combination of three phases for detection of hypervascular hepatocellular carcinomas, and the delayed phase becomes superfluous (CHOI et al. 1997). However, in this series of patients only hypervascular hepatocellular carcinoma was included, whilst in clinical practice, there are also cases of hypovascular hepatocellular carcinoma. This concept has been confirmed by other authors, who stated that portal venous-phase images are inferior to late phase images for detecting HCC nodules; in the same paper sensitivity of the unenhanced phase was also evaluated and it was demonstrated not to be necessary (KIM et al. 1999).

Even with regard to the use of an unenhanced phase opinions are controversial with papers demonstrating no additionally detected lesions (hepatomas or metastases) compared with other phases and other experiences showing a 3% increase in the detection rate for hepatocellular carcinomas compared with arterial and portal venous phases (MILLER et al. 1998; OLIVER et al. 1996).

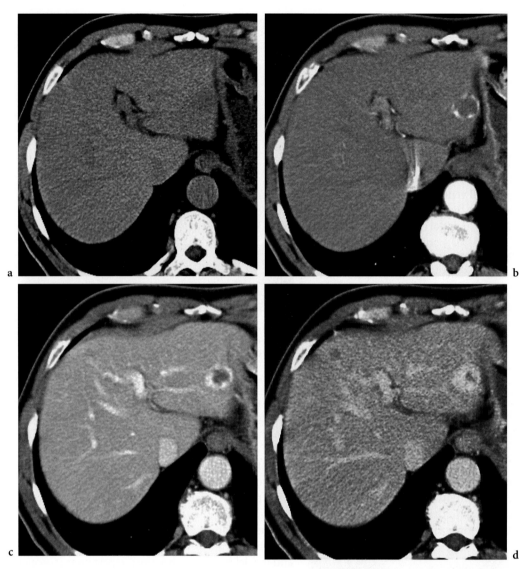

Fig. 2.8a–d. Typical haemangioma. **a** In the basal scan it appears as slightly hypodense area. **b** The lesion presents an initial peripheral enhancement during the arterial phase. **c** In the portal venous phase a globular centripetal enhancement is observed. **d** In the delayed phase the lesion shows an almost complete filling

2.2.4
Suggestions for Scanning Protocols

As noted earlier, several options for liver scanning are available. Theoretically a complete liver examination might include a pre-contrast scan, followed by contrast-enhanced acquisition obtained during the arterial (sometimes split into early and late arterial passes) and portal venous phases and a delayed equilibrium phase. For several reasons, including radiation exposure, data explosion with complex image viewing and storing, all the five phases are not acquired in each patient. Although there is not a clear consensus over this issue, the selection and combina-tion of acquisition phases depends on clinical questions (Table 2.1).

In non-hepatopathic patients, with no history of neoplasia, our protocol includes a pre-contrast scan followed by late arterial and portal venous phases. The acquisition of a late arterial phase is justified by the relatively high percentage of hypervascular benign lesions (see focal nodular hyperplasia) which might be easily missed only on pre-contrast and portal venous phase (Fig. 2.9). A delayed scan is used only in cases of suspected haemangiomas if arterial and portal venous patterns are doubtful and there is the need to confirm complete and delayed enhancement.

Table 2.1. Suggested MDCT imaging protocols, according to clinical indication

	UN	EAP	LAP	PVP	EP
Non-hepatopathic patient No history of neoplasia	+	–	+	+	±
Non-hepatopathic patient History of neoplasia (suspected hypovascular metastases)	+	–	–	+	–
Non-hepatopathic patient History of neoplasia (suspected hypervascular metastases)	–	–	+	+	±
Hepatopathic patient	?	±	+	+	+

UN, unenhanced scan; EAP, early arterial phase; LAP, late arterial phase; PVP, portal venous phase; EP, equilibrium phase.

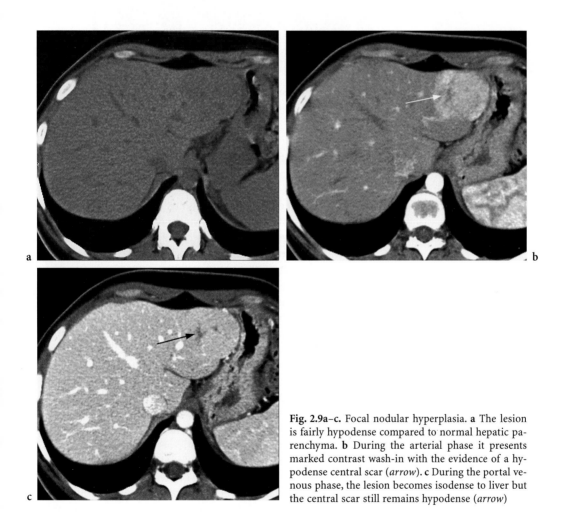

a

b

c

Fig. 2.9a–c. Focal nodular hyperplasia. **a** The lesion is fairly hypodense compared to normal hepatic parenchyma. **b** During the arterial phase it presents marked contrast wash-in with the evidence of a hypodense central scar (*arrow*). **c** During the portal venous phase, the lesion becomes isodense to liver but the central scar still remains hypodense (*arrow*)

In non-hepatopathic patients, with a previous history of neoplasia with typical hypovascular liver lesions (i.e. colon cancer) the CT protocol is limited to a pre-contrast scan followed by a contrast-enhanced scan obtained during the portal venous phase (Fig. 2.10). If patients have a history of tumour with possible hypervascular liver metastases (kidney, breast, islet cell tumours) a late arterial phase is added to the previous scanning protocol.

A completely different approach is dedicated to hepatopathic patients. A pre-contrast scan is questionable since no benefit was obtained in terms of identification of hepatocellular carcinoma compared with a dynamic contrast-enhanced study. Mandatory

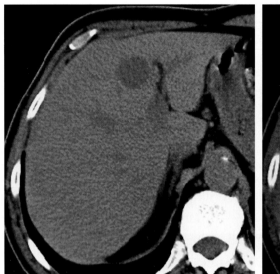
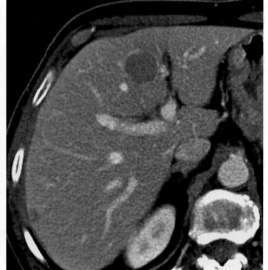

Fig. 2.10a,b. Typical pattern of hypovascular colorectal cancer metastasis. **a** Lesion is hypodense on unenhanced image. **b** Lesion remains hypodense 60 s after i.v. administration of contrast medium

are late arterial, portal venous and delayed phases, since they contribute to the identification of both hypervascular and well-differentiated hypovascular hepatocellular carcinomas. An early arterial phase is indicated only in cases where a vascular map is required (i.e. before chemoembolization, surgery, etc.).

2.2.5
Timing and Intravenous Administration of Contrast Medium

In order to take full advantage of MDCT capabilities adequate timing and flow rate of injection should be carefully evaluated. Hepatic arterial enhancement is primarily influenced by the rate of iodine injection and timing of contrast bolus, whereas venous phase enhancement is determined by total dose of iodine administered to patients.

Different circulatory phases can only be separated by precisely timing the scanning delay to the patient's individual circulation time; timing can be determined by using fixed delay, a test bolus, or a computer auto-mated scanner technology (CAST) (bolus tracking) (FLEISCHMANN 2003b).

The use of fixed delay time cannot guarantee opti-mal separation between early and late arterial phases, due to inherent variability among individuals, such as patient size and cardiovascular status. A good bi-phasic study, including late arterial and portal ve-nous phases can be reliably obtained in most cases using fixed delays of respectively 35–40 s and 60–70 s (SHEIMAN et al. 1996).

But a more rational use of MDCT can be accom-plished by using a test bolus or by using bolus track-ing software (HITTMAIR and FLEISCHMANN 2001). The test bolus enables calculation of the circulation time and planning of the optimal scanning delay. It consists in the administration of 20–30 ml of contrast medium at the same flow rate to be used during spiral scanning (i.e. 3.5–5 ml/s) followed by the acquisition of a series of single-level, low dose (120 kVp, 10 mA), CT scans acquired every 2 s for around 40 s and start-ing immediately after the injection. Although test bo-lus is accurate in determining the optimal delay time, it does require additional contrast and increases the occupation time of the scanner room.

Automatic software is now very accurate at track-ing aortic and liver enhancement curves. It simpli-fies timing of the hepatic arterial phase, regardless of whether a single or double pass is required, and may reduce the volume of contrast required. The au-tomatic bolus-tracking program is used to automati-cally start the first arterial phase scan after the injec-tion of contrast material. This technique is capable of real-time monitoring, automatic calculation of CT values in a region of interest (ROI), and automatic initiation of diagnostic CT after the CT value of the ROI has reached a trigger threshold level after the in-jection of contrast material (KIM et al. 2002).

The main factor in relation to arterial enhance-ment is iodine flux (mg of iodine entering the circulation per second), which depends on flow rate (ml/s) and concentration of contrast medium (mg of iodine/ml).

Faster injection rates increase maximum enhancement of the aorta and arterial enhancement of liver. Although faster injection rates reduce time from injection to the beginning and the end of the arterial phase, faster injection rates do not decrease the duration of the arterial phase itself, but they increase temporal separation of arterial and portal scan phases, which is important to produce unique phases of imaging; the optimal flow rate should be considered equal to or higher than 3.5 ml/s (KIM et al. 1998). High infusion rates are often limited by intravenous access and an effective alternative is a higher-concentration contrast medium (370 and 400 mg of iodine/ml); it is also advantageous in patients in whom there is a reduced signal/noise ratio on CT (heavy individuals and those requiring thin slices or reduced radiation dose). Several data in the literature support the hypothesis that an increase in contrast medium concentration results in a greater degree of enhancement and diagnostic efficacy for hypervascular lesions; AWAI et al. (2002) compared two iodine concentrations of Iopamidol (300 mg/ml and 370 mg/ml) with the same total iodine load per patient per body weight and a total lower volume of contrast material and shorter duration of injection time in patients with more concentrated contrast medium; no difference was observed in liver enhancement in all the contrasted passes, but during the first arterial phase aortic enhancement and the attenuation differences between the hepatic parenchyma and hepatic tumours were significantly higher with more concentrated contrast medium; the same results were obtained in different experiences (MARCHIANÒ 2003).

Venous phase enhancement is not modified by changes in flow rate since it is determined by the total given dose of iodine. So when total iodine dose is fixed but higher concentration and lower volume of contrast medium is used, an earlier and higher arterial enhancement and an improved depiction of hypervascular HCCs is obtained; this results in a greater diagnostic efficacy, employing an equal iodine dose without an increase in cost, because the cost of contrast material for CT examinations depends on the total amount of iodine in the contrast material (AWAI et al. 2002).

Because of the rapid scanning times of multidetector scanners, the entire liver may be scanned when a substantial volume of the injected contrast material remains in the dead space of the injector tubing, peripheral veins, right heart or pulmonary circulation, and central arteries. Enhancement of liver parenchyma is predominantly from contrast material delivered via the portal vein; therefore, the contrast material still in the dead space can be considered wasted for the purpose of hypovascular liver lesion detection. It was reported that the use of 50 ml of saline chaser to replace the last third (50 ml) of the standard contrast material bolus in order to push the bolus into the heart and further along in the circulation, reduces the amount of contrast material remaining in the brachiocephalic vein and superior vena cava (DORIO et al. 2003). Other benefits of this technique are the substantial cost savings and potential increase in safety (reduction of nephrotoxicity) inherent in replacing 50 ml of non-ionic contrast material with 50 ml of sterile saline solution. It is important to remark that liver enhancement and tumour conspicuity were not adversely affected by lower dose of contrast material. In another study, other authors showed that saline solution flush following low dose contrast material bolus improves parenchymal (the liver, the spleen, the pancreas and the renal cortex) and vascular (the portal vein, the inferior vena cava and the abdominal aorta) enhancement during abdominal MDCT study (SCHOELLNAST et al. 2004).

2.2.6
Collimation and Slice Thickness

With MDCT the same acquired raw dataset can be used to reconstruct two or more datasets of varying thickness. The optimal slice thickness for MDCT of the liver and its value for detection and characterization of focal liver lesions was extensively investigated. In a preliminary experience scans were achieved during hepatic arterial and portal venous phases using a detector configuration of 4×1 mm with a pitch factor of 1.4 (KOPKA et al. 2001). Slice thicknesses of 1, 2, 4, 6, 8, and 10 mm were retrospectively reconstructed and evaluated. It Was observed that slice thicknesses of 2 or 4 mm proved to be most effective for the detection of focal liver lesions, with an identical detection rate of 96%. Thinner (1 mm) and thicker (6, 8 and 10 mm) slice thicknesses showed significantly lower detection rates (85%, 84%, 75% and 70%, respectively). Moreover, 1-mm slice thickness generated the highest number of false positive findings. Lesion characterization was also significantly higher using 2 and 4 mm slice thicknesses. Results of 1-mm slice thickness were lower due to increased image noise which hindered the judgement of specific contrast material enhancement patterns; moreover,

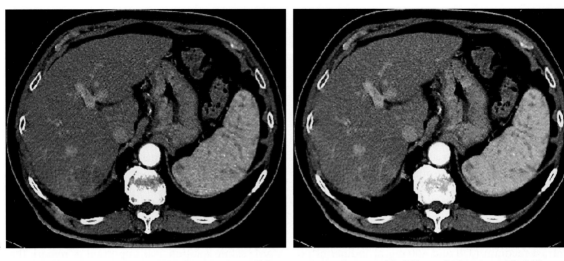

a   b

Fig. 2.11a,b. Image noise. From MDCT data set it is possible to reconstruct images with different thickness. **a** With thickness of 1.8 mm the noise is high and image is grainy. **b** A 5-mm thick slice is affected by lower noise and reduced artefacts

1-mm slice thickness has longer acquisition times, increases patient radiation exposure and produces a high number of images (Fig. 2.11). Correct characterization decreased with thicker (>4 mm) slices due to partial-volume artefacts. The most significant differences between different protocols were recorded for lesions smaller than 11 mm. Sensitivity and positive predictive value (PPV) in lesion identification were investigated with a detector configuration of 4×2.5 mm and reconstruction thickness of 2.5 mm, 5.0 mm and 7.5 mm. No statistically significant differences in terms of sensitivities and PPV for slice thickness of 2.5 mm and 5 mm (76% and 73% of sensitivity; 69% of PPV) were observed; but a significantly lower sensitivity was demonstrated if 7.5 mm slice thickness is used (KAWATA et al. 2002).

2.2.7
Radiation Issues

Phantom studies have revealed a possible increase in radiation exposure when imaging protocols of MDCT scanners have been compared to those of single-slice CT scanners. In general, energy dose values of the abdomen increased by a factor of 2.6 with multislice CT compared to single-slice CT. To take full advantage of the potentials of MDCT, imaging protocols must be adapted and optimized but the radiation dose must also be taken into consideration (FENCHEL et al. 2002). With MDCT there is a dramatic increase in radiation dose to the patient if mAs settings similar to those used for single-slice scanning are chosen. This can be due to either differences in scanner geometry (that result

in higher CT dose index per milliamperes, CTDI), different pre-filtering or due to the fact that the effective mAs (=mAs/pitch; by definition independent of pitch and therefore better indicator of patient dose) settings are displayed instead of the real mAs settings on the user interface; thus, if the protocol used for MDCT has the same mAs setting as the single-slice scanner protocol, the user will administer a higher radiation dose to the patient, proportional to the pitch used on the single-slice scanner. For these reasons, scanning protocols should be designed not on the basis of previous milliampere settings but on actual dose values as indicated by the CTDI, that can be displayed on the user interface of all MDCT scanners and represents the local dose quantity that indicates irradiation intensity inside the limits of the body regions as defined by the operator (FLEISCHMANN 2003a). It is a measure of the intensity of irradiation at a specified slice location and does not represent total radiation exposure. Dose-length product (DLP) is an integral dose quantity that describes total amount of absorbed radiation and represents the intensity and extent of irradiation for the entire series of CT examination. As different organs have different radiation sensitivity, normalizing the DLP on the basis of the specific organ, the effective DLP is obtained, which is the most relevant descriptor for assessing cancer risk. The result of DLP and effective DLP provide an estimate of effective dose with CT scanning. Dose reduction strategies may involve modifying scanning parameters or protocols to reduce radiation dose for individual patients or specific clinical situations and, technologic developments for improving scanner efficiency or improving image quality at low-dose CT scanning (KALRA et al. 2003).

2.3
Data Review Post-Processing

Due to the large number of slices generated by a single liver examination, especially if performed using a multiphasic study protocol, images should be analysed interactively by the operator on a secondary console (RUBIN 2000). Today all the MDCT scanners are equipped with two separate consoles, one for data acquisition and the second for data viewing and processing.

This approach requires powerful computers and user-friendly software in order to have a smooth data workflow. Real time interaction between operator and dataset is a mandatory pre-requisite. It is also important to have an absolutely seamless scrolling that lets the radiologist forget that he/she is reviewing several hundred images. Scrolling should be mouse-controlled in a way that lets the user move from top to bottom of the dataset within a single move but also lets him finely evaluate a particular abnormality. Slice thickness should interactively be chosen thick enough to reduce noise to a reasonable level but as thin as possible to keep partial volume effects low. It should be easy (one mouse click) to shift the image plane from axial to coronal or sagittal, or to change the viewing mode from thick multiplanar reformations to thin-slab maximum intensity projection (MIP) or even thin-slab volume rendering (VR) (KAMEL et al. 2003).

Image post-processing is based on more complex algorithms and is used for generating vascular reconstructions or for calculating hepatic volumetry.

Three-dimensional vascular reconstructions can be obtained by using either maximum intensity projection (MIP), or surface-rendering or volume-rendering algorithms.

For better anatomic representation and evaluation of spatial relationships, as well as for a faster and easier interaction with 3D datasets, volume rendering is the preferred reconstruction algorithm, although the diagnosis is derived from a combined evaluation of source and reconstructed images. With volume rendering, selective vessel representation is obtained using different rendering curves. A panoramic overview of the entire major abdominal branches can be obtained using a preset opacity curve showing only the vascular surface. The evaluation of minor vessels (i.e. second, third, and more distal orders of collateral branches) requires the analysis of 3D datasets using interactive multiplanar cut planes ("oblique trim") and by modulating the opacity of the anatomical structures under evaluation and window/level parameters in order to see vessels "through" abdominal organs. A complete analysis of arterial and venous vessels can be obtained within a mean interpretation time of 10 min.

Hepatic volumetry is another indication for post-processing liver datasets. Determination of liver volume is necessary in case of liver transplantation from a living donor (for both patient selection and surgical planning) and to evaluate the feasibility of hepatectomy, especially in the case of atypical resections (Fig. 2.12) (ABDALLA et al.

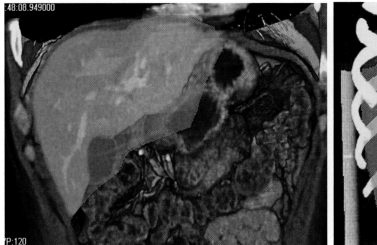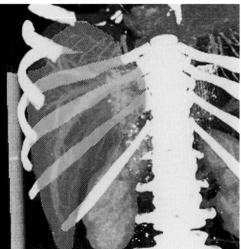

a · · · · · b

Fig. 2.12a,b. Volumetric rendering of liver parenchyma. **a** Calculation of the entire liver. **b** Following virtual left hepatectomy, the volume of the remaining right liver lobe is calculated

2004). An insufficient remnant liver volume calculated preoperatively might lead to performing iatrogenic occlusion of right or left portal vein in order to determine a lobar liver hypertrophy, making the resection feasible. Software for the calculation of liver volume is under development. From completely manual software where it was necessary to manually outline liver contour slice by slice, there are now semi-automatic and completely automatic programs (MEIER et al. 2004). The latter are able to highlight different liver segments and to create vascular maps for arterial and portal afferences and for hepatic vein drainage. The volume of each single segment can be calculated and a simulation of surgical resection can be performed. Information can be displayed using coloured maps or 3D movies (Fig. 2.13).

2.4
Conclusions

The development of spiral CT technology had a significant impact on liver imaging, further improved by the introduction of MDCT. Multiphasic and multiplanar capabilities of MDCT are the key issues representing the real added value of this technique. The possibility to acquire images during different pure vascular phases may improve the lesion detection rate, and may contribute to better characterization of focal liver lesions. Improved spatial resolution along the z-axis and the availability of almost-isotropic volumetric datasets offer high-quality multiplanar reconstructions as well as detailed vascular maps, especially useful before surgical and interventional therapeutic procedures.

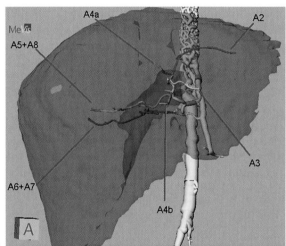

a

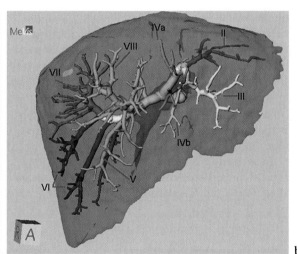

b

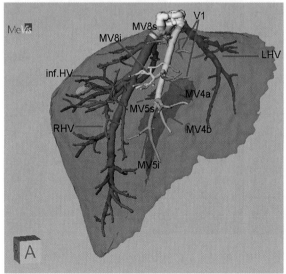

c

Fig. 2.13a–c. Automatic segmentation of hepatic parenchyma by means of liver vessels definition. **a** Three-dimensional reconstruction of different segments of hepatic artery. **b** Three-dimensional view of portal vein segmentation. **c** Similar view of segmental distribution of hepatic veins

References

Abdalla EK, Denys A, Chevalier P, et al (2004) Total and segmental liver volume variations: implications for liver surgery. Surgery 135:404–410

Altmann HW (1978) Pathology of human liver tumors. In: Remmer H, Bolt HM, Bannasch P (eds) Primary liver tumors. MTP, Lancaster, pp 53–71

Awai K, Takada K, Onishi H et al (2002) Aortic and hepatic enhancement and tumor to liver contrast: analysis of the effect of different concentrations of contrast material at multi-detector row helical CT. Radiology 224:757–763

Baron RL, Oliver JH 3rd, Dodd GD 3rd, et al (1996) Hepatocellular carcinoma: evaluation with biphasic, contrast enhanced, helical CT. Radiology 199:505–511

Berland LL, Smith JK (1998) Multidetector-array CT: once again, technology creates new opportunities. Radiology 209:327–329

Bernardino ME, Galambos JT (1989) Computed tomography and magnetic resonance imaging of the liver. Semin Liver Dis 9:32–49

Brink JA (2003) Contrast optimization and scan timing for single- and multidetector-row computed tomography. J Comput Assist Tomogr 27 [Suppl 1]:S3–8

Cademartiri F, Luccichenti G, Marano R, et al (2003) Spiral CT-angiography with one, four, and sixteen slice scanners. Technical note. Radiol Med 106:269–283

Choi BI, Lee HJ, Han JK et al (1997) Detection of hypervascular nodular hepatocellular carcinomas: value of triphasic helical CT compared with iodized-oil CT. AJR Am J Roentgenol 168:219–224

Dorio PJ, Lee FT Jr., Henseler KP et al (2003) Shock SA. Using a saline chaser to decrease contrast media in abdominal CT. AJR Am J Roentgenol 180:929–934

Fenchel S, Fleiter TR, Merkle EM (2002) Multislice helical CT of the abdomen. Eur Radiol 12:S5–S10

Ferrucci JT (1991) Liver tumor imaging: current concepts. Keio J Med 40:194–205

Fleischmann D (2003a) Future prospects in MDCT imaging. Eur Radiol 13 [Suppl 5]:M127–M128

Fleischmann D (2003b) Use of high-concentration contrast media in multiple-detector-row CT: principles and rationale. Eur Radiol 13:M14–M20

Flohr T, Stierstorfer K, Bruder H, et al (2002) New technical developments in multislice CT. Part 1: approaching isotropic resolution with sub-millimeter 16-slice scanning. Rofo Fortschr Geb Rontgenstr Neuen Bildgeb Verfahr 174:839–845

Foley WD, Mallisee TA, Hohenwalter MD, et al (2000) Multiphase hepatic CT with a multirow detector CT scanner. AJR Am J Roentgenol 175:679–685

Hittmair K, Fleischmann D (2001) Accuracy of predicting and controlling time-dependent aortic enhancement from a test bolus injection. J Comput Assist Tomogr 25:287–294

Hollett MD, Jeffrey RB Jr, Nino-Murcia M et al (1995) Dual-phase helical CT of the liver: value of arterial phase scans in the detection of small (≤1.5 cm) malignant hepatic neoplasms. AJR Am J Roentgenol 164:879–884

Honda O, Johkoh T, Yamamoto S et al (2002) Comparison of quality of multiplanar reconstructions and direct coronal multidetector CT scans of the lung. AJR Am J Roentgenol 179:875–879

Hu H, He HD, Foley WD, et al (2000) Four multidetector-row helical CT: image quality and volume coverage speed. Radiology 215:55–62

Hwang GJ, Kim MJ, Yoo HS et al (1997) Nodular hepatocellular carcinomas: detection with arterial-, portal-, and delayed-phase images at spiral CT. Radiology 202:383–388

Ichikawa T, Kitamura T, Nakajima H et al (2002) Hypervascular hepatocellular carcinoma: can double arterial phase imaging with Multidetector CT improve tumor depiction in the cirrhotic liver? AJR Am J Roentgenol 179:751–758

Ji H, Ros PP (2001) Application of multislice computed tomography in liver and pancreas. In: Marincek B, Ros PP, Reiser M, Baker ME (eds) Multislice CT: a practical guide. Springer, Berlin Heidelberg New York, pp 195–203

Ji H, McTavish GD, Mortele KJ et al (2001) Hepatic imaging with multidetector CT. Radiographics 21:S71–S80

Kalender WA, Seissler W, Klotz E, et al (1990) Spiral volumetric CT with single breath-hold technique, continuous transport, and continuous scanner rotation. Radiology 176:181–183

Kalra MK, Maher MM, Saini S (2003) Future prospects in MDCT imaging. Eur Radiol 13 [Suppl 5]:M129–M133

Kamel IR, Georgiades C, Fishman EK (2003) Incremental value of advanced image processing of multislice computed tomography data in the evaluation of hypervascular liver lesions. J Comput Assist Tomogr 27:652–656

Kang BK, Lim JH, Kim SH et al (2003) Preoperative depiction of hepatocellular carcinoma: ferumoxides-enhanced MR imaging versus triple-phase helical CT. Radiology 226:79–85

Kawata S, Murakami T, Kim T et al (2002) Multidetector CT: diagnostic impact of slice thickness on detection of hypervascular hepatocellular carcinoma. AJR Am J Roentgenol 179:61–66

Kim T, Murakami T, Takahashi S et al (1998) Effects of injection rates of contrast material on arterial phase hepatic CT. AJR Am J Roentgenol 171:429–432

Kim T, Murakami T, Takahashi S et al (1999) Optimal phases of dynamic CT for detecting hepatocellular carcinoma: evaluation of unenhanced and triple-phase images. Abdom Imaging 24:473–480

Kim T, Murakami T, Hori M et al (2002) Small hypervascular hepatocellular carcinoma revealed by double arterial phase CT performed with single breath-hold scanning and automatic bolus tracking. AJR Am J Roentgenol 178:899–904

Klingenbeck-Regn K, Schaller S, Flohr T et al (1999) Subsecond multi-slice computed tomography: basics and applications. Eur J Radiol 31:110–124

Kopka L, Rodenwaldt J, Hamm B (2001) Biphasic multi-slice helical CT of the liver: intraindividual comparison of different slice thicknesses for the detection and characterization of focal liver lesions. Radiology 217:367

Kopp AF, Heuschmid M, Claussen CD (2002) Multidetector helical CT of the liver for tumor detection and characterization. Eur Radiol 12:745–752

Laghi A, Iannaccone R, Rossi P et al (2003) Hepatocellular carcinoma: detection with triple-phase multi-detector row CT in patients with chronic hepatitis. Radiology 226:543–549

Laniado M, Kopp AF (1997) Liver specific contrast media: a magic bullet or a weapon for dedicated targets? Radiology 205:319–322

Liang Y, Kruger RA (1996) Dual-slice spiral versus single-slice spiral scanning: comparison of the physical performance of two computed tomography scanners. Med Phys 23:205–220

Lim JH, Choi D, Kim SH et al (2002) Detection of hepatocellular carcinoma: value of adding delayed phase imaging to
dual-phase helical CT. AJR Am J Roentgenol 179:67–73

Marchianò A (2003) MDCT of primary liver malignancies. Eur
Radiol 13:M26-M30

Meier S, Schenk A, Mildenberger P et al (2004) Evaluation of a
new software tool for the automatic volume calculation of
hepatic tumors. First results. Rofo Fortschr Geb Rontgenstr
Neuen Bildgeb Verfahr 176:234–238

Miller FH, Butler RS, Hoff FL et al (1998) Using triphasic helical CT to detect focal hepatic lesions in patients with neoplasms. AJR Am J Roentgenol 171:643-649

Murakami T, Kim T, Takamura M, et al (2001) Hypervascular
hepatocellular carcinoma: detection with double arterial
phase multi-detector row helical CT. Radiology 218:763–767

Oliver JH 3rd, Baron RL, Federle MP et al (1996) Detecting
hepatocellular carcinoma: value of unenhanced or arterial phase CT imaging or both used in conjunction with
conventional portal venous phase contrast-enhanced CT
imaging. AJR Am J Roentgenol 167:71–77

Oliver JH 3rd, Baron RL, Federle MP et al (1997) Hypervascular liver metastases: do unenhanced and hepatic arterial phase CT images affect tumor detection? Radiology
205:709–715

Prokop M (2003a) Multislice CT: technical principles and
future trends. Eur Radiol 13 [Suppl 5]:M3–M13

Prokop M (2003b) Image processing and display techniques.
In: Prokop M, Galanski M (eds) Spiral and multislice computed tomography of the body. Thieme, Stuttgart, pp 131–
160

Prokop M (2003c) General Principles of MDCT. Eur J Radiol
45:S4–S10

Rubin GD (2000) Data explosion: the challenge of multidetector-row CT. Eur J Radiol 36:74–80

Saini S, Dsouza RV (2003) Optimizing technique for multislice CT. Eur Radiol 13:M21–M24

Schoellnast H, Tillich M, Deutschmann HA et al (2004)
Improvement of parenchymal and vascular enhancement
using saline flush and power injection for multiple-detector-row abdominal CT. Eur Radiol 14:659–664

Sheiman RG, Raptopoulos V, Caruso P, et al (1996) Comparison of tailored and empiric scan delays for CT
angiography of the abdomen. AJR Am J Roentgenol
167:725–729

Uggowitzer MM (2003) What is the current situation in liver
imaging? Eur Radiol 13 [Suppl 3]:N65–69

Valls C, Cos M, Figueras J et al (2004) Pretransplantation diagnosis and staging of hepatocellular carcinoma in patients
with cirrhosis: value of dual-phase helical CT. AJR Am J
Roentgenol 182:1011–1017

Wang G, Vannier MW (1999) The effect of pitch in multislice
spiral/helical CT. Med Phys 26:2648–2653

3 Magnetic Resonance

Carlo Bartolozzi, Clotilde Della Pina, Dania Cioni, Laura Crocetti, Elisa Batini, and Riccardo Lencioni

CONTENTS

3.1
Introduction

Technical advances in magnetic resonance (MR) hardware and software have allowed the introduction of faster pulse sequences void of motion artifacts that previously posed limitations to abdominal MR imaging. Plain imaging is useful to point out the morphology and the inherent structure of focal liver lesions and provides essential information for the diagnosis. However, in most cases, these features are not enough to correctly detect and characterize liver tumors (Bartolozzi et al. 1999; Bartolozzi et al. 2001). MR imaging contrast agents are currently used to accentuate the differences in signal intensity between the liver lesion and the adjacent tissue and to highlight different enhancement patterns. Thus there is now a consensus that use of contrast media is mandatory in liver MR imaging. A variety of contrast agents, including extracellular, hepatobiliary, and reticuloendothelial system (RES)-targeted contrast agents, is used to improve the diagnostic capability of MR imaging (Lencioni et al. 2004). Furthermore, MR can also provide functional information in addition to morphological information: new techniques such as diffusion and perfusion imaging have been developed and now are assuming an increasing role in clinical practice.

3.2
Methodology

The technical equipment of the MR scanner, the choice of pulse sequence and the use of the most appropriate contrast agent should be taken into consideration to obtain high quality liver MR examinations. The use of high field strength MR scanners (≥ 1.0 T) with fast gradients and phased-array surface coils is now standard for liver MR imaging (Keogan and Edelman 2001; Morrin and Rofsky 2001). Phased-array coils provide a great improvement in the signal to noise ratio (SNR) and a better image quality (Schwartz et al. 1997). The recently developed parallel imaging exploits the intrinsic different sensitivity of phased-array coils to speed the acquisition time. Rapidly switched gradient systems are needed to obtain fast sequences as echo-planar imaging, true fast imaging with steady state free precession (true FISP) or sequences with short repetition time (TR) and echo time (TE). Nevertheless the selection of the MR sequence and the manipulation of parameters are fundamental to avoid motion artifacts and increase the SNR and contrast to noise (CNR) ratio.

3.2.1
Technical Issues

Motion artifacts have been traditionally considered as an important limitation in performing liver MR. Two strategies have been pursued to obtain high quality MR images: (1) suppression of the movement artifacts; (2) reduction of the acquisition time.

C. Bartolozzi, MD; C. Della Pina, MD; D. Cioni, MD; L. Crocetti, MD; E. Batini, MD; R. Lencioni, MD
Division of Diagnostic and Interventional Radiology, Department of Oncology, Transplants, and Advanced Technologies in Medicine, University of Pisa, Via Roma 67, 56126 Pisa, Italy

To avoid motion artifacts, respiratory triggered imaging was introduced. Images are acquired in a fixed point of the expiratory breathing phase; the limitation of this kind of sequence is its inefficacy in patients with irregular breathing and its long acquisition time, which is related also to the respiratory frequency of the patient (Fig. 3.1) (Low et al. 1997). Fat suppression is another tool to reduce motion artifacts, in particular to eliminate those concentric hyperintense lines superimposed on abdominal organs produced by movement of the abdominal wall (BARISH and JARA 1999; Low et al. 1994).

On the other hand, strong gradients accelerate image encoding times and enable fast and ultrafast imaging, including fast dynamic, parallel and echo-planar imaging. Fast imaging with breath hold sequences allows the elimination of the respiratory artifacts and blurring, and greatly reduces the acquisition time. To improve the SNR, fat sup-

pression is needed when fast images are performed (Fig. 3.2) (KANEMATSU et al. 1999). More recently, parallel acquisition techniques have allowed two to four times faster acquisition of the entire liver if compared to other pulse sequences. Most important, the parallel MR approach may accelerate any imaging sequence (HEIDEMANN et al. 2003). The accelerated image acquisition derives from an array of surface coils that are used as independent elements elaborating MR echoes simultaneously (each coil detects only a part of the object). To decrease the acquisition time a certain fraction of phase-encoding steps are skipped and images are reconstructed by means of dedicated parallel MR algorithms (SENSE, SMASH, GRAPPA, etc.). However, the shorter total acquisition time slightly decreases the SNR, making this new approach especially useful in non-cooperative patients (McKENZIE et al. 2004).

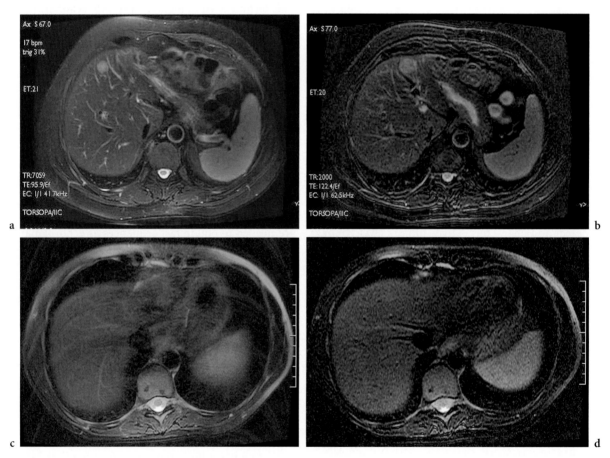

Fig. 3.1a–d. T2-weighted respiratory triggered and breath-hold FRFSE imaging. **a** Respiratory triggered FRFSE has a longer acquisition time (3 min and 39 s) in comparison with breath-hold imaging (40 s) (**b**). **c** If the patient is unable to produce a regular respiratory waveform, triggering may be unsuccessful with evident motion artifacts. **d** Breath-hold examination allows high quality images to be obtained even in patients with irregular breathing

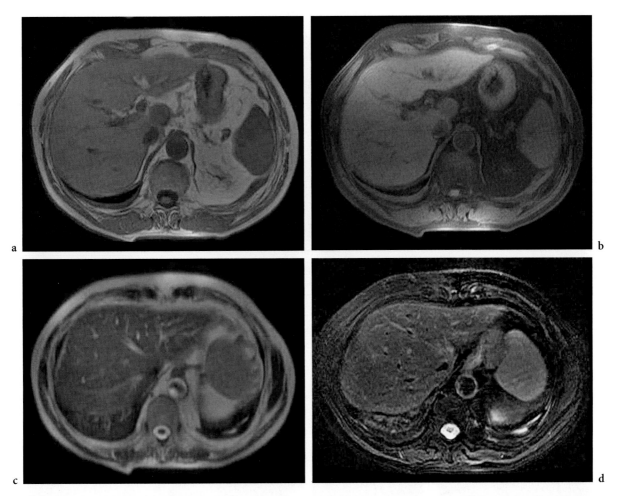

Fig. 3.2a–d. T1-weighted FSPGR and T2-weighted FRFSE without and with fat saturation protocol. Comparison between T1-weighted FSPGR without (**a**) and with fat saturation (**b**), and between T2-weighted FRFSE without (**c**) and with fat saturation (**d**), shows that fat suppression is needed to improve SNR when fast images are performed

3.2.2
Fast and Ultrafast Imaging

Improvements in gradient performance allow the application of very short TR and TE, enabling subsecond acquisition (NITZ 2002). The more widely used sequences for T1-weighted images are fast spoiled gradient recalled acquisition into steady state (FSPGR) and fast low angle shot (FLASH) sequences, with short TR and short TE. To evaluate lipid compounds in focal lesions, fatty sparing or fatty infiltration, TE may be set in phase (4.4 ms at 1.5 T) or out of phase (2.2 ms at 1.5 T). Signal intensity decrease is present in out of phase images if fat and water are in the same voxel. In phase and out of phase images can be acquired simultaneously with a double-echo gradient echo (GRE) sequence (Fig. 3.3) (ROFSKY et al. 1996; SOYER et al. 1997).

T1-weighted bidimensional (2D) GRE sequences are used to perform dynamic studies throughout the liver. The need to acquire enough sections to cover the whole liver during a breath-hold requires sections of no more than 8–10 mm. Volumetric interpolated breath-hold examination (VIBE) permits the acquisition of isotropic pixels of approximately 2 mm in all dimensions with an acquisition time of less than 25 s. The volumetric data set can be reconstructed in any plane, producing MR angiography and venography that can be useful in the assessment of liver vascular anatomy (Fig. 3.4) (HAWIGHORST et al. 1999; LEE et al. 2000; ROFSKY et al. 1999).

Turbo spin-echo/fast spin-echo (TSE/FSE) is the well accepted sequence for obtaining breath-hold T2-weighted images (KANEMATSU et al. 1999). The TSE/FSE technique shows a tissue contrast similar to that of conventional T2-weighted SE images, but

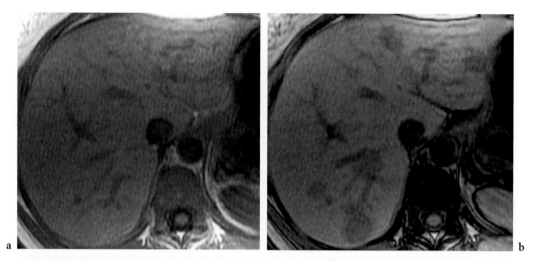

Fig. 3.3a,b. GRE in phase and out of phase. **a** GRE in phase (TE:4.4 ms): no focal lesions are visible. **b** GRE out of phase (TE:2.2 ms): some focal fat infiltrations are visible as hypointense lesions, because fat and water spins are in opposed phase, then their signal cannot be summed up

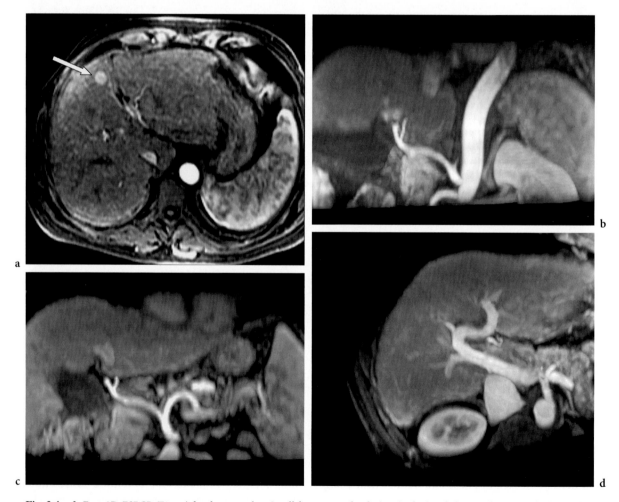

Fig. 3.4a–d. Fast 3D FSPGR T1-weighted protocol. **a** Small hypervascular lesion is depicted during the arterial phase after paramagnetic contrast media administration (*arrow*). **b–d** Coronal maximum intensity projection images of arterial (**b, c**) and venous (**d**) phase can be useful in the assessment of vascular anatomy

with faster acquisition time. The potential reduction in acquisition time with TSE/FSE is directly proportional to the number of echoes: to reduce the duration of breath-hold, a long echo train should be used (>17 echoes). The reduction in the acquisition time can be converted into an improved contrast setting a longer TR, or into an improved spatial resolution increasing the matrix size. Fat suppression is necessary, because the short interecho spacing increases fat signal intensity. The respiratory-triggered FSE can be useful in patients who are unable to hold the breath also for a few seconds. The limitation of this sequence is the long acquisition time, also influenced by the respiratory frequency of the patient.

A modified FSE technique with fast recovery (FRFSE) was developed to allow full coverage of the liver in one or two breath holds with high quality T2-weighted images (AUGUI et al. 2002). The FRFSE technique guides the recovery of longitudinal magnetization instead of leaving it to recover with the T1 process. This results in better SNR for liver and CNR for hepatic lesions than those obtained with FSE T2-weighted images. The half-Fourier single-shot turbo spin echo (HASTE) sequence is helpful in uncooperative, medically unstable or claustrophobic patients; another acronym is single-shot FSE (SSFSE) (HELMBERGER et al. 1999). With HASTE only half the K-space is filled, with a few additional lines to correct the imperfections, the remaining part being reconstructed by software. The time saving, however, has its price as the SNR is decreased (KIM et al. 1998).

Sequences that are sensitive to magnetic susceptibility, such as T2*-weighted sequences, are useful for the study of hemochromatosis or for focal liver lesions following the injection of superparamagnetic iron oxide (SPIO) contrast agents. T2*-weighted GRE images are more sensitive to the effects of SPIO in comparison to T2-weighted FSE, because they lack a 180° refocusing pulse, so the effect of susceptibility from local field inhomogeneities is increased (Fig. 3.5) (WARD et al. 2003).

Single-shot echo-planar imaging (EPI), which allows the acquisition of a T2-weighted image in a very short time, is useful for new applications such as diffusion and perfusion imaging. In addition to providing information for morphologic diagnosis, EPI is widely used for functional and qualitative diagnosis (YAMASHITA et al. 1998). Diffusion is the thermally induced motion of water molecules in biologic tissues. The abdominal organs have unique diffusion characteristics, as measured with the apparent diffusion coefficient (ADC). The results of some recent studies have shown that benign lesions, such as hepatic cysts and hemangiomas, have higher ADCs than malignant lesions (hepatocellular carcinoma and metastases), where the large amount of tumoral cells restricts the water diffusion (Fig. 3.6) (ICHIKAWA et al. 1998a; KIM et al. 1999). TAOULI et al. (2003) showed that, for the diagnosis of malignant lesions, the use of a threshold ADC value less than 1.5×10^{-3} mm^2/s, with a diffusion factor ("b") of 0 and 500 s/mm^2, would result in sensitivity, specificity, positive predictive value, and accuracy of 84%, 89%, 87% and 86% respectively. Moreover, with single-shot echo-planar technique, it is possible to perform a perfusion study of the liver by obtaining images at 1–2 s intervals after a bolus injection of paramagnetic contrast agent. On perfusion-weighted images (which are T2*-weighted images) gadolinium chelates serve as negative contrast agents decreasing the signal in the enhancing lesions (PADHANI and HUSBAND 2001). ICHIKAWA et al. (1998b) were able to discriminate between metastases, hepatocellular carcinoma (HCC) and hemangiomas on the basis of different signal intensity changes on EPI. In HCC and hemangiomas, a signal intensity decrease was observed as the contrast agent reaches the tumor; in contrast in metastases the decrease in signal intensity was minimal (ICHIKAWA et al. 1998b). Negative T2*-weighted enhancement may be advantageous in the evaluation of perfusion in tumors that are hyperintense on T1 images, such as well differentiated HCC.

Ultrafast imaging of the liver can be performed by using the true fast imaging with steady state free precession (true FISP), that is a GRE sequence with fully refocused transverse magnetization. Another acronym for this technique is fast imaging employing steady-state acquisition (FIESTA) (Fig. 3.7). True FISP imaging keeps TR and TE as short as possible to minimize motion and susceptibility artifacts. In true FISP imaging the contrast is related to the T2/T1 ratio; thus the tissues with a high T2/T1 ratio like blood, fat and bile appear bright. Acquisition time is approximately 10 s; thus it is possible to scan the liver in a breath-hold. This type of sequence permits detailed information of the vascular system to be gained without contrast agents and is under investigation for the characterization of focal liver lesions (NUMMINEM et al. 2003; HERBON et al. 2003).

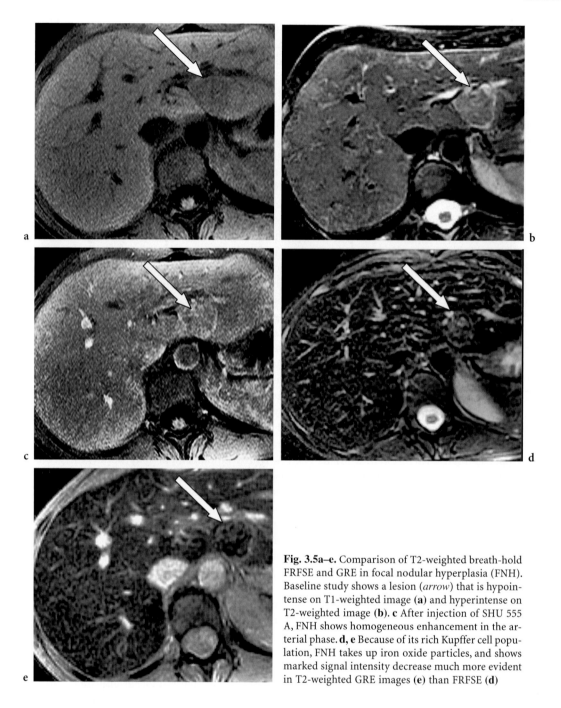

Fig. 3.5a–e. Comparison of T2-weighted breath-hold FRFSE and GRE in focal nodular hyperplasia (FNH). Baseline study shows a lesion (*arrow*) that is hypointense on T1-weighted image (**a**) and hyperintense on T2-weighted image (**b**). **c** After injection of SHU 555 A, FNH shows homogeneous enhancement in the arterial phase. **d, e** Because of its rich Kupffer cell population, FNH takes up iron oxide particles, and shows marked signal intensity decrease much more evident in T2-weighted GRE images (**e**) than FRFSE (**d**)

Fig. 3.6a–f. Diffusion-weighted imaging in benign and malignant tumors. In hemangioma single-shot echoplanar images at b=500 s/mm^2 (**a**) and b=0 s/mm^2 (**b**) show hyperintense lesion. **c** Mapping image had an ADC of 1.9×10^{-3} mm^2/s. **d, e** In metastasis single-shot echoplanar images at b=500 s/mm^2 (**d**) and b=0 s/mm^2 (**e**) show hyperintense lesion (*arrows*). **f** Mapping image had an ADC of 1×10^{-3} mm^2/s. Benign lesions, such as hemangiomas, have higher ADCs than malignant lesions, where the large amount of tumoral cells restricts the water diffusion

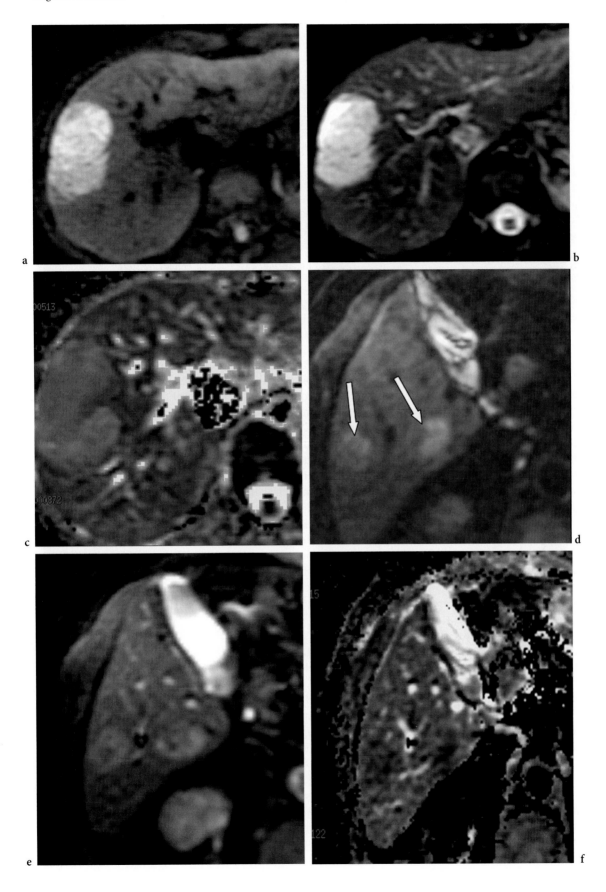

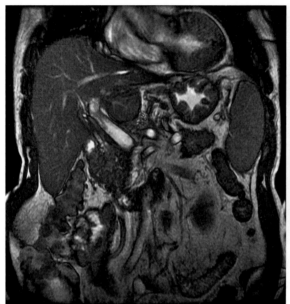

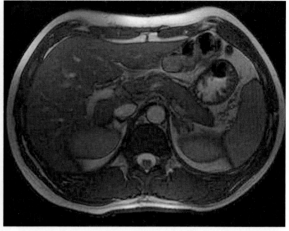

Fig. 3.7a,b. Fast imaging employing steady-state acquisition (FIESTA) sequence. Anatomic features can be visualized in a single breath-hold using coronal (**a**) and axial plane (**b**). Tissues like blood, fat and bile appear bright because of their high T2/T1 ratio

3.3
Contrast Agents

According to the biodistribution, the contrast agents available for liver imaging can be divided into three categories: (a) extracellular contrast agents; (b) hepatobiliary contrast agents; and (c) RES-targeted contrast agents (SEMELKA and HELMBERGER 2001; LENCIONI et al. 2004).

3.3.1
Extracellular Contrast Agents

Extracellular contrast agents are hydrophilic, small-molecular-weight gadolinium chelates. After intravenous administration these substances are rapidly cleared from the intravascular space to the interstitial space. They do not penetrate into intact cells and are eliminated via the urinary system. Several gadolinium complexes are currently available including gadopentetate dimeglumine (Gd-DTPA, Magnevist, Schering AG/Berlex Laboratoires), gadoterate meglumine (Gd-DOTA, Dotarem, Laboratoires Guerbet), gadodiamide (Gd-DTPA-BMA, Omniscan, Amersham Health), and gadoteridol (Gd-HP-DO3A, ProHance, Bracco). The usual clinical dose of these gadolinium chelates is 0.1 mmol/kg.

Extracellular contrast agents provide information on vascularization and perfusion similar to that of iodinated contrast media used for CT. Following the introduction of breath-hold T1-weighted GRE sequences, a dynamic contrast-enhanced study of the liver is performed during the arterial (20–30 s after injection), portal venous (70–80 s after injection), and the delayed phase (2–3 min after injection) of enhancement (Figs. 3.8, 3.9) (BELLIN et al. 2003; HAMM et al. 1994; MAHFOUZ et al. 1993; YU et al. 1999). Fat saturation is recommended to decrease motion artifacts and to homogenize the images.

The timing of image acquisition has a key role: arterial phase imaging may be inadequate if fixed image delays are used. To overcome this problem, some approaches may be used such as a timing bolus of 1–2 ml of a Gd-chelate, automatic triggering based on the detection of vessel enhancement (Smartprep, Carebolus), and fluoroscopic imaging (HUSSAIN et al. 2003).

3.3.2
Hepatobiliary Contrast Agents

Hepatobiliary or hepatocyte-selective contrast agents are paramagnetic compounds that are partially taken up by the hepatocytes and excreted in the biliary tract (REIMER et al. 2004). Two hepatobiliary agents are currently available on the market: gadobenate dimeglumine (Gd-BOPTA/Dimeg, MultiHance, Bracco) and mangafodipir trisodium (MnDPDP, Teslascan, Amersham Health). A third hepatobiliary contrast agent, gadolinium ethoxybenzyl diethylenetriaminepentaacetic acid (Gd-EOB-DTPA, Primovist, Schering AG), is likely to get approval shortly.

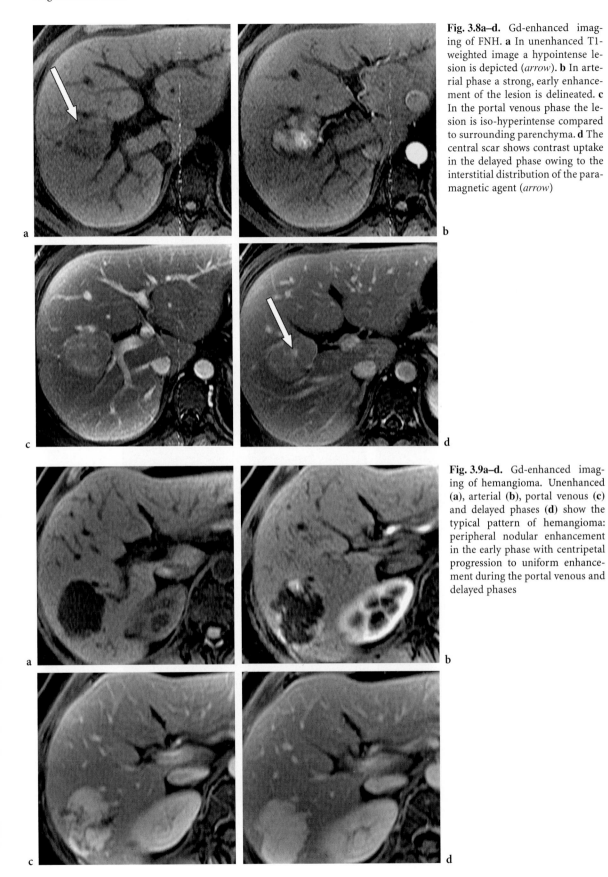

Fig. 3.8a–d. Gd-enhanced imaging of FNH. **a** In unenhanced T1-weighted image a hypointense lesion is depicted (*arrow*). **b** In arterial phase a strong, early enhancement of the lesion is delineated. **c** In the portal venous phase the lesion is iso-hyperintense compared to surrounding parenchyma. **d** The central scar shows contrast uptake in the delayed phase owing to the interstitial distribution of the paramagnetic agent (*arrow*)

Fig. 3.9a–d. Gd-enhanced imaging of hemangioma. Unenhanced (**a**), arterial (**b**), portal venous (**c**) and delayed phases (**d**) show the typical pattern of hemangioma: peripheral nodular enhancement in the early phase with centripetal progression to uniform enhancement during the portal venous and delayed phases

Gd-BOPTA consists of a hydrophilic Gd-DTPA moiety covalently coupled to a lipophilic benzene ring; this contrast agent is intravenously administered in a lower dose of 0.05 mmol/kg compared to other extracellular contrast agents. Gd-EOB-DTPA is a highly water-soluble contrast agent with an ethoxybenzyl group attached to the gadolinium ion. The agent can be administered as a bolus in the dose of 25 μmol/kg. These compounds undergo both hepatobiliary and renal excretion. Approximately 50% of the administered dose of Gd-EOB-DTPA is excreted in the bile, which is much higher than the biliary ex-cretion of Gd-BOPTA (approximately 5%). The remainder undergoes renal glomerular filtration and excretion. It is thought that the hepatic uptake occurs through the organic anion transport system located on the hepatocytes' membrane. These Gd-chelates are both a non-specific extracellular contrast agent on early post-contrast images and a hepatospecific contrast agent on delayed images: these agents can be administered as a bolus injection allowing dynamic study; then they provide a persistent enhancement of normal hepatic parenchyma due to their uptake by hepatocytes (Figs. 3.10, 3.11). Hepatospecific phase

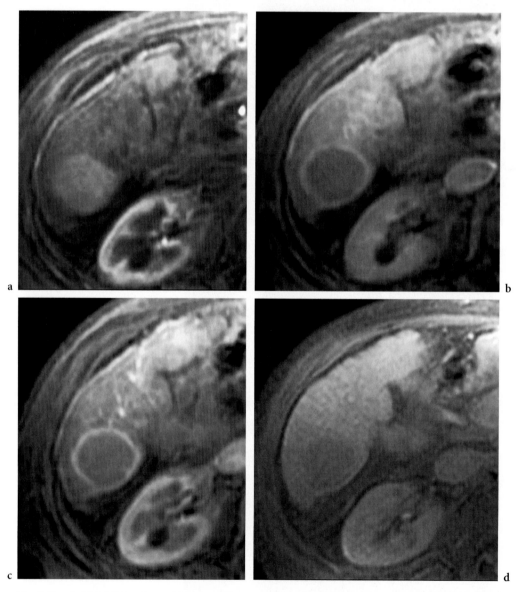

Fig. 3.10a–d. Gd-BOPTA-enhanced imaging of hepatocellular carcinoma (HCC). **a** T1-weighted 3D FSPGR in the arterial phase delineates the HCC with early uptake of contrast. **b, c** In the portal and delayed phase the lesion shows wash-out of contrast material and hyperintense pseudocapsule. **d** In the hepatospecific phase no uptake of contrast is seen

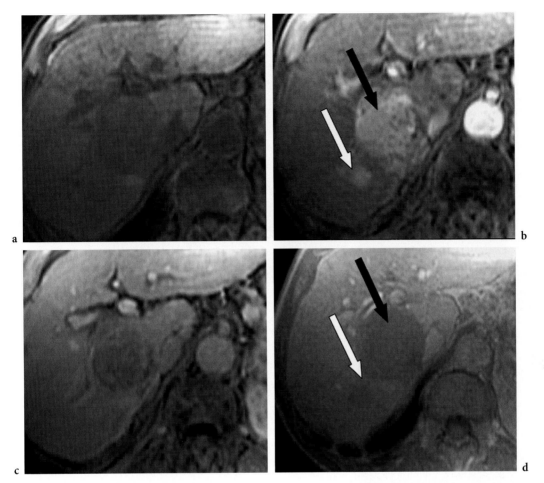

Fig. 3.11a–d. Gd-EOB-DTPA-enhanced imaging of HCC. **a** Unenhanced T1-weighted image delineates a large hypointense lesion. **b** T1-weigheted 3D FSPGR in the arterial phase delineates the large HCC with early uptake of contrast (*black arrow*) and a tiny hypervascular satellite nodule (*white arrow*). **c** In the portal phase the main lesion shows wash-out of contrast material. **d** In the hepatospecific phase both lesions do not show uptake of contrast (*arrows*)

imaging can be performed at 20 min after the injection of Gd-EOB-DTPA and at 40 min after the injection of Gd-BOPTA (Huppertz et al. 2004; Spinazzi et al. 1998).

On the other hand, Mn-DPDP is a weak chelate of the Mn ion, and dissociates in vivo to give free Mn, which is taken up by the hepatocytes and excreted into the bile. The contrast agent is injected at a dose of 0.5 ml/kg as a slow drop infusion with an injection speed of 2–3 ml/min. Scans following Mn-DPDP are obtained 20 min after the start of the injection (Figs. 3.12, 3.13) (Reimer et al. 2004).

Besides the dynamic scanning feasible with those contrast agents injected as a bolus, these agents produce strong and sustained enhancement of liver parenchyma on T1-weighted images (Huppertz et al. 2004; Oudkerk et al. 2002; Petersein et al. 2000; Tsuda et al. 2004). Because of the selective increase in the signal intensity of normal hepatocytes compared with tumor cells of malignant focal lesions, CNR between lesions and healthy liver is usually increased, and lesion detectability and conspicuity are improved on T1-weighted images (Bartolozzi et al. 2000; Bartolozzi et al. 2004; Kim et al. 2004; Reimer et al. 1997).

Due to the strong biliary excretion of Mn-DPDP and Gd-EOB-DTPA, enhancement of the biliary system is visualized 20 min after administration. This effect gives additional information to MR cholangiography T2-weighted pulse sequences. For visualization of the contrast-enhanced biliary system, a T1-weighted 3D GRE pulse sequence in the coro-

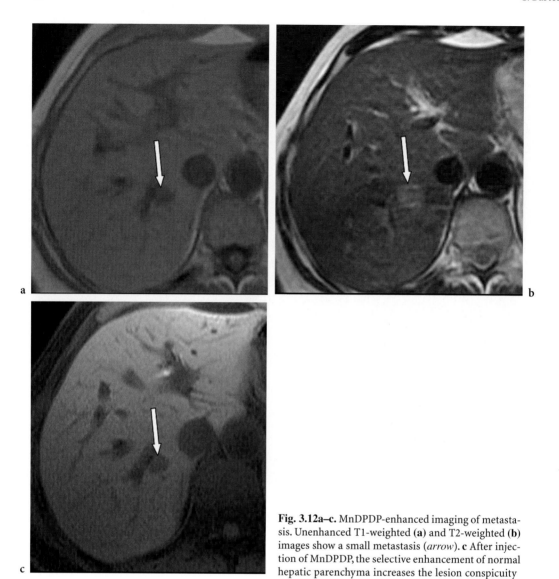

Fig. 3.12a–c. MnDPDP-enhanced imaging of metastasis. Unenhanced T1-weighted (**a**) and T2-weighted (**b**) images show a small metastasis (*arrow*). **c** After injection of MnDPDP, the selective enhancement of normal hepatic parenchyma increases the lesion conspicuity

nal/oblique plane provides the best spatial resolution (Carlos et al. 2002; Lee et al. 2001).

3.3.3
RES-Targeted Contrast Agents

RES-targeted contrast agents are superparamagnetic particles of iron oxide (SPIO) which produce distortions of local magnetic field. The inhomogeneous field causes dephasing of hydrogen spins in tissues that take up the iron oxide particles, resulting in signal loss on T2-weighted images. Once injected intravenously, these agents are rapidly removed from the circulation by the RES system. Kupffer cells in the liver play a dominant role in this process, taking up more than 80% of circulating particles. Two of these agents are currently available for clinical use: AMI-25 (Endorem, Laboratoires Guerbet; or Feridex, Advanced Magnetics) and SH U 555 A (Resovist, Schering AG).

The iron oxide AMI-25 is administered in a dosage of 10–15 µmol/kg and infused over 30 min. Static post-contrast T2-weighted images are obtained 30 min after the infusion. SHU 555 A is administered via intravenous bolus injection in a fixed dose of 0.9 ml per patient with a body weight ranging from 35 to 60 kg and 1.4 ml per patients above

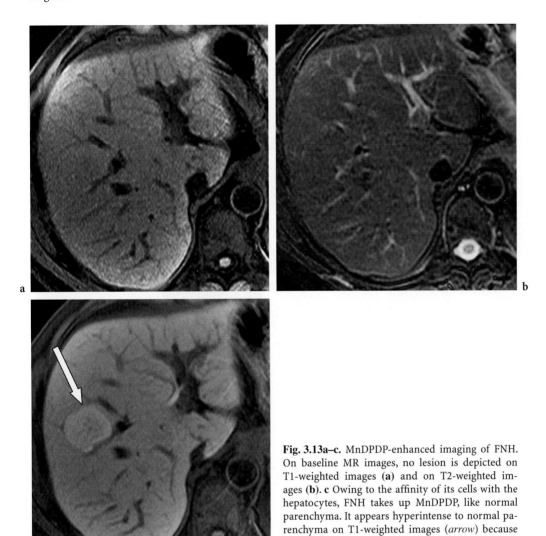

Fig. 3.13a–c. MnDPDP-enhanced imaging of FNH. On baseline MR images, no lesion is depicted on T1-weighted images (**a**) and on T2-weighted images (**b**). **c** Owing to the affinity of its cells with the hepatocytes, FNH takes up MnDPDP, like normal parenchyma. It appears hyperintense to normal parenchyma on T1-weighted images (*arrow*) because the contrast agent is trapped within the lesion, since FNH is unable to effectively eliminate the compound via biliary excretion

60 kg. The diameters of the particles range between 45 and 60 nm: the larger particles are quickly taken up by Kupffer cells; the smaller ones remain longer in the vessels, displaying blood pool characteristics. Therefore peculiar features of SHU 555 A include bolus administration, which can deliver dynamic imaging using the T1 effect of the vascular phase, and early Kupffer cell uptake, which allows liver-specific phase imaging 10 min after the injection (Fig. 3.14) (Reimer and Balzer 2003; Kopp et al. 1997). Breathhold T1-weighted dynamic imaging can be obtained either using 2D sequences or 3D protocols with fat saturation.

The reduction in signal intensity of liver parenchyma on T2-weighted images increases lesion detectability and conspicuity, since malignant focal lesions, that usually do not contain Kupffer cells, do not change their signal intensity after injection of RES-targeted agents and therefore appear as bright nodules (Fig. 3.15) (Reimer and Tombach 1998; Lencioni et al. 1998; Ros et al. 1995; Vogl et al. 2003).

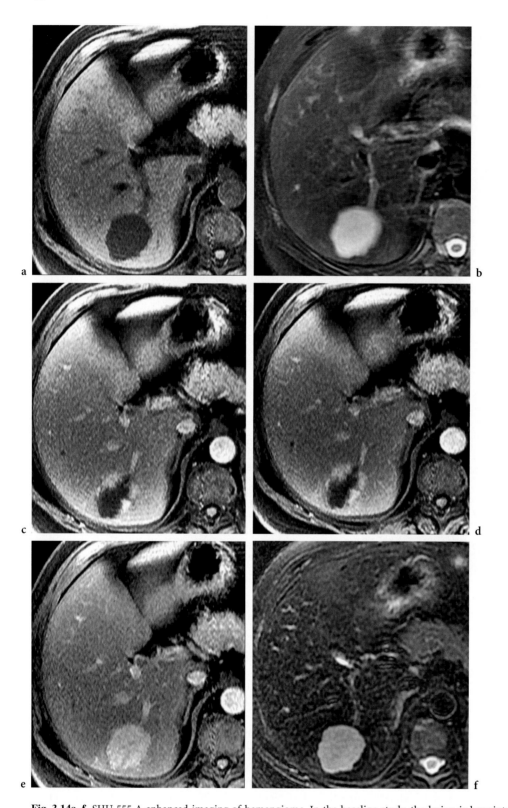

Fig. 3.14a–f. SHU 555 A-enhanced imaging of hemangioma. In the baseline study, the lesion is hypointense on T1-weighted image (**a**) and hyperintense on T2-weighted image (**b**). **c, d** Dynamic SHU 555 A-enhanced study shows the centripetal filling of the hemangioma similar to Gd-enhanced studies. **e** Hemangiomas show a peculiar feature, which is lesion hyperintensity on T1-weighted images performed 10 min after the injection of Resovist due to a blood pool effect. **f** On post-contrast T2-weighted images no signal decrease of the lesion is visible

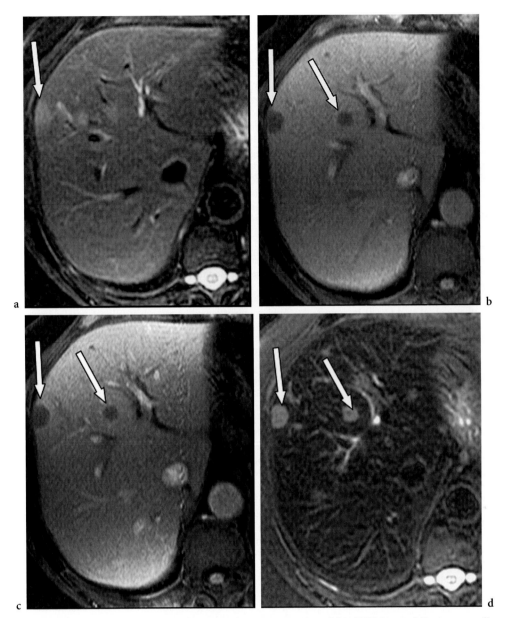

Fig. 3.15a–d. SHU 555 A-enhanced imaging of metastases. **a** T2-weighted FSE image delineates a small metastasis (*arrow*). **b, c** During the dynamic study two small metastases are visible (*arrows*). **d** On SHU 555 A-enhanced FSE image no uptake of contrast agent is documented in both metastases. Of interest, the uptake of SPIO particles in the peripheral zone of the metastases allows the better demarcation of the lesions

References

Augui J, Vignaux O, Argaud C, et al (2002) Liver: T2-weighted MR imaging with breath-hold fast-recovery optimized fast spin-echo compared with breath-hold half-Fourier and non-breath-hold respiratory-triggered fast spin-echo pulse sequences. Radiology 223:853–859

Barish MA, Jara H (1999) Motion artefact control in body MR imaging. Magn Reson Imaging Clin N Am 7:289–301

Bartolozzi C, Lencioni R, Donati F, et al (1999) Abdominal MR: liver and pancreas. Eur Radiol 9:1496–1512

Bartolozzi C, Donati F, Cioni D, et al (2000) MnDPDP-enhanced MRI vs dual-phase spiral CT in the detection of hepatocellular carcinoma in cirrhosis. Eur Radiol 10:1697–1702

Bartolozzi C, Cioni D, Donati F, et al (2001) Focal liver lesions: MR imaging-pathologic correlation. Eur Radiol 11:1374–1388

Bartolozzi C, Donati F, Cioni D, et al (2004) Detection of colorectal liver metastases: a prospective multicenter trial comparing unenhanced MRI, MnDPDP-enhanced MRI, and spiral CT. Eur Radiol 14:14–20

Bellin MF, Vasile M, Morel-Precetti S (2003) Currently used

non-specific extracellular MR contrast media. Eur Radiol 13:2688–2698

Carlos RC, Branam JD, Dong Q, et al (2002) Biliary imaging with Gd-EOB-DTPA: is a 20-minute delay sufficient? Acad Radiol 9:1322–1325

Hamm B, Thoeni RF, Gould RG, et al (1994) Focal liver lesions: characterization with nonenhanced and dynamic contrast material-enhanced MR imaging. Radiology 190:417–423

Hawighorst H, Schoenberg SO, Knopp MV, et al (1999) Hepatic lesions: morphologic and functional characterization with multiphase breath-hold 3D gadolinium-enhanced MR angiography–initial results. Radiology 210:89–96

Heidemann RM, Özsarlak Ö, Parizel PM, et al (2003) A brief review of parallel magnetic resonance imaging. Eur Radiol 13:2323–2337

Helmberger TK, Schroder J, Holzknecht N, et al (1999) T2-weighted breathhold imaging of the liver: a quantitative and qualitative comparison of fast spin echo and half Fourier single shot fast spin echo imaging. MAGMA 9:42–51

Herbon CU, Vogt FM, Lauenstein TC, et al (2003) MRI of the liver: can true FISP replace HASTE? J Magn Reson Imaging 17:190–196

Huppertz A, Balzer T, Blakeborough A, et al (2004) Improved detection of focal liver lesions in MRI. A multicenter comparison of Gd-EOB-DTPA with intraoperative findings. Radiology 230:266–275

Hussain HK, Londy FJ, Francis IR, et al (2003) Hepatic arterial phase MR imaging with automated bolus-detection three-dimensional fast gradient-recalled-echo sequence: comparison with test-bolus method. Radiology 226:558–566

Ichikawa T, Haradome H, Hachiya J, et al (1998a) Diffusion-weighted MR imaging with a single-shot echoplanar sequence: detection and characterization of focal hepatic lesions. AJR Am J Roentgenol 170:397–402

Ichikawa T, Haradome H, Hachiya J, et al (1998b) Characterization of hepatic lesions by perfusion-weighted MR imaging with echoplanar sequence. AJR Am J Roentgenol 170:1029–1034

Kanematsu M, Hoshi H, Itoh K, et al (1999) Focal hepatic lesion detection: comparison of four fat-suppressed T2-weighted MR imaging pulse sequences. Radiology 211:363–371

Keogan MT, Edelman RR (2001) Technologic advances in abdominal MR imaging. Radiology 220:310–320

Kim TK, Lee HJ, Jang HJ, et al (1998) T2-weighted breath-hold MRI of the liver at 1.0 T: comparison of turbo spin-echo and HASTE sequences with and without fat suppression. J Magn Reson Imaging 8:1213–1218

Kim T, Murakami T, Takahashi S, et al (1999) Diffusion-weighted single-shot echoplanar MR imaging for liver disease. AJR Am J Roentgenol 173:393–398

Kim KW, Kim AY, Kim TK, et al (2004) Small (<or= 2 cm) hepatic lesions in colorectal cancer patients: detection and characterization on mangafodipir trisodium-enhanced MRI. AJR Am J Roentgenol 182:1233–1240

Kopp AF, Laniado M, Dammamm F, et al (1997) MR imaging of the liver with Resovist: safety, efficacy, and pharmaco-dynamic properties. Radiology 204:749–756

Lee VS, Lavelle MT, Rofsky NM, et al (2000) Hepatic MR imaging with a dynamic contrast-enhanced isotropic volumetric interpolated breath-hold examination: feasibility, reproducibility, and technical quality. Radiology 215:365–372

Lee VS, Rofsky NM, Morgan GR, et al (2001) Volumetric mangafodipir trisodium-enhanced cholangiography to define intrahepatic biliary anatomy. AJR Am J Roentgenol 176:906–908

Lencioni R, Donati F, Cioni D, et al (1998) Detection of colorectal liver metastases: prospective comparison of unenhanced and ferumoxides-enhanced magnetic resonance imaging at 1.5 T, dual-phase spiral CT, and spiral CT during arterial portography. MAGMA 7:76–87

Lencioni R, Cioni D, Crocetti L, et al (2004) Magnetic resonance imaging of liver tumors. J Hepatol 40:162–171

Low RN, Hinks RS, Alzate GD, et al (1994) Fast spin-echo MR imaging of the abdomen: contrast optimization and artefact reduction. J Magn Reson Imaging 4:637–645

Low RN, Alzate GD, Schimakawa A (1997) Motion suppression in MR imaging of the liver: comparison of respiratory-triggered and nontriggered fast spin-echo sequences. AJR Am J Roentgenol 168:225–231

Mahfouz AE, Hamm B, Taupitz M (1993) Hypervascular liver lesions: differentiation of focal nodular hyperplasia from malignant tumors with dynamic gadolinium-enhanced MR imaging. Radiology 186:133–138

McKenzie CA, Lim D, Ransil BJ, et al (2004) Shortening MR image acquisition time for volumetric interpolated breath-hold examination with a recently developed parallel imaging reconstruction technique: clinical feasibility. Radiology 230:589–594

Morrin MM, Rofsky NM (2001) Techniques for liver MR imaging. Magn Reson Imaging Clin N Am 9:675–696

Nitz WR (2002) Fast and ultrafast non-echo-planar MR imaging techniques. Eur Radiol 12:2866–2882

Numminem K, Halavaara J, Isoniemi H, et al (2003) Magnetic resonance imaging of the liver: true fast imaging with steady state free precession sequence facilitates rapid and reliable distinction between hepatic hemangiomas and liver malignancies. J Comput Assist Tomogr 27:571–576

Oudkerk M, Torres CG, Song B, et al (2002) Characterization of liver lesions with mangafodipir trisodium-enhanced MR imaging: multicenter study comparing MR and dual-phase spiral CT. Radiology 223:517–524

Padhani AR, Husband JE (2001) Dynamic contrast-enhanced MRI studies in oncology with an emphasis on quantification, validation and human studies. Clin Radiol 56:607–620

Petersein J, Spinazzi A, Giovagnoni A, et al (2000) Focal liver lesions: evaluation of the efficacy of gadobenate dimeglumine in MR imaging. A multicenter phase III clinical study. Radiology 215:727–736

Reimer P, Balzer T (2003) Ferucarbotran (Resovist): a new clinically approved RES-specific contrast agent for contrast-enhanced MRI of the liver: properties, clinical development, and applications. Eur Radiol 13:1266–1276

Reimer P, Tombach B (1998) Hepatic MRI with SPIO: detection and characterization of focal liver lesions. Eur Radiol 8:1198–1204

Reimer P, Rummeny EJ, Daldrup HE, et al (1997) Enhancement characteristics of liver metastases, hepatocellular carcinomas, and hemangiomas with Gd-EOB-DTPA: preliminary results with dynamic MR imaging. Eur Radiol 7:257–280

Reimer P, Schneider G, Schima W (2004) Hepatobiliary contrast agents for contrast-enhanced MRI of the liver: properties, clinical development and applications. Eur Radiol 14:559–578

Rofsky NM, Weinreb JC, Ambrosino MM, et al (1996) Comparison between in-phase and opposed-phase T1-weighted breath-hold FLASH sequences for hepatic imaging. J Comput Assist Tomogr 20:230–235

Rofsky NM, Lee VS, Laub G, et al (1999) Abdominal MR imaging with a volumetric interpolated breath-hold examination. Radiology 212:876–884

Ros PR, Freeny PC, Harms SE, et al (1995) Hepatic MR imaging with ferumoxide: a multicentric clinical trial of the safety and efficacy in the detection of focal hepatic lesions. Radiology 196:481–488

Schwartz LH, Panicek DM, Thomson E, et al (1997) Comparison of phased-array and body coils for MR imaging of liver. Clin Radiol 52:745–749

Semelka RC, Helmberger TK (2001) Contrast agents for MR imaging of the liver. Radiology 218:27–38

Soyer P, Rondeau Y, Dufresne A, et al (1997) T1-weighted spoiled gradient-echo MR imaging of focal hepatic lesion: comparison of in-phase vs opposed-phase pulse sequence. Eur Radiol 7:1048–1053

Spinazzi A, Lorusso V, Pirovano G, et al (1998) Multihance clinical pharmacology: biodistribution and MR enhancement of the liver. Acad Radiol 5(Suppl 1):S86–S89

Taouli B, Vilgrain V, Dumont E, et al (2003) Evaluation of liver diffusion isotropy and characterization of focal hepatic lesions with two single-shot echo-planar MR imaging sequences: prospective study in 66 patients. Radiology 226:71–78

Tsuda N, Kato N, Murayama C, et al (2004) Potential for differential diagnosis with gadolinium-ethoxybenzyl-diethylenetriamine pentaacetic acid-enhanced magnetic resonance imaging in experimental hepatic tumors. Invest Radiol 39:80–88

Vogl TJ, Schwarz W, Blume S, et al (2003) Preoperative evaluation of malignant liver tumors: comparison of unenhanced and SPIO (Resovist)-enhanced MR imaging with biphasic CTAP and intraoperative US. Eur Radiol 13:262–272

Ward J, Guthrie JA, Wilson D, et al (2003) Colorectal hepatic metastases: detection with SPIO-enhanced breath-hold MR imaging–comparison of optimized sequences. Radiology 228:709–718

Yamashita Y, Tang Y, Takahashi M (1998) Ultrafast MR imaging of the abdomen: echo planar imaging and diffusion-weighted imaging. J Magn Reson Imaging 8:367–374

Yu JS, Kim KW, Kim EK, et al (1999) Contrast enhancement of small hepatocellular carcinoma: usefulness of three successive early image acquisitions during multiphase dynamic MR imaging. AJR Am J Roentgenol 173:597–604

Liver Anatomy

4 Segmental Anatomy of the Liver

Pietro Majno, Pierre Loubeyre, Gilles Mentha, Philippe Morel, Christoph Becker, and Jean Fasel

CONTENTS

4.1
Introduction

The liver is formed by eight independent functional units, each with specific vascular and biliary connections. The identification of these units or segments – first described in its current naming by the French surgeon and anatomist Claude Couinaud – in each individual organ is the key to a reproducible and clinically meaningful description of where liver lesions are localized, and to modern liver surgery. We present a simple way to identify liver segments in radiological examinations based on constant anatomical landmarks, and to memorize their numbering.

The anatomy of the liver can be detailed based on the external appearance of the organ (external or de-

P. Majno, MD; G. Mentha, MD; P. Morel, MD
Departments of Surgery and Transplantation, University Hospitals of Geneva, 24, Rue Micheli du Crest, 1211 Geneva 14, Switzerland
P. Loubeyre, MD; C. Becker, MD
Department of Radiology, University Hospitals of Geneva 24, Rue Micheli du Crest, 1211 Geneva 14, Switzerland
J. Fasel, MD
Department of Anatomy, University Hospitals of Geneva 24, Rue Micheli du Crest, 1211 Geneva 14, Switzerland

scriptive anatomy) or based on its vascular and biliary architecture (vascular or functional anatomy). The descriptive anatomy was sufficient until abdominal surgeons had to perform liver resection, when it became important to respect the vascular integrity and the biliary drainage of the portion of the gland that would be spared. Two problems had to be addressed. The first was to simplify the intricacy of the vascular architecture of the liver to a relatively constant pattern to which even variations can be related (an "ideal" functional anatomy). The second was to relate this ideal pattern to the individual anatomy of each liver (the "real" functional anatomy) and to follow this real anatomy in describing the location of liver lesions and in planning and performing the operations. We will see in the following paragraphs how these problems were solved and how the solution – segmental liver anatomy – is easily accessible to the radiologist. For the sake of clarity, Arabic numerals will be used in the following paragraphs and in the illustrations.

4.2
Descriptive Anatomy of the Liver

The anatomy of the liver according to its external appearance identifies a superior or diaphragmatic surface and an inferior or ventral surface. On the superior aspect the falciform ligament separates the gland into a larger right lobe and a smaller left lobe (Fig. 4.1). The inferior surface is more varied: the round ligament continues into with the umbilical portion of the left portal vein (at an anatomical landmark called Rex's recessus) (Fig. 4.2). The "hepatic pedicle" containing the portal vein, the hepatic artery and the bile duct spreads out, near the liver, in a space called the "porta hepatis or hepatic hilum" (defined by the bifurcation of the portal vein) and divides into a shorter right pedicle and a longer left pedicle.

The left pedicle runs almost horizontal and separates a quadrate lobe anteriorly and a caudate lobe

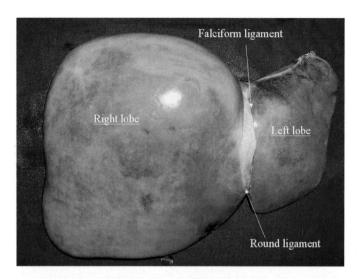

Fig. 4.1. Superior (diaphragmatic) aspect of the liver. The only landmarks that can be recognized are the falciform and the round ligament, separating the left lobe from the right lobe

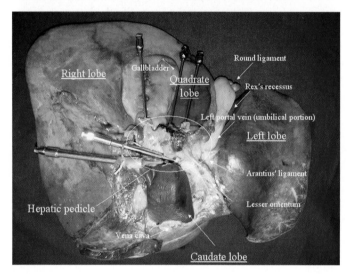

Fig. 4.2. Inferior aspect of the liver: the round ligament continues into the umbilical portion of the left portal vein (at an anatomical landmark called Rex's recessus). The "hepatic pedicle" spreads out, near the liver, as a virtual space called the "porta hepatis or hepatic hilum" (defined by the bifurcation of the portal vein) and divides into a shorter right pedicle and a longer left pedicle. The left pedicle separates a quadrate lobe anteriorly and a round caudate lobe posteriorly and arches up as an umbilical portion to join the round ligament. Arantius' ligament runs from the angle between the transverse portion and the umbilical portion of the left portal vein to the confluence of the left and middle hepatic veins. The right hepatic pedicle is in contact with the gallbladder that defines the right border of the quadrate lobe. Posteriorly the right hepatic pedicle is separated from the vena cava by a rim of liver tissue that corresponds to the right portion of the caudate lobe

posteriorly. Further on the left, the left hepatic pedicle arches up as an umbilical portion to join the round ligament. The lesser omentum extends from the left border of the hepatic pedicle, along the left hepatic pedicle, abandons the umbilical portion to follow Arantius' ligament up to the vena cava and the diaphragm. It separates the left lobe anteriorly from the caudate lobe posteriorly. In 10%–20% of the cases an accessory hepatic artery (left hepatic artery) originating from the left gastric artery runs into the lesser omentum to join the left hepatic pedicle. Arantius' ligament is the remnant of Arantius' duct, or "ductus venosus", that in the fetal circulation connects the left portal vein to the caval system, and that runs from the angle between the transverse portion and the umbilical portion of the left portal vein to the confluence of the left and middle hepatic veins (MAJNO et al. 2002).

The right hepatic pedicle is in contact with the gallbladder that defines the right border of the quadrate lobe. Posteriorly the right hepatic pedicle is separated from the vena cava by a rim of liver tissue that corresponds to the right portion of the caudate lobe.

4.3
The Functional or Vascular Anatomy

The merit of recognizing and of popularizing a (relatively) simplified pattern of the vascular structure of the liver has to be credited to the French anatomist and surgeon Claude Couinaud (COUINAUD 1957). A summary of this work was presented in two landmark articles by the French surgeon Henri Bismuth (BISMUTH 1982; BISMUTH et al. 1982).

The simplified scheme assumes that the blood enters the liver from the portal vein (the arteries and the bile ducts follow the branches of the portal vein, so only the portal anatomy will be described henceforth) and is collected by three hepatic veins (left, middle and right) inserting into the inferior vena cava (Fig. 4.3). The main portal vein divides into two branches, right and left, defining a right liver and a left liver. The middle hepatic vein drains the liver from the main bifurcation.

On the right, the right portal vein divides into two second order sectorial branches defining a right anterior sector and a right posterior sector, separated by the right hepatic vein. The third-order division of the (sectorial) portal branches will separate each sector into two segments.

On the left, although sectors can be recognized on embryological grounds, it is simpler to remember that the portal vein describes an arch towards the round ligament, and that the concavity of this arch embraces one segment (limited on the right by the middle hepatic vein), and the convexity of the arch two segments, separated by the left hepatic vein.

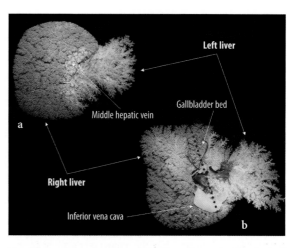

Fig. 4.4a,b. Corrosion cast of the liver shown in Fig. 4.1 and Fig. 4.2. The portal vein has been injected with acrylic resin coloured green for the right branch and blue for the left branch. The hepatic veins have been injected retrogradely from the vena cava with white resin. The main hepatic artery has been injected with red resin and the bile duct with yellow resin. a Superior (diaphragmatic) aspect. The right liver-defined as the portion of the gland perfused by the right branch of the portal vein-is coloured green, and the left liver, perfused by the left portal vein, is coloured blue. The middle hepatic vein surfaces in between as a white watershed. This landmark is *not* visible on the surface of the liver and does not correspond to the falciform ligament. b Ventral aspect. The border between the left and the right liver can be approximated to a plane that joins the gallbladder bed-visible on this cast as the branches of the cystic artery-to the inferior vena cava (*blue dots*)

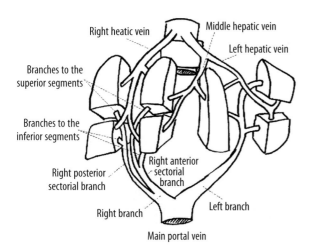

Fig. 4.3. Simplified scheme of the liver segments. The main portal vein divides into two branches, right and left, defining a right liver and a left liver. The median hepatic vein drains the liver from the main bifurcation. On the right, the right portal vein divides into two second order branches defining a right anterior and a right posterior sector, separated by the right hepatic vein. The third-order division of the (sectorial) portal branches will separate each sector into two segments. On the left, the portal vein describes an arch towards the round ligament; the concavity of this arch embraces one segment (limited on the right by the median hepatic vein), and the convexity of the arch two segments, separated by the left hepatic vein. A last segment is constituted by the liver tissue that lies between the posterior aspect of the portal bifurcation and the vena cava

A last segment is constituted by the liver tissue that lies between the posterior aspect of the portal bifurcation and the vena cava. This segment extends from the left (where it has a recognizable external identity in the form of the caudate lobe) to the right, around the vena cava, up to the confluence of the hepatic veins. This segment is fed by a series of smaller portal branches originating from the portal bifurcation before the takeoff of the right and left portal branches, and its parenchyma is drained by a variable number of separate hepatic veins directly into the vena cava.

The separation between the right and the left liver is evident when the right branch and the left branch of the portal vein are injected with dyes of different colours (Fig. 4.4). The plane of separation between the right and the left liver can be approximated as a plane going from the gallbladder fossa to the vena cava in which runs the middle hepatic vein.

Couinaud named the eight segments of the liver from the centre (segment 1) clockwise when a cast of the liver vessels is seen from in front, allegedly reproducing the distribution of the *arrondissements* of Paris (Bismuth H, personal communication) (Fig. 4.5).

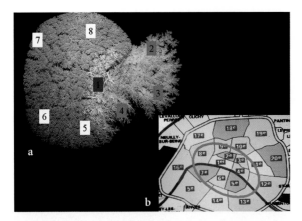

Fig. 4.5a,b. Numbering of the segments of the liver according to Couinaud. **a** Segment 1 is in the centre and the numbers will progress clockwise, similar to the *Arrondissements* of Paris (**b**)

Whether this story is true or apocryphal, the concept is appealing and helps memorizing the progression of the segments, bearing in mind that the clockwise pattern refers to the liver as seen by an anatomist or a radiologist on traditional contrast studies, from in front, while in the new era of axial imaging the liver is seen from below, the numbering progresses anti-clockwise and not all segments of the right liver are visible on all slices: the superior segments will appear on slices above the portal bifurcation and the inferior segments on slices below the portal bifurcation (Fig. 4.6). A more

detailed view of the liver as seen from below, with the observer able to see the whole organ, is illustrated in Fig. 4.7; the reader will notice that the position of the segments can only be approximated, and that the boundaries between the segments can not be defined, with the exception of segment 3 and 4 (the round ligament), of segment 4 and 5 (the gallbladder bed) and of the left part of segment 1, corresponding to the Spigel's lobe (Fig. 4.8).

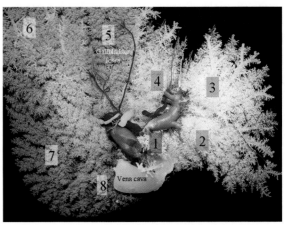

Fig. 4.7. Inferior view of a liver cast, with the numbering of the segments. The borders between the segments can not be recognized, with the exception of segments 3 from segment 4 (the round ligament), the left part of segment 1 (Spigel's lobe), and to some extent segment 4 from segment 5 (the gallbladder fossa, or more precisely, somewhere in the gallbladder fossa, because – as shown in the illustration – the plane may not correspond to the middle of the fossa)

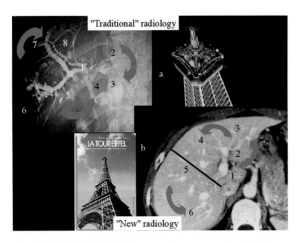

Fig. 4.6.**a** The similarities between the progression of the segments and the *Arrondissements* of Paris holds for radiological investigations and observers that see the liver – and Paris – from above, such as the percutaneous cholangiogram depicted in the illustration. **b** As modern axial imaging sees the patient from below, the similarity requires to imagine Paris as if looking to the sky coming out from a Metrò station. Also, because of the cephalad-caudal development of the right liver, not all segments will appear on axial slices: the superior segments (7 and 8) will be visible on slices above the portal bifurcation and the inferior segments (5 and 6) below the portal bifurcation

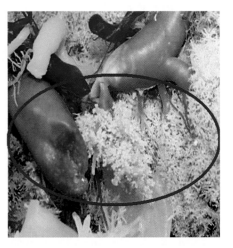

Fig. 4.8. Detail of the left part of segment 1, corresponding to Spigel's lobe. The right part is hidden by the right portal vein (*green*). This segment is perfused by small independent branches from the posterior aspect of the portal vein, and is drained by independent hepatic veins opening directly into the inferior vena cava

4.4
The Correspondence Between the Descriptive Anatomy and the Functional Anatomy

Only few landmarks on the external surface of the liver correspond to the functional (vascular) anatomy, and the eye of the surgeon is blind to the inner architecture of the liver. These landmarks are limited to the round ligament inserting into the umbilical portion of the left portal vein, the left portion of segment 1 (Spigel's lobe) separated from the left liver by the lesser omentum inserting along Arantius' ligament, and the gallbladder fossa, separating segment 4 from segment 5, therefore the right from the left liver (Fig. 4.2). Also, in the rim of tissue between the portal vein and the vena cava, a notch on the surface separates a left portion of segment 1 (supplied mainly by the left half of the portal bifurcation) from a right portion, supplied by the corresponding part of the portal bifurcation. The importance of the division of segment 1 into two parts is questionable, although the notch offers a landmark to start right liver resections (KOGURE et al. 2000).

4.5
The Correlation Between the Radiological Anatomy and the Functional Anatomy

As opposed to the surgeon, the modern radiologist has the privilege of seeing the blood vessels within the liver and can easily find the landmarks of the segmental anatomy, and to use liver segments as an agreed-upon format on which the location of pathological lesions can be reported.

Bearing in mind the pattern of the segmental anatomy detailed above, and a conceptualized representation of the main vascular landmarks, it is straightforward to describe in which segment a lesion is located (Fig. 4.9).

The right and the left liver: the plane separating the right and the left liver runs from the middle hepatic vein, to the inferior vena cava, to the gallbladder.

The segments in the right liver: the first landmark is the right hepatic vein. All that is anterior and to the left of the right hepatic vein will be in the right anterior sector (segments 5 and 8), all that is posterior and to the right will be in the right posterior sector (segments 6 and 7). The second landmark should be

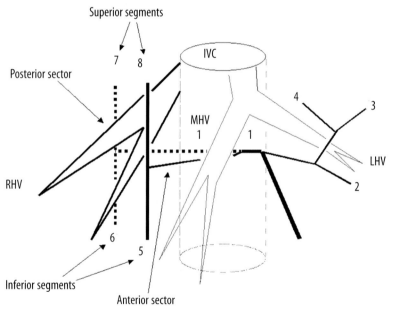

Fig. 4.9. Schematic representation of the vascular landmarks in the liver. The observer sees the organ as an anatomist looking into the abdomen (Fig. 4.1). The main landmark is the middle hepatic vein (*MHV*) separating the right liver from the left liver. On the right, the main landmark is the right hepatic vein (*RHV*), inserting into the inferior vena cava (*IVC*). All that is anterior and to the left of the right hepatic vein will be in the right anterior sector (segments 5 and 8), all that is posterior and to the right will be in the right posterior sector (segments 6 and 7). Because the plane where the segmental branches originate can be approximated to the plane passing by the main portal bifurcation, this plane can be taken as the second landmark. In each sector the inferior segments (5 and 6) will lie caudal to the portal bifurcation, and the superior segments (7 and 8) will be cranial to it. Therefore in the right anterior sector segment 5 will be below and segment 8 above, and in the posterior sector segment 6 below and segment 7 above. On the left, the main landmark is the left portal vein that describes an arch towards the round ligament. All that is between the concavity of the arch and to the left of the MHV is segment 4. On the convexity of the arch, the first branches will be feeding segment 2 and the more distal branches segment 3. The distal branches of the left hepatic vein (*LHV*) will separate segment 2 from segment 3

the third order bifurcation of the portal vein (where the right sectorial branches separate into segmental branches). Normally, however, it is not necessary to follow the sectorial into the segmental branches, and as the portal vein divides into the sectorial and the segmental branches very close to the hepatic hilum, the plane where the segmental branches originate can be approximated to the plane passing by the main portal bifurcation: in each sector the inferior segments (5 and 6) will lie caudal to the portal bifurcation, and

the superior segments (7 and 8) will be cranial to it. Therefore in the right anterior sector segment 5 will be below and segment 8 above, and in the posterior sector segment 6 below and segment 7 above.

In the left liver: the main landmark is the left portal vein, and the second landmark is the left hepatic vein. The left portal vein describes a smooth arch from the main bifurcation to the umbilical ligament. All liver tissue comprised by the concavity of the arch and the middle hepatic vein will be segment 4. On the convex-

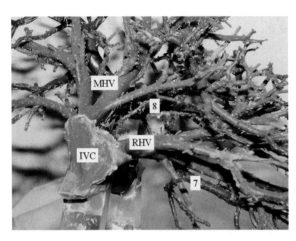

Fig. 4.10. The superior segments of the right liver. Resin cast of a liver seen from above and to the right (the observer is looking at the liver from the right diaphragm). The right hepatic vein (*RHV*) and the inferior vena cava (*IVC*) can be identified, and taken as the landmark to separate the superior segments: *8* anterior to the *RHV*, and *7*, posterior to the *RHV*

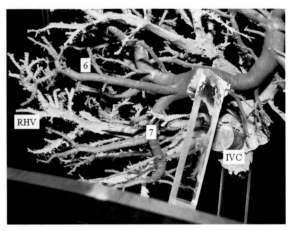

Fig. 4.11. The posterior sector of the right liver. The observer is looking on the liver from the pancreas. The RHV can be identified and posterior to it lie segment *6* inferiorly and segment *7* superiorly. The anterior sector of the right liver, with branches to segment 5 and 8, can be seen anterior to the *RHV*

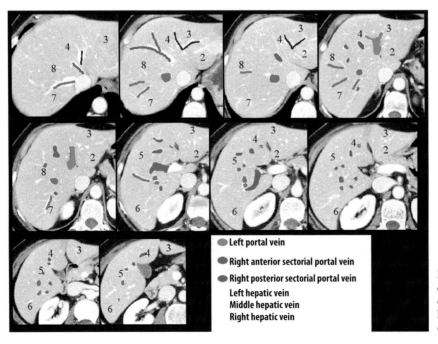

Fig. 4.12. Computerized tomography of the liver. The vessels can be recognized and used as landmarks to define the different segments

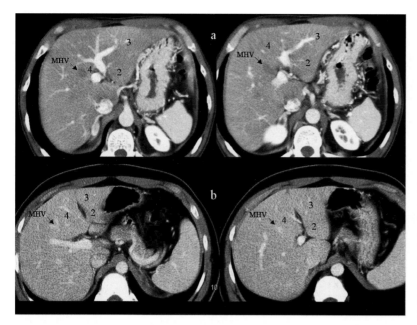

Fig. 4.13a,b. Using the vessels as landmarks to divide segments adjusts for the variable size of liver segments. **a** Segments *3* and *2* are hypertrophic, while segment *4* is small. **b** Segment *4* is well developed in this patient, while the left lobe is atrophic. This variation can be easily recognized and described in radiological reports, and lesions in the different segments localized without ambiguity. *MHV*, middle hepatic vein

ity of the arch, on the left side (the left lobe of the descriptive anatomy) the distal part of the left hepatic vein will separate segment 2 (posteriorly and superiorly) from segment 3 (more anteriorly and inferiorly).

After this ideal pattern is drilled, it is easy to apply it to the real anatomy on radiological investigations, on anatomical casts or on surgical-dissection specimen (Figs. 4.10–4.14).

4.6
The Correlation Between the Functional Anatomy and the Surgical Anatomy

The lack of external landmarks that relate the surface anatomy to the vascular anatomy of the liver can be a problem for the surgeon who has to perform liver resections, and several solutions can be devised. The main hepatectomies (right and left hepatectomy, right posterior sectoriectomy, left lobectomy) can be performed simply by occlusion of the inflow at the hilum and seeing a demarcation plane appear (Fig. 4.15). The resection plane can then be refined with intraoperative ultrasound to spare or remove the hepatic veins according to the needs of the surgery. More elegant approaches, completely based on intraoperative ultrasound, can be used when resections limited to a segment are required, such as injecting dye in the corresponding portal branch, or test-occluding the flow with an intravascular balloon or with other

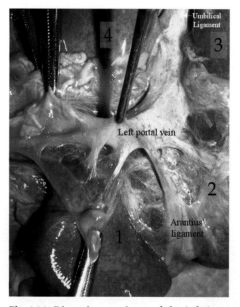

Fig. 4.14. Dissection specimen of the inferior aspect of the left liver. The organ is seen as in Fig. 4.7. The left portal vein has been exposed by opening the peritoneum of the left hepatic pedicle. A horizontal portion and a vertical (umbilical) portion can be recognized. The two portions are separated by *Arantius' ligament*, joining the left portal vein to the left hepatic vein

devices (TORZILLI and MAKUUCHI 2003; CASTAING et al. 1986). Alternatively, the segmental branches can be dissected high in the hepatic hilum. More details on these techniques can be found in the specialized surgical literature (BLUMGART and FONG 2000).

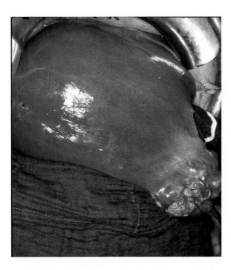

Fig. 4.15. Vascular demarcation after temporary occlusion of the posterior sectorial vessels in a patient with several lesions in segments 6 and 7

4.7
Beyond the Ideal View

A more realistic analysis of the anatomy of the liver-beyond the idealized scheme given above-will show that, to some extent, the division of he portal vein into segmental branches is observer dependent, and arbitrary (FASEL et al. 1998). In addition, there is a relatively high variability of the sectorial and even the main portal branches on the right such in cases of a portal trifurcation, or of separate segmental branches for segment 6, for instance (Fig. 4.16). As for the hepatic veins, the most common variation is the presence of an accessory right inferior hepatic vein draining segment 6 or segments 5 and 6. Also, the relative importance of the right and of the middle hepatic vein can vary, from a very large dominant tight hepatic vein, to a small right hepatic vein and a large, dominant and bifurcated middle hepatic vein (Fig. 4.16). On the left the anatomy is much more constant, the main variability being in the number of the portal branches feeding segment 4 from the concavity of the left portal vein, or of additional branches arising from the convexity of the curve, in theory defining more than two segments in the left lobe in these cases. The pattern of the left portal vein, giving off segmental and sub-segmental branches directly, however, is constant, possibly because the variability in this region is restricted by the importance of the umbilico-portal-caval circuit in the fetal circulation. The predictability of the anatomy of the left portal vein is a major asset in transplantation surgery, in which a procedure to produce a small left graft and a large right graft (segment 2–3 split) is virtually always possible.

An additional shortcut of the scheme given above is that it considers that the hepatic veins almost as flat structures running in planes, while in reality they are more like trees, or cones converging into the vena cava. Despite these limitations, however, the authors believe that Couinaud's segmental anatomy is reasonable compromise between useless detail and unrealistic simplification.

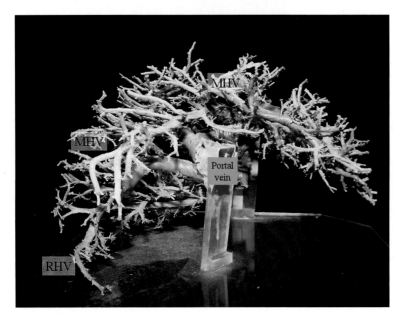

Fig. 4.16. Liver cast of an organ showing different abnormalities. The portal vein trifurcates rather than bifurcates. The right hepatic vein (*RHV*) is hypoplastic and the middle hepatic vein (*MHV*) is hypertrophic. Despite the variations, the different abnormalities can be reconciled with the usual segmental pattern, with segments of different sizes

4.8
Conclusions

A systematic approach to identify the main vascular structures of the liver at the beginning of a radiological investigation will allow in virtually all the cases to reconcile the real anatomy of the liver to the pattern of the segmental anatomy described by Couinaud. This will serve as the basis to describe where liver lesions are localized, and as a common ground where further treatments can be planned with the interventional radiologist and the liver surgeon.

References

Bismuth H (1982) Anatomical surgery and surgical anatomy of the liver. World J Surg 6:3–9

Bismuth H, Houssin D, Castaing D (1982) Major and minor segmentectomies "reglees" in liver surgery. World J Surg 6:10–24

Blumgart L, Fong Y (2000) Surgery of the liver and the biliary tract, 5th edn. Saunders, pp 1785–1795

Castaing D, Emond J, Kunstlinger F, et al. (1986) Utility of operative ultrasound in the surgical management of liver tumors. Ann Surg 204:600–605

Couinaud C (1957) Le foie: etudes anatomiques et chirurgicales. Masson, Paris, pp 13–33

Fasel JH, Selle D, Evertsz CJ, et al. (1998) Segmental anatomy of the liver: poor correlation with CT. Radiology 206:151–156

Kogure K, Kuwano H, Fujimaki N, et al. (2000) Relation among portal segmentation, proper hepatic vein, and external notch of the caudate lobe in the human liver. Ann Surg 231:223–228

Majno PE, Mentha G, Morel P, et al. (2002) Arantius' ligament approach to the left hepatic vein and to the common trunk. J Am Coll Surg 195:737–739

Torzilli G, Makuuchi M (2003) Intraoperative ultrasonography in liver cancer. Surg Oncol Clin N Am 12:91–103

5 Imaging Landmarks for Segmental Lesion Localization

Laura Crocetti, Clotilde Della Pina, Erika Rocchi, Sara Montagnani, Jacopo Lera, and Carlo Bartolozzi

CONTENTS

5.1
Introduction

Segmental anatomy of the liver is a matter of interest to the radiologist, in view of the need for an accurate localization of focal hepatic lesions. Segmental anatomy is in fact the basis of modern hepatic surgery and the type of surgical resection depends largely on the segmental localization of the hepatic lesion (Sugarbaker 1990; Soyer et al. 1994). The careful assessment of segmental localization of a focal liver lesion is also the basis for the precise planning of radiologic interventional procedures. Furthermore, the use of a system for lesion localization that is anatomically based and shared by the medical community is a prerequisite for the correct management and follow-up of patients who are bearing liver tumors (Dodd 1993; Soyer 1993; Fasel et al. 1996). Procedures for delineating segmental anatomy on ultrasound (US), CT, and MR images have, therefore, been the subject of several studies over the past decade (Lafortune et al. 1991; Jung et al. 1996; Soyer et al. 1991). In this

chapter, after a review of the anatomical landmarks, a method for segmental liver localization in different imaging modalities will be examined together with future prospects for three-dimensional renderings and image fusion.

5.2
Anatomical Landmarks and Nomenclature

Segmental anatomy of the liver is based essentially on the internal vascular and biliary architecture of the organ. In Europe and Japan the nomenclature most commonly used by surgeons and radiologists is based on the description introduced by Couinaud (1957) and Bismuth (1982). In American and British publications the terminology proposed by Goldsmith and Woodburne (1957) has generally been employed; however, Couinaud's classification has recently also permeated the English North American radiology and surgery literature (Dodd 1993; Ferrucci 1990).

The segmental anatomy described by Couinaud and modified by Bismuth is based on the three-dimensional concept that all hepatic segments except for the caudate lobe are defined by three vertical scissurae and a single transverse scissura. The middle hepatic vein (corresponding to the main scissura) divides the liver into right and left hemilivers. The right hemiliver is divided by the right hepatic vein into anterior and posterior sectors. The left hemiliver is divided by the left hepatic vein into medial and lateral sectors. There are four sectors (right anterior, right posterior, left medial, and left lateral). Each of these is divided into superior and inferior segments by a transverse line drawn through the right and left portal branches, the so-called transverse scissura. The eight segments are numbered clockwise in frontal view and counterclockwise from the inferior vena cava on a caudal to cranial view. Although convenient for daily radiologic practice, use of this concept is highly questionable from an anatomic point of view

L. Crocetti, MD; C. Della Pina, MD; E. Rocchi, MD; S. Montagnani, MD; J. Lera, MD; C. Bartolozzi, MD
Division of Diagnostic and Interventional Radiology, Department of Oncology, Transplants, and Advanced Technologies in Medicine, University of Pisa, Via Roma 67, 56126 Pisa, Italy

(Fasel et al. 1998; Fischer et al. 2002; Strunk et al. 2003).

Using cross-sectional imaging, the following anatomic landmarks are used to divide the liver into segments: hepatic veins, portal system, gallbladder fossa, falciform/round ligament, and ligamentum venosum. The falciform ligament contains at its base the obliterated umbilical vein (ligamentum teres or round ligament) and separates the right from the left liver lobe. It is seen between the umbilical portion of the left portal vein and the outer surface of the liver. The ligamentum venosum carries the obliterated ductus venosus, which until birth shunts blood from the umbilical vein to the inferior vena cava and therefore runs from the umbilical portion of the left portal vein to the confluence of the left and middle hepatic veins (Majno et al. 2002).

5.3
Imaging Landmarks: CT and MR Imaging

Computed tomography and MR are traditionally considered as cross-sectional axial imaging modalities, and the concept of three vertical planes that divide the liver into four sectors and of a transverse scissura that further subdivides the sectors into two segments each, is applied to localize liver lesions (Bismuth 1982; Couinaud 1957; Soyer et al. 1994).

The hepatic veins separate the following segments: the left hepatic vein separates segment 2 from segment 4; the middle hepatic vein separates segment 4 from segments 5 and 8; and the right hepatic vein separates the anteriorly situated segments 5 and 8 from the more posteriorly situated segments 6 and 7.

The main portal vein divides into right and left branches. The right portal vein has an anterior branch that lies centrally within the anterior segment of the right lobe and a posterior branch that lies centrally within the posterior segment of the right lobe. As the portal vein divides into the sectorial and the segmental branches very close to the hepatic hilum, the plane where the segmental branches originate can be approximated to the plane passing by the main portal bifurcation: in each sector the inferior segments (5 and 6) will lie caudal to the portal bifurcation, and the superior segments (7 and 8) will be cranial to it. Therefore in the right anterior sector segment 5 will be below and segment 8 above, and in the posterior sector segment 6 below and segment 7 above.

The left portal vein initially courses anterior to the caudate lobe and describes a smooth arch from the main bifurcation to the round ligament. All liver tissue consisting of the concavity of the arch and the middle hepatic vein will be segment 4. On the convexity of the arch, on the left side (the left lobe of the descriptive anatomy) the distal part of the left hepatic vein will separate segment 2 (posteriorly and superiorly) from segment 3 (more anteriorly and inferiorly).

A CT "road map" to identify all the imaging landmarks and therefore liver segments is given in Fig. 5.1.

Anatomical landmarks, represented by hepatic and portal veins, can be represented on CT only after contrast media injection. These vessels are in fact hardly visible on baseline scans and during the arterial phase of a liver CT scan. A precise match between arterial phase and portal-venous phase images is needed to assign the correct segment, also considering that some lesions are best depicted during the arterial phase (Fig. 5.2).

Magnetic resonance imaging has some inherent advantages in its segmental lesion localization, due to the natural high contrast between vessels and liver parenchyma also in the plain images (Fig. 5.3). After injection of paramagnetic contrast media the segmental delineation is almost the same as that described for portal-venous phase CT (Fig. 5.4).

Recent advances in MR imaging allow fast sequences (true-FISP, FIESTA) to be performed which are less sensitive to motion artifacts and in which blood has high signal intensity also in the absence of contrast material (Fig. 5.5) (Nitz 2002).

An additional point that has to be taken into consideration is that in the scheme previously described the hepatic veins are considered almost as flat structures running in planes, while in reality they are like branches of a tree, the vena cava. Because of the cross-sectionality of CT and MR, all these anatomical landmarks are not contained in a single image and a meticulous evaluation of the overlapping transverse slices in an interactive cine-mode at a workstation allows the appreciation of the individual vascular anatomy. Multiplanar and three-dimensional reconstructions are not necessarily needed to provide insight into the segmental anatomy, but may often better convey to the surgeon the complex relationship between lesions and individual vascular anatomy (Fig. 5.6) (van Leeuwen et al. 1994a; van Leeuwen 1994b).

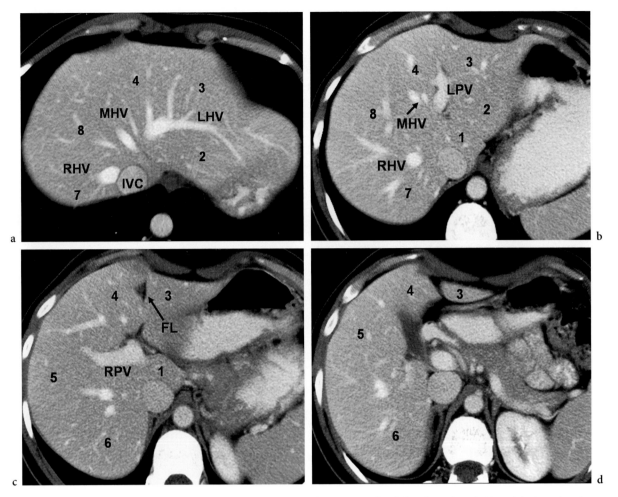

Fig. 5.1a–d. Sequential CT scan through the liver with Couinaud's segments divided and numbered. *RHV,* right hepatic vein; *MHV,* middle hepatic vein; *LHV,* left hepatic vein; *IVC,* inferior vena cava; *RPV,* right portal vein; *LPV,* left portal vein; *FL,* falciform ligament

5.4
Imaging Landmarks: Ultrasound

The multiplanar imaging capability of US is well suited to the identification of the anatomical landmarks and therefore to the precise localization of focal liver lesions to hepatic segments (LAFORTUNE et al. 1991; SMITH et al. 1998). Even landmarks placed along oblique plans can be visualized in the same image, differently from axial CT and MR. Usually subcostal oblique, intercostal oblique and sagittal approaches are all used to explore liver parenchyma and to subdivide it into the described Coinaud's segments.

5.4.1
US Approach to the Left Hemiliver

Using cranial to caudal scans in the subxiphoid region, all the imaging landmarks of the left lobe can be visualized. First of all the three hepatic veins can be depicted. As far as the left liver lobe is concerned, it must be taken into consideration that the left hepatic vein separates segment 2 from segment 3 and that the middle hepatic vein separates segment 4 from segment 8. The left portal vein, the branch entering segment 2, and the branches to segments 3 and 4 can be visualized with an oblique, upwardly tilted subxiphoid view (also called recur-

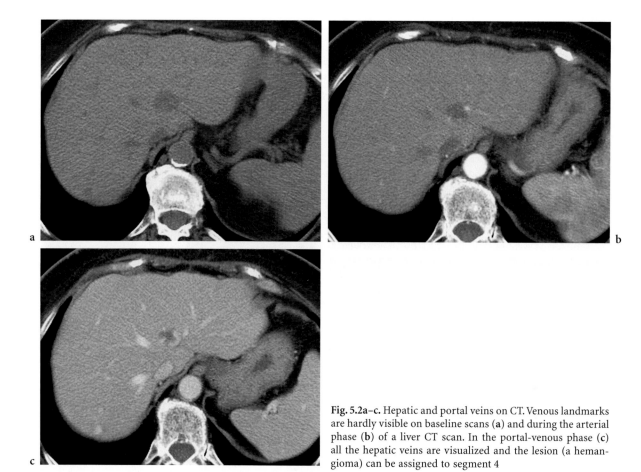

Fig. 5.2a–c. Hepatic and portal veins on CT. Venous landmarks are hardly visible on baseline scans (a) and during the arterial phase (b) of a liver CT scan. In the portal-venous phase (c) all the hepatic veins are visualized and the lesion (a hemangioma) can be assigned to segment 4

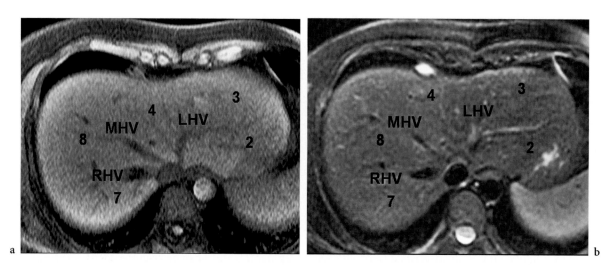

Fig. 5.3a,b. Plain MR images. On T1 (a) and T2 (b) weighted plain images anatomical landmarks are visible

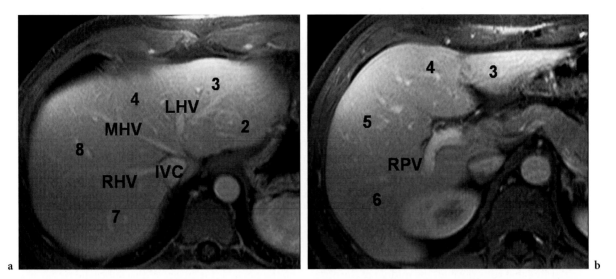

Fig. 5.4a,b. MR of the liver after paramagnetic contrast media administration. In the portal venous phase the segmental delineation is almost the same as that described for portal-venous phase CT

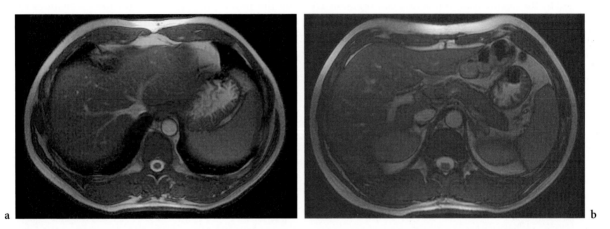

Fig. 5.5a,b. Fast imaging employing steady-state acquisition (FIESTA). Anatomical landmarks are precisely delineated without motion artifacts

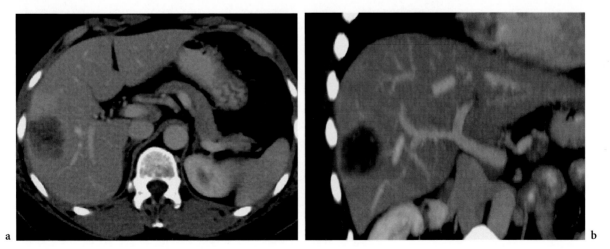

Fig. 5.6a,b. Multiplanar reconstruction of a CT scan. The localization of a metastatic lesion placed in segments 5–6 (**a**) is demonstrated in a more immediate way by means of multiplanar reconstruction (**b**)

rent oblique view by Weill 1989). With a subxiphoid transverse scan segment 1 is shown. Segment 1 is bordered posteriorly by the inferior vena cava and anteriorly by the left portal vein. Laterally, the ligamentum venosum divides segment 1 and segment 2. Segments 2 and 3 are located to the left of the umbilical portion of the left portal vein, the ligamentum venosum, and the falciform ligament. Segment 4 is situated to the right of the umbilical portion of the left portal vein and the falciform ligament. Segment 4 is separated from segments 5 and 8 by the middle hepatic vein and it is separated from segment 1 by the left portal vein.

Using a sagittal approach and scanning to the left of the round ligament, segments 2 and 3 can be visualized. They can be divided by an imaginary perpendicular line that runs through the middle of the outer surface of the liver. With a sagittal view between the round ligament and the gallbladder, segment 4, separated by the ligamentum venosum from segment 1, is visualized (Fig. 5.7)

5.4.2
US Approach to the Right Hemiliver

Scanning in the subcostal region with a cranial to caudal direction and an oblique approach, the three hepatic veins form a "W", with its base on the inferior vena cava. In the right lobe the middle hepatic vein separates segment 8 from segment 4; and the right hepatic vein separates segment 8 from segment 7. Segment 7 is bordered laterally and cephalad by the rib cage and the dome of the diaphragm. With this subcostal oblique view the right portal vein is seen in face, which helps to separate the superficial segment 5 from the more deeply situated segment 8 (Lafortune et al. 1991). All the hepatic segments can be visualized by means of a subcostal oblique view on the portal bifurcation. With a subcostal transverse scan conducted caudally to the portal bifurcation, segments 5 and 6 can be seen. Segment 5 is bordered by the middle hepatic vein and the gallbladder on the left, and segment 6 is delimited laterally by the ribcage. These two segments are separated one from

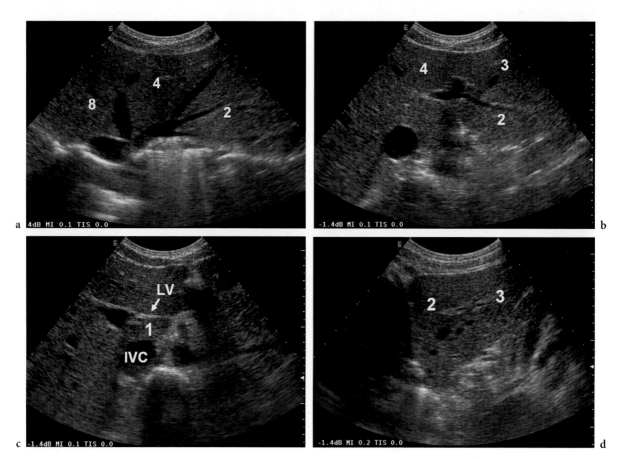

Fig. 5.7a–d. US approach to the left hemiliver. By means of subxiphoid (**a–c**) and sagittal (**d**) views left liver segments can be visualized. *LV*, ligamentum venosum; *IVC*, inferior vena cava

the other by a plane running through the right hepatic vein.

The right portal vein and its branches can be seen using sagittal or oblique midaxillary intercostal approaches. The right portal vein follows an oblique or vertical course, directed anteriorly. The branch for segments 5 and 8 is directed anteriorly and superiorly, while the branch for segments 6 and 7 is directed posteriorly and inferiorly. The branches of segments 6 and 7 are more obliquely oriented and the transducer should be rotated slightly upward for segment 7 and

downward in the direction of the right kidney for segment 6 (Fig. 5.8) (LAFORTUNE et al. 1991)

5.5
Normal Variants

Generally, a constant relationship between external liver anatomy, hepatic veins, and the intrahepatic branches of the portal veins is presumed. However,

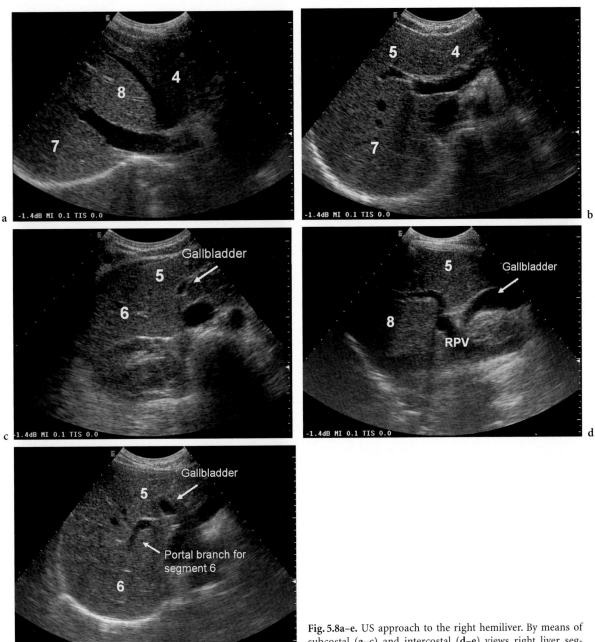

Fig. 5.8a–e. US approach to the right hemiliver. By means of subcostal (**a–c**) and intercostal (**d–e**) views right liver segments can be visualized. *RPV*, right portal vein

each of these systems is subject to marked individual variation. As a result of this variability, inconsistency in the position of the different landmarks indicating the anatomic and segmental boundaries can occur (VAN LEEUWEN et al. 1994a; VAN LEEUWEN et al. 1994b).

A large right inferior hepatic vein draining segment 6 is found in 15–20% of normal subjects (Fig. 5.9). When a right inferior hepatic vein is present, the right hepatic vein is usually smaller, as it does not drain segment 6. In some cases, the right hepatic vein is absent, or limited to a very small vessel, when a large inferior right hepatic vein is associated with a predominant middle hepatic vein (CHENG et al. 1997).

Portal vein variants occur in 20% of cases. The most usual and important abnormalities are represented by portal trifurcation or separate segmental branches for segment 6 or left portal vein arising from the right portal vein or from the anterior branch of the right portal vein (Figs. 5.10, 5.11). Rarely, the right portal vein arises from the intrahepatic left portal vein; usually, the anterior branch of the right portal vein arises from the segment 4 branch of the left portal vein (CHENG et al. 1996; KO et al. 2004).

On the left the anatomy is much more constant, the main variation being the number of portal branches feeding segment 4 or accessory branches in theory defining more than two segments in the left lobe.

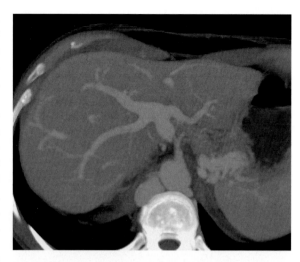

Fig. 5.10. Portal trifurcation. Multiplanar imaging reconstruction of a CT data set showing portal trifurcation

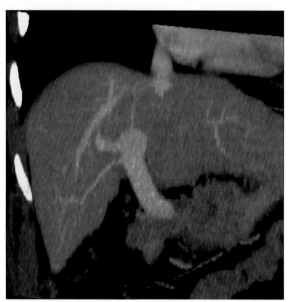

Fig. 5.11. Separate portal branch for segment 6 is shown by CT multiplanar reconstruction

5.6
Future Prospects

Segmental anatomy of the liver is all but an obsolete topic. Advances in hepatic oncologic surgery require that radiologists precisely specify location of tumors according to the segmental anatomy of the liver. Despite the localization of liver segments in some sense being observer dependent and the existence of interindividual anatomic variability, Couinaud's segmental anatomy is a useful, if imperfect, method

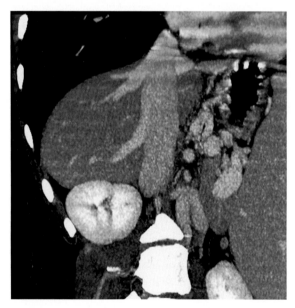

Fig. 5.9. A right inferior hepatic vein, draining segment 6, is shown by CT multiplanar reconstruction

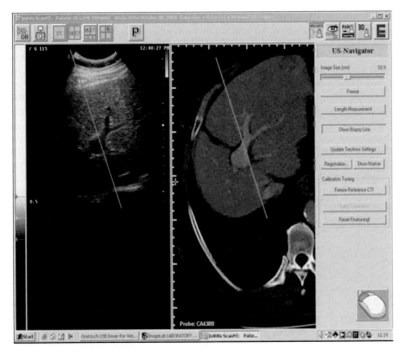

Fig. 5.12. Real-time visualization of US and CT. The NaviSuite platform (Esaote, Bracco, Milan, Italy) allows real-time visualization of US scans with corresponding CT scans, allowing the precise localization of anatomical landmarks (in this case LPV)

for conveying precise information concerning lesion localization. Couinaud's system continues to have validity as a model but has to be individualized for differentiated surgical or interventional planning. With the aid of modern computer technology and newly introduced three-dimensional systems, a preoperative quantitative statement can be made with respect to size, shape, and location of liver segments and their relative share of overall liver volume (FISCHER et al. 2002; WAGGENSPACK et al. 1993).

Another new horizon is represented by tools that allow fusion or real-time matching of images coming from different phases of acquisition with the same technique, or from different imaging modalities. The accuracy of lesion localization can therefore be increased and the spatial correspondence of findings obtained with multiple techniques verified (Fig. 5.12).

References

Bismuth H (1982) Surgical anatomy and anatomical surgery of the liver. World J Surg 6:3–9

Cheng YF, Huang TL, Lee TY, et al (1996) Variation of the intrahepatic portal vein; angiographic demonstration and application in living-related hepatic transplantation. Transplant Proc 28:1667–1668

Cheng YF, Huang TL, Chen CL, et al (1997) Variations of the middle and inferior right hepatic vein: application in hepatectomy. J Clin Ultrasound 25:175–182

Couinaud C (1957) Le foie. In: Couinaud C (ed) Etudes anatomiques et chirurgicales. Masson, Paris

Dodd GD 3rd (1993) An American's guide to Couinaud's numbering system. AJR Am J Roentgenol 161:574–575

Fasel JH, Gailloud P, Terrier F, et al (1996) Segmental anatomy of the liver: a review and proposal for an international working nomenclature. Eur Radiol 6:834–837

Fasel JH, Selle D, Evertsz C, et al (1998) Segmental anatomy of the liver: poor correlation with CT. Radiology 206:151–156

Ferrucci JT (1990) Liver tumor imaging: current concepts. AJR Am J Roentgenol 155:473–484

Fischer L, Cardenas C, Thorn M, et al (2002) Limits of Couinaud's liver segment classification: a quantitative computer-based three dimensional analysis. J Comput Assist Tomogr 26:962–967

Goldsmith NA, Woodburne RT (1957) The surgical anatomy pertaining to liver resection. Surg Gynecol Obstet 105:310–318

Jung G, Krahe T, Krug B, et al (1996) Delineation of segmental liver anatomy. Comparison of ultrasonography, spiral CT and MR imaging for preoperative localization of focal liver lesions to specifc hepatic segments. Acta Radiol 37:691–695

Ko S, Murakami G, Kanamura T, et al (2004) Cantlie's palne in major variations of the primary portal vein ramification at the porta hepatis: cutting experiment using cadaveric livers. World J Surg 28:13–18

Lafortune M, Madore E, Patriquin H, et al (1991) Segmental anatomy of the liver: a sonographic approach to the Couinaud nomenclature. Radiology 181:443–448

Majno PE, Mentha G, Morel P, et al (2002) Arantius' ligament approach to the left hepatic vein and to the common trunk. J Am Coll Surg 195:737–739

Nitz WR (2002) Fast and ultrafast non-echo-planar MR imaging techniques. Eur Radiol 12:2866–2882

Smith D, Downey D, Spouge A, et al (1998) Sonographic demonstration of Couinaud's liver segments. J Ultrasound Med 17:375–381

Soyer P (1993) Segmental anatomy of the liver: utility of a nomenclature accepted worldwide. AJR Am J Roentgenol 161:572–573

Soyer P, Roche A, Gad M, et al (1991) Preoperative segmental localization of hepatic metastases: utility of three-dimensional CT during arterial portography. Radiology 180:653–658

Soyer P, Bluemke DA, Bliss DF, et al (1994) Surgical segmental anatomy of the liver: demonstration with spiral CT during arterial portography and multiplanar reconstruction. AJR Am J Roentgenol 163:99–103

Strunk H, Stuckmann G, Textor J, et al (2003) Limitations and pitfalls of Couinaud's segmentation of the liver in trans-axial imaging. Eur Radiol 13:2472–2482

Sugarbaker PH (1990) En bloc resection of hepatic segments 4b, 5 and 6 by transverse hepatectomy. Surg Gynecol Obstet 170:250–252

van Leeuwen MS, Noordzij J, Femandez MA, et al (1994a) Portal venous and segmental anatomy of the right hemiliver: observations based on three dimensional spiral CT renderings. AJR Am J Roentgenol 163:1395–1404

van Leeuwen MS, Fernandez MA, van Es HW, et al (1994b) Variations in venous and segmental anatomy of the liver: two- and three-dimensional MR imaging in healthy volunteers. AJR Am J Roentgenol 162:1337–1345

Waggenspack GA, Tabb RD, Tiruchelvam V, et al (1993) Three-dimensional localization of hepatic neoplasms with computer generated scissurae recreated from axial CT and MR images. AJR Am J Roentgenol 160:307–309

Weill FS (1989) Ultrasound diagnosis of digestive disease. Springer-Verlag, New York, pp 38–39

Benign Liver Lesions

6 Clinico-Pathological Classification

Fabio Piscaglia, Antonia D'Errico, Simona Leoni, Annamaria Venturi, and Luigi Bolondi

6.1 Introduction

Benign lesions of the liver may present clinically with symptoms due to mass effect or to vascular complications, or may be discovered incidentally during surgical exploration or imaging evaluation for other clinical indications. Given the increased access to medical care, the latter instance, namely discovery of incidental focal lesions of the liver at imaging techniques, is steadily increasing and the statement that they are less commonly encountered than metastatic or primary liver malignant tumors does not stand true anymore. As a consequence, benign liver lesions are becoming a subject of great interest, both for specialists and primary care physicians, because they may present a challenge for differential diagnosis with malignant lesions and secondly because of decisions on their therapeutic management.

These tumors may be epithelial or mesenchymal in nature. The knowledge of their cellular origin, macro- and microscopic presentations, tissue composition and of the condition of the surrounding parenchyma are the prerequisites for a correct interpretation of the findings at imaging techniques and hence for an accurate diagnosis.

This presentation will cover the classification of non-infective benign liver lesions: these may be dysplastic/neoplastic or non-neoplastic (mainly regenerative).

Several authors used to divide these lesions into tumoral and pseudotumoral, considering the term "tumor" with the meaning of neoplastic. However, a "tumor", according to the Latin origin of the word, is a pathological enlargement of a portion of the body or, in other words, a mass. Focal nodular hyperplasia, which according to that classification should be considered, for instance, a pseudotumoral lesion, but is instead a real mass, despite being non-neoplastic. Again, various non-neoplastic masses may present a very difficult differential diagnosis with malignant lesions, so that their precise nature is determined only at histological examination on the resected specimen. In these case the term pseudotumoral does not reflect, therefore, a completely benign, risk-free management.

Taking all these observations together, we prefer the following approach: focal liver lesions can be classified from a pathological point of view in pseudotumoral (which include only focal fatty changes, not constituting a mass) and in tumoral (true masses). These latter may have two origins: neoplastic and non-neoplastic (Table 6.1). Within each group, tumors are eventually subgrouped according to their cellular origin: this can be hepatocellular, biliary or mesenchymal. The latter origin gives rise to several different types of lesions, following the complexity of the stromal compartment in the liver, which includes endothelial cells, stellate cells, smooth muscle cells,

F. Piscaglia, MD; S. Leoni, MD; A. Venturi, MD;
L. Bolondi MD
Division of Internal Medicine, Department of Internal Medicine and Gastroenterology, University of Bologna, Via Albertoni 15, 40138, Bologna, Italy
A. D'Errico, MD,
Department of Pathology, Institute of Oncology F. Addarii, University of Bologna, Via Massarenti 9, 40138, Bologna, Italy

Table 6.1. Benign non-infectious focal liver lesions. Pathological classification

Tumoral lesions

1) Hepatocellular
   Adenoma
   Macroregenerative nodules[a]
   Focal nodular hyperplasia[a]
   Adenomatosis
   Nodular regenerative hyperplasia[b]
2) Biliary
   Cholangiocellular adenoma (or peribiliary duct hamartoma)
   Bile-duct cystadenoma
   Papillomatosis[c]
3) Stromal
   Angiomyolipoma
   Angiomyelolipoma
   Benign hemangioendothelioma
   Hemangioma
   Infantile hemangioma
   Inflammatory pseudotumor[a]
   Isolated hepatic splenosis[a]
   Lymphangioma
   Leiomyoma
   Lipoma
   Mesenchymal hamartoma[a]
   Pseudolipoma[a]
   Peliosis hepatis[a]
   Schwannoma
   Solitary necrotic nodule[a]
Pseudotumors
   Focal fatty sparing
   Focal fatty change

[a] These lesions are not neoplastic.
[b] May cause portal hypertension leading up to orthotopic liver transplant in selected cases.
[c] This type of lesion is a benign tumor of the liver but does not show as a focal liver lesion, but rather with signs related to bile-duct obstruction.

adipocytes, nerve terminations, Pitt cells, Kupffer's cells, monocytes and lymphatic cells.

Hepatocellular nodules may be neoplastic or non-neoplastic. The latter usually correspond to a regenerative response to injury. The size and structure of regenerative nodules varies with the distribution and severity of the hepatic injury, leading to a complex classification. Biliary and stromal cells also produce neoplastic or regenerative lesions (YEUNG et al. 2003).

The clinical approach and classification of focal liver lesions partially differs from the pathological one. The classification in tumoral and pseudotumoral remains appropriate also from a clinical point of view, since pseudotumoral lesions, i.e. fatty changes, have no clinical impact at all, apart from the possible

difficulty in their correct diagnosis at imaging. This is particularly true in patients with a history of carcinoma (especially breast carcinoma), who have undergone chemotherapy, in whom the differentiation between focal fatty changes and infiltrating metastatic disease may be very difficult at imaging techniques. On the contrary, for all the benign tumoral lesions, the clinical approach depends upon three main factors: (1) whether they have arisen in a normal or cirrhotic liver, (2) whether a definitive diagnosis can be reached preoperatively and (3) the type of benign tumor, which, according to its neoplastic nature may eventually or may not at all proceed to malignant transformation.

As a consequence, following a practical approach, focal liver lesions arising in a normal liver can be divided in those requiring intervention (either for a diagnostic or therapeutic purpose) or not requiring any treatment (Table 6.2).

Table 6.2. Benign non-infectious focal liver lesions. Clinical classification

Tumoral lesions

Arising in normal liver (or with fatty liver):
   it may be any type of lesion.

Lesions, however, can be divided into:
(1) Those requiring curative intervention (either resection, ablation or liver transplant) to prevent malignant degeneration or hemorrhagic complications and in
(2) those which do not require any treatment.
The former group comprises (large) adenomas, adenomatosis, biliary adenomas – cystadenomas and papillomatosis, hemangioendothelioma. In selected cases an intervention may also be needed in other tumors in the presence of compression of nearby structures. An intervention, however, may also be necessary in those other lesions in which imaging techniques are not able to reach a diagnosis, which can be properly ascertained, instead, only on the resected specimen (e.g. solitary necrotic nodule, pseudolipoma, isolated hepatic splenosis, mesenchymal hamartoma, inflammatory pseudotumor, and possibly also schwannoma, lymphangioma, infantile hemangioma).

Arising in a cirrhotic liver:

If not an HCC, first think of a macroregenerative nodule. Secondly, think of a hemangioma or lymphatic lesion (malignant). Any other type of benign lesion may be present but this possibility should be regarded as extremely remote.

Pseudotumoral lesions (usually seen only at ultrasound, with no contrast perfusion defects)

Focal fatty sparing
Focal fatty change

The main clinical differentiation in connection with the background liver condition occurs in hepatocellular lesions. In fact, in this field, it is very relevant, whether the lesion has arisen on a healthy normal liver or on chronic liver disease with cirrhosis.

For instance, in normal livers, especially in young females with a history of use of contraceptive pills, the diagnosis should be directed towards an adenoma. On the other hand, in cirrhosis, the most likely finding for the same type of nodule would a macroregenerative/dysplastic nodule. Any possible adenoma in a male, especially if no specific hormonal risk factor is present, should be regarded with great caution for not misdiagnosing a malignant lesion.

6.2
Pathological Features

Assessment of a tissue sample by light microscopy is regarded as the gold standard for diagnosis of focal liver lesions. However, several considerations should be taken into account, leading to the conclusion that pathological assessment plays the major role in various instances, but provides maximal accuracy only when integrated with all the pertinent clinical and radiological information. Major problems concern the quality of the material to be analyzed. Whereas whole tumor samples, as those deriving from surgical resection, provide everything requested for a definite diagnosis, biopsy specimens may be far less adequate. Limitations may be due to: (1) small specimens, preventing the possibility of performing enough different stainings or not including enough tumoral tissue, (2) absence of any portion of the perilesional parenchymal tissue, which usually acts as internal reference standard. In these cases the pathological diagnosis may become uncertain. As regards the size, a biopsy sample should be considered adequate if at least 15 mm in length and 0.8 mm in diameter (corresponding to samples obtained with at least a 19-Gauge biopsy needle).

Provided that a sufficient specimen has been obtained and all relevant clinical and radiological information was sent to the pathologist, the latter bases his/her final judgment upon the following features. Finally, it is worth noting that making a definite diagnosis of benign liver lesion, possibly involves greater responsibility for the medical team, than suspecting a malignant disease. In fact, a diagnosis of a benign mass excludes, in most cases, the need of any treatment; this might have serious consequences on the prognosis if, instead, a malignant lesion has been missed. On the contrary the suspicion of a malignant lesions, when this is not a case, may lead to over treatment, but does not modify the prognosis. All efforts should be made therefore to support the diagnosis of benign liver lesions, especially in atypical cases.

6.2.1
Hepatocellular Adenoma and Adenomatosis

Adenoma is a benign neoplastic lesions made of morphologically normal hepatocytes. It arises in normal (i.e. non-cirrhotic) livers. The very large majority is detected in young females. Malignant progression has been reported, but it is rare (GYORFFY et al. 1989; NEUBERGER et al. 1986). Medical history nearly always reveals a setting of hepatocellular stimulation, usually with oral contraceptives for several years (especially of the first generation type), but the pathophysiological relationship between hormones and neoplasm development still remains unclear (TORBENSON et al. 2002). Affected males usually report a history of anabolic hormones. The concurrent appearance of several (usually more than ten) adenomas is named adenomatosis (GRAZIOLI et al. 2000). The disease may complicate other conditions of hepatocellular stimulation, such as a glycogenosis type Ia or III, a Klinefelter syndrome, familial diabetes or have a familial history (BACQ et al. 2003; LERUT et al. 2003; REZNIK et al. 2004; VOLMAR et al. 2003). Adenomas may vary in size from small (1 cm) to very large (30 cm) masses. They are hypervascular and often present areas of intralesional hemorrhages, which can be detected at imaging techniques and are rather typical of this neoplasm. At gross inspection adenomas are soft, well demarcated and usually without a fibrous capsule (Fig. 6.1). Large adenomas (>5 cm in diameter) are prone to rupture with intraabdominal bleeding (hemoperitoneum), if located in a subcapsular position. Scientific clinical literature reports a low accuracy of fine needle biopsy in the diagnosis of adenomas, but often all the clinical and radiological information contributing to an appropriate pathological judgment was lacking. Great caution should be taken in puncturing adenoma due to their proneness to bleeding. A safe approach should include various centimeters of normal liver parenchyma before reaching the lesion. The most challenging differential diagnosis is that with well differentiated hepatocellular carcinoma (Edmondson G1). Pathological features of adenoma include: morphologically normal hepatocytes distributed along single

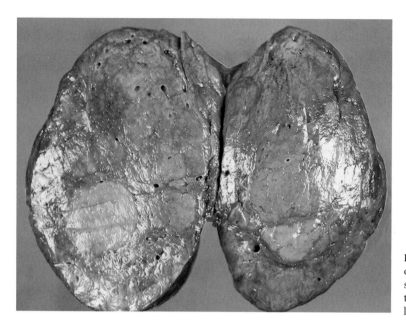

Fig. 6.1. Gross appearance at cut surface of a resected hepatic adenoma. The lesion is yellowish, also due to its fat content, well demarcated but not encapsulated and does not show fibrous septa

or double layers without acinar distribution, portal spaces and ductular structures. The nuclei present all the same appearance (nuclear monomorphism). The nuclear/cytoplasmic ratio is low. The cytoplasm is large and clear and, in focal areas of the tumor, contains fat deposition which may be an additional clue to diagnosis, together with intralesional hemorrhage, at imaging techniques. Mib-1 proliferation index is usually lower than that observed in G1 hepatocellular carcinoma.

6.2.2
Focal Nodular Hyperplasia

It is not a truly neoplastic lesion, but rather a regenerative mass caused by a vascular abnormality: indeed hepatocytes are not monoclonal (IWP 1995; FUKUKURA et al. 1998; GAIANI et al. 1999; SCOAZEC et al. 1995). It is more common in females (with a F/M ratio of 10/1 in our experience) and often is associated with a history of hormone consumption (usually contraceptive pills). It may significantly increase in size during pregnancy. It may be detected at any age, since the majority (over 80%) are asymptomatic. It is commonly not associated with any alteration of blood liver enzymes.

In most cases it is a solitary lesion, but sometimes may appear multiple: this was the case in 16% of our patients, who showed from two to four nodules at imaging techniques (personal observation) and up to 30% in other case series. Pathological fea-

tures typically include the presence of a central (or sometimes eccentric) large fibrous scar, containing an artery that is larger than expected for the native artery of the portal tract and for the accompanying ducts. The artery is usually visible also just outside the nodule where it has the meaning of a feeding artery (Fig. 6.2). The scar is surrounded by hyperplastic small nodules, with fibrous septa containing ductular proliferation, whereas major bile ducts are usually absent. The vascular disorder causing formation of the nodule is characterized by loss of the terminal central hepatic vein and by capillarization of the sinusoids (FUKUKURA et al. 1998). The smallest arteries supply monoacinar nodules approximately 1 mm in diameter. Portal veins are usually absent. This peculiar vascularization justifies the typical appearance at contrast imaging techniques. A chronic cholestasis may derive locally from these alterations. A deposition of copper may also be detected when specifically searched for. The differentiation with adenoma relies on the presence of fibrous septa and ductular proliferation with inflammation. The differential diagnosis may be particularly challenging in small specimens as those obtained with fine needle biopsy.

FNH has been subgrouped in the solid type and telangiectatic type. The differentiation has no clinical impact, but the latter type usually occur in the multiple FNH syndrome. This syndrome is present if at least two FNH lesions and one or more other type of lesion are present (including hepatic hemangioma, arterial structural defects, central nervous system vascular malformation, SNC tumors) (IWP 1995).

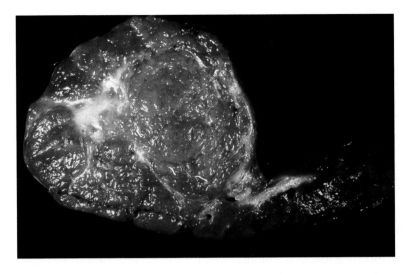

Fig. 6.2. Gross appearance at cut surface of a nodule of focal nodular hyperplasia 6 cm in diameter, which was partially exophytic from the liver. The lesions typically show the central (eccentric) large fibrous (*white*) scar connected to the periphery by fibrous septa which contain relatively large arteries

6.2.3
Diffuse Nodular Regenerative Hyperplasia

Diffuse nodular regenerative hyperplasia (NHR) occurs with similar frequency in males and females. Mild to moderate elevation of alkaline phosphatase is often present. It is characterized by small (1–10 mm) hepatocellular nodules distributed throughout the liver, usually in periportal areas, in the absence of fibrous septa (or with very limited extent of fibrosis) associated with surrounding acinar atrophy. Nodules may be monoacinar, in other words containing no more than one portal tract, located centrally, or multiacinar (IWP 1995). Multiple adjacent nodules usually appear grossly as large nodules, possibly affecting the whole liver. As a consequence NHR may resemble micronodular cirrhosis grossly, but the nodules are less well defined and the parenchyma is softer than in cirrhosis (Fig. 6.3). The margin of the nodule is poorly demarcated because the transition is gradual and the hepatocytes inside and outside the nodule differ only in size and plate arrangement. Hepatocytes, in fact, are large, with light cytoplasm (due to glycogen/lipid storage). Large nodules may occasionally show pseudoacinar features, pseudoxanthomatous transformation, copper deposition and, rarely, large cell dysplasia, these characteristic being absent in the usual small nodules. A differential diagnosis with hepatocellular adenoma based merely on histology may be difficult on fine needle biopsy specimens. Obliteration of small (<50 μm) portal and hepatic veins, usually as a consequence of compression by nearby nodules, is characteristic of diffuse NRH but not of adenomas; it is thought to be the mechanism causing portal hypertension (NABER

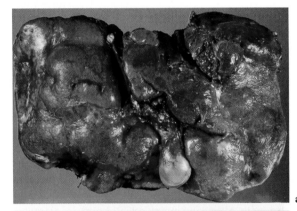
a

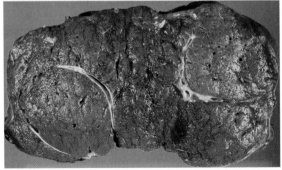
b

Fig. 6.3. a Gross appearance of an explanted liver with nodular regenerative hyperplasia (NRH) of a patient submitted to transplantation for untreatable portal hypertension. NRH may resemble cirrhosis grossly, but at cut surface the nodules, which affect the whole liver, are less well defined and the parenchyma is softer than in cirrhosis and fibrous septa are lacking. **b** The margins of large nodules are poorly demarcated, but a mass effect, compressing hepatic veins is clearly evident. The portal system is not enlarged, since portal hypertension is caused by compression of the intrahepatic (mainly smallest) portal veins

et al. 1991; WANLESS 1990). Signs of the latter, however, although usually held as a typical manifestation of NHR, were evident only in a small minority of patients described in a large autopsy series (WANLESS 1990). Furthermore, NHR, despite possibly showing up at any age, was found to be histologically present at necroscopy in 5.6% of individuals over age 80. Apart from older age, it is more frequent in patients with rheumatic and hematologic diseases (MATSUMOTO et al. 2000; WANLESS et al. 1980). As a consequence, NHR was proposed to encompass a broad spectrum of lesions being not a primary neoplastic disease or a specific entity, but a secondary tissue adaptation to heterogeneous distribution of blood flow (WANLESS 1990).

A single case was reported in a patient under azathioprine treatment, in whom hepatocellular carcinoma was detected in a background of NHR (RUSSMANN et al. 2001). However, no direct evidence that NHR may undergo malignant transformation exists to date.

6.2.4
Cirrhotic Nodule

A regenerative nodule composed of hepatocytes that is largely or completely surrounded by fibrous septa and contains more than one terminal portal tract is termed cirrhotic nodule. This entity occurs in the background of cirrhotic chronic liver disease. Regenerative nodules are respectively defined micro- or macronodules by size, with a division point set at 3 mm in diameter (IWP 1995) and their relative prevalence defines the micronodular or macronodular pattern of cirrhosis. When the size is greater than 10 mm, macronodules are termed macroregenerative nodules. These nodules are benign masses, which, however, may regress, remain stationary or progress in size. The presence of a region of hepatocytes at least 1 mm in diameter with dysplasia within a cirrhotic nodules, but without definite histologic criteria of malignancy, lets the nodules be termed "dysplastic nodule", low or high-grade (respectively when atypia is mild or at least moderate). As the size of the lesion increases, there is a greater likelihood that high-grade or malignant lesions are present; benign lesions are seldom greater than 20 mm in diameter. A dysplastic nodule is a pre-malignant lesion, but the time to progression is unpredictable and may last several years or decades.

New genetic markers will probably be introduced in clinical practice in the near future to differentiate small focal liver lesions in cirrhosis.

6.2.5
Nodules in Budd-Chiari Syndrome

Livers affected by Budd-Chiari syndrome often develop focal liver lesions, which, at pathology performed on the explants of transplanted patients are 0.5–4 cm in diameter. Those larger than 1 cm are usually seen also at imaging and may raise questions about their nature, especially in hematological patients and, as a consequence, on the possibility of liver transplantation. These nodules were initially classified as part of the spectrum of nodular regenerative hyperplasia, since constituted of essentially normal hepatocytes (DE SOUSA et al. 1991). However, they can develop on a background of cirrhosis due to chronic hepatic outflow obstruction and may variably contain fibrous septa, the latter including neoductules and large, mostly dysmorphic arteries. Hence, they were classified as large regenerative nodules (TANAKA and WANLESS 1998; BRANCATELLI et al. 2002; ZHOU et al. 2000). Further recent works in this field, showed that hepatocellular nodules seen in livers from patients with Budd-Chiari syndrome share indeed morphological characteristics with large regenerative nodules, but in other cases resemble focal nodular hyperplasia or hepatocellular adenomas and were respectively termed FNH-like and adenoma-like (IBARROLA et al. 2004; MAETANI et al. 2002). Nodules of the various categories may coexist in the same liver. Patchy or diffuse monoacinar regeneration was seen in most cases (six out of seven cases) in the macroscopically non-nodular liver parenchyma studied by IBARROLA et al. (2004). Their multiplicity, the existence of mixed lesions, the frequent hepatocellular regenerative background as well as the frequently associated portal venous obstructions suggest that these nodules are regenerative in nature and conditioned by an uneven blood perfusion throughout the liver. In their differential diagnosis, the clinicopathological context in which they occur is of paramount importance and should allow recognition that those resembling adenomas may not be true neoplasms (IBARROLA et al. 2004).

6.2.6
Cholangiocellular Adenoma (or Peribiliary Gland Hamartoma)

Cholangiocellular adenoma of the liver is usually a single mass (commonly small, 0.5–2 cm), well circumscribed but not encapsulated, constituted of disorganized, mature peribiliary gland acini, with basal small nuclei and tubules within a variable amount of stroma, with a more or less intense inflammatory infiltration. Small granulomas are seldom observed at the periphery. The lumen of the tubules does not contain bile. It is hypothesized to derive from a reactive process to a focal injury (inflammatory or traumatic). As a consequence it has been renamed peribiliary gland hamartoma (BHATHAL et al. 1996). It has a very benign clinical behavior and, since asymptomatic, is practically always discovered by chance, either intra-operatively or during imaging (ALLAIRE et al. 1988; VARNHOLT et al. 2003; WOHLGEMUTH et al. 1998). Unfortunately, the pathological differential diagnosis with metastatic well-differentiated adenocarcinomas or intrahepatic/peripheral cholangiocellular carcinoma may sometimes be difficult, especially in frozen sections. Recently a new entity was described, named atypical bile duct adenoma (ALBORES-SAAVEDRA et al. 2001). An interesting pathological finding is the von Meyenburg complexes, an entity, generally less than 2 mm in size, comprising dilated small bile ducts containing bile plugs, surrounded by mature fibrous stroma, without inflammatory infiltrate; it can be found in around 5% of adult patients at autopsy, particularly in those harboring renal cysts (GOVINDARAJAN and PETERS 1984; REDSTON and WANLESS 1996). Their very small size make these lesions interesting for the pathologist, but less so for the radiologist, apart from exceptional cases.

6.2.7
Cystic Lesions

Cystic lesions comprise simple bile duct cysts, ciliated hepatic foregut cysts and bile duct cystadenoma.

6.2.7.1
Simple Bile Duct Cysts

The majority of simple bile duct cysts present between the 4th and the 6th decade and are encountered rather frequently (up to 1% prevalence in autopsy series). They are unilocular cysts lined by a single layer of columnar or cuboidal benign epithelium of biliary originally with functional properties similar to that of the epithelium of the bile ducts (EVERSON et al. 1990). The cysts contain serous fluid, not communicating with the intrahepatic biliary tree. There is no septation. In 50% of affected adults there is one single cyst. In the remaining half of patients there are two or more cysts. They are regarded as a congenital malformation, but often become evident only in adult life. Liver cysts are found also in the adult polycystic kidney disease.

Caroli's disease is, instead, a congenital malformation consisting of multifocal dilatation of segmental bile ducts. It is a diffuse liver disease, but should be considered in the differential diagnosis of cystic lesions of the liver, since it may resemble this condition.

6.2.7.2
Ciliated Hepatic Foregut Cysts

Less than 100 case have been reported in the literature (VICK et al. 1999). On average they are around 5 cm in diameter, usually bilocular. Sometimes they are associated with elevated levels of CA19-9. One case of malignant transformation was described. Histopathological features include lining of pseudostratified columnar epithelium.

6.2.7.3
Bile Duct Cyst Adenoma or Hepatobiliary Cystadenoma

It is a solitary multilocular cystic lesion, lined by a layer of columnar or flat epithelial cells. Size varies from 2 to 28 cm. The preoperative diagnosis is largely based on imaging studies, but the definitive diagnosis of benignity is not possible with certainty by the sole imaging work-up (CHOI et al. 1989; D'ERRICO et al. 1998). Malignant transformation has been described (WHEELER and EDMONDSON 1985a; WEE et al. 1993).

6.2.8
Mesenchymal Lesions

Apart from hemangioma, other benign mesenchymal lesions of the liver are relatively rare and do not show pathological features that are of value for a sufficiently specific diagnosis at imaging techniques. Hence histology assessment (either on an adequate biopsy specimen or on the resected lesions) is usually unavoidable. Some mesenchymal lesions are more frequent in children. Specific aspects are described in the pertinent literature, mostly as single case reports due to the limited number of observed cases or, in a few instances, summarized in short reviews.

These lesions include mesenchymal hamartoma, infantile hemangioma angiomyolipoma, inflammatory pseudotumor pseudolipoma, isolated hepatic splenosis, leiomyoma, schwannoma, solitary necrotic nodules, coelomic fat ectopia, lymphangioma (LEE and DuBois 2001; QUINN and GUZMAN-HARTMAN 2003; WHEELER and EDMONDSON 1985b; ASCH et al. 1974; BOON et al. 1996; BRUNELLO et al. 1994; D'ANGELICA et al. 1998; GRAZI et al. 1998; HAWKINS et al. 1980; O'SULLIVAN et al. 1998; PAPASTRATIS et al. 2000; REN et al. 2003; SAKAI et al. 2001; SCHMID et al. 1996; STROTZER et al. 1999; WADA et al. 1998; YEN et al. 2003). Hemangioendothelioma is more frequent in children and usually has an uncertain malignant potential (MANI and VAN THIEL 2001; MEYERS and SCAIFE 2000).

6.2.9
Hemangioma

Being detected in the past at autopsy and more recently at ultrasound in up to 5% of the population, hemangioma is the most common benign tumor of the liver. Size is on average larger in women, but these do not show a greater incidence of the disease. Hemangiomas are commonly small (<4 cm) and single, but may also be multiple and may occasionally occupy the largest part of the liver. On microscopic examination they are composed of large vascular channels, lined by mature flattened endothelial cells, enclosed in loose fibroblastic stroma with a variable amount of collagenization. Usually they do not increase in size with time, although it has been reported that during pregnancy or during estrogenic therapy the tumor may grow (READING et al. 1988). The prognosis is excellent, apart from exceptionally giant lesions.

6.2.10
Pseudotumoral Lesions

Focal fatty changes and focal fatty sparing usually are believed to correspond respectively to areas with fatty infiltration in a normal liver or areas preserved from fatty deposition in a steatotic liver. However, the division appears not so clear cut in all cases, since often the different appearance at imaging techniques, and particularly at ultrasound, seems rather to correspond to a similar quantity of deposited fat, but contained in fewer droplets within the pseudotumor (when it appears "hypoechoic") or in larger numbers of fat-filled vacuoles with respect to that of the surrounding parenchyma ("hyperechoic" lesions or fatty changes) (CATURELLI et al. 1991).

References

Albores-Saavedra J, Hoang MP, Murakata LA, et al (2001) Atypical bile duct adenoma, clear cell type: a previously undescribed tumor of the liver. Am J Surg Pathol 25:956–960

Allaire GS, Rabin L, Ishak KG, et al (1988) Sesterhenn IA. Bile duct adenoma. A study of 152 cases. Am J Surg Pathol 12:708–715

Asch MJ, Cohen AH, Moore TC (1974) Hepatic and splenic lymphangiomatosis with skeletal involvement: report of a case and review of the literature. Surgery 76:334–339

Bacq Y, Jacquemin E, Balabaud C, et al (2003) Familial liver adenomatosis associated with hepatocyte nuclear factor 1alpha inactivation. Gastroenterology 125:1470–1475

Bhathal PS, Hughes NR, Goodman ZD (1996) The so-called bile duct adenoma is a peribiliary gland hamartoma. Am J Surg Pathol 20:858–864

Boon LM, Burrows PE, Paltiel HJ, et al (1996) Hepatic vascular anomalies in infancy: a twenty-seven-year experience. J Pediatr 129:346–354

Brancatelli G, Federle MP, Grazioli L, et al (2002) Benign regenerative nodules in Budd-Chiari syndrome and other vascular disorders of the liver: radiologic-pathologic and clinical correlation. Radiographics 22:847–862

Brunello F, Caremani M, Marcarino C, et al (1994) Inflammatory pseudotumour of the liver: diagnosis by fine needle biopsy in two cases and a review of the literature. Ital J Gastroenterol 26:151–153

Caturelli E, Costarelli L, Giordano M, et al (1991) Hypoechoic lesions in fatty liver. Quantitative study by histomorphometry. Gastroenterology 100:1678–1682

Choi BI, Lim JH, Han MC, et al (1989) Biliary cystadenoma and cystadenocarcinoma: CT and sonographic findings. Radiology 171:57–61

D'Angelica M, Fong Y, Blumgart LH (1998) Isolated hepatic splenosis: first reported case. HPB Surg 11:39–42

de Sousa JM, Portmann B, Williams R (1991) Nodular regenerative hyperplasia of the liver and the Budd-Chiari syndrome. Case report, review of the literature and reappraisal of pathogenesis. J Hepatol 12:28–35

D'Errico A, Deleonardi G, Fiorentino M, et al (1998) Diagnostic implications of albumin messenger RNA detection and cytokeratin pattern in benign hepatic lesions and biliary cystadenocarcinoma. Diagn Mol Pathol 7:289–294

Everson GT, Emmett M, Brown WR, et al (1990) Functional similarities of hepatic cystic and biliary epithelium: studies of fluid constituents and in vivo secretion in response to secretin. Hepatology 11:557–565

Fukukura Y, Nakashima O, Kusaba A, et al (1998) Angioarchitecture and blood circulation in focal nodular hyperplasia of the liver. J Hepatol 29:470–475

Gaiani S, Piscaglia F, Serra C, et al (1999) Hemodynamics in focal nodular hyperplasia. J Hepatol 31:576

Govindarajan S, Peters RL (1984) The bile duct adenoma. A lesion distinct from Meyenburg complex. Arch Pathol Lab Med 108:922–924

Grazi GL, Mazziotti A, Gruttadauria S, et al (1998) Solitary necrotic nodules of the liver. Am Surg 64:764–767

Grazioli L, Federle MP, Ichikawa T, et al (2000) Liver adenomatosis: clinical, histopathologic, and imaging findings in 15 patients. Radiology 2000 216:395–402

Gyorffy EJ, Bredfeldt JE, Black WC (1989) Transformation of hepatic cell adenoma to hepatocellular carcinoma due to oral contraceptive use. Ann Intern Med 110:489–490

Hawkins EP, Jordan GL, McGavran MH (1980) Primary leio-myoma of the liver. Successful treatment by lobectomy and presentation of criteria for diagnosis. Am J Surg Pathol 4:301–304

Ibarrola C, Castellano VM, Colina F (2004) Focal hyperplastic hepatocellular nodules in hepatic venous outflow obstruc-tion: a clinicopathological study of four patients and 24 nodules. Histopathology 44:172–179

International Working Party (1995) Terminology of nodular hepatocellular lesions. Hepatology 22:983–993

Lee SL, DuBois JJ (2001) Hepatic inflammatory pseudotumor: case report, review of the literature, and a proposal for morphologic classification. Pediatr Surg Int 17:555–559

Lerut JP, Ciccarelli O, Sempoux C, et al (2003) Glycogenosis storage type I diseases and evolutive adenomatosis: an indi-cation for liver transplantation. Transpl Int 16:879–884

Maetani Y, Itoh K, Egawa H, et al (2002) Benign hepatic nod-ules in Budd-Chiari syndrome: radiologic-pathologic cor-relation with emphasis on the central scar. AJR Am J Roent-genol 178:869–875

Mani H, Van Thiel DH (2001) Mesenchymal tumors of the liver. Clin Liver Dis 5:219–257, viii

Matsumoto T, Kobayashi S, Shimizu H, et al (2000) The liver in collagen diseases: pathologic study of 160 cases with particular reference to hepatic arteritis, primary biliary cirrhosis, autoimmune hepatitis and nodular regenerative hyperplasia of the liver. Liver 20:366–373

Meyers RL, Scaife ER (2000) Benign liver and biliary tract masses in infants and toddlers. Semin Pediatr Surg 9:146–155

Naber AH, Van Haelst U, Yap SH (1991) Nodular regenerative hyperplasia of the liver: an important cause of portal hyper-tension in non-cirrhotic patients. J Hepatol 12:94–99

Neuberger J, Forman D, Doll R, et al (1986) Oral contracep-tives and hepatocellular carcinoma. Br Med J (Clin Res Ed) 292:1355–1357

O'Sullivan DA, Torres VE, de Groen PC, et al (1998) Hepatic lymphangiomatosis mimicking polycystic liver disease. Mayo Clin Proc 73:1188–1192

Papastratis G, Margaris H, Zografos GN, et al (2000) Mesen-chymal hamartoma of the liver in an adult: a review of the literature. Int J Clin Pract 54:552–554

Quinn AM, Guzman-Hartman G (2003) Pseudolipoma of Glis-son capsule. Arch Pathol Lab Med 127:503–504

Reading NG, Forbes A, Nunnerley HB, et al (1988) Hepatic haemangiomas: a critical review of diagnosis and manage-ment. Quart J Med 67:431–445

Redston MS, Wanless IR (1996) The hepatic von Meyenburg complex: prevalence and association with hepatic and renal cysts among 2843 autopsies. Mod Pathol 9:233–237

Ren N, Qin LX, Tang ZY, et al (2003) Diagnosis and treatment of hepatic angiomyolipoma in 26 cases. World J Gastroen-terol 9:1856–1858

Reznik Y, Dao T, Coutant R, et al (2004) Hepatocyte nuclear factor-1alpha gene inactivation: cosegregation between liver adenomatosis and diabetes phenotypes in two matu-rity-onset diabetes of the young (MODY)3 families. J Clin Endocrinol Metab 89:1476–1480

Russmann S, Zimmermann A, Krahenbuhl S, et al (2001) Veno-occlusive disease, nodular regenerative hyperplasia and hepatocellular carcinoma after azathioprine treatment in a patient with ulcerative colitis. Eur J Gastroenterol Hepatol 13:287–290

Sakai M, Ikeda H, Suzuki N, Takahashi A, et al (2001) Inflam-matory pseudotumor of the liver: case report and review of the literature. J Pediatr Surg 36:663–666

Schmid A, Janig D, Bohuszlavizki A, et al (1996) Inflamma-tory pseudotumor of the liver presenting as incidentaloma: report of a case and review of the literature. Hepatogastro-enterology 43:1009–1014

Scoazec JY, Flejou JF, D'Errico A, et al (1995) Focal nodular hyperplasia of the liver: composition of the extracellular matrix and the expression of cell-cell and cell-matrix adhe-sion molecules. Hum Pathol 26:1114–1125

Strotzer M, Paetzel C, Feuerbach S (1999) Multiple hepatic angiolipomas: a case report and review of literature. Eur Radiol 9:259–261

Tanaka M, Wanless IR (1998) Pathology of the liver in Budd-Chiari syndrome: portal vein thrombosis and the histogen-esis of veno-centric cirrhosis, veno-portal cirrhosis, and large regenerative nodules. Hepatology 27:488–496

Torbenson M, Lee JH, Choti M, et al (2002) Hepatic adenomas: analysis of sex steroid receptor status and the Wnt signal-ing pathway. Mod Pathol 15:189–196

Varnholt H, Vauthey JN, Cin PD, et al (2003) Biliary adenofi-broma: a rare neoplasm of bile duct origin with an indolent behavior. Am J Surg Pathol 27:693–698

Vick DJ, Goodman ZD, Deavers MT, et al (1999) Ciliated hepatic foregut cyst: a study of six cases and review of the literature. Am J Surg Pathol 23:671–677

Volmar KE, Burchette JL, Creager AJ (2003) Hepatic adenoma-tosis in glycogen storage disease type Ia: report of a case with unusual histology. Arch Pathol Lab Med 127:402–405

Wada Y, Jimi A, Nakashima O, et al (1998) Schwannoma of the liver: report of two surgical cases. Pathol Int 48:611–617

Wanless IR (1990) Micronodular transformation (nodular regenerative hyperplasia) of the liver: a report of 64 cases among 2,500 autopsies and a new classification of benign hepatocellular nodules. Hepatology 11:787–797

Wanless IR, Godwin TA, Allen F, et al (1980) Nodular regen-erative hyperplasia of the liver in hematologic disorders: a possible response to obliterative portal venopathy. A mor-phometric study of nine cases with an hypothesis on the pathogenesis. Medicine (Baltimore) 59:367–379

Wee A, Nilsson B, Kang JY, et al (1993) Biliary cystadenocarci-noma arising in a cystadenoma. Report of a case diagnosed by fine needle aspiration cytology. Acta Cytol 37:966–970

Wheeler DA, Edmondson HA (1985a) Cystadenoma with mes-enchymal stroma (CMS) in the liver and bile ducts. A clini-copathologic study of 17 cases, 4 with malignant change. Cancer 56:1434–1445

Wheeler DA, Edmondson HA (1985b) Coelomic fat ectopia in the liver. Arch Pathol Lab Med 109:783–785

Wohlgemuth WA, Bottger J, Bohndorf K (1998) MRI, CT, US and ERCP in the evaluation of bile duct hamartomas (von Meyenburg complex): a case report. Eur Radiol 8:1623–1626

Yen JB, Kong MS, Lin JN (2003) Hepatic mesenchymal hamar-toma. J Paediatr Child Health 39:632–634

Yeung YP, AhChong K, Chung CK, et al (2003) Biliary papil-lomatosis: report of seven cases and review of English lit-erature. J Hepatobiliary Pancreat Surg 10:390–395

Zhou H, Wolff M, Pauleit D, et al (2000) Multiple macrore-generative nodules in liver cirrhosis due to Budd-Chiari syndrome. Case reports and review of the literature. Hepa-togastroenterology 47:522–527

7 Cysts and Cystic-Like Lesions

Chiara Del Frate , Roberto Pozzi-Mucelli, Giuseppe Brancatelli, Koenraad Mortelè, Chiara Zuiani, and Massimo Bazzocchi

CONTENTS

C. Del Frate, MD; C.Zuiani, MD; M. Bazzocchi, MD
Institute of Radiology, University of Udine, Via Colugna 50, 33100 Udine, Italy
R. Pozzi-Mucelli, MD
Department of Radiology, University of Trieste, Cattinara's Hospital, Via Strada di Fiume 447, 34149 Trieste, Italy
G. Brancatelli, MD
Department of Radiology, Policlinico Universitario, Via del Vespro 127, 90127 Palermo, Italy
K. Mortelè, MD
Division of Abdominal Imaging and Intervention, Department of Radiology, Brigham and Women's Hospital, Francis Street 75, 02115 Boston MA, USA

software in sonography such as compound imaging, dynamic spiral and multi-detector computed tomography (CT), and fast magnetic resonance (MR) imaging, make it possible to identify several imaging features of these lesions which, when associated with clinical parameters such as age, gender, clinical history, and symptoms may help to characterize and classify cystic and cyst-like lesions (Mergo and Ros 1998; Mortelé and Ros 2001; Murphy et al. 1989; Singh et al. 1997).

These lesions include simple (bile duct) cyst, autosomal dominant polycystic liver disease, biliary hamartoma, Caroli's disease, pyogenic and amoebic abscesses, intrahepatic hydatid cyst, biliary cystadenoma and cystadenocarcinoma, cystic subtypes of primary liver neoplasms, cystic metastases, and intrahepatic hematoma and biloma.

7.1 Introduction

Cystic and cyst-like lesions of the liver in the adult can be classified as developmental, inflammatory, neoplastic, or miscellaneous. The ability to differentiate these types of cystic tumors non-invasively is extremely relevant, since their nature and origin influence the clinical management or the treatment. The rapid advances in imaging techniques over the past two decades, including the development of new

7.2 Developmental Lesions

7.2.1 Hepatic (Bile Duct) Cyst

Simple hepatic or congenital cysts are benign developmental lesions that do not communicate with the biliary tree (van Sonnenberg et al. 1994). They seem to originate from hamartomatous tissue (van Sonnenberg et al. 1994). Hepatic cysts are a common finding, being found in 1%–3% of routine liver examinations (Mathieu et al. 1997). They are more often discovered in women and are usually asymptomatic (Mathieu et al. 1997; van Sonnenberg et al. 1994); rarely they may cause pain, and symptoms disappear after percutaneous aspiration. Simple hepatic cysts can be solitary or multiple. Their size is very variable, although they are frequently less than 5 cm. They tend to increase in number and size with age. Usually they have a serous content, rarely they may present as "complicated" cysts due to the presence of hemorrhage or inflammation.

The typical appearance of a single cyst at sonography is of an anechoic, round or ellipsoid structure, characterized by the absence of an own wall, by an increased acoustic signal behind and, sometimes, by the presence of subtle lateral acoustic shadows (Fig. 7.1a). Rarely, septa or calcifications may be present. They may sometimes behave as space-occupying masses, displacing intrahepatic vessels and sometimes the biliary tree leading to jaundice, and causing swelling of the hepatic margin. Color Doppler analysis may be helpful in excluding the presence of vessels.

On non-enhanced CT scans a hepatic cyst appears as a round or ovoid well-defined lesion, with no evident wall. It has a homogeneous and hypoattenuating content with attenuation values similar to water (<20 HU) (Fig. 7.1c). After contrast media injection, both the wall or its content do not show any enhancement (Fig. 7.1b) (Mathieu et al. 1997). Higher attenuation values (>20 HU) are present in cyst with hemorrhage or inflammation inside; in these cases "complicated" cysts are difficult to differentiate from metastases arising from cystic carcinomas (as pancreatic or ovarian ones) (Figs. 7.2, 7.3).

At MR imaging, hepatic cysts have homogeneous very low signal intensity on T1-weighted images and homogeneous very high signal intensity on T2-weighted images, similar to the water signal intensity. Owing to their fluid content, an increase in signal intensity is seen on heavily T2-weighted images. This increase allows differentiation of these lesions from metastatic disease. The wall is never seen and no enhancement is present after administration of gadolinium chelates.

The intracystic hemorrhage, a rare complication in simple hepatic cysts, is usually demonstrated by high signal intensity, sometimes with a fluid–fluid level, on both T1- and T2-weighted images when mixed blood products are present (Mathieu et al. 1997); the hemorrhage may be dated thanks to the different appearance of the different phases of degradation of hemoglobin. Fat-saturation sequences may be helpful in confirming the blood content.

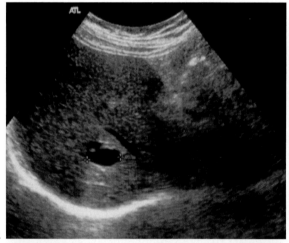

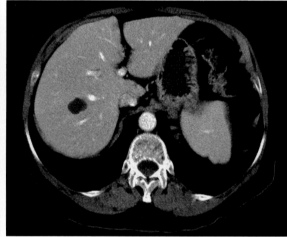

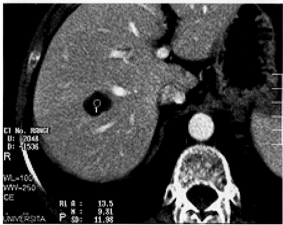

Fig. 7.1a–c. Hepatic (bile duct) cyst. Simple hepatic cyst in patient with colon cancer. **a** US examination (ascending oblique scan) shows an oval, anechoic structure, characterized by the absence of an own wall and increased acoustic signal behind. **b** Axial enhanced CT image in portal-venous phase shows a non-enhancing hypoattenuating regular cystic lesion in the right hepatic lobe. **c** The density value of the cystic lesion described above (around 10 HU) is measured positioning the region of interest inside the lesion

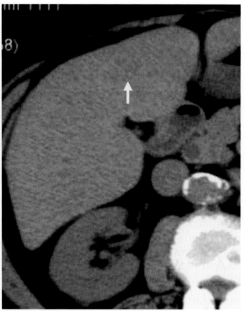

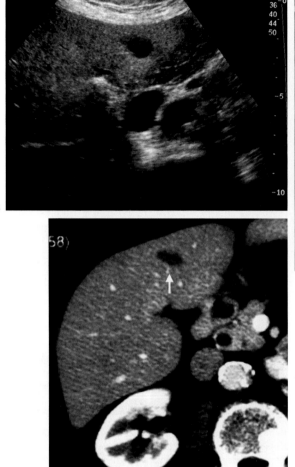

Fig. 7.2a–c. Hepatic dense cyst. 75-year-old woman in follow-up for a HCV-related chronic hepatitis. **a** Sonographic axial image on the left hepatic lobe shows an oval hypo-anechoic lesion with ill-defined borders and increased acoustic signal behind. **b** Axial non-enhanced CT image shows an hypo-attenuating lesion with ill-defined borders (*arrow*). **c** Axial portal phase CT image: no enhancement is present after contrast media administration and it always persists hypodense with higher attenuating values than water (30–35 HU) (*arrow*)

7.2.2
Polycystic Liver Disease

Hepatic cysts can also be part of polycystic liver disease, an autosomal dominant disorder often found in association with renal polycystic disease (VAN SONNENBERG et al. 1994). It is due to a ductal plate malformation of the small intrahepatic bile ducts, which loses communication with the biliary tree. It is characterized by the presence of multiple, sometimes innumerable cysts ranging in size from less than 1 cm to more than 12 cm; spontaneous intracystic hemorrhage, infection, and rupture may occur. Usually, patients with autosomal dominant polycystic liver disease are asymptomatic and liver dysfunction occurs rarely

(VAN SONNENBERG et al. 1994). However, advanced disease may cause hepatomegaly, which may result in abdominal pain and dyspnea. Hepatic cysts are found in 40% of cases of autosomal dominant polycystic disease involving the kidneys; nevertheless, they may be seen without identifiable renal involvement at imaging (MORTELÉ and ROS 2001; MURPHY et al. 1989).

Polycystic liver at sonography is characterized by the presence of multiple round or ovoid anechoic lesions, often grouped, which cause a diffuse inhomogeneity of the liver parenchyma. Polycystic liver disease typically appears as multiple homogeneous and hypoattenuating cystic lesions with regular borders on non-enhanced CT scans, with no enhancement after contrast media adminis-

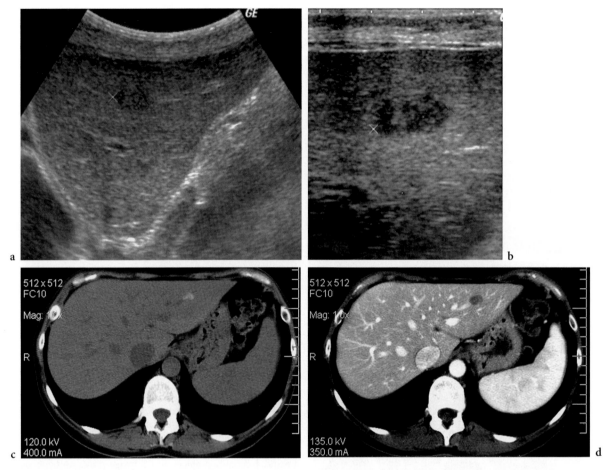

Fig. 7.3a–d. Hepatic hemorrhagic cyst. A 38-year-old woman with polyserositis, leukopenia, platelet disorder, retrobulbar neuritis and suspected SLE. Recent onset of ascites. **a** Sonographic longitudinal image on the third hepatic segment shows an ovoid, slightly hypoechoic lesion with ill-defined borders. **b** Sonographic image obtained with an high-frequency linear probe (7.5 MHz) better shows the heterogeneity of the lesion described in Fig. 7.3a. **c** Axial non-enhanced CT image shows a small ovoid hyper-attenuating lesion, probably due to the presence of fresh blood within it. **d** Axial portal phase CT image shows no enhancement of the lesion described, resulting hypoattenuating in this phase

tration (Fig. 7.4). Generally, the attenuation level may be greater than the water one, due to hemorrhage more frequently encountered than in cases of simple hepatic cysts thanks to the great number of cysts; at the same time on non-enhanced CT, calcification of the cyst walls, due to old hemorrhage, may be detected. At MR imaging, hepatic cysts in polycystic liver disease have very low signal intensity on T1-weighted images and high signal intensity on T2-weighted images, and do not enhance after administration of gadolinium contrast material. The intracystic hemorrhage is characterized by signal intensity inhomogeneity (Fig. 7.5) (MATHIEU et al. 1997).

7.2.3
Biliary Hamartoma

Bile duct hamartomas, also called von Meyenburg complexes, arise owing to failure of involution of embryonic bile ducts (MAHER et al. 1999; MARTINOLI et al. 1992; MORTELÉ et al. 2002; SEMELKA et al. 1999; SLONE et al. 1993; WEI et al. 1997; WOHLGEMUTH et al. 1998). They are usually encountered as an incidental finding at imaging, laparotomy, or autopsy, with an estimated incidence of 0.69%–2.8% in autopsy series (MORTELÉ et al. 2002). Generally they are asymptomatic; over-infection with micro-abscesses is very rare such as degeneration into cholangiocarcinoma (MAHER et al. 1999; MARTINOLI et al. 1992; SEMELKA et al. 1999; SLONE et al. 1993; WEI et al. 1997;

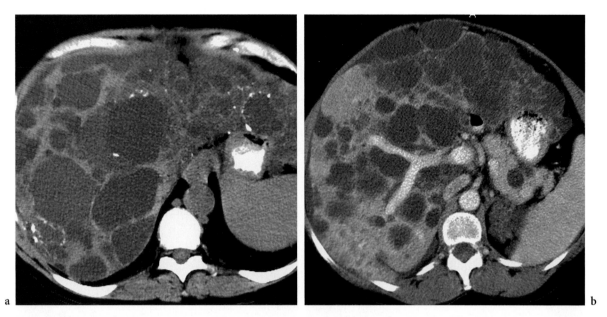

Fig. 7.4a,b. Polycystic liver disease on CT. **a** Axial non-enhanced CT image shows innumerable cysts of varying size in both liver lobes. Cysts are thin-walled, with regular margins. Some of the cysts have calcified walls, while some other have higher density due to the presence of blood or proteinaceous material. **b** Axial portal phase CT image of the same patient: multiple non-enhancing, regular cystic lesions. There is also a cyst in the body of the pancreas

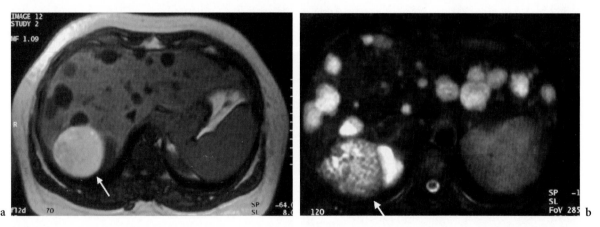

Fig. 7.5a,b. Polycystic liver disease and hemorrhagic cyst on MR. A 42-year-old woman, with known history of polycystic liver disease and recent onset of abdominal pain. **a** Axial T1-weighted MR image shows multiple low signal intensity lesions scattered throughout the liver, corresponding to simple cysts, and a large round hyperintense lesion (*arrow*). **b** Axial STIR T2-weighted MR image shows as the multiple simple cysts become hyperintense while the large lesion persists hyperintense (*arrow*), due to intra-cystic hemorrhage

Wohlgemuth et al. 1998). They are composed of one or multiple small spherical masses lined by biliary epithelium with variable amounts of fibrous stroma. At pathologic analysis, they appear as grayish-white nodular lesions 0.1–1.5 cm in diameter that do not communicate with the biliary tree and are scattered throughout the liver parenchyma (Wei et al. 1997).

Sonographic findings in biliary hamartomas have been described as either hypoechoic or anechoic small nodules with distal acoustic enhancement (Gallego et al. 1995; Martinoli et al. 1992; Salo et al. 1992). Hyperechoic biliary hamartomas or a combination of hypo- and hyperechoic lesions, however, have also been reported (Eisenberg et al. 1986; Martinoli et al. 1992; Mortelé et al. 2002; Salo et al. 1992).

In almost all reported cases, non-enhanced CT showed hypodense small hepatic nodules, scattered throughout the liver and typically measuring between 0.5 and 1.0 cm in diameter (MARTINOLI et al. 1992; MORTELÉ et al. 2002; WOHLGEMUTH et al. 1998). The latter feature is the most essential one in the differential diagnosis from multiple simple cysts. Furthermore, simple cysts are typically regularly outlined, whereas bile duct hamartomas have a more irregular outline. Although homogeneous enhancement of these lesions has been noted in some cases, in most reports, however, no enhancement was seen after contrast media administration (Fig. 7.6a) (MORTELÉ et al. 2002; SEMELKA et al. 1999; SLONE et al. 1993; WOHLGEMUTH et al. 1998.

The MR appearance of bile duct hamartomas has been reported sporadically (MAHER et al. 1999; MORTELÉ et al. 2002; SEMELKA et al. 1999; SLONE et al. 1993. All lesions were hypointense compared with liver parenchyma on T1-weighted images and markedly hyperintense on T2-weighted images (MORTELÉ and Ros 2001; MORTELÉ et al. 2002; SEMELKA et al. 1999; MURPHY et al. 1989. On heavily T2-weighted images, the signal intensity increases further, nearly reaching the signal intensity of fluid (SEMELKA et al. 1999; WOHLGEMUTH et al. 1998. Biliary hamartomas also do not exhibit a characteristic pattern of enhancement after administration of

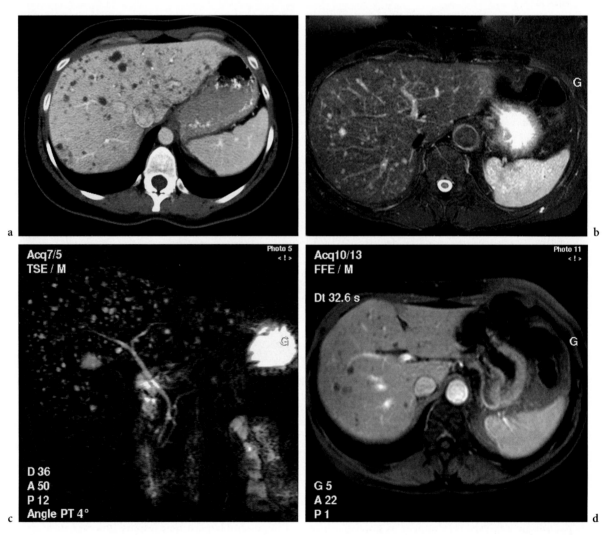

Fig. 7.6a–d. Biliary hamartomas. **a** Axial portal phase CT image shows multiple, nonenhancing, hypoattenuating irregular cystic lesions, measuring up to 10 mm and located in both lobes of the liver. **b** Fat-suppressed, turbo spin-echo T2-weighted MR image shows numerous, markedly hyperintense cystic lesions. Intensity of the lesions nearly reaches that of cerebrospinal fluid. **c** Single-shot coronal projection MR cholangiogram shows innumerable high signal intensity liver cysts and normal intra- and extrahepatic biliary duct. Lesions do not show communication with the biliary tree. *G*, gastric. **d** Axial T1-weighted MR image shows multiple low signal intensity lesions scattered throughout the liver

Gadolinium chelates; some authors observed homogeneous enhancement of these lesions, some others a thin rim enhancement, whereas others did not find any enhancement (MORTELÉ and ROS 2001; MAHER et al. 1999; MARTINOLI et al. 1992; MURPHY et al. 1989; SLONE et al. 1993; WOHLGEMUTH et al. 1998). At MR cholangiography, bile duct hamartomas appear as multiple tiny cystic lesions that do not communicate with the biliary tree, helping in the differential diagnosis with Caroli's disease (Fig. 7.6b–d) (LUO et al. 1998).

7.2.4
Caroli's Disease

Caroli's disease, also known as congenital communicating cavernous ectasia of the biliary tract, is a rare, autosomal recessive developmental abnormality due to a ductal plate malformation of the large intrahepatic bile ducts. The abnormal ducts retain their communication with the biliary tree. The disease results from the arrest of or a derangement in the normal embryologic remodeling of ducts and causes varying degrees of destructive inflammation and segmental dilatation. If the large intrahepatic bile ducts are affected, the result is Caroli's disease, whereas abnormal development of the small interlobular bile ducts results in congenital hepatic fibrosis. If all levels of the biliary tree are involved, features of both congenital hepatic fibrosis and Caroli's disease are present. This condition has been termed "Caroli's syndrome" (LEVI et al. 2002; ZANGGER et al. 1995). Complications include multiple intrahepatic calculi, cholangitis, and rarely cholangiocarcinoma (PAVONE et al. 1996). It may be associated with cystic renal disease (CHOI et al. 1990; PAVONE et al. 1996; ZANGGER et al. 1995). The abnormality may be segmental or diffuse. Clinical symptoms are usually related to recurrent attacks of right upper quadrant pain, fever, and, more rarely, jaundice (MORTELÉ and ROS 2001; MURPHY et al. 1989).

Sonograms of the liver may show, besides bile duct dilatations, intraluminal bulbar protrusions, bridge formation across dilated lumina, and portal radicles partially or completely surrounded by dilated bile ducts (MARCHAL et al. 1986). The cholangiographic features of Caroli's disease are well established as saccular or fusiform dilatation of the intrahepatic bile ducts. Irregular bile duct walls, strictures, and stones may be present (LUCAYA et al. 1978). Segmental ductal dilatation is more common than diffuse ductal dilatation. Alternating areas of

stricture and dilatation are a common observation with cholangiograms (LEVI et al. 2002). Inside the dilated segments echoes with shadowing may be present and referred to calculi or small hyperechoic deposits may be seen.

CT typically shows hypoattenuating dilated cystic structures that communicate with the biliary tree (Fig. 7.7) (PAVONE et al. 1996). The "central dot sign", or the presence of tiny dots with strong contrast enhancement within the dilated intrahepatic bile ducts, is considered very suggestive of Caroli's disease (CHOI et al. 1990). Intraluminal biliary calculi may be demonstrated.

At MR imaging, the dilated and cystic biliary system appears hypointense on T1-weighted images and strongly hyperintense on T2-weighted images (ZANGGER et al. 1995). The intraluminal portal vein radicals present marked enhancement after administration of gadolinium chelates (ZANGGER et al. 1995). MR imaging may show bridges across dilated intrahepatic ducts, which resemble internal septa (ZANGGER et al. 1995). MR cholangiography can be extremely valuable in diagnosis of Caroli's disease by demonstrating the pathognomonic feature of saccular dilated and non-obstructed intrahepatic bile ducts that communicate with the biliary tree (PAVONE et al. 1996). Furthermore, stones, when present, are evident as signal voids within ducts and cystic spaces. Sludge or debris may be evident within dependent cysts.

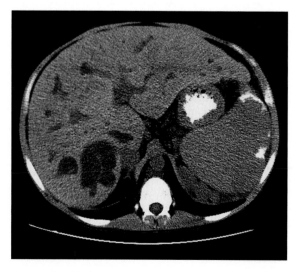

Fig. 7.7. Caroli's disease in a 34-year-old male. Nonenhanced CT shows a hypoattenuating saccular dilatation that communicates with the intrahepatic biliary tree

7.2.5
Choledochal Cyst

A choledochal cyst is a rare congenital dilation of the hepatic duct of the liver and is due to a ductal plate malformation of the large bile ducts. They maintain continuity with the biliary tree. These cysts can be intrahepatic and/or extrahepatic (KIM et al. 1995).

Choledochal cysts have been classified by Modani into five types:

- The type 1 is the most common type, making up about half of all choledochal cysts. This type is a cystic dilation of the extrahepatic biliary duct.
- The type 2 is an abnormal pouch or sac (diverticulum) opening from the main duct.
- The type 3 involves a cyst that is located within the duodenal wall.
- The type 4 refers to cystic dilations of both the intrahepatic and extrahepatic biliary tracts.
- The type 5 is the least common type of hepatic duct cyst, which involves multiple intrahepatic cysts. This type of clustering of cysts is also known as Caroli's disease.

Symptoms and signs include right upper quadrant pain, jaundice, abdominal mass, nausea, and fever. Possible complication are calculi, cholangitis, pancreatitis, and rarely malignant degeneration into cholangiocarcinoma.

At imaging the shape of the choledochal cyst depends on the type, appearing as a fusiform or cystic dilatation of the bile duct. For example, the type 1 cyst appears as a fusiform dilatation of the common duct.

Choledochal cysts present water echogenicity/ density/intensity in sonography, CT, or MR. In CT and MR, coronal or reformatted imaging shows better the shape and nature of the biliary anomaly.

Direct cholangiography is anyway the best method for detailed anatomy of the biliary tract, often showing aberrant entry of the common bile duct into the side of the pancreatic duct.

7.3
Inflammatory Lesions

7.3.1
Abscess

Abscesses can be defined as intrahepatic single or multiple collections and they are classified, based on the etiology, as pyogenic, amebic, or fungal (MERGO and ROS 1997). Clinical symptoms of abscesses are related to the coexistence of sepsis and the presence of one or more space-occupying lesions (MORTELÉ and ROS 2001; MURPHY et al. 1989).

Pyogenic hepatic abscesses, actually not very common, are related to five principal mechanism of diffusion:

- Biliary: ascending cholangitis due to neoplastic or lithiatic biliary obstruction; retrograde bacterial diffusion from bowel in post-surgical patients
- Portal: pylephlebitis from appendicitis or other inflammatory pathologies of bowel (Crohn, Meckel, or colonic diverticula) or pancreas
- Arterial: septicemia from other systemic infections (i.e. bacterial endocarditis)
- Direct extension from adjacent organs (i.e. perforated ulcer, sub-phrenic abscess)
- Traumatic: due to penetrating lesions

Pyogenic abscesses are most commonly caused by *Clostridium* species and gram-negative bacteria, such as *Escherichia coli* and *Bacteroides* species (MERGO and ROS 1997). Ascending cholangitis and portal phlebitis are the most frequent causes of pyogenic hepatic abscesses (MORTELÉ and ROS 2001; MURPHY et al. 1989). The abscesses related to the portal mechanism are usually single, while those related to biliary mechanism are typically multiple and localized in both lobes.

The sonographic pattern of pyogenic abscesses is correlated with its evolution. In the initial phase it may appear as a hypoechoic area with irregular and ill-defined borders, without specific characteristics. In this phase color-Doppler may demonstrate an hypervascularization of the surrounding liver parenchyma. The colliquative phase presents as an anechoic area with hyperechoic spots in suspension, with irregular borders; increased posterior acoustic transmission and lateral acoustic shadows may be present. The appearance may vary from anechoic, to hyperechoic, depending on the concentration of the necrotic content. The resolution phase is characterized by a progressive reduction of the liquid component; the lesion will tend to reduce in size becoming hypo-hyperechoic (RALLS et al. 1987).

The overall appearance of a hepatic abscess at cross-sectional imaging varies according to the pathologic stage of the infection (MERGO and ROS 1997). Abscesses have a unilocular cystic appearance in subacute stages, in which necrosis and liquefaction predominate (MERGO and ROS 1997). In more acute stages, abscesses frequently manifest as a cluster of small low-attenuation or high-signal-intensity lesions, which represent different locations of contamination (MORTELÉ and ROS 2001; MURPHY et al. 1989). This coalescent, grouped appearance is especially suggestive of pyogenic infection (cluster sign) (MORTELÉ and ROS 2001; MURPHY et al. 1989). At CT the pyogenic abscess appears as an irregularly round, inhomogeneously hypodense area, with density values ranging from 0 to 50 HU, usually higher than simple cysts. In most cases, the lesion is well demarcated with a thick wall, sometimes with a papillary aspect. After contrast media administration, the lesion presents a characteristic rim-enhancement. In general, the presence of microbubbles within a lesion, although uncommon, is diagnostic of a gas-forming organism if there is no history of instrumentation or rupture into a hollow viscus. Air is easily recognizable at CT by measuring the Hounsfield units (range −1000 to −100 HU) (Fig. 7.8).

On MR imaging, pyogenic abscesses appear as thick-walled lesions, with homogeneous usually low signal intensity on T1-weighted MR images, and homogeneous high signal intensity on T2-weighted MR images (MERGO and ROS 1997; MENDEZ et al. 1994). On enhanced images, MR imaging typically shows increased peripheral rim enhancement, which is secondary to increased capillary permeability in the surrounding liver parenchyma ("double target sign") (MORTELÉ and ROS 2001; MENDEZ et al. 1994; MURPHY et al. 1989). Perilesion edema is seen on T2-weighted MR images in 50% of abscesses, although it may also be seen in 20%–30% of patients with primary or secondary hepatic malignancies (MENDEZ et al. 1994). Therefore, the presence of perilesion

edema can be used to differentiate a hepatic abscess from a benign cystic hepatic lesion (MENDEZ et al. 1994).

An amebic abscess results from infection with the protozoan *Entamoeba histolytica* and is the most commonly encountered hepatic abscess on a worldwide basis (MERGO and ROS 1997).

The sonographic pattern of amebic abscesses is also correlated with its evolution. In the pre-suppurative phase the sonographic examination is negative; indirect signs such as edematous acute pancreatitis or non-lithiatic cholecystitis may be present in 50% of cases. From the fourth or fifth day, a homogeneous hypoechoic area with ill-defined borders may be seen. The suppurative phase is characterized initially by necrosis, appearing as homogeneous hypoechoic areas with regular borders, and in a second phase by liquefaction, appearing as an anechoic area with ill-defined borders (Fig. 7.9a) (RALLS et al. 1987).

The CT appearance of the amebic abscess is nonspecific, characterized by a homogeneous hypodense, round or oval, lesion with a slightly hyperdense border, which enhances after contrast media injection, remaining hypodense nevertheless in relation to the surrounding liver parenchyma. The abscess is usually located in peripheral liver and appears frequently as a multiloculated lesion (Fig. 7.9b) (RADIN et al. 1988).

The MR appearance is related to the size of the lesion; usually it appears hypointense in T1-weighted images and markedly hyperintense in T2-weighted images, with a thick pseudocapsule without significant enhancement after contrast media administration. In amebic granulomatous hepatitis, multiple

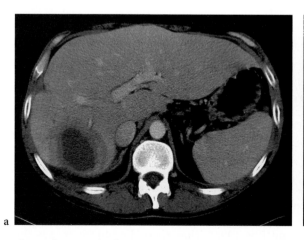
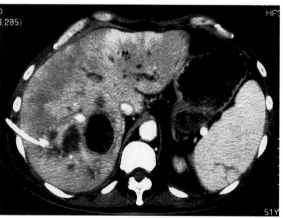

a   b

Fig. 7.8a,b. Pyogenic abscess. **a** Pyogenic abscess in a 35-year old man status post laparoscopic right hepatectomy due to an hydatid cyst. Portal venous-phase contrast-enhanced CT scan shows a thick-walled cystic lesion with homogeneous low attenuation. **b** Pyogenic abscess with presence of gas within the lesion in a 52-year-old man with fever, head of pancreas neoplasia (not resectable due to superior mesenteric vein infiltration) and recent portal thrombosis. An axial portal phase CT scan shows an hypoattenuating lesion with non-homogeneous content and gas inside

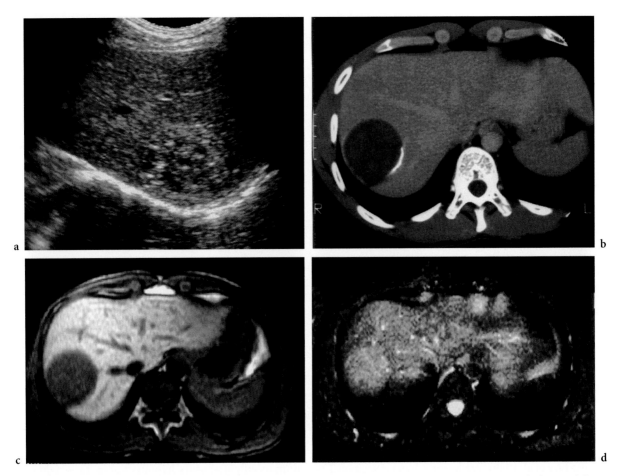

Fig. 7.9a–d. Amebic abscess in a 40-year-old man, with abdominal pain. **a** Sonographic longitudinal scan on right hepatic lobe shows an hypoechoic, heterogeneous lesion with ill-defined margins. **b** Axial nonenhanced CT image shows a round, homogeneously hypodense lesion with partially calcified wall. **c** GE T1-weighted MR image shows a round homogeneously hypointense lesion. **d** TSE STIR T2-weighted MR image shows the same lesion as isointense to the surrounding liver parenchyma

lesions appear hyperintense in T2-weighted images, showing the characteristic double perilesional rim (internal hyperintense, external hypointense) (Fig. 7.9c, d) (Giovagnoni et al. 1993).

Fungal abscesses are most often caused by *Candida albicans* (Mergo and Ros 1997).

The sonographic appearance in the initial phase is pathognomonic: the "wheel inside wheel sign" consists of a hypoechoic area (edema) which surrounds a hyperechoic area (inflammatory cells), and a central hypoechoic necrotic area (Ralls et al. 1987). The CT and MR appearance of fungal abscesses are similar to those of pyogenic ones; therefore, only a sample of the lesion enables definition of the pathogen.

In immunodepressed patients multiple small hypoechoic lesions less than 1 cm in diameter may be spread throughout the liver. The liquid component is not present in these cases and only parenchymal

phlogosis is detectable. These lesions are visible only in contrast-enhanced CT as hypodense lesions.

7.3.2
Intrahepatic Hydatid Cyst

Hepatic echinococcosis is an endemic disease in the Mediterranean basin and other sheep-raising countries (Mergo and Ros 1997). Humans become infected by ingestion of eggs of the tapeworm Echinococcus granulosus, either by eating contaminated food or from contact with dogs (Mergo and Ros 1997). The ingested embryos invade the intestinal mucosal wall and proceed to the liver by entering the portal venous system (Mergo and Ros 1997). Although the liver filters most of these embryos, those that are not destroyed then become hepatic hydatid cysts (MERGO and ROS 1997). The more frequent location of hydatid cysts is the liver (70%), followed by lung (20%) and other parenchymas, as spleen, kidney, heart, brain, and muscle. At biochemical analysis, there is usually eosinophilia, and a serologic test is positive in 25% of patients (MORTELÉ and ROS 2001; MURPHY et al. 1989). At histopathological analysis, a hydatid cyst is composed of three layers: the outer pericyst, which corresponds to compressed liver tissue; the endocyst, an inner germinal layer; and the ectocyst, a translucent thin interleaved membrane (MERGO and ROS 1997). Maturation of a cyst is characterized by the development of daughter cysts in the periphery as a result of endocyst invagination (MERGO and ROS 1997). Peripheral calcifications are not uncommon in viable or nonviable cysts (MERGO and ROS 1997).

The sonographic appearance of hydatid cysts is correlated with its evolution and six classes may be identified: type 1: simple cyst; type 2: septate cyst; type 3: cyst with membrane detachment; type 4: cyst with mixed echo structure; type 5: heterogeneous cyst; type 6: calcified cyst. Type 1 appears as a single, round, anechoic lesion, with regular borders, indistinguishable from a dysplastic cyst. The diagnosis of hydatid cyst may be considered when focal thickening of the wall is present or when fine hyperechoic spots, due to the hydatid sand, appear in the dependent areas. The type 2 is a multilocular lesion, due to the development of daughter cysts in the periphery, which present the same characteristics as the primary cysts, even though with thinner walls. The type 3 cyst is related to the detachment of the germinating membrane. Type 4 presents a mixed, solid and cystic, echo structure. Type 5 is characterized by inconstant echo structure, with progressive reduction of the liquid component, with thickening of the wall, that becomes hyperechoic. Type 6 presents as a hyperechoic lesion with strong shadowing (Fig. 7.10b).

At CT, a hydatid cyst usually appears as a well-defined hypoattenuating lesion with a distinguishable wall (Fig. 7.10a) (DE DIEGO CHOLIZ et al. 1982). Coarse calcifications of the wall are present in 50% of cases, and daughter cysts are identified in approximately 75% of patients (MORTELÉ and ROS 2001; DE DIEGO CHOLIZ et al. 1982; MURPHY et al. 1989). MR imaging clearly demonstrates the pericyst, the matrix, and daughter cysts (Fig. 7.10c) (MARANI et al. 1990). The pericyst is seen as a hypointense rim on both T1- and T2-weighted images because of its fibrous composition and the presence of calcifica-

tions (MERGO and ROS 1997; MARANI et al. 1990). The hydatid matrix (hydatid "sand") appears hypointense on T1-weighted images and markedly hyperintense on T2-weighted images; when present, daughter cysts are more hypointense than the matrix on T2-weighted images (MARANI et al. 1990). After contrast media administration, no enhancement is seen either in CT or MR.

7.4
Neoplasms

7.4.1
Biliary Cystadenoma and Cystadenocarcinoma

Biliary cystadenoma and cystadenocarcinoma are considered two aspects of the same pathology, having the former malignant potential and the latter real malignant characteristics. Biliary cystadenomas are rare, usually slow growing, multilocular cystic tumors and represent less than 5% of intrahepatic cystic masses of biliary origin (BUETOW and MIDKIFF 1997; MORTELÉ and ROS 2001; MURPHY et al. 1989; PALACIOS et al. 1990; VILGRAIN et al. 2000). They are generally intrahepatic (85%), even though some extrahepatic lesions have been reported (PALACIOS et al. 1990). Among intrahepatic cystadenomas, 55% occur in the right lobe, 29% in the left lobe, and 16% in both lobes (LUNDSTEDT et al. 1992). Biliary cystadenomas range in diameter from 1.5 to 35 cm. A total of 90% of cystadenocarcinomas occur in middle-aged women (mean age 38 years) (BUETOW and MIDKIFF 1997). Symptoms are usually related to the mass effect of the lesion and consist of intermittent pain or biliary obstruction (MORTELÉ and ROS 2001; MURPHY et al. 1989). At microscopy, a single layer of mucin-secreting cells lines the cyst wall. Proteinaceous, mucinous, and occasionally gelatinous, purulent, or hemorrhagic fluid may be present inside the tumor (BUETOW and MIDKIFF 1997; PALACIOS et al. 1990).

At sonography, cystadenocarcinoma appears as a cyst-like multilocular, hypoechoic lesion, with internal septa and small nodules at the level of the cystic wall.

At CT, a biliary cystadenoma appears as a solitary cystic mass (5–25 HU) with a well-defined thick fibrous capsule, mural nodules, internal septa, and rarely capsular calcification (BUETOW and MIDKIFF 1997; PALACIOS et al. 1990). Polypoid, pedunculated excrescences are seen more commonly in biliary

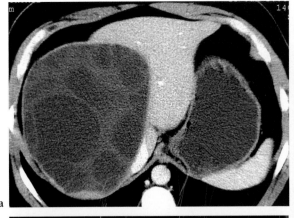

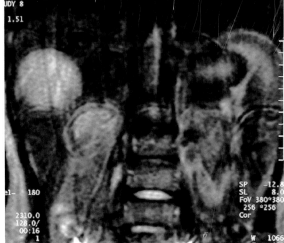

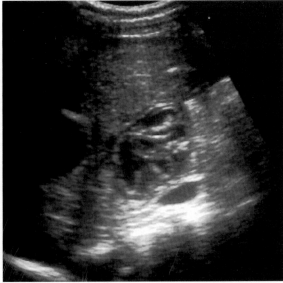

Fig. 7.10a-c. Intrahepatic hydatid cyst. **a** Portal venous-phase contrast-enhanced CT scan shows well defined, hypoattenuating cystic lesion in the right lobe of the liver. Multiple daughter cyst are noted within the cystic lesions. **b** Sonographic longitudinal scan on the right hepatic lobe shows a multilocular septate lesion, due to the development of daughter cysts, with thickened walls and increased acoustic signal behind. **c** Coronal T2-weighted MR image shows an heterogeneous round lesion for the presence of hypointense curvilinear rim due to the fibrotic tissue of the pericyst and hyperintense material inside due to the hydatid "sand"

cystadenocarcinoma than in cystadenoma, although papillary areas and polypoid projections have been reported in cystadenomas without frank malignancy (KOROBKIN et al. 1989). After contrast media administration, septa, mural nodules, and pedunculated excrescences show enhancement (Fig. 7.11) (KOROBKIN et al. 1989).

The MR imaging characteristics of an uncomplicated biliary cystadenoma correlate well with the pathologic features: the appearance of the content is typical for a fluid-containing multilocular mass, with homogeneous low signal intensity on T1-weighted images and homogeneous high signal intensity on T2-weighted images (BUETOW and MIDKIFF 1997; PALACIOS et al. 1990). Variable signal intensities on both T1- and T2-weighted images depend on the presence of solid components, hemorrhage, and protein content (BUETOW and MIDKIFF 1997; PALACIOS et al. 1990).

7.4.2
Cystic Subtypes of Primary Liver Neoplasms

Cystic subtypes of primary liver neoplasms are rare and are usually related to internal necrosis due to disproportionate growth or systemic and loco-regional treatment. The two most common primary neoplasms of the liver, that rarely manifest as an entirely or partially cystic mass, are hepatocellular carcinoma and giant cavernous hemangioma.

Whenever a predominant cystic lesion, with well-defined intrinsic tumor characteristics of hepatocellular carcinoma, such as hypervascularity of the solid parts, a capsule, and vascular or biliary invasion, is detected in a cirrhotic liver, the diagnosis of hepatocellular carcinoma should be considered (MORTELÉ and ROS 2001; MURPHY et al. 1989). In fact, in about 70% of patients with hepatocellular carcinoma, CT or MR imaging demonstrate signs

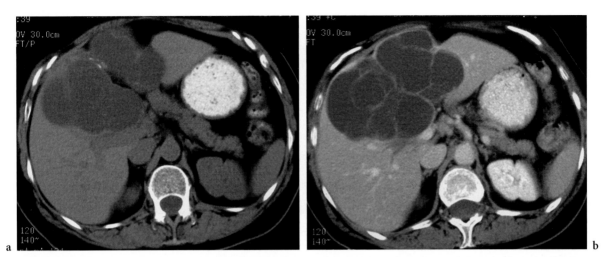

Fig. 7.11a,b. Biliary cystadenoma **a** Nonenhanced axial CT shows a lobulated hypoattenuating lesion with some parietal calcifications. **b** Portal venous phase CT shows a multiseptate cystic lesion. Intralesional septa are better seen after contrast administration

or complications of underlying liver cirrhosis, such as hypertrophy of the left hepatic lobe and caudate lobe, regeneration nodules, splenomegaly, and recanalization of the umbilical vein (KOROBKIN et al. 1989).

Central cystic degeneration in giant cavernous hemangioma may occur whenever the lesion outgrows its blood supply (CASILLAS et al. 2000). At CT and MR imaging, a central nonenhancing area is demonstrated within the lesion (VILGRAIN et al. 2000). Since hemangioma has a characteristic peripheral nodular enhancement pattern at both contrast-enhanced CT and contrast-enhanced MR imaging, even lesions with extensive central necrosis are easily diagnosed correctly with both imaging modalities (SEMELKA and SOFKA 1997).

7.4.3
Cystic Metastases

Metastases to the liver are common, and a variety of often nonspecific appearances have been reported (LEWIS and CHEZMAR 1997). The majority of hepatic metastases are solid, but some have a complete or partially cystic appearance (LEWIS and CHEZMAR 1997). The cyst-like appearance of hepatic metastases may be related to two different pathologic mechanisms. First, hypervascular metastatic tumors with rapid growth may lead to necrosis and cystic degeneration. This mechanism is frequently demonstrated in metastases from neuro-

endocrine tumors, sarcoma, melanoma, and certain subtypes of lung and breast carcinoma (LEWIS and CHEZMAR 1997). Second, mucinous adenocarcinomas, such as colorectal or ovarian carcinoma, may present cystic metastases (SUGAWARA et al. 2000). Moreover, ovarian metastases commonly spread by means of peritoneal seeding rather than hematogenously, appearing on cross-sectional images as cystic serosal implants on both the visceral peritoneal surface of the liver and the parietal peritoneum of the diaphragm (LUNDSTEDT et al. 1992). At ultrasound, these metastases appear as anechoic nodules; the elements which help in the differential diagnosis between a simple cyst and a cystic metastases are the presence of a thick wall, mural nodules, irregular border, or a plurianular aspect (peripheral hypoechoic rim, echogenic intermediate rim, and central anechoic area). Contrast-enhanced CT and MR imaging typically demonstrate multiple lesions with strong enhancement of the peripheral viable and irregularly defined tissue (Figs. 7.12, 7.13) (LEWIS and CHEZMAR 1997).

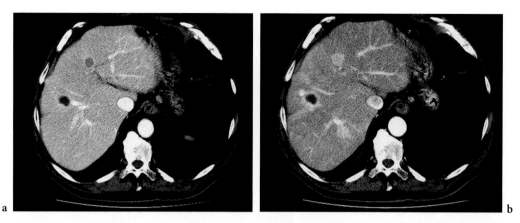

Fig. 7.12a,b. Cystic metastases from colon cancer. A 70-year-old man with colon cancer. **a** Portal venous-phase contrast-enhanced CT scan shows a cyst-like, hypoattenuating lesion, without peripheral enhancement. **b** The arterial phase CT image alone shows a peripheral rim-enhancement, typical of a metastatic lesion. The rapid growth of these metastases leads to cystic degeneration

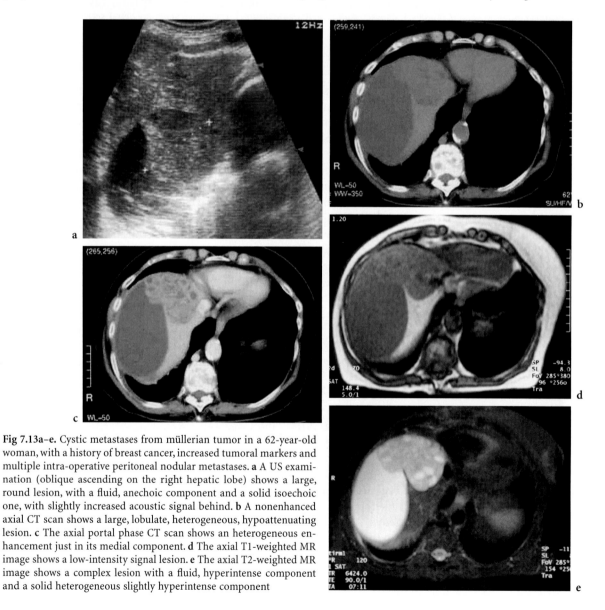

Fig 7.13a–e. Cystic metastases from müllerian tumor in a 62-year-old woman, with a history of breast cancer, increased tumoral markers and multiple intra-operative peritoneal nodular metastases. **a** A US examination (oblique ascending on the right hepatic lobe) shows a large, round lesion, with a fluid, anechoic component and a solid isoechoic one, with slightly increased acoustic signal behind. **b** A nonenhanced axial CT scan shows a large, lobulate, heterogeneous, hypoattenuating lesion. **c** The axial portal phase CT scan shows an heterogeneous enhancement just in its medial component. **d** The axial T1-weighted MR image shows a low-intensity signal lesion. **e** The axial T2-weighted MR image shows a complex lesion with a fluid, hyperintense component and a solid heterogeneous slightly hyperintense component

7.5
Miscellaneous lesions

7.5.1
Hematoma

Hepatic hematoma is a lesion characterized by bleeding inside the liver parenchyma, under the capsule, with or without free rupture. Surgery and trauma are the two most common causes of hepatic bleeding. Hemorrhage within a solid liver neoplasm, especially a hepatocellular adenoma, is a third well-known mechanism by which intra- or perihepatic hematoma can be induced (CASILLAS et al. 2000). Symptomatic manifestations depend on the severity of the bleeding, the location, and the time frame during which the hemorrhage occurred.

The sonographic appearance of hematoma is extremely variable, depending on the time elapsed from the bleeding. In the initial phase (12–24 h) hematoma is hyperechoic; then it becomes hypo-anechoic with ill-defined borders. At CT, the appearance of an intrahepatic hemorrhage depends on the cause of the bleeding and the lag time between the traumatic event and the imaging procedure. In an acute or subacute setting, hemorrhage shows a higher attenuation value than pure fluid due to the presence of aggregated fibrin components (MERRINE et al. 1988). The hematoma is usually better seen in enhanced than non-enhanced CT, since the difference in density increases after contrast media administration due to the lack of enhancement of the hematoma (when active bleeding is not present). In chronic cases, a hematoma has

attenuation identical to that of pure fluid. Frequently, the cause of the hemorrhage can be detected at CT. In post-traumatic cases, coexistent features such as hepatic lacerations, rib fractures, or perihepatic fluid will be present. In hemorrhage induced by surgery, the location of the hematoma is usually along the surgical plane. Because of the paramagnetic effect of methemoglobin, MR imaging is even more suitable than CT for detection and characterization of hemorrhage. A subacute hematoma appears as a heterogeneous mass with pathognomonic high signal intensity on T1-weighted images and intermediate signal intensity on T2-weighted images (BALCI et al. 1999).

7.5.2
Biloma

Bilomas result from rupture of the biliary system, which can be spontaneous, traumatic, or iatrogenic following surgery or interventional procedures (MORTELÉ and ROS 2001; MURPHY et al. 1989). Bilomas can be intrahepatic or perihepatic. Extravasation of bile into the liver parenchyma generates an intense inflammatory reaction, thereby inducing formation of a well-defined pseudocapsule. Clinical manifestations depend on the location and size of the biloma (MORTELÉ and ROS 2001; MURPHY et al. 1989).

At sonography, a biloma appears as a juxtahepatic anechoic collection, sometimes with fine echoes inside (Fig. 7.14a). At both CT and MR imaging, a biloma usually appears as a well-defined or slightly irregular cystic mass without septa or calcifications

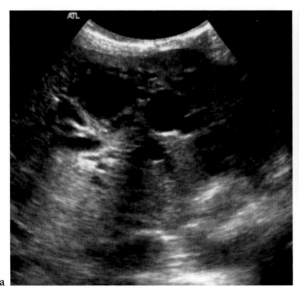

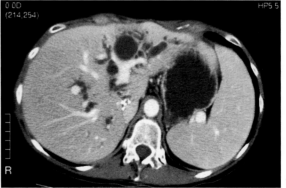

Fig. 7.14a,b. Biloma in a 37-year-old woman with chronic stenosis of the main hepatic artery, fever. **a** Sonographic axial image on the left hepatic lobe shows two anechoic round lesions communicating with the dilated biliary tree. **b** Axial contrast-enhanced CT image shows two hypodense well-defined round lesions, communicating with the biliary tree

(Mortelé and Ros 2001; Murphy et al. 1989). Also, the pseudocapsule is usually not readily identifiable (Fig. 7.14b) (Mortelé and Ros 2001; Murphy et al. 1989). This imaging appearance, in combination with the clinical history and location, should enable correct diagnosis.

References

Balci NC, Semelka RC, Noone TC, et al (1999) Acute and subacute liver-related hemorrhage: MRI findings. Magn Reson Imaging 17:207–211

Buetow PC, Midkiff RB (1997) Primary malignant neoplasms in the adult. Magn Reson Imaging Clin N Am 5:289–318

Casillas VJ, Amendola MA, Gascue A, et al (2000) Imaging of nontraumatic hemorrhagic hepatic lesions. Radiographics 20:367–378

Choi BI, Yeon KM, Kim SH, et al (1990) Caroli's disease: central dot sign in CT. Radiology 174:161–163

De Diego Choliz J, Lecumberri FJ, Francquet T, et al (1982) Computed tomography in hepatic echinococcosis. AJR Am J Roentgenol 13:699–702

Eisenberg D, Hurwitz L, Yu AC (1986) CT and sonography of multiple bile duct hamartomas simulating malignant liver disease (case report). AJR Am J Roentgenol 147:279–280

Gallego JC, Suarez I, Soler R (1995) Multiple bile duct hamartomas: US, CT and MR findings. A case report. Acta Radiol 36:273–275

Giovagnoni A, Gabrielli O, Coppa GV et al (1993) MRI appearance in amoebic granulomatous hepatitis: a case report. Pediatr Radiol 23:536–537

Kim OH, Chung HJ, Choi BG (1995) Imaging of the choledochal cyst. Radiographics 15:69–89

Korobkin MT, Stephens DH, Lee JKT et al (1989) Biliary cystadenoma and cystadenocarcinoma: CT and sonographic findings. AJR Am J Roentgenol 153:507–511

Levi AD, Rohrmann CA Jr, Murakata LA, et al (2002) Caroli's disease: radiologic spectrum with pathologic correlation. AJR Am J Roentgenol 179:1053–1057

Lewis KH, Chezmar JL (1997) Hepatic metastases. Magn Reson Imaging Clin N Am 5:319–330

Lucaya J, Gomez JL, Molino C, et al (1978) Congenital dilatation of the intrahepatic bile ducts (Caroli's disease). Radiology 127:746–778

Lundstedt C, Holmin T, Thorvinger B (1992) Peritoneal ovarian metastases simulating liver parenchymal masses. Gastrointest Radiol 17:250-252

Luo TY, Itai Y, Eguchi N, et al (1998) Von Meyenburg complexes of the liver: imaging findings. J Comput Assist tomogr 22:372–378

Maher MM, Dervan P, Keogh B, et al (1999) Bile duct hamartomas (von Meyenburg complexes): value of MR imaging in diagnosis. Abdom Imaging 24:171–173

Marani SA, Canossi GC, Nicoli FA, et al (1990) Hydatid disease: MR imaging study. Radiology 175:701–706

Marchal GJ, Desmet VJ, Proesmans WC, et al (1986) Caroli disease: high-frequency US and pathologic findings. Radiology 158:507–511

Martinoli C, Cittadini GJr, Rollandi GA, et al (1992) Case report:

imaging of bile duct hamartomas. Clin Radiol 45:203–205

Mathieu D, Vilgrain V, Mahfouz A, et al (1997) Benign liver tumors. Magn Reson Imaging Clin N Am 5:255-288

Mendez RJ, Schiebler ML, Outwater EK, et al (1994) Hepatic abscesses: MR imaging findings. Radiology 190:431–436

Mergo PJ, Ros PR (1997) MR imaging of inflammatory disease of the liver. Magn Reson Imaging Clin N Am 5:367–376

Mergo PJ, Ros PR (1998) Benign lesions of the liver. Radiol Clin North Am 36:319–331

Merrine D, Fishman EK, Zerhouni EA (1988) Spontaneous hepatic hemorrhage: clinical and CT findings. J Comput Assist Tomogr 12:397–400

Mortelé K, Ros PR (2001) Cystic focal liver lesions in the adult: differential CT and MR Imaging features. Radiographics 21:895–910

Mortelé B, Mortelé K, Seynaeve P et al (2002) Hepatic bile duct hamartomas (von Meyenburg complexes): MR and MR colangiography findings. J Comput Assist Tomogr 26:438–443

Murphy BJ, Casillas J, Ros PR, et al (1989) The CT appearance of cystic masses of the liver. Radiographics 9:307–322

Palacios E, Shannon M, Solomon C, et al (1990) Biliary cystadenoma: ultrasound, CT, and MRI. Gastrointest Radiol 15:313–316

Pavone P, Laghi A, Catalano C, et al (1996) Caroli's disease: evaluation with MR cholangiopancreatography (MRCP). Abdom Imaging 21:117–119

Radin RD, Ralls PW, Colletti PM, et al (1988) CT of amebic liver abscesses. AJR Am J Roentgenol 150:1297–1301

Ralls PW, Barnes PF, Radin DR, et al (1987) Sonographic features of amebic and pyogenic abscesses: a blinded comparison. AJR Am J Roentgenol 149:499–501

Salo J, Bru C, Vitella A, et al (1992) Bile duct hamartomas presenting as multiple focal lesions on hepatic ultrasonography. Am J Gastroenterol 2:221-223

Semelka RC, Sofka CM (1997). Hepatic hemangiomas. Magn Reson Imaging Clin N Am 5:241–253

Semelka RC, Hussain SM, Marcos HB, et al (1999) Biliary hamartomas: solitary and multiple lesions shown on current MR techniques including gadolinium enhancement. J Magn Reson Imaging 10:196–201

Singh Y, Winick AB, Tabbara SO (1997) Multiloculated cystic liver lesions: radiologic-pathologic differential diagnosis. Radiographics 17:219–224

Slone HW, Bennett WF, Bova JG (1993) MR findings of multiple biliary hamartomas. AJR Am J Roentgenol 161:581–583

Sugawara Y, Yamamoto J, Yamasaki S, et al (2000) Cystic liver metastases from colorectal cancer. J Surg Oncol 74:148–152

van Sonnenberg E, Wroblicka JT, D'Agostino HB, et al (1994) Symptomatic hepatic cysts: percutaneous drainage and sclerosis. Radiology 190:387–392

Vilgrain V, Boulos L, Vullierme MP, et al (2000) Imaging of atypical hemangiomas of the liver with pathologic correlation. Radiographics 20:379–397

Wei SC, Huang GT, Chen CH, et al (1997) Bile duct hamartomas: a report of two cases. J Clin Gastroenterol 25:608–611

Wohlgemuth WA, Böttger J, Bohndorf K (1998) MRI, CT, US and ERCP in the evaluation of bile duct hamartomas (von Meyenburg complex): a case report. Eur Radiol 8:1623–1626

Zangger P, Grossholz M, Mentha G, et al (1995) MRI findings in Caroli's disease and intrahepatic pigmented calculi. Abdom Imaging 20:361–364

8 Liver Hemangioma

Valérie Vilgrain and Giuseppe Brancatelli

CONTENTS

V. Vilgrain, MD
Department of Radiology, Hospital Beaujon, Avenue Du
General Leclerc 100, 92118 Clichy, France
G. Brancatelli, MD
Department of Radiology, Policlinico Universitario, Via del
Vespro 127, 90127 Palermo, Italy

8.1
Introduction

Hemangioma is the most common benign hepatic tumor. The prevalence of hemangioma in the general population ranges from 1%–2% to 20% (Semelka and Sofka 1997). The female-to-male ratio varies from 2:1 to 5:1. They occur at all ages. The vast majority of hemangiomas remain clinically silent. Few patients are symptomatic due to a mass lesion, complications or compression of adjacent structures. Most of these symptoms are observed in large hemangiomas. The natural history of hemangiomas is variable: most of them remain stable, some may grow or involute. The role of sex hormones in causing enlargement during pregnancy or recurrence is disputed.

Hemangiomas are usually solitary, less than 5 cm in size and appear as well-delineated lesions of red color that partially collapse on sectioning. A few are pedunculated. Giant hemangiomas (often defined as 10 cm or larger) are heterogeneous and show varying degrees of fibrosis and calcification. Some hemangiomas may become entirely fibrous.

Microscopically, hemangiomas are composed of blood-filled spaces of variable size and shape and are lined by a single layer of flat endothelium. The septa between the spaces are often incomplete. Blood vessels and arteriovenous shunting may be seen in large septa (Craig et al. 1988).

8.2
Sonography

The classic sonographic appearance of hemangioma is that of an echogenic mass of uniform-density, less than 3 cm in diameter with acoustic enhancement and sharp margins (Fig. 8.1). A hypoechoic center may be present. Typically hemangiomas do not have a hypoechoic halo (Bree et al. 1987). Liver hemangiomas may present an atypical pattern on sonography, usually if larger than 3 cm, appearing hypo- or isoechoic.

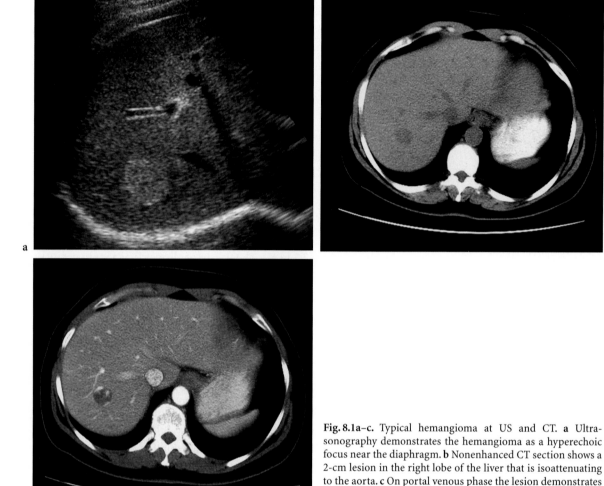

Fig. 8.1a–c. Typical hemangioma at US and CT. **a** Ultrasonography demonstrates the hemangioma as a hyperechoic focus near the diaphragm. **b** Nonenhanced CT section shows a 2-cm lesion in the right lobe of the liver that is isoattenuating to the aorta. **c** On portal venous phase the lesion demonstrates centripetal enhancement that is isoattenuating to the hepatic vessels

On color Doppler no vascular pattern is identified because intralesional flows are too slow to be revealed but few peripheral flow signals may be seen (Tano et al. 1997).

Power Doppler is more sensitive in revealing venous flows within hemangiomas. Recent papers have highlighted the potential of contrast enhanced harmonic ultrasound (US) to characterize liver lesions. In hemangiomas, the absence of intratumoral vessels in the arterial phase and peripheral nodular enhancement in the portal phase are the most typical patterns and were observed in 76% and 88%, respectively (Fig. 8.2) (Isozaki et al. 2003). The sensitivity, specificity, and accuracy of diagnosis based on this combination of enhancement pattern were 88%, 99%, and 98% (Isozaki et al. 2003). Peripheral globular enhancement in the portal phase and isoechoic pattern on late phase are also observed in most atypical hemangiomas larger than 3 cm (Quaia et al. 2002).

8.3
Computed Tomography

Strict criteria for the diagnosis of hemangioma were described before the most recent technical advances in computed tomography (CT). These criteria were:
- Low attenuation on non-contrast CT
- Peripheral enhancement of the lesion followed by a central enhancement on contrast CT
- Contrast enhancement of the lesion on delayed scans (Freeny and Marks 1986)

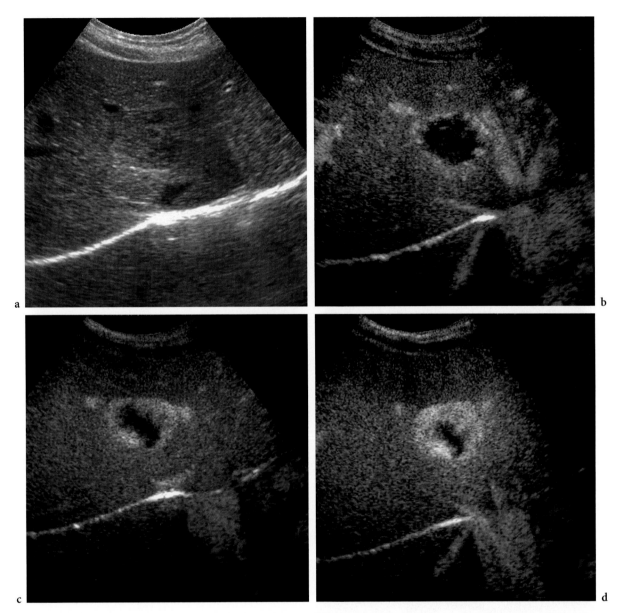

Fig. 8.2a–d. Typical hemangioma at contrast enhanced US. **a** Oblique ascending right subcostal baseline image in a 63-year-old man shows a hypo-isoechoic lesion in the right liver. **b** On the oblique ascending right subcostal image obtained in the arterial phase (25 s after SonoVue injection), the lesion shows peripheral globular enhancement. **c,d** In the portal-venous and delayed phases (60 s and 120 s after SonoVue injection, respectively) a progressive but incomplete centripetal fill-in is depicted. (Courtesy of Bartolotta)

These criteria have been updated with the helical CT technique and the multiphasic examination. Three-phase helical CT is the most suitable technique. Presence of peripheral puddles at arterial phase has a sensitivity of 67%, a specificity of 99%, and a positive predictive value of 86% for hemangioma (Nino-Murcia et al. 2000).

In a series of 100 focal liver lesions, the only false positive case (lesion with peripheral puddles) was a melanoma metastasis (Nino-Murcia et al. 2000).

With triphasic spiral CT, results are even better for characterization of liver hemangioma. In a series of 375 liver lesions, 86% (51/59) of the hemangiomas had peripheral nodular enhancement of vascular attenuation on arterial and portal phase imaging and were hyperattenuating with possible central hypoattenuation or isoattenuation to vascular space in the equilibrium phase (van Leeuwen et al. 1996). In this series, there were no false-positive cases. Conversely 13.6% of the hemangiomas were atypical: hypoattenuating on all phases or hypoattenuating on both arterial and portal venous phases and hyperattenuating in the equilibrium phase, which probably correspond to fibrosed hemangiomas (VAN LEEUWEN et al. 1996).

One of the hallmarks of liver hemangiomas is the isoattenuation with the arterial system (Fig. 8.1) (VAN LEEUWEN et al. 1996). Among the hemangiomas, those which are the most difficult to characterize are lesions smaller than 3 cm, because they may not demonstrate nodular enhancement but often enhance homogeneously during the hepatic arterial or portal venous phase (Fig. 8.3) (KIM et al. 2001a). KIM et al. (2001a) has compared small hepatic hemangiomas with hypervascular malignant tumors and has shown that at arterial phase CT, enhancement similar to aortic enhancement was observed in 19%–32% of hemangiomas and 0%–2% of malignant tumors;

globular enhancement in 62%–68% and 4%–12%, respectively. At portal venous phase, enhancement similar to blood pool enhancement was observed in 43%–54% hemangiomas and 4%–14% of malignant tumors; globular enhancement in 46%–49% and 0%–2%, respectively (KIM et al. 2001a). So, small hemangiomas frequently show atypical appearances at CT resulting in a decrease in sensitivity compared to larger hemangiomas but specificity remains high.

8.4
Magnetic Resonance

Two major papers published in 1985 in the radiologic literature have underlined the potential impor-

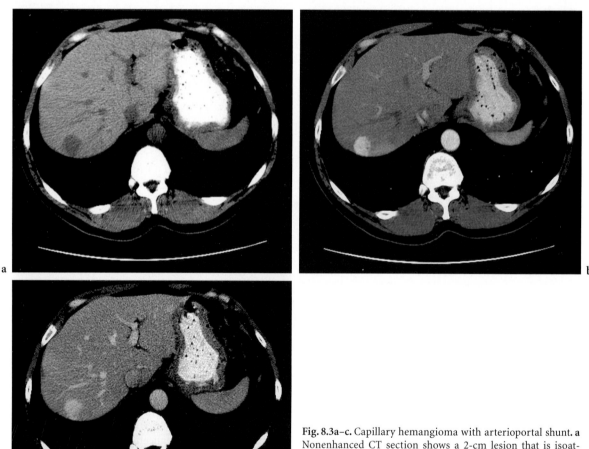

Fig. 8.3a–c. Capillary hemangioma with arterioportal shunt. **a** Nonenhanced CT section shows a 2-cm lesion that is isoattenuating to the aorta in the right liver. **b** On hepatic arterial phase image the lesion demonstrates bright uniform enhancement almost isodense with the aorta. Note the wedge-shaped homogeneous hyperattenuating area adjacent to the tumor, due to an arterioportal shunt. **c** Portal venous phase image shows that the hemangioma remains isodense to the aorta and hepatic veins. The arterioportal shunt is no longer seen

tance of magnetic resonance (MR) imaging in the characterization of liver hemangiomas (ITAI et al. 1985; STARK et al. 1985). These papers have shown that:

- Most hemangiomas have a homogeneous appearance and smooth, well defined margins (STARK et al. 1985).
- Hemangiomas have a significantly greater contrast-to-noise ratio than cancer, especially on long T2-weighted sequences (STARK et al. 1985).
- MR imaging detects more hemangiomas than any other technique (STARK et al. 1985).
- MR allows detection of almost all hemangiomas over 1 cm in diameter with 90% sensitivity, 92% specificity, and an overall accuracy of 90% (ITAI et al. 1985; STARK et al. 1985).

Both reports and an editor's note emphasized the role of T2-weighted sequences and suggested that MR imaging may become the procedure of choice for distinguishing liver hemangiomas from liver cancer.

Many other papers were published afterwards discussing the role of low vs high field strengths, conventional spin-echo (SE) T2-weighted imaging vs fast imaging techniques, fast SE imaging with and without fat suppression and serial gadolinium-enhanced gradient echo (GE) images (SOYER et al. 1997).

The routine MR protocol for characterizing liver lesions includes a gradient echo (GE) T1-weighted sequence, a fast spin-echo (FSE) T2-weighted sequence preferably with fat suppression technique (because it increases the contrast to noise ratio of liver hemangiomas) and gadolinium-enhanced triphasic dynamic GE images (which may be acquired in 2D or in 3D). The classical appearance of liver hemangiomas is that of hypointense lesion on T1-weighted sequences and strongly hyperintense lesion on heavily T2-weighted sequences with a "light bulb" pattern (Fig. 8.4). This strong hypersignal on T2 is due to long T2 values (greater than 88 ms). Numerous articles have attempted to determine a cut-off T2 value allowing discrimination between hemangiomas and malignant tumors. However, in most of the centers, the lesion characterization is obtained with qualitative assessment and rarely with quantitative measures (McFARLAND et al. 1994). More recently, other sequences have been used to facilitate rapid and reliable distinction between hemangiomas and other lesions. Single-shot fast spin echo sequences are a half-Fourier technique that enable acquisition of heavily T2-weighted images within a few seconds

per slice and are helpful for differentiation between liver lesions. By using a short TE (90 ms) and a long TE (600–700 ms) they may also differentiate hemangiomas from cysts (KIRYU et al. 2002). True fast imaging with steady state free precession is an ultrafast gradient echo sequence with a balanced structure that compensates first-order phase shifts produced by flow. Echo and repetition times are short. Image contrast is related to the T2*/T1 ratio. Comparison between this sequence and HASTE sequence has shown that distinction between hemangiomas and liver malignancies was more often correct with the balanced sequence (NUMMINEN et al. 2003).

Today, gadolinium chelate administration with dynamic serial postcontrast MR imaging is performed in all cases and is an analogous technique to multiphasic contrast-enhanced CT. Hemangiomas have the following features:

- Peripheral hyperintense nodules with a non-intact ring immediately after contrast administration
- Progressive centripetal enhancement that is most intense at 90 s
- Undulating nodular contour of the inner ring margin
- Persistent homogeneous enhancement without heterogeneous or peripheral washout (SEMELKA et al. 1994)

Most of the medium (1.5–5 cm), and large hemangiomas (>5 cm) had initial peripheral nodular enhancement whereas uniform enhancement was observed in 35 of 81 small lesions in Semelka's paper (SEMELKA et al. 1994).

Interestingly, the rapid enhancing hemangiomas tend to be hypoechoic on sonography whereas lesions that are slow-enhancing tend to be hyperechoic (YU et al. 1998). Rapid-enhancing hemangiomas may mimic other lesions at the arterial phase such as hepatocellular tumors or hypervascular metastases (Fig. 8.5). However, most of them show hyperintense complete fill-in in the equilibrium phase and very high signal intensity with T2-weighted sequences (KATO et al. 2001). Therefore, combination of T2-weighted images with serial dynamic postgadolinium MR sequences is a reliable imaging modality for the diagnosis of hemangiomas.

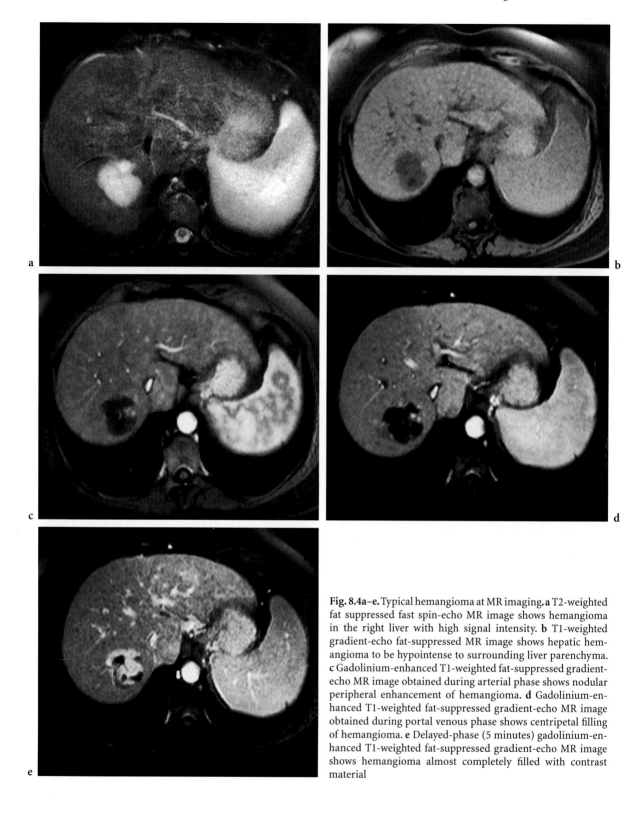

Fig. 8.4a–e. Typical hemangioma at MR imaging. **a** T2-weighted fat suppressed fast spin-echo MR image shows hemangioma in the right liver with high signal intensity. **b** T1-weighted gradient-echo fat-suppressed MR image shows hepatic hemangioma to be hypointense to surrounding liver parenchyma. **c** Gadolinium-enhanced T1-weighted fat-suppressed gradient-echo MR image obtained during arterial phase shows nodular peripheral enhancement of hemangioma. **d** Gadolinium-enhanced T1-weighted fat-suppressed gradient-echo MR image obtained during portal venous phase shows centripetal filling of hemangioma. **e** Delayed-phase (5 minutes) gadolinium-enhanced T1-weighted fat-suppressed gradient-echo MR image shows hemangioma almost completely filled with contrast material

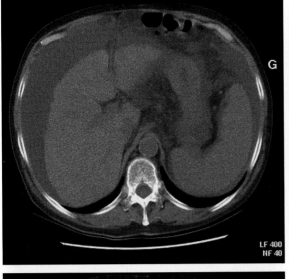

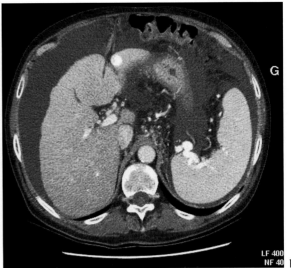

a

b

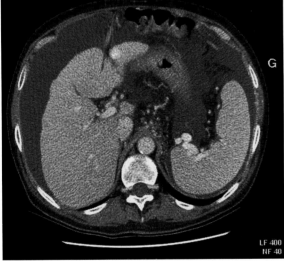

c

Fig. 8.5a–c. Capillary flash-filling hemangioma in a cirrhotic liver. **a** Nonenhanced transverse CT. The hemangioma is sub-capsular and isoattenuating to blood. **b** Hepatic arterial phase image at the same level. The hemangioma enhances homogeneously and equally compared with splenic artery. **c** On portal venous phase the lesion remains isoattenuating to vessels, a finding that confirm blood-pool characteristics for the lesion. The lack of contrast material washout in the portal venous phase allows differentiation of capillary hemangioma from hepatocellular carcinoma in this cirrhotic liver

8.5
Scintigraphy

[99m]Tc-pertechnetate-labeled red blood cell scintigraphy is a relatively specific examination for identifying hemangiomas. Using this method, there is a decreased activity on early dynamic images and increased activity on delayed blood pool images. Comparison between ^{99m}Tc-pertechnetate-labeled red blood cell single-photon emission CT (SPECT) and MR imaging has shown that MR had a higher sensitivity and specificity than SPECT, especially for lesions less than 2 cm in diameter (BIRNBAUM et al. 1990).

8.6
Percutaneous Biopsy

Liver hemangioma has been considered a contraindication to needle biopsy for many years because of the high risk of hemorrhage. Recently, several series of percutaneous biopsy in liver hemangiomas have been reported and the contraindications should be reconsidered. No serious complications were observed in two large series: one in 47 biopsy specimens obtained using a core-needle biopsy and one in 114 patients having fine-needle aspiration biopsy (HEILO and STENWIG 1997; CALDIRONI et al. 1998). In the latter, two minor accidents were observed due to profuse bleeding of giant hemangioma and resolved with medical care. However, as in other tumors, a cuff of normal hepatic parenchyma should be interposed between the capsule and the margin of hemangioma. Indications of percutaneous biopsy should be restricted to atypical cases despite a combination of imaging modalities. Sensitivity and overall accuracy are reported in more than 90% (CALDIRONI et al. 1998; NAKAIZUMI et al. 1990).

Interestingly, both core-needle biopsy and fine-needle aspiration biopsy are useful in diagnosing liver hemangioma.

8.7
Atypical Patterns

8.7.1
Hemangioma with Echoic Border

An atypical but suggestive appearance of hemangiomas at US is the following: the lesion has an echoic border, which is seen as a thick echoic rind or a thin echoic rim (MOODY and WILSON 1993). Unlike typical hemangiomas, this type of hemangioma has an internal echo pattern that is at least partially hypoechoic. The central low echogenicity is assumed to correspond to previous hemorrhagic necrosis, scarring, or myxomatous changes. Although, the real percentage is unknown, some authors have reported that 40% of all hemangiomas could have this atypia (MOODY and WILSON 1993).

8.7.2
Large, Heterogeneous Hemangioma

Large hemangiomas are often heterogeneous (YAMASHITA et al. 1994). They are termed giant hemangiomas when they exceed 4 cm in diameter (NELSON and CHEZMAR 1990; VALLS et al. 1996). However, some authors define giant hemangiomas as lesions greater than 6 cm or 12 cm in diameter (CHOI et al. 1989; DANET et al. 2003). Large hemangiomas may be responsible for liver enlargement and abdominal discomfort.

At US, large hemangiomas often appear heterogeneous. On non-enhanced CT scans, lesions appear hypoattenuating and heterogeneous with marked central areas of low attenuation. After intravenous administration of contrast material, the typical early, peripheral, globular enhancement is observed. However, during the venous and delayed phases, the progressive centripetal enhancement of the lesion,

although present, does not lead to complete filling (Fig. 8.6). At MR imaging, T1-weighted sequences show a sharply marginated, hypointense mass with a cleft-like area of lower intensity and sometimes with hypointense internal septa. T2-weighted images show a markedly hyperintense cleft-like area and some hypointense internal septa within a hyperintense mass. The enhancement is equivalent to that seen at CT, with incomplete filling of the lesion; the cleft-like area remains hypointense, as do the internal septa (Fig. 8.7) (CHOI et al. 1989). The MR imaging findings of giant hemangiomas are closely correlated with the macroscopic appearance, which demonstrates changes such as hemorrhage, thrombosis, extensive hyalinization, liquefaction, and fibrosis. The central cleft-like area may be due to cystic degeneration, liquefaction or myxoid tissue (CHOI et al. 1989; DANET et al. 2003).

Modifications of internal components such as thrombosis and hemorrhage may induce compression of biliary and vascular structures (COUMBARAS et al. 2002).

8.7.3
Rapidly Filling Hemangioma

Rapidly filling hemangiomas are not very frequent (16% of all hemangiomas). However, rapid filling seems to occur significantly more often in small hemangiomas (42% of hemangiomas <1 cm in diameter) (Figs. 8.3, 8.5) (HANAFUSA et al. 1995).

CT and MR imaging show a particular enhancement pattern: immediate homogeneous enhancement at arterial-phase CT or contrast-enhancement T1-weighted MR imaging (Figs. 8.3, 8.5) (SEMELKA and SOFKA 1997). This feature makes differentiation from other hypervascular tumors difficult. T2-weighted images may be helpful, but hypervascular tumors such as islet cell metastases are also hyperintense on such images. Accurate diagnosis is made with delayed-phase CT or MR imaging because hemangiomas remain hyperattenuating or hyperintense, whereas hypervascular metastases do not (Figs. 8.3, 8.5). Another important finding in diagnosis of hemangioma is attenuation equivalent to that of the aorta during all phases of CT (Figs. 8.3, 8.5) (QUINN and BENJAMIN 1992). At Doppler US, unusual arterial flow may be present.

Because histopathologic confirmation is usually not performed, the mechanism of the enhancement is not clearly understood; however, the difference in enhancement patterns may be due to a difference in the size of the blood spaces. It is likely that the smaller

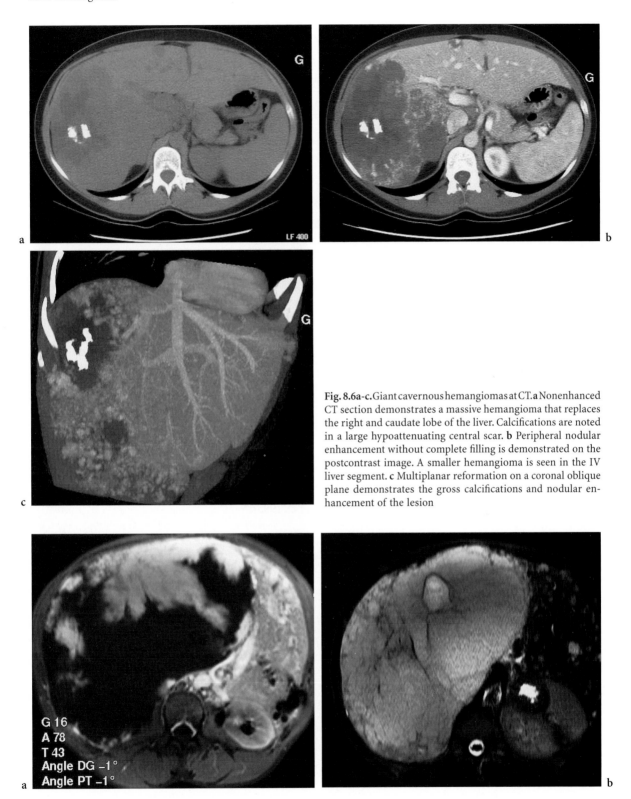

Fig. 8.6a-c. Giant cavernous hemangiomas at CT. **a** Nonenhanced CT section demonstrates a massive hemangioma that replaces the right and caudate lobe of the liver. Calcifications are noted in a large hypoattenuating central scar. **b** Peripheral nodular enhancement without complete filling is demonstrated on the postcontrast image. A smaller hemangioma is seen in the IV liver segment. **c** Multiplanar reformation on a coronal oblique plane demonstrates the gross calcifications and nodular enhancement of the lesion

Fig. 8.7a,b. Giant cavernous hemangiomas at MR. **a** Fat-suppressed T1-weighted gradient-echo MR image shows a giant cavernous hemangioma replacing the right liver with nodular, centripetal, cloud-like enhancement. **b** T2-weighted fat suppressed fast spin-echo MR image shows hemangioma to be of high signal intensity to normal liver. The central hyperintense area corresponds to a central scar. Multiple hypointense linear elements corresponding to internal fibrotic septa are noted within the lesion. Numerous other hyperintense lesions, corresponding to smaller hemangiomas, are seen in the left lobe of the liver

the lesion, the more rapid is the spread of contrast material within it (HANAFUSA et al. 1995). This theory could explain the high proportion of small hemangiomas with rapid and complete filling.

8.7.4
Very Slow Filling Hemangioma

They appear as hypoattenuating lesions on multiphasic examination or they have tiny enhancing dots that do not progress to the classic globular enhancement (Fig. 8.8). Their incidence is estimated at between 8%–16% of cases. They are problematic in patients with malignancy (JANG et al. 2003).

8.7.5
Calcified Hemangioma

Although hemangiomas in the soft tissue, gastrointestinal tract, retroperitoneum, and mediastinum may show calcifications (phleboliths, which are pathognomonic for the tumor), hepatic hemangiomas rarely demonstrate calcifications (DARLAK et al. 1990; SCATARIGE et al. 1983). Calcified hemangiomas are mostly found incidentally.

Calcifications may occur in the marginal or central portion of the lesion (MITSUDO et al. 1995). A particular pattern consists of multiple spotty calcifications, which correspond to phleboliths. However, large, organized calcifications are also possible. Some calcified hemangiomas may demonstrate poor enhancement, especially at CT (MITSUDO et al. 1995).

The finding of a nonenhancing hepatic tumor with calcifications should not preclude the diagnosis of hemangioma. High signal intensity in non-calcified areas of the lesion on T2-weighted MR images can help in diagnosis.

8.7.6
Hyalinized Hemangioma

Hyalinized hepatic hemangiomas are rare (CHENG et al. 1995; TUNG et al. 1994). Some authors have suggested that hyalinized hemangiomas represent an end stage of hemangioma involution. Such hemangiomas do not demonstrate any particular symptoms.

Hyalinization of a hemangioma changes its radiological features, thus making diagnosis before biopsy virtually impossible. Hyalinized hemangiomas show only slight high signal intensity on T2-weighted MR images (CHENG et al. 1995). Moreover, there is lack of early enhancement on dynamic contrast-enhanced images. Slight peripheral enhancement may occur in the late phase (CHENG et al. 1995). MR imaging does not allow differentiation of hyalinized hemangiomas from malignant hepatic tumors.

Pathologic examination reveals extensive fibrous tissue and obliteration of vascular channels (CHENG et al. 1995).

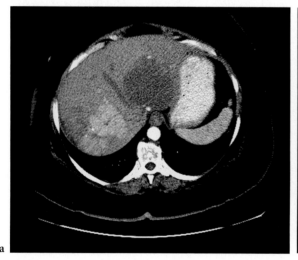
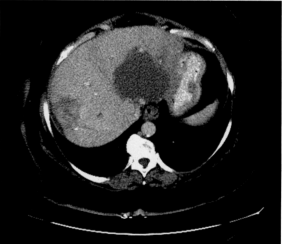

a   b

Fig. 8.8a,b. Hemangioma associated with focal nodular hyperplasia. **a** Hepatic arterial-phase image shows two focal nodular hyperplasia lesions with strong and homogeneous hyperattenuation in comparison to adjacent liver parenchyma. A central scar is noted in the largest lesion. Hemangioma shows nodular peripheral enhancement. **b** On portal venous-phase image the focal nodular hyperplasia lesions are isoattenuating to liver, while hemangioma shows progressive nodular, centripetal enhancement that is unusually slow

8.7.7
Cystic or Multilocular Hemangioma

Cavernous hemangiomas with a large central cavity that contains fluid are very rare. To our knowledge, only one hemangioma with a multilocular cystic component has been reported in the literature (HIHARA et al. 1990). This entity does not demonstrate any particular symptoms.

Definite diagnosis of such hemangiomas with imaging is difficult. This atypia may be due to cystic degeneration caused by central thrombosis and hemorrhage.

8.7.8
Hemangioma with Fluid–Fluid Level

Fluid–fluid levels within hemangiomas are very rare. To our knowledge, only three articles on this entity have been published (AZENCOT et al. 1993; ITAI et al. 1987; SOYER et al. 1998). The patient may present with abdominal pain.

US shows a hyperechoic or hypoechoic pattern. The fluid–fluid level is not seen at US (AZENCOT et al. 1993; SOYER et al. 1998). CT and especially MR imaging easily demonstrate this feature (ITAI et al. 1987).

8.7.9
Pedunculated Hemangioma

Pedunculated hemangiomas are very rare. To our knowledge, only two cases have been reported in the literature (ELLIS et al. 1985; TRAN-MINH et al. 1991). They can be asymptomatic or complicated by subacute torsion and infarction.

At US, the origin of the lesion may be difficult to recognize. The lesion can be attached to the liver by a thin pedicle, which is nearly undetectable at imaging. Multiplanar reconstruction of CT scans and coronal or sagittal MR imaging can be helpful. At CT and MR imaging, the diagnosis is made by demonstrating the typical enhancement pattern and the typical signal intensities on both T1- and T2-weighted images.

Complicated pedunculated hemangiomas must be resected.

8.7.10
Hemangioma with Arterial-Portal Venous Shunt

Arterial-portal venous shunts are mainly associated with hepatic malignancy but can also be seen in benign liver masses, in particular hemangiomas (WINOGRAD and PALUBINSKAS 1977; SHIMADA et al. 1994). This entity is usually asymptomatic.

An arterial-portal venous shunt can be detected with helical CT or dynamic contrast-enhanced MR imaging. The findings consist of early parenchymal enhancement associated with early filling of the portal vein (HANAFUSA et al. 1995). Arterio-portal shunts are found in 25% of hemangiomas. They are not related to the lesion size but they are more frequently seen in hemangiomas with rapid enhancement (Fig. 8.3) (KIM et al. 2001b).

8.7.11
Hemangioma with Capsular Retraction

Capsular retraction is usually associated with malignant tumors such as cholangiocarcinoma, epithelioid hemangioendothelioma, or metastases. This finding is very rare in benign liver tumors and has been described in very few hemangiomas (Fig. 8.9) (YANG et al. 2001).

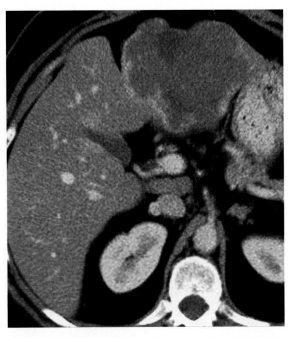

Fig. 8.9. Hemangioma with capsular retraction. Portal-phase CT demonstrates a large mass in the left lobe of the liver with a central hypoattenuating scar and associated capsular retraction

8.8
Hemangioma Developing in Abnormal Liver

8.8.1
Hemangioma in Fatty Liver

Diffuse fatty infiltration of the liver is a common finding and may change the typical appearances of lesions, making them more difficult to characterize at imaging.

At US, a hemangioma may appear slightly hyperechoic, isoechoic, or hypoechoic relative to a fatty liver (MARSH et al. 1989). Posterior acoustic enhancement is usually observed. At non-enhanced CT, the lesion may be hyperattenuating relative to the liver or may not seen (Fig. 8.10). Contrast-enhanced CT shows peripheral enhancement and delayed filling, an appearance similar to that of a hemangioma in a normal liver (FREENY and MARKS 1986). However, at arterial-phase imaging, the hemangioma may be iso-attenuating relative to the liver. MR imaging is more helpful than CT and allows reliable detection and differentiation of hemangiomas from other hepatic masses (Fig. 8.11) (STARK et al. 1985). Hemangiomas may also be accompanied by a focal spared zone as seen in malignant tumors in fatty liver (JANG et al. 2003).

8.8.2
Hemangioma in Liver Cirrhosis

With progressive cirrhosis, hemangiomas are likely to decrease in size and become more fibrotic and difficult to diagnose radiologically (BRANCATELLI et al. 2001).

8.9
Association with Other Lesions

8.9.1
Multiple Hemangiomas

Hemangiomas are multiple in 10% of cases (ISHAK and RABIN 1975). Multiple hemangiomas generally consist of a few scattered lesions (YAMASHITA et al. 1994). They often have typical imaging features.

8.9.2
Hemangiomatosis

Hemangiomas, even giant ones, are usually well defined (VALLS et al. 1996). In rare cases, the lesion may be large and ill defined, replacing almost the whole hepatic parenchyma. This entity is seen more often

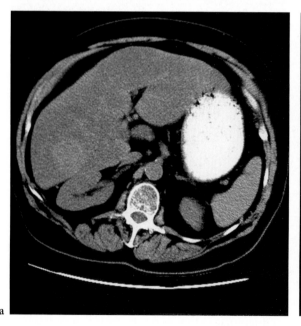
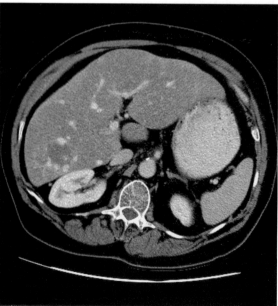

a   b

Fig. 8.10a,b. Hemangioma in a fatty liver at CT. **a** Nonenhanced CT scan shows a hyperattenuating lesion in a hypoattenuating fatty liver parenchyma. **b** Portal-phase CT scan shows nodular centripetal enhancement of the lesion

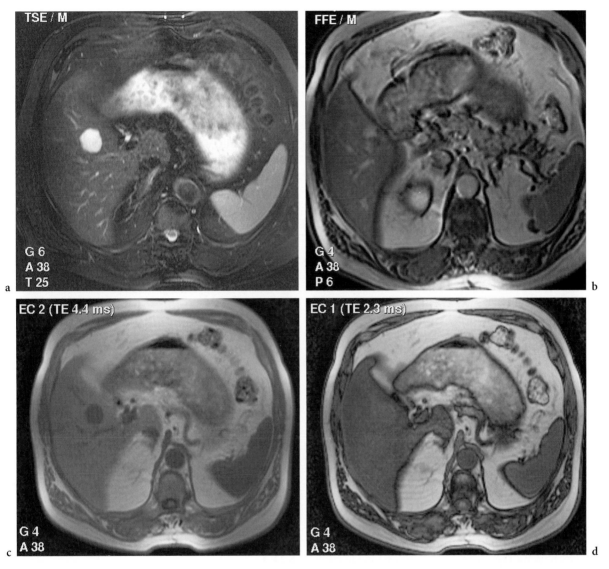

Fig. 8.11a–d. Hemangioma in fatty liver at MR imaging. **a** T2-weighted fat suppressed fast spin-echo MR image shows hemangioma with signal intensity almost as strong as that of the cerebrospinal fluid. **b** Gadolinium-enhanced T1-weighted gradient-echo MR image obtained during portal venous phase shows nodular peripheral enhancement of hemangioma. **c** Axial T1-weighted in-phase gradient echo image shows normal intermediate to high signal intensity liver in comparison to spleen. The hemangioma is seen as hypointense to surrounding liver. **d** Corresponding axial T1-weighted opposed-phase gradient echo image shows loss of signal intensity of the liver compared with the spleen, representing hepatic steatosis. Hemangioma is hyperintense to liver

in infants than in adults and may be associated with cardiac failure and high mortality. In adults, hemangiomatosis can be asymptomatic.

8.9.3
Focal Nodular Hyperplasia

Association of hepatic hemangioma and focal nodular hyperplasia is quite frequent (23% of cases) and

not fortuitous (Fig. 8.8) (MATHIEU et al. 1989). It has also been suggested that the association is more frequent in cases of multiple focal nodular hyperplasia (33%) (VILGRAIN et al. 2003). Focal nodular hyperplasia is considered to be a hyperplastic response due to focal increased arterial flow in the hepatic parenchyma and, like hemangioma, is thought to have a vascular origin.

When the tumors have typical imaging features, the diagnosis can be made with confidence.

8.9.4
Angiosarcoma

To our knowledge, there is only one report of malignant transformation of a hepatic hemangioma in the literature (BERTRAND et al. 1980). Another report described a cavernous hemangioma surrounded by angiosarcoma, and the authors raised the hypothesis of malignant transformation of a hemangioma (TOHME et al. 1991).

8.10
Atypical Evolution

Most hemangiomas remain stable in size or demonstrate minimal increase in diameter over time (NGHIEM et al. 1997; TAKAYASU et al. 1990). Very few observations of significant enlargement of a hemangioma have been reported (SCHWARTZ and HUSSER 1987; NGHIEM et al. 1997; TAKAYASU et al. 1990). They include cases of enlargement during pregnancy and during estrogen use.
Enlarged hemangiomas can be asymptomatic or may manifest as an abdominal mass or pain. The US, CT, and MR imaging features are identical to those of typical hemangiomas.

The mechanism of enlargement is believed to be vascular ectasia (FOUCHARD et al. 1994). A role for estrogen in hemangioma enlargement is suspected but has never been proved (SCHWARTZ and HUSSER 1987; FOUCHARD et al. 1994). Despite the growth of the lesion, if imaging features are characteristic of hemangioma, the diagnosis can still be made confidently with imaging.

8.11
Complications

The overall complication rate varies from 4.5% to 19.7% (FREENY et al. 1979). Complications are mostly observed in large hemangiomas and can be divided into alterations of internal architecture such as inflammation; coagulation, which could lead to systemic disorders; hemorrhage, which can cause hemoperitoneum, volvulus, and compression of adjacent structures.

8.11.1
Inflammatory Process

Some cases of inflammatory processes complicating giant hemangiomas have been reported (TAKAYASU et al. 1990). The prevalence is probably underestimated. Signs and symptoms of an inflammatory process include low-grade fever, weight loss, abdominal pain, accelerated erythrocyte sedimentation rate, anemia, thrombocytosis, and increased fibrinogen level.

The imaging features are those of giant hemangioma. Histological signs of inflammation may not be detected. A possible explanation is the release of immune mediators by hepatic endothelial cells lining the hemangioma. Clinical and laboratory abnormalities may disappear after surgical excision of the hemangioma.

8.11.2
Kasabach-Merritt Syndrome

Kasabach-Merritt syndrome is a rare complication of hepatic hemangiomas in adults. It is a coagulopathy consisting of intravascular coagulation, clotting, and fibrinolysis within the hemangioma (ABOUT et al. 1994). The initially localized coagulopathy may progress to secondary increased systemic fibrinolysis and thrombocytopenia, leading to a fatal outcome in 20%–30% of patients (MACEYKO and CAMISA 1991).

8.11.3
Intratumoral Hemorrhage

Intratumoral hemorrhage is rarely encountered in hepatic hemangiomas. It can occur spontaneously or after anticoagulation therapy. The symptoms consist of acute-onset vomiting and epigastric pain (GRAHAM et al. 1993).

The bleeding is suggested by intratumoral high attenuation on non-enhanced CT scans and high signal intensity on T1-weighted MR images. When the typical enhancement features of hemangioma are present in association with marked high signal intensity on T2-weighted MR images, the diagnosis can be made. If not, histopathological examination allows correct diagnosis.

8.11.4
Hemoperitoneum Due to Spontaneous Rupture of Hemangioma

Spontaneous rupture of a hemangioma is unusual. Clinical symptoms include acute abdominal pain.

Imaging procedures reveal hemoperitoneum. Intraperitoneal clotting may be seen adjacent to the bleeding hemangioma. MR imaging is very sensitive in detection of bleeding by showing high signal intensity on T1-weighted images. Angiography can be useful for diagnosis, and embolization can be performed, thus allowing planned hepatic resection (SOYER and LEVESQUE 1995).

8.12
Diagnostic Work Up

The diagnostic evaluation of hemangiomas varies with different clinical and imaging scenarios (NELSON and CHEZMAR 1990). Typical appearance of a hemangioma at US imaging does not require any work up in a patient with no malignancy or chronic liver disease. Conversely, in patients with atypical imaging or at high risk for developing hepatic malignancies, diagnostic confirmation is mandatory. Although overall accuracy of CT for diagnosing hemangioma is high, MR imaging is the recommended modality with both T2 and postgadolinium information. If the diagnosis remains inconclusive, then percutaneous biopsy is indicated.

In conclusion, radiologists have to face two problems in diagnosing liver hemangiomas. First, to differentiate typical hemangiomas from other liver lesions, especially liver malignancies. The impact is so important that we should keep in mind getting a 100% specificity for hemangiomas which implies that doubtful cases should not be considered as hemangiomas. False positive hemangiomas are much more dramatic than false negative cases. Second, to recognize atypical hemangiomas. Although atypical hemangiomas are rare, many radiologists will encounter atypical findings due to the high prevalence of hepatic hemangiomas. In some cases, such as large heterogeneous hemangiomas, calcified hemangiomas, pedunculated hemangiomas, or hemangiomas developing in diffuse fatty liver, a specific diagnosis can be established with imaging, especially MR imaging. However, in other atypical cases, the diagnosis will remain uncertain at imaging, and these cases will require histopathological examination.

References

About I, Capdeville J, Bernard P, et al (1994) Hémangiome hépatique géant non résécable et syndrome de Kasabach-Merritt. Rev Med Interne 15:846–850

Azencot M, Soyer P, Laissy J-P, et al (1993) Niveaux liquide-liquide dans des angiomes multiples du foie: aspect en IRM et en TDM. Rev Im Med 5:703–705

Bertrand L, Puyeo J, Pages A, et al (1980) Hémangiosarcome du foie secondaire à un angiome caverneux calcifié: mort en coagulopathie de consommation. Ann Gastroenterol Hepatol 16:19–27

Birnbaum BA, Weinreb JC, Megibow AJ (1990) Definitive diagnosis of hepatic hemangiomas: MR vs Tc-99m labeled red blood cell SPECT. Radiology 176:95–105

Brancatelli G, Federle MP, Blachar A, et al (2001) Hemangioma in the cirrhotic liver: diagnosis and natural history. Radiology 219:69–74

Bree RL, Schwab RE, Glazer GM, et al (1987) The varied appearances of hepatic cavernous hemangiomas with sonography, computed tomography, magnetic resonance imaging and scintigraphy. Radiographics 7:1153–1175

Caldironi MW, Mazzucco M, Aldinio MT, et al (1998) Echo-guided fine-needle biopsy for the diagnosis of hepatic angioma. A report on 114 cases. Minerva Chir 53:505–509

Cheng HC, Tsai SH, Chiang JH, et al (1995) Hyalinized liver hemangioma mimicking malignant tumor at MR imaging. AJR Am J Roentgenol 165:1016–1017

Choi BI, Han MC, Park JH, et al (1989) Giant cavernous hemangioma of the liver: CT and MR imaging in 10 cases. AJR Am J Roentgenol 152:1221–1226

Coumbaras M, Wendum D, Monnier-Cholley L, et al (2002) CT and MR imaging features of pathologically proven atypical giant hemangioma of the liver. AJR Am J Roentgenol 179:1457–1463

Craig JR, Peters RL, Edmondson HA (1988) Tumors of the liver and intrahepatic bile ducts. AFIP, Washington, pp 64–75

Danet IM, Semelka, RC, Braga L, et al (2003) Giant hemangioma of the liver: MR imaging characteristics in 24 patients. Magn Res Img 21:95–101

Darlak JJ, Moshowitz M, Kattan KR (1990) Calcifications in the liver. Radiol Clin North Am 18:209–219

Ellis JV, Salazar JE, Gavant ML (1985) Pedunculated hepatic hemangioma: an unusual cause for anteriorly displaced retroperitoneal fat. J Ultrasound Med 4:623–624

Fouchard I, Rosenau L, Calès P, et al (1994) Survenue d'hémangiomes hépatiques au cours de la grossesse. Gastroenterol Clin Biol 18:512–515

Freeny PC, Marks WM (1986) Hepatic hemangioma: dynamic bolus CT. AJR Am J Roentgenol 147:711–719

Freeny PC, Vimont TR, Barnett DC (1979) Cavernous hemangioma of the liver: ultrasonography, arteriography, and computed tomography. Radiology 132:143–148

Graham E, Cohen AW, Soulen M, et al (1993) Symptomatic liver hemangioma with intra-tumor hemorrhage treated by angiography and embolization during pregnancy. Obstet Gynecol 81:813–816

Hanafusa K, Ohashi I, Himeno Y, et al (1995) Hepatic hemangioma: findings with two-phase CT. Radiology 196:465–469

Heilo A, Stenwig AE (1997) Liver hemangioma: US-guided 18-Gauge core-needle biopsy. Radiology 204:719–722

Hihara T, Araki T, Katou K, et al (1990) Cystic cavernous hemangioma of the liver. Gastrointest Radiol 15:112–114

Ishak KG, Rabin L (1975) Benign tumors of the liver. Med Clin North Am 59:995–1013

Isozaki T, Numata K, Kiba T (2003) Differential diagnosis of hepatic tumors by using contrast enhancement patterns at US. Radiology 229:798–805

Itai Y, Ohtomo K, Furui S, et al (1985) Noninvasive diagnosis of small cavernous hemangioma of the liver: advantage of MRI. AJR Am J Roentgenol 145:1195–1199

Itai Y, Ohtomo K, Kokubo T, et al (1987) CT demonstration of fluid–fluid levels in nonenhancing hemangiomas of the liver. J Comput Assist Tomogr 11:763–765

Jang HJ, Kim TK, Lim HK, et al (2003) Hepatic hemangioma: atypical appearances on CT, MR imaging, and sonography. AJR Am J Roentgenol 180:135–141

Kato H, Kanematsu M, Matsuo M, et al (2001) Atypically enhancing hepatic cavernous hemangiomas: high-spatial-resolution gadolinium-enhanced triphasic dynamic gradient-recalled-echo imaging findings. Eur Radiol 11:2510–2515

Kim T, Federle MP, Baron RL, et al (2001a) Discrimination of small hepatic hemangiomas from hypervascular malignant tumors smaller than 3 cm with three-phase helical CT. Radiology 219:699–706

Kim KW, Kim TK, Han JK, et al (2001b) Hepatic hemangiomas with arterio-portal shunt: findings at two-phase CT. Radiology 219:707–711

Kiryu S, Okada Y, Ohtomo K (2002) Differentiation between hemangiomas and cysts of the liver with single-shot fast-spin echo image using short and long TE. Abdom Imaging 26:687–690

Maceyko RF, Camisa C (1991) Kasabach-Merritt syndrome. Pediatr Dermatol 8:113–136

Marsh JI, Gibney RG, Li DK (1989) Hepatic hemangioma in the presence of fatty infiltration: an atypical sonographic appearance. Gastrointest Radiol 14:262–264

Mathieu D, Zafrani ES, Anglade MC, et al (1989) Association of focal nodular hyperplasia and hepatic hemangioma. Gastroenterology 97:154–157

McFarland EG, Mayo-Smith WW, Saini S, et al (1994) Hepatic hemangiomas and malignant tumors: improved differentiation with heavily T2-weighted conventional spin-echo MR imaging. Radiology 193:43–47

Mitsudo K, Watanabe Y, Saga T, et al (1995) Nonenhanced hepatic cavernous hemangioma with multiple calcifications: CT and pathologic correlation. Abdom Imaging 20:459–461

Moody AR, Wilson SR (1993) Atypical hepatic hemangioma: a suggestive sonographic morphology. Radiology 188:413–417

Morley JE, Myers JB, Sack FS, et al (1974) Enlargement of cavernous haemangioma associated with exogenous administrations of oestrogens. S Afr Med J 48:695–697

Nakaizumi A, Iishi H, Yamamoto R (1990) Diagnosis of hepatic cavernous hemangioma by fine-needle aspiration biopsy under ultrasonic guidance. Gastrointest Radiol 15:39–42

Nelson RC, Chezmar JL (1990) Diagnostic approach to hepatic hemangiomas. Radiology 176:11–13

Nghiem HV, Bogost GA, Ryan JA, et al (1997) Cavernous hemangiomas of the liver: enlargement over time. AJR Am J Roentgenol 169:137–140

Nino-Murcia M, Olcott EW, Brooke Jeffrey R, et al (2000) Focal liver lesions: pattern-based classification scheme for enhancement arterial phase CT. Radiology 215:746–751

Numminen K, Halavaara J, Isoniemi H, et al (2003) Magnetic resonance imaging of the liver: true fast imaging with steady state free precession sequence facilitates rapid and reliable distinction between hepatic hemangiomas and liver malignancies. Abdom Imaging 27:571–576

Quaia E, Bertolotto M, Dalla Palma L (2002) Characterization of liver hemangiomas with pulse inversion harmonic imaging. Eur Radiol 12:537–544

Quinn SF, Benjamin GG (1992) Hepatic cavernous hemangiomas: simple diagnostic sign with dynamic bolus CT. Radiology 182:545–548

Scatarige JC, Fishman EK, Saksouk FA, et al (1983) Computed tomography of calcified liver masses. J Comput Assist Tomogr 7:83–89

Schwartz SI, Husser WC (1987) Cavernous hemangioma of the liver. A single institution report of 16 resections. Ann Surg 205:456–462

Semelka RC, Sofka CM (1997) Hepatic hemangiomas. Magn Reson Imaging Clin N Am 5:241–253

Semelka RC, Brown ED, Ascher SM, et al (1994) Hepatic hemangiomas: a multi-institutional study of appearance on T2-weighted and serial gadolinium-enhanced gradient-echo MR images. Radiology 192:401–406

Shimada M, Matsumata T, Ikeda Y, et al (1994) Multiple hepatic hemangiomas with significant arterioportal venous shunting. Cancer 73:304–307

Soyer P, Levesque M (1995) Haemoperitoneum due to spontaneous rupture of hepatic haemangiomatosis: treatment by superselective arterial embolization and partial hepatectomy. Australas Radiol 39:90–92

Soyer P, Dufresne AC, Somveille E, et al (1997) Hepatic cavernous hemangioma appearance on T2-weighted fast spin echo MR imaging with and without fat suppression. AJR Am J Roentgenol 168:461–465

Soyer P, Bluemke DA, Fishman EK, et al (1998) Fluid-fluid levels within focal hepatic lesions: imaging appearance and etiology. Abdom Imaging 23:161–165

Stark DD, Felder RC, Wittenberg J et al (1985) Magnetic resonance imaging of cavernous hemangioma of the liver: tissue-specific characterization. AJR Am J Roentgenol 145:213–222

Takayasu K, Makuuchi M, Takayama T (1990) Computed tomography of a rapidly growing hepatic hemangioma. J Comput Assist Tomogr 14:143–145

Tano S, Veno N, Tomiyama T, et al (1997) Possibility of differentiating small hyperechoic liver tumors using contrast enhanced colour Doppler ultrasonography: a preliminary study. Clin Radiol 52:41–45

Tohme C, Drouot E, Piard F, et al (1991) Hémangiome caverneux du foie associé à un angiosarcome: transformation maligne? Gastroenterol Clin Biol 15:83–86

Tran-Minh VA, Gindre T, Pracros J-P, et al (1991) Volvulus of a pedunculated hemangioma of the liver. AJR Am J Roentgenol 156:866–867

Tung GA, Vaccaro JP, Cronan JJ, et al (1994) Cavernous hemangioma of the liver: pathologic correlation with high-field MR imaging. AJR Am J Roentgenol 162:1113–1117

Valls C, Reñe M, Gil M, et al (1996) Giant cavernous hemangioma of the liver: atypical CT and MR findings. Eur Radiol 6:448–450

van Leeuwen MS, Noordzij J, Feldberg MAM, et al (1996) Focal liver lesions: characterization with triphasic spiral CT. Radiology 201:327–336

Vilgrain V, Uzan F, Brancatelli G, et al (2003) Prevalence of hepatic hemangioma in patients with focal nodular hyperplasia: MR imaging analysis. Radiology 229:75–79

Winograd J, Palubinskas J (1977) Arterial-portal venous shunting in cavernous hemangioma of the liver. Radiology 122:331–332

Yamashita Y, Hatanaka Y, Yamamoto H, et al (1994) Differential diagnosis of focal liver lesions: role of spin-echo and contrast-enhanced dynamic MR imaging. Radiology 193:59–65

Yang DM, Yvon MH, Kim HS, et al (2001) Capsular retraction in hepatic giant hemangioma: CT and MR features. Abdom Imaging 26:36–38

Yu JS, Kim MJ, Kim KW et al (1998) Hepatic cavernous hemangioma: sonographic patterns and speed of contrast enhancement on multiphase dynamic MR imaging. AJR Am J Roentgenol 171:1021–1025

9 Focal Nodular Hyperplasia

Antonella Filippone, Raffaella Basilico, Francesca Di Fabio, and Lorenzo Bonomo

CONTENTS

9.1
Introduction

Focal nodular hyperplasia (FNH) is the second most common benign hepatic tumor after hemangioma and has a prevalence that in different studies ranges from 1% to 3% (Karhunen 1986).

It can occur in both sexes but it is most frequently found in young and middle aged women during the third to fifth decade of life (Mathieu et al. 1997). Although a relationship between the use of oral contraceptives and FNH has never been proven, endogenous or exogenous estrogens play a role in the growth of the lesions by increasing the size of the nodule and inducing vascular change thanks to a trophic effect on FNH. Approximately 20% of the patients have multiple FNH lesions (Fig. 9.1) (Nguyen et al. 1999).

FNH is always asymptomatic, incidentally discovered during imaging studies performed for other reasons. When present, the clinical symptoms are due to the large diameter of the lesion which may expand the Glisson capsule and/or may compress adjacent structures (Fig. 9.2).

A. Filippone, MD; R. Basilico, MD; F. Di Fabio, MD
Department of Radiology, University G. d'Annunzio, Via dei Vestini, 66013 Chieti, Italy
L. Bonomo, MD
Department of Radiology, Imaging Sciences Department, Catholic University of Rome, Largo A. Gemelli, 00168 Rome, Italy

The absence of a malignant potential, the unlikely modifications of internal structure due to hemorrhage or necrosis and the reduction in size of these nodules, make it possible to conservatively manage FNH (Di Stasi et al. 1996). Only in symptomatic cases, surgical resection of the nodule can be considered.

9.2
Histopathological Findings

FNH is considered a hyperplastic response of the liver to a pre-existing arteriovenous malformation (Wanless et al. 1985). The arteries of FNH arise from the hepatic artery and the vein drains into the hepatic vein. Therefore, FNH does not contain portal vessels.

There are two types of FNH: typical (80%) and atypical (20%).

The gross appearance of typical FNH is characterized by lobulated contours and by nodules surrounded by radiating fibrous septa originating from a central scar that contains a large artery from which blood flows centrifugally to the periphery of the lesion. Histologically, the typical FNH is characterized by a proliferation of hepatocytes, Kupffer cells, bile ductules and blood vessels arranged in abnormal pattern.

Differently from typical FNH which is a lobulated, well-circumscribed solid, hypervascular mass, with a central scar and peripheral fibrous septa, atypical FNH is more heterogeneous and the central scar is always absent at gross appearance.

Both typical and atypical FNH contains hepatocytes and Kupffer cells; however, in atypical FNH there is only bile ductular proliferation with a lack of malformed vessels or nodular architecture that are always present in typical FNH. Wanless et al. (1989) and Nguyen et al. (1999) reported the pathologic features of a form of atypical FNH, called telangiectatic FNH. According to these authors, there are two differences between classic and telangiectatic FNH:

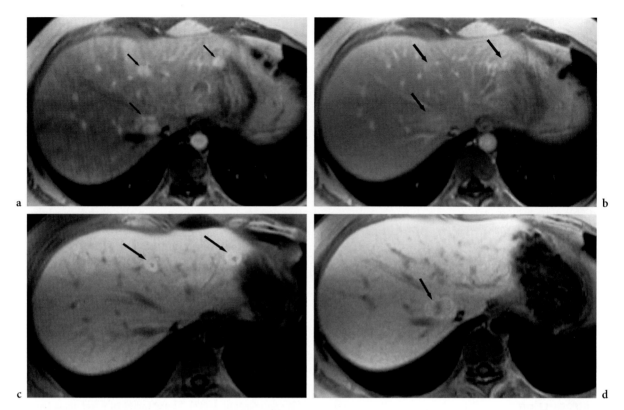

Fig. 9.1a–d. Multiple focal nodular hyperplasia. **a** Arterial phase image acquired after Gd-BOPTA bolus injection shows strong hypervascularization of all lesions (*arrows*) and a hypointense central scar in the biggest of them. **b** In the portal venous phase the lesions are slightly hyperintense. **c,d** T1-weighted images acquired during the hepatobiliary phase show enhancement of the liver lesions which appear slightly hyperintense with a clear evidence of hypointense central scar in all lesions

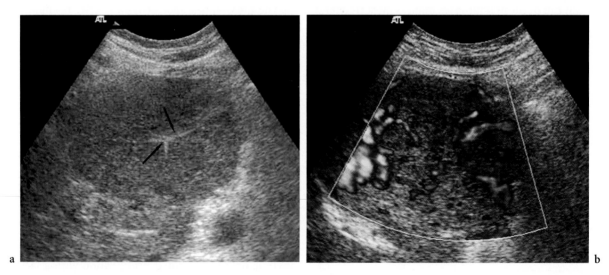

Fig. 9.2a–h. Chronic right upper abdominal pain in a 25 year-old woman. **a** Conventional transverse US scan through the lateral segment of the left hepatic lobe shows a 10-cm hypoechoic solid lesion. A subtle hyperechoic central scar is seen (arrows). **b** Power Doppler US scan shows the central stellate aspect of the scar. **c** Contrast-enhanced US scan with low MI pulse inversion and a second generation contrast agent: in the arterial phase the macrocirculation of the FNH is very well depicted. **d** The portal phase scan highlights the microcirculation of the lesion that enhances homogeneously apart from the central scan which is hypoechoic. **e** Non-enhanced CT scan shows a homogeneously hypodense lesion. **f** Enhanced dynamic CT scans reveal intense and homogeneous enhancement during the arterial phase.   ▷ ▷ ▷

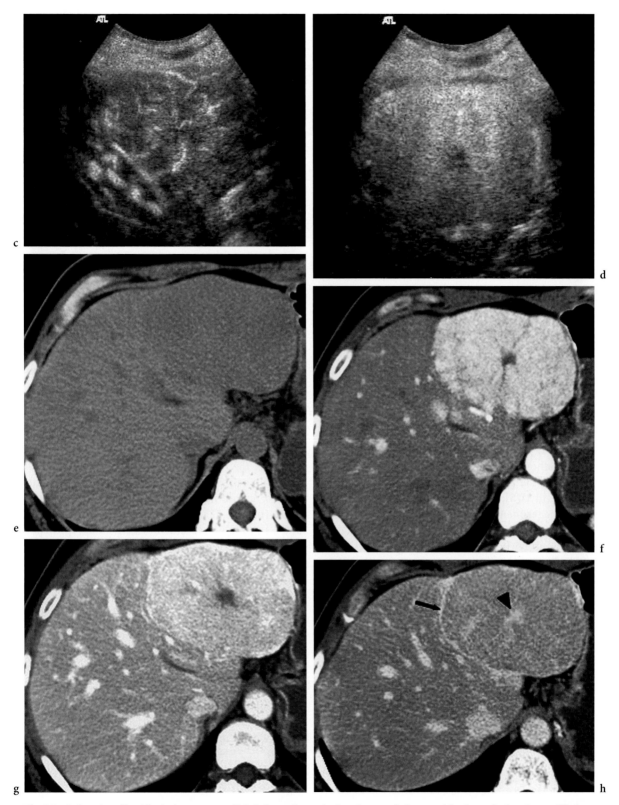

Fig. 9.2a–h *(continued).* **g** The lesion appears slightly hyperdense during the portal phase and isodense during the equilibrium phase (**h**). The central scar is typically hypodense on arterial and portal venous phases, whereas it appears hyperdense in the equilibrium phase (*arrowhead*). Nodule appears delimited by a thin hyperdense rim, detectable during the equilibrium phase (*arrow*), due to the compression of normal surrounding vascular structures

a) In telangiectatic FNH, arteries have hypertrophied muscular media but no intimal proliferation well documented in the classic form.

b) In telangiectatic FNH, these abnormal vessels drain directly into the adjacent sinusoids, while in classic FNH, connection to the sinusoids are almost never seen.

9.3
Diagnostic Imaging

Histopathologic features determine findings at diagnostic imaging. Imaging modality that are best able to characterize FNH are those that can distinguish Kupffer cell activity or can delineate the central scar. The ability to show Kupffer cell activity has historically been made by technetium (Tc)-99m sulfur colloid scintigraphy, which is a diagnostic modality of choice for this lesion. A total of 80% of FNH show uptake of Tc-99m sulfur colloid with scintigraphic evaluation (WELCH et al. 1985). Unfortunately, other hepatocellular neoplasms, such as hepatocellular adenoma (HCA) and hepatocellular carcinoma (HCC), can also have Kupffer cells and can subsequently show sulfur colloid uptake. Thus, the uptake of sulfur colloid can suggest the diagnosis of FNH, but it is not pathognomonic.

During the past few years, technical advances in ultrasound (US), computed tomography (CT) and magnetic resonance (MR) imaging and research into contrast agents have led to a marked increase in diagnostic accuracy in the detection and characterization of FNH.

Familiarity with the spectrum of US, CT and MR imaging findings makes it possible to differentiate FNH from other primary and secondary hepatic hypervascular lesions and to avoid invasive procedures such as biopsy and surgery.

In the following paragraphs the features of typical and atypical FNH at US, CT and MR imaging are discussed.

9.3.1
Typical Findings

9.3.1.1
Ultrasound

FNH is usually incidentally found during an abdominal US examination. Although US is a sensitive mo-

dality, it is not specific due the wide range of echo-patterns. FNH may be slightly hypoechoic, isoechoic or slightly hyperechoic (Fig. 9.3a). Some lesions may be detected only because they lead to the displacement of normal hepatic surrounding vessels. On the contrary, some lesions may have well defined lobulated contours or may show a hypoechoic halo which is more evident around FNH with fatty infiltration and located in liver with steatosis. This halo, also present around other benign lesions such as hemangiomas or adenomas, as well as around malignant lesions, most likely represents compressed hepatic parenchyma or vessels surrounding the lesion.

The conspicuity of FNH at US may improve with the detection of a hyperechoic or hypoechoic scar, located in the lesion's center or, less frequently, at the lesion's periphery (Fig. 9.2a). This scar is found in 20% of cases (SHAMSI et al. 1993). Sometimes the central scar is so small in size that it is not detectable by means of US. The use of color and power Doppler, providing information about the vascularization of FNH, makes it possible to visualize the vessels located in the central scar, improving not only the characterization but also the detection of these lesions. Typical findings at color/power Doppler US include the presence of a central feeding artery with a stellate or spoke-wheel pattern determined by vessels running into radiating fibrous septa originating from the central scar (Figs. 9.2b, 9.3b). Doppler spectral analysis can show an intralesional pulsatile waveform with high diastolic flow and low resistive index (mean 0.51), consisting of malformed arteries, and a continuous waveform which could represent a draining vein of the lesion (Fig. 9.3c) (UGGOWITZER et al. 1997; WANG et al. 1997).

The specificity of ultrasonography in the diagnosis of FNH has improved thanks to the introduction of ultrasound contrast agents (UCA) and non-linear imaging techniques. The characterization of FNH may be achieved by exploiting both the vascular and the late phase of first and second generation contrast agents.

Using second generation UCA and any of the non-linear continuous imaging modes at low-mechanical index (MI) or first generation UCA and high-MI intermittent imaging, the characteristic vascular pattern of FNH is represented by a central vascular supply with centrifugal filling to the periphery at the very early arterial phase (the so-called stellate or spoke-wheel pattern). Within 15 s of the bolus injection of contrast agent, in the late arterial phase, the lesion shows an uniform or lobulated dense stain and becomes homogeneously hyperechoic compared

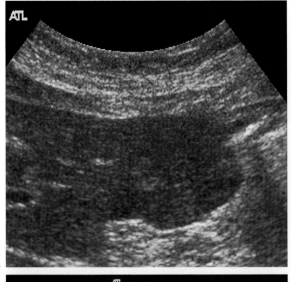

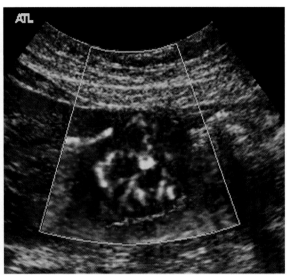

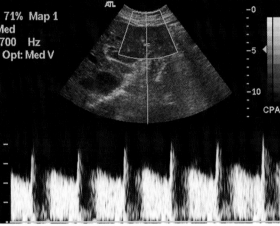

Fig. 9.3. a Conventional transverse US scan through the left hepatic lobe shows an isoechoic solid lesion barely differentiating from the surrounding liver. **b** Power Doppler US scan shows a typical *spoke-wheel pattern*, determined by vessels radiating from a vascularized central area. **c** Doppler spectral analysis of one of these radiating vessels shows the presence of pulsatile waveform with high diastolic flow

with the surrounding liver parenchyma. During the portal phase the lesion remains hyperechoic relative to the enhanced normal liver tissue. In the late portal and sinusoidal phases the lesion has usually the same vascular behavior of the adjacent liver parenchyma, being slightly hyperechoic against the background of the enhanced liver tissue.

During both the arterial and portal phases, the central scar becomes more easily detectable as a hypo-anechoic area (Figs. 9.2c, d, 9.4).

There are some non-linear US techniques that make it possible to visualize, at the same time, macro- and microcirculation using one bolus administration of US contrast agent (Fig. 9.5).

By using microbubble destructive techniques, such as stimulated acoustic emission (SAE), or agent detection imaging (ADI), it is possible to exploit the liver specific phase of some agents, which is probably mediated by Kupffer cell uptake. Interaction with

Kupffer cells would explain the enhancement that BLOMLEY et al. (2001) observed in FNH at 5 min after injection of a first generation contrast agent. In their series, strong late-phase SH U 508A uptake was detected by means of SAE in all FNHs, at a level similar or identical to that of the adjacent liver (Fig. 9.6). On the contrary, malignancies showed significant low late-phase uptake, with a complete separation between FNH and malignancies. Comparable results have been obtained by BRYANT et al. (2004) with ADI and the same contrast agent. These encouraging results might improve the potential of ultrasonography in the characterization of FNH.

9.3.1.2
Computed Tomography

With the introduction of multislice technology CT has become an excellent tool for the detection and

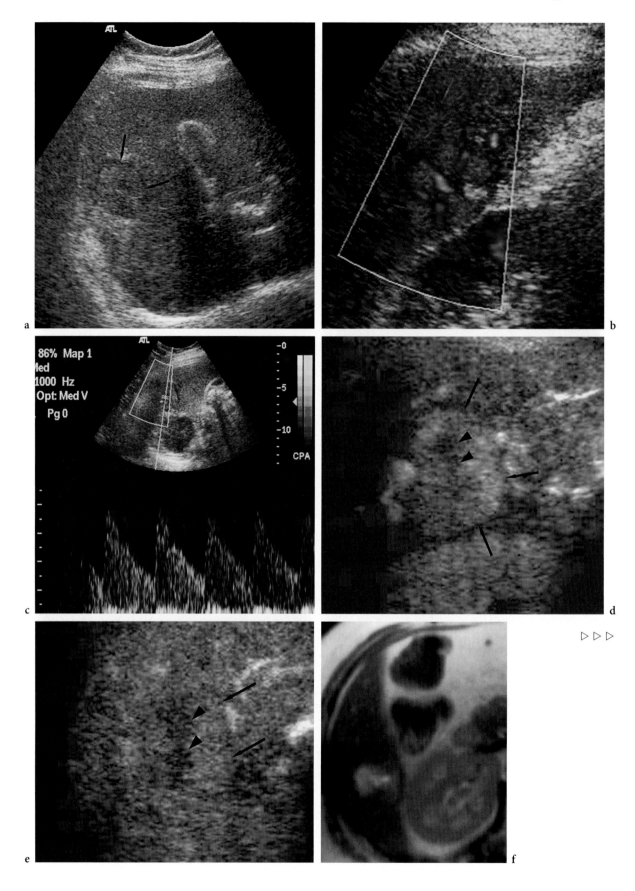

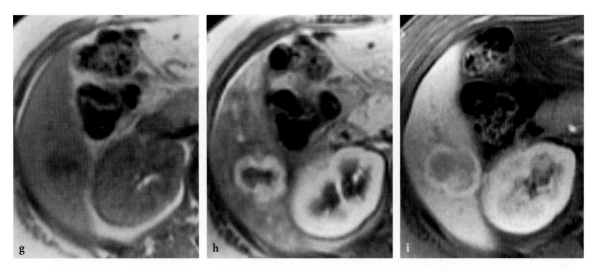

Fig. 9.4. a Conventional subcostal US scan shows an inhomogeneous slightly hyperechoic lesion, with subtle halo (*arrows*). **b** Power Doppler US scan shows radiating vessels. **c** Doppler spectral analysis of Power signals reveals pulsatile and continuous intratumoral waveform. **d** Contrast-enhanced US images: during the arterial phase the lesion appears hypervascular and becomes hyperechoic against the background of the unenhanced liver parenchyma (*arrows*). A hypoechoic central scar is visible (*arrowheads*). **e** During the portal phase the FNH is isoechoic to the surrounding liver (*arrows*), unlike the central scar which remains hypoechoic (*arrowheads*). **f** Non-enhanced MR images show small lesion in the segment VI with a thick central scar which appears typically hyperintense on T2-weighted image and hypointense (**g**) on T1-weighted image. **h** After administration of Gd-BOPTA T1-weighted MR image shows the typical hypervascularization during the arterial phase with hypointense central scar. **i** The delayed hepatobiliary phase reveals a peripheral rim enhancement with a central hypointensity due to the thick central scar

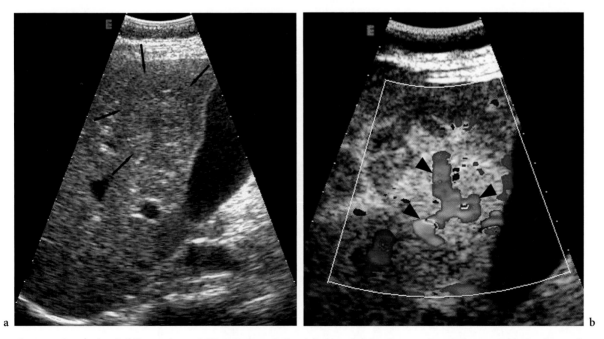

Fig. 9.5. a Conventional oblique subcostal US scan through the right hepatic lobe shows an isoechoic rounded lesion (*arrows*). **b** Contrast-enhanced US scan obtained at the same time with both color Doppler mode and non-linear contrast specific mode: color Doppler shows the macrocirculation of the lesion due to the central artery and some radiating vessels (*arrowheads*) and the microcirculation depicted during the portal phase

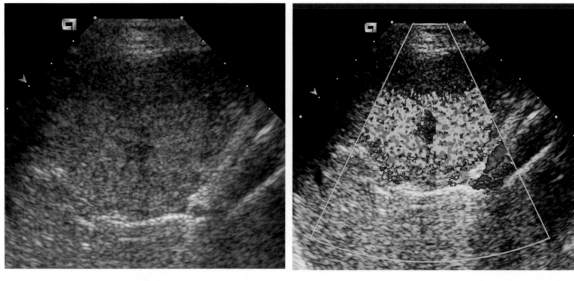

Fig. 9.6. a Oblique US scan through the right lobe of the liver shows a hyperechoic lesion with a hypoechoic central scar. **b** The same lesion is depicted with color SAE data 5 min after the administration of contrast agent: there is a large amount of SAE within the lesion, apart from the central scar. (Courtesy of Blomley et al. 2001)

characterization of FNH because it allows greater spatial and temporal resolution than conventional or single-detector helical CT.

CT examination includes the acquisition of non-enhanced and enhanced images; the latter are performed during the arterial, portal and delayed hepatic phases, with a start delay of 25–35 s, 60–70 s and 5–10 min, respectively, after the intravenous bolus injection of iodinated contrast material. High concentration contrast medium (370–400 mgI/ml), administered with a flow rate of 4–5 ml/s by means of a power injector, is usually preferred.

On non-enhanced CT scans FNH is usually iso-attenuating or hypoattenuating to the surrounding liver (Fig. 9.2e). When FNH is isodense to the liver, it may be detectable only because of its mass effect or its hypoattenuating central scar. The detection of a central scar is related to the size of FNH and can be identified in about 60% of nodules larger than 3 cm. In fatty liver FNH is usually hyperattenuating to non-enhanced liver.

On enhanced images, FNH shows a homogeneous strong enhancement during arterial phase: the degree of enhancement reflects the arterial hypervascularity and the homogeneous distribution is related to the uniform internal architecture of the tumor. The central scar, if present, remains hypodense during the arterial phase (Fig. 9.7a).

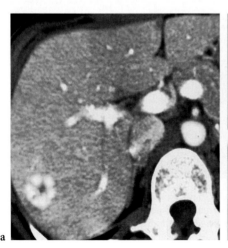

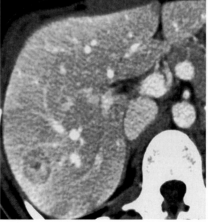

Fig. 9.7a–h. Typical CT and MR findings of focal nodular hyperplasia. **a** Arterial phase contrast-enhanced CT scan shows strong homogeneous enhancement of lesion, caused by arterial vascular supply; focal central area of low attenuation represents the central scar. **b** Contrast-enhanced CT scan during the portal venous phase shows lesion being slightly hypoattenuating compared with surrounding liver because of rapid contrast material washout. ▷ ▷ ▷

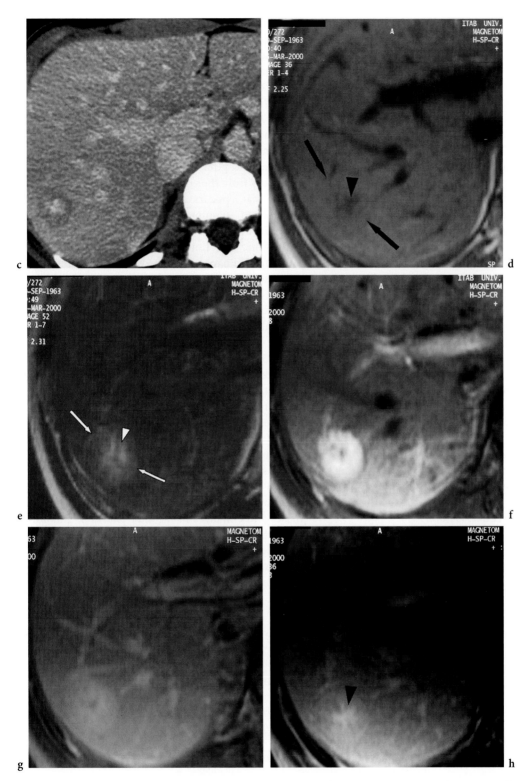

Fig. 9.7a–h *(Continued)*. **c** Delayed phase contrast-enhanced CT scan shows persistent enhancement of central scar. **d** T1-weighted MR image shows isointense lesion (*arrows*) with more hypointense central scar (*arrowhead*). **e** Fat suppressed T2-weighted HASTE image shows slightly hyperintense lesion (*arrows*) with obvious hyperintense central scar (*arrowhead*). **f** Arterial phase after i.v. injection of Gadolinium shows strong hyperintensity of the lesion whereas central scar remains hypointense. **g** During the portal phase the lesion appears slightly hyperintense to normal liver and during the equilibrium phase (**h**) central scar is highly enhanced (*arrowhead*)

During the portal venous phase there is the normal enhancement of the liver and FNH becomes isoattenuating or slightly hypoattenuating to the hepatic parenchyma (Fig. 9.7b).

On delayed images the FNH nodule is isoattenuating while the central scar becomes hyperattenuating in 81% of cases because of its content of myxomatous stroma (Fig. 9.7c).

On transverse CT scans it is not easy to identify the origin and the path of vessels; 3D multidetector CT angiography can be used in order to display angioarchitecture of FNH. This information has also a benefit in planning for embolization or ligation of vessels in symptomatic patients. Moreover, another potential benefit of the 3D display of hepatic vasculature provided by CT angiography is to noninvasively improve the differential diagnosis with other hypervascular lesions, thanks to the visualization of typical FNH vascular features which are characterized by the hepatic venous drainage and by the absence of portal vein supply (BRANCATELLI et al. 2002).

9.3.1.3
Magnetic Resonance

MR imaging has higher sensitivity (70%) and specificity (98%) for FNH than CT and US (MORTELÈ et al. 2000). The sensitivity and specificity of MR can be related to the higher capability of MR imaging to characterize soft-tissue. Thus, MR imaging is able to detect the central scar in 78% of cases (MORTELÈ et al. 2000, HUSSAIN et al. 2004).

MR examinations are usually performed using a high magnetic field MR imager (1.5 T) with phased array body coil and breath-hold sequence for high-resolution MR images.

Before administration of contrast agent T1-weighted GRE and T2-weighted HASTE or FSE or TSE images are acquired. Typical FNH nodules are iso- or hypointense on T1-weighted images and iso- or slightly hyperintense on T2-weighted images (Fig. 9.7d, e) (Table 9.1).

The minimal differences in signal intensity between normal liver parenchyma and FNH depend on the components of this lesion which are represented by normal Kupffer cells and hepatocytes arranged differently from the normal hepatic architecture. The central scar appears hyperintense on T2-weighted images and hypointense on T1-weighted images (Fig. 9.7d, e).

Dynamic gadolinium-enhanced MR imaging is performed with multisection 2D or 3D Gradient-echo (GRE) sequences that in a short time (5 s) are able to acquire the central K space profiles which determine the contrast of the image.

Usually T1-weighted GRE images are acquired at 20–25 s (arterial phase), 60–70 s (portal venous phase) and 3–5 min (equilibrium phase) following the administration of contrast medium. The 10-min post-contrast images are useful to evaluate the retention of contrast material within fibrous tissue and, therefore, are necessary in order to pick up the central scar.

FNH shows intense and homogeneous enhancement during the arterial phase, followed by isointensity or slight hypointensity during portal and equilibrium phases (Fig. 9.7f, g). Otherwise, the central scar is hypointense during arterial and portal venous phases and enhances in the later phases of gadolinium-enhanced imaging (3–5 and 10 min) (Fig. 9.7h).

Therefore, MR imaging offers similar dynamic changes as CT but provides additional information with non-enhanced T1- and T2-weighted images.

Table 9.1. Typical MR findings in FNH

Features	Signal intensity to health liver parenchyma	
	Lesion	Central scar
Nonenhanced T1w	*Iso- or sligthly hypointense*	*Hypointense*
Nonenhanced T2w	*Iso- or slightly hyperintense*	*Hyperintense*
Dynamic Gd-enhanced T1w		
– Arterial	*Homogeneously hyperintense*	*Hypointense*
– Portal	*Iso- or slightly hypointense*	*Slightly hypointense*
– Equilibrium phase	*Iso- or slightly hypointense*	*Hyperintense*
Hepatobiliary agents (Gd-BOPTA, Gd-EOB, Mn-DPDP)	*iso or hyperintense*	*hypointense*
Reticuloendothelial agents (SHU 555A, AMI 25)	*iso or slightly hyperintense*	*hyperintense*

9.3.2
Atypical Findings

FNH is usually characterized by a homogeneous structure. Nevertheless, although rare and only sporadically mentioned in literature, fatty infiltration of FNH is described and it was thought to be a result of the extension of the patient's underlying hepatic steatosis (MORTELÈ et al. 2000).

Hemorrhage as well as necrosis are unusual findings and may be related to a history of oral contraceptive use.

Although the central scar was thought to not calcify in FNH, a review by CASEIRO-ALVES et al. (1996) demonstrated calcification (central or peripheral) in 1.4% of their 357 cases of FNH.

In some cases the central scar may be extremely small and, therefore, undetectable on CT (16%–40%) and on MR imaging (22%) (Fig. 9.8) (HUSSAIN et al. 2004; MORTELÈ et al. 2000).

Although the central scar is usually hyperintense on T2-weighted images and hypointense on T1-weighted images and shows a delayed contrast enhancement on both CT and MR imaging, in some atypical FNH the central scar can appear hypointense on precontrast T2-weighted images or in T1-weighted post-contrast equilibrium phase MR images and hypodense on delayed enhanced CT images for the

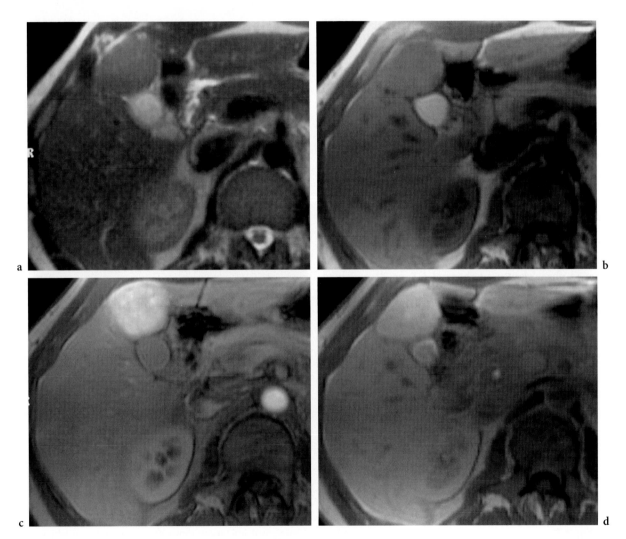

Fig. 9.8a–d. Atypical MR finding in focal nodular hyperplasia: non-visualization of central scar. **a** Non-enhanced images show a slightly hyperintense lesion on T2-weighted image and **a** isointense lesion on T1-weighted image (**b**) in segment IV without evidence of central scar. **c** Arterial phase image shows homogeneous and intense enhancement. No central scar is evident. **d** Image obtained 3 h after administration of Gd-BOPTA shows a homogeneously hyperintense lesion without evidence of central scar. Although central scar is not visualized, intense and homogeneous enhancement during the arterial and delayed hepatobiliary phases allows to differentiate FNH from hepatic adenoma

obliterative vascular hyperplasia of central arteries (MATHIEU et al. 1997; VILGRAIN et al. 1992).

In some cases color/power Doppler examinations do not show the characteristic "spoke-wheel pattern" but vessels randomly distributed in the lesion and at its periphery, without a clear central artery. In these lesions, the detection of an arterial Doppler signal with high diastolic flow can help in differentiating FNH from malignant lesions, such as hypervascular metastases and HCCs.

A pseudocapsule has also been reported as an atypical feature of FNH. BA-SSALAMAH et al. (2002) detected a pseudocapsule in 9% of the lesion on non-enhanced images and in 18% of the lesions on contrast-enhanced images. Dilated vessels and sinusoids around FNH lesions are well-documented sources of the pseudo-capsule. As in other type of lesions, the pseudocapsule may show enhancement on delayed contrast-enhanced images, but typically shows high signal intensity on T2-weighted images (Fig. 9.2h).

Telangiectatic FNH represents an example of atypical lesions and its imaging features has been recently described in the radiology literature (ATTAL et al. 2003). According to these authors, atypical findings in telangiectatic FNH were represented by heterogeneous pattern, seen in 43% of lesions, hyperintensity on T1-weighted MR images, seen in 53% of lesions, strong hyperintensity on T2-weighted MR images, seen in 44% of lesions, absence of a central scar, seen in 92% of lesions, and persistent enhancement on delayed-phase contrast-enhanced CT or T1-weighted images, seen in 61% of lesions.

The development of MR imaging liver specific contrast agents with hepatobiliary (Gd-BOPTA, Gd-EOB-DTPA, MnDPDP) or reticuloendothelial (SPIO or USPIO) effect has greatly increased the utility of MR imaging for the diagnosis of typical and mostly atypical FNH. MR imaging diagnosis of FNH with the extracellular gadolinium chelates is based on the early hyperintensity of the lesion and delayed contrast enhancement of the central scar. However, other hepatocellular tumors can show similar contrast behavior. On the other hand, BA-SSALAMAH et al. (2002) reported that 12% of FNH lesions showed only modest or minimal contrast enhancement during the arterial phase, which is an additional atypical finding (Fig. 9.9).

Gd-BOPTA and Gd-EOB-DTPA are molecules with a vascular-interstitial phase like the other gadolinium-based contrast agents and liver-specific properties in a later delayed phase in which the molecule accumulates selectively in hepatocytes.

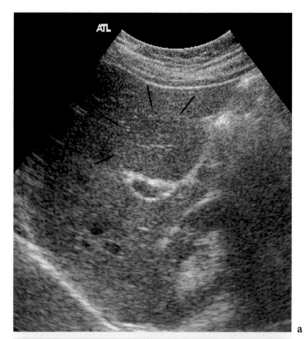

a

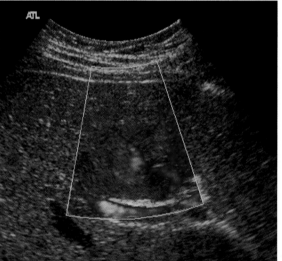

b ▷

Fig. 9.9a–h. Atypical finding in focal nodular hyperplasia: minimal contrast enhancement during the arterial phase. **a** Longitudinal US scan through the left hepatic lobe shows an isoechoic solid lesion with a subtle hyperechoic scar (*arrows*). **b** Power Doppler US shows few vessels radiating from a central one. **c** At contrast-enhanced US the lesion appears slightly hyperechoic in the arterial phase, due to a minimal enhancement. **d** Contrast-enhanced CT scan acquired during the arterial phase does not show a significant enhancement of lesion located in segment IV with hyperattenuating central scar during the equilibrium phase (*arrow*) (**e**). **f** Non-enhanced T2-weighted MR image shows an isointense lesion which is only detectable thanks to central scar hyperintensity (*arrow*). **g** Arterial phase T1-weighted image confirms the absence of a significant enhancement of the lesion, whereas the hepatobiliary phase (**h**) makes it possible to characterize the lesion as FNH thanks to Gd-BOPTA uptake with the evidence of a thin hypointense central scar (*arrow*)

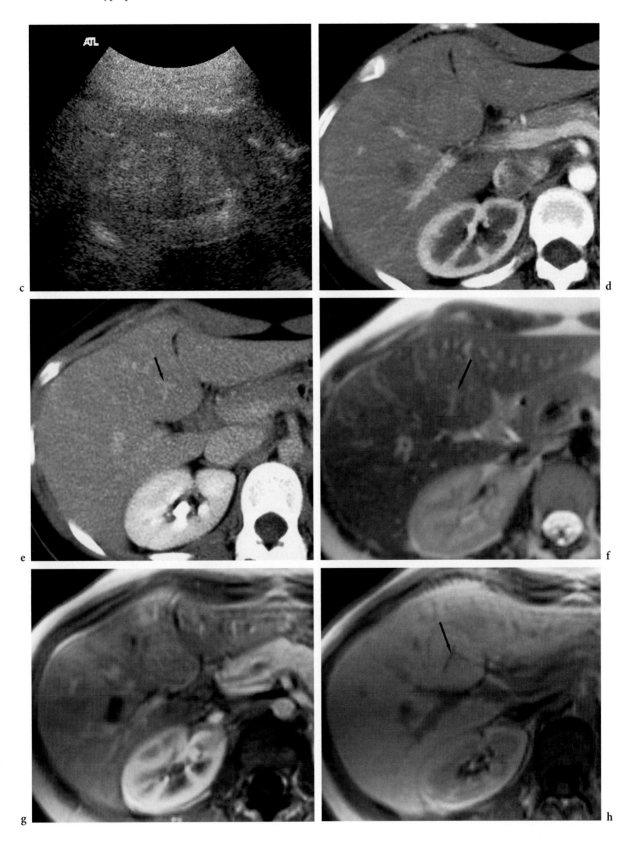

The FNH nodule appears hyperintense or isointense during the delayed phase after administration of Gd-BOPTA because FNH lacks a well-formed bile canalicular system to permit normal excretion. Thus, Gd-BOPTA gives morphologic and functional information of FNH nodules (Figs. 9.8d, 9.9h) (GRAZIOLI et al. 2001).

Similarly, FNH lesions typically enhance following MnDPDP. On early phase imaging (start delay of 20 min) lesions may appear isointense or hyperintense to normal liver and are usually hyperintense to normal liver parenchyma on delayed imaging (start delay of 24 h) (KING et al. 2002). Non-enhancing central scar or septa are frequently demonstrated.

Using superparamagnetic iron oxide (SPIO) based media, FNH nodules show a signal loss on T2 and T2*-weighted images related to the uptake of iron oxide particles by Kupffer cells within the lesion. Therefore, the central scar appears more conspicuous when these contrast agents are used (Fig. 9.10). The decrease in signal intensity of FNH, however, may be less than that of the hepatic parenchyma for the different content of Kupffer cells. Liver tissue after administration of SPIO shows a signal loss of 68%, while in FNH the signal loss intensity is approximately 30% (BEETS-TAN et al. 1998).

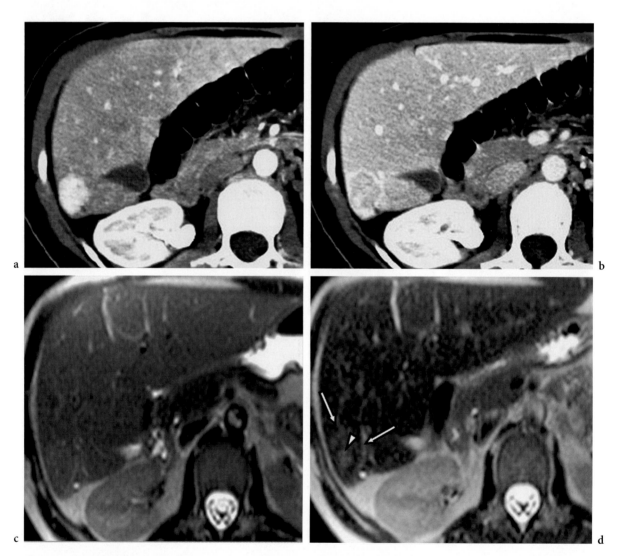

Fig. 9.10a–d. Focal nodular hyperplasia in a 35-year-old woman with a history of ileum carcinoid. **a** Contrast-enhanced CT scan shows in the right lobe a hypervascular lesion during the arterial phase with a rapid wash-out and a peripheral capsule during the portal phase (**b**). **c,d** MR findings after SPIO contrast agent administration. **c** Unenhanced T2-weighted image reveals a slightly hyperintense lesion which after i.v. bolus injection of SPIO agent (SHU 555A-Resovist). **d** Shows contrast uptake (*arrows*) with clear evidence of hyperintense central scar (*arrowhead*)

9.4
Associated Lesions

FNH has been associated with benign or malignant hypervascular liver tumors: knowledge and recognition of this association is important because the presence of multiple hypervascular lesions may be erroneously suggestive of hepatic malignancy.

Several authors reported that there is a significant non random association between FNH and hemangioma in the liver (23%) (Fig. 9.11) (Mathieu et al. 1997; Vilgrain et al. 2003). Both lesions, FNH and hemangioma, may be caused by the same factors, including focal disturbance of the hepatic blood supply that somehow facilitates the hyperplastic development of these benign lesions.

FNH has also be described in association with hepatocellular adenoma: in a series of 168 patients with 305 lesions FNH lesions the association with adenoma was observed in 3.6% of cases (Nguyen et al. 1999). Other investigations have noted that FNH and hepatic adenomas occur more often in patients who have coexisting vascular tumors, portal venous absence or occlusion, or portohepatic venous shunts (Ishak and Rabin 1975; Di Stasi et al. 1996; Grazioli et al. 2000; Lalonde et al. 1992).

FNH has also been described in association with the fibrolamellar type of hepatocellular carcinoma (Saul et al. 1987; Saxema et al. 1994).

9.5
Differential Diagnosis

The differential diagnosis of FNH includes other hypervascular tumors such as hepatocellular adenoma, hepatocellular carcinoma (particularly fibrolamellar hepatocellular carcinoma), and hypervascular metastases (Table 9.2).

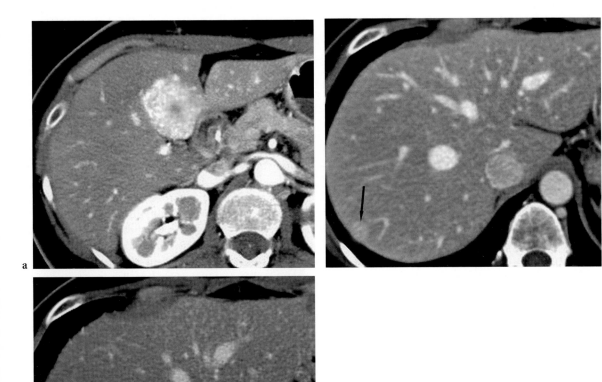

Fig. 9.11a–c. Focal nodular hyperplasia associated with hemangioma. **a** Contrast-enhanced arterial phase shows typical FNH nodule which appears as hyperdense lesion with a small hypodense central scar. **b,c** In segment VII of the same patient portal (**b**) and equilibrium phase (**c**) CT scans show a hyperdense small nodule whose imaging pattern is consistent with that of hemangioma (*arrows*)

Table 9.2. Findings to differentiate FNH from hepatocellular adenoma

Features	FNH	HCA
Sex	Female	Female
Hormone therapy	–/+	+++
Symptoms	Rare	Occasional
Multiple	+++	++
Central arterial scar	Yes	No
Internal hemorrhage or necrosis	–/+	+++
Calcification	–/+	+
Arterial phase enhancement	Homogeneous	Inhomogeneous
MR liver contrast behaviour		
Hepatobiliary agents		
– Gd-BOPTA,	Uptake	No significant uptake
– Mn-DPDP	Uptake	Uptake
Reticuloendothelial agents	Uptake	Uptake
(SHU 555A, AMI 25)	iso or slightly hyperintense	hyperintense

Hepatocellular adenoma shows no central scar, may bleed spontaneously and, therefore, contains areas of heterogeneity, fat, necrosis, hemorrhage, and calcification. At US examination hepatocellular adenoma appears more inhomogeneous than FNH and at color/power Doppler it shows peripheral and peritumoral vessels, most of them with a continuous waveform (BARTOLOZZI et al. 1997). At contrast-enhanced US, this lesion enhances inhomogeneously at arterial phase, remains slightly hypoechoic compared to the surrounding liver parenchyma in portal phase and becomes isoechoic to the normal liver tissue in the late phase. During the arterial phase, CT attenuation is significantly different between FNH and hepatocellular adenoma: the latter shows lower and heterogeneous enhancement. Some authors investigated not only qualitative, but also quantitative parameters of triphasic helical CT attenuation and enhancement patterns of FNH and hepatocellular adenoma (RUPPERT-KOHLMAYR et al. 2001). According to their results, relative enhancement of FNH and hepatocellular adenoma for the arterial phase was significantly higher in FNH than in hepatocellular adenoma: if relative enhancement was greater than 1.6 in the arterial phase, then FNH was most probable.

Whenever dynamic CT or MR study is not enough to indicate the diagnosis, Gd-BOPTA delayed (3 h) enhanced MR images provide additional information by showing a markedly hypointense appearance of hepatic adenoma, whereas FNH usually appear isointense or slightly hyperintense (GRAZIOLI et al. 2001).

After Mn-DPDP the differentiation of adenoma from FNH is more difficult because both lesions show contrast uptake with an iso or slightly hyperintense appearance to the normal liver.

The use of SPIO could show the same limitation of MN-DPDP as in some cases adenoma may take up SPIO, although BEETS-TAN et al. (1998) measured only 20% of signal loss on T2 weighted images in the adenoma, while the signal loss in FNH was as high as 70%.

Fibrolamellar carcinoma is another hypervascular tumor that occurs in young adults and contain a fibrotic scar. Fibrolamellar carcinoma usually appears as a large (>10 cm), heterogeneous, lobulated mass, with calcification (68% of cases). Because of its purely fibrous nature, the scar is hypointense on both T1- and T2-weighted images. The lack of enhancement of liver specific contrast agent on delayed images is useful in differentiating fibrolamellar carcinoma and FNH.

Hypervascular metastases occur in patients with known malignancy, are more often multiple, heterogeneous, hypointense on T1 weighted and hyperintense on T2-weighted non-enhanced MR images. At contrast-enhanced US hypervascular metastases, unlike FNH, show rapid wash out in portal phase and remain hypoechoic in the late phase. During the dynamic study, metastatic lesions appear hypodense on portal and equilibrium phases CT images, and hypointense on portal and equilibrium phases MR images. Furthermore, the lack of MR liver specific contrast agent uptake is an obvious sign of malignancy.

References

Attal P, Vilgrain V, Brancatelli G, et al (2003) Teleangiectatic focal nodular hyperplasia: US, CT and MR imaging findings with histopathologic correlation in 13 cases. Radiology 228:465–472

Bartolozzi C, Lencioni R, Paolicchi A et al (1997) Differentiation of hepatocellular adenoma and focal nodular hyperplasia of the liver: comparison of power Doppler imaging and conventional color Doppler sonography. Eur Radiol 7:1410–1415

Ba-Ssalamah A, Schima W, Schmook MT, et al (2002) Atypical focal nodular hyperplasia of the liver: imaging features of nonspecific and liver-specific MR contrast agents. AJR Am J Roentgenol 179:1447–1456

Beets-tan RGH, Van Engelshoven JMA, Greve JWM (1998) Hepatic adenoma and focal nodular hyperplasia: MR findings with superparamagnetic iron oxide enhanced MRI. Clin Imaging 22:211–215

Blomley MJK, Sidhu PS, Cosgrove DO et al (2001) Do different types of liver lesions differ in their uptake of the microbubble contrast agent SH U 508A in the late liver phase? Early experience. Radiology 220:661–667

Brancatelli G, Federle MP, Katyal S, et al (2002) Hemodynamic characterization of focal nodular hyperplasia using three-dimensional volume-rendered multidetector CT angiography. AJR Am J Roentgenol 179:81–85

Bryant TH, Blomley MJK, Albrecht T et al (2004) Liver phase uptake of a liver specific microbubble improves characterization of liver lesions: a prospective multicentre study. Radiology (in press)

Caseiro-Alves F, Zins M, Mahfouz AE, et al (1996) Calcification in focal nodular hyperplasia: a new problem for differentiation from fibrolamellar hepatocellular carcinoma. Radiology 198:889–892

Di Stasi M, Caturelli E, De Sio I et al (1996) Natural history of focal nodular hyperplasia of the liver: an ultrasound study. J Clin Ultrasound 24:345–350

Grazioli L, Federle MP, Jchaikawa T, et al (2000) Liver adenomatosis: clinical, histopathologic, and imaging findings in 15 patients. Radiology 216:395–402

Grazioli L, Morana G, Federle MP, et al (2001) Focal nodular hyperplasia: morphological and functional information from MR imaging with gadobenate dimeglumine. Radiology 221:731–739

Hussain SM, Terkivatan T, Zondervan PE, et al (2004) Focal nodular hyperplasia: findings at state-of-the-art MR imaging, US, CT, and pathologic analysis. Radiographics 24:3–17

Ishak KG, Rabin L (1975) Benign tumors of the liver. Med Clin North Am 59:995–1013

Karhunen PJ (1986) Benign hepatic tumor and tumor-like conditions in man. J Clin Pathol 39:183–188

King LJ, Burkill GJC, Scurr ED, et al (2002) MnDPDP enhanced magnetic resonance imaging of focal liver lesions. Clin Radiol 57:1047–1057

Lalonde L, Van Beers B, Trigaux J-P et al (1992) Focal nodular hyperplasia in association with spontaneous intrahepatic portosystemic venous shunt. Gastrointestinal Radiol 17:154–156

Mathieu D, Vilgrain V, Mahfouz AE, et al (1997) Benign liver tumors. Magn Reson Imaging Clin N Am 5:255–288

Mortelè KJ, Praet M, Van Vlierberghe H, Kunnen M, Ross PR (2000) CT and MR imaging findings in focal nodular hyperplasia of the liver: radiologic-pathologic correlation. AJR Am J Roentgenol 175:687–692

Nguyen BN, Flejou JF, Terris B, et al (1999) Focal Nodular hyperplasia of the liver : a comprehensive pathologic study of 305 lesions and recognition of new histologic forms. Am J Surg Pathol 23:1441–1454

Ruppert-Kohlmayr AJ, Uggowitzer MM, Kugler C, et al (2001) Focal nodular hyperplasia and hepatocellular adenoma of the liver: differentiation with multiphasic helical CT. AJR Am J Roentgenol 176:1493–1498

Saul SH, Titelbaum DS, Gansler TS, et al (1987) The fibrolamellar variant of hepatocellular carcinoma: its association with FNH. Cancer 60:3049–3055

Saxema R, Humphreys S, Williams R, et al (1994) Nodular hyperplasia surrounding fibrolamellar carcinoma: a zone of arterialized liver parenchyma. Hystopathology 25:275–278

Shamsi K, De Schepper A, Degryse H, et al (1993) Focal nodular hyperplasia of the liver: radiologic findings. Abdom Imaging 18:32–38

Uggowitzer M, Kugler C, Machan L, et al (1997) Power Doppler imaging and evaluation of the resistive index in focal nodular hyperplasia of the liver. Abdom Imaging 22:268–273

Vilgrain V, Flejou JF, Arrive L, et al (1992) Focal nodular hyperplasia of the liver: MR imaging and pathologic correlation in 37 patients. Radiology 184:699–703

Vilgrain V, Uzan F, Brancatelli G, et al (2003) Prevalence of hepatic hemangioma in patients with focal nodular hyperplasia: MR imaging analysis. Radiology 229:75–79

Wang LY, Wang JH, Lin ZY et al (1997) Hepatic focal nodular hyperplasia: findings on color Doppler ultrasound. Abdom Imaging 22:178–181

Wanless IR, Mawdsley C, Adams R (1985). On the pathogenesis of focal nodular hyperplasia of the liver. Hepatology 5:1194–1200

Welch TJ, Sheedy PF, Johnson CM, et al (1985) Focal nodular hyperplasia and hepatic adenoma: comparison of angiography, CT, US and scintigraphy. Radiology 156:593–595

10 Hepatocellular Adenoma

Luigi Grazioli, Marie Pia Bondioni, and Giuseppe Brancatelli

10.1
Introduction

Hepatocellular adenoma (HA) is a rare, benign neoplasm of hepatocellular origin that is frequently found in middle-aged women. The pathogenesis of the tumor is not yet clear, but is likely caused by multiple factors. The use of estrogen-containing or androgen-containing steroid clearly increases the incidence, number, and size of adenomas (Walness and Medline 1982; Soe et al. 1992). Moreover, this casual relationship is related to dose and duration, with the greatest risk encountered in patients taking large doses of estrogen or androgen for prolonged periods of time compared with the population without a history of oral contraceptive use (Soe et al. 1992). In particular in women who have never used oral contraceptives, the annual incidence of this tumor is 1 per million; conversely, this increases to 30-40 per million in long-term users of oral contraceptives (Reddy and Schiff 1993).

Another risk group for hepatocellular adenoma are patients affected by glycogenosis, in particular

L. Grazioli, MD; M.P. Bondioni, MD
Department of Radiology, University of Brescia, Spedali Civili di Brescia, Piazzale Spedali Civili 1, 25023 Brescia, Italy
G. Brancatelli, MD
Department of Radiology, Policlinico Universitario, Via del Vespro 127, 90127 Palermo, Italy

the type I glycogen storage disease (Labrune et al. 1997). In these patients the possible pathogenetic mechanism includes glucagon/insulin imbalance, cellular glycogen overload, and proto-oncogene activation (Bianchi 1993). Patients with diabetes mellitus have decreased circulating insulin levels and elevated serum glucose; therefore they share a similar pathogenetic mechanism with patients affected by glycogenesis. Hepatocellular adenomas can occur sporadically in patients without known predisposing factors. A recently recognized association is that of congenital or acquired abnormalities of the hepatic vasculature, such as portal vein absence, occlusion or portohepatic venous shunts; these vascular abnormalities have been noted, particularly in patients with liver adenomatosis (LA) (Nakasaki et al. 1989; Kawakatsu et al. 1994). This entity is considered a separate form characterized by the presence of more than ten adenomas within an otherwise normal liver, without a history of glycogen storage disease or chronic anabolic steroid use (Flejou et al. 1985; Grazioli et al. 2000).

Although the adenomas in liver adenomatosis are histologically similar to other adenomas, they are not steroid dependent, but are multiple, progressive, symptomatic, and more likely to lead to impaired liver function, hemorrhage, and perhaps malignant degeneration (Grazioli et al. 2000). An association with pregnancy has also been described, probably due to increased levels of endogenous steroid hormones (Terkivatan et al. 2000).

Recently, some authors have suggested a genetic alteration in the hepatocellular adenoma origin; they found respectively a β-catenin mutation and a deletion locus on chromosome 12 in patients with this neoplasm (Bluteau et al. 2002; Chen et al. 2002).

A new classification of adenomas has been proposed according to which anabolic steroid associated type HA is considered separately from the classical form (Kew 1998). This is due to its distinct histological appearance, which often resembles that of hepatocellular carcinoma.

10.2
Histopathologic Features

Hepatic adenomas are reported to be solitary in 70–80% of cases, but it is not unusual to encounter two or three adenomas in one patient. Adenomas are usually well-circumscribed lesions, varying in size from less than 1 cm to more than 15 cm. The typical steroid-related adenoma often comes to clinical attention when it reaches about 5 cm in diameter. Histologically, hepatic adenoma is defined as a tumor composed of cells closely resembling normal hepatocytes, but larger than normal liver cells, the cytoplasm containing variable amounts of glycogen and lipid; a typical yellow appearance of the cut surface of the tumor is related to lipid accumulation.

Adenoma cells are arranged in cords and separated by sinusoids (ISHAK 1994). The tumor lacks portal tracts or bile ducts, a key histological feature that helps distinguish hepatocellular adenoma from focal nodular hyperplasia (BOULAHDOUR et al. 1993). Kupffer's cells are found in adenomas but probably they are often decreased in number or less functional than normal liver tissue, as reflected by absent or diminished uptake of technetium (Tc)-99m sulfur colloid (Fig. 10.1) (RUBIN and LICHTENSTEIN 1993). Because this neoplasm has no portal tracts, the tumor perfusion occurs solely by peripheral arterial feeders; therefore the hypervascular nature of adenoma, related to sinusoids and feeding arteries, associated with poor connective tissue support, can lead frequently to hemorrhage. Because a tumor capsule is usually absent or incomplete, hemorrhage may spread into the liver or abdominal cavity (MOLINA and SCHIFF 1999).

Many or most patients with no more than a few adenomas are asymptomatic and almost invariably have normal liver function and no elevation of serum "tumor markers" such as α-fetoprotein. Large adenomas may cause a sensation of right upper quadrant fullness or discomfort. However, the classic clinical manifestation of hepatic adenoma, especially in large neoplasm, is spontaneous rupture or hemorrhage, leading to acute abdominal pain and possibly progressing to hypotension and even death (Fig. 10.2) (LEESE et al. 1998).

10.3
Imaging Features

10.3.1
Ultrasound

On US examination, HA has variable sonographic appearances, depending on changes in the lesion. The neoplasm is described in many cases as a large mixed echoic lesion, mainly hypoechoic with anechoic areas, corresponding to zones of internal hemorrhage. Adenomas may undergo extensive necrotic and hemorrhagic changes, and the ultrasound appearance is that of a complex mass with large cystic components (Fig. 10.3). This US appearance is basically found in large, more than 5 cm, adenomas. The high lipid content of adenomas may contribute to the hyperechoic appearance of some of these lesions (Fig. 10.4). Noncomplicated and "non-fat" adenomas may appear as homogeneous isoechoic or hypoechoic lesions with or without a surrounding hypoechoic rim (Fig. 10.5). Using the color Doppler technique the arterial hypervascularity is well demonstrated

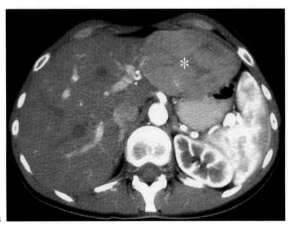
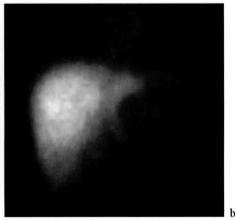

a   b

Fig. 10.1a,b. Non-complicated hepatocellular adenoma. **a** On CT scan during the arterial phase after contrast medium administration the neoplasm becomes homogeneously hyperdense (*asterisk*) compared to the surrounding liver parenchyma. **b** Nuclear medicine shows absent uptake of technetium (Tc)-99m sulfur colloid, and the lesion is seen as "cold defect"

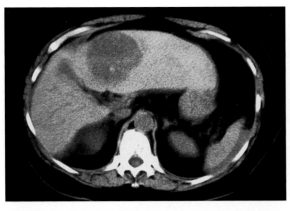
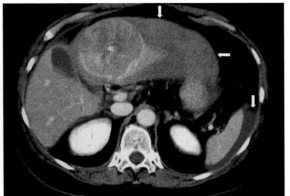

a b

Fig. 10.2a,b. Complicated hemorrhagic hepatocellular adenoma: CT evaluation. **a** The precontrast and portal venous CT (**b**) scans show a large and inhomogeneous mass located in the left lobe of the liver (*asterisk*). The rupture of the neoplasm determined abundant subcapsular hematoma and hemoperitoneum (*arrows*)

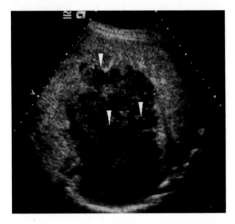

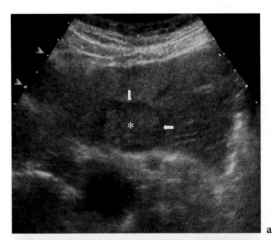

a

Fig. 10.3. Hemorrhagic hepatocellular adenoma: ultrasound evaluation. Ultrasound examination reveals a large and dishomogeneous lesion characterized by a peripheral solid portion and central heterogeneous hypoechoic zone with multiple anechoic areas (*arrowheads*) related to hemorrhage

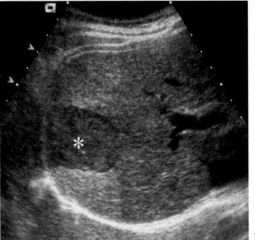

b

Fig. 10.5a,b. Non-complicated hepatocellular adenoma: ultrasound findings. **a** Ultrasound examination shows a well-defined isoechoic nodule (*asterisk*) delimited by a hypoechoic rim (*arrows*) in the left lobe of the liver. **b** Hepatocellular adenoma may show a different pattern and appears as a homogeneous slightly hypoechoic lesion (*asterisk*)

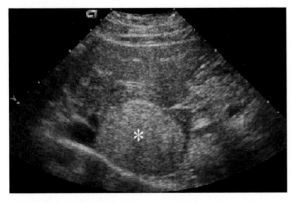

Fig. 10.4. Non-complicated fatty adenoma: ultrasound examination. Ultrasound scan shows, in segment I of the liver, a well-delimited, round and homogeneously hyperechoic lesion (*asterisk*) due to abundant fatty infiltration

directly by the arterial vessels within the lesion and with the typical arterial spectrum (Fig. 10.6). Color ultrasound also demonstrates intratumoral and peripheral peritumoral vessels; the former may have a flat continuous or, less commonly, a triphasic waveform. Peritumoral arteries and intratumoral veins are often present in HA and this finding may be useful to discriminate features distinguishing HA from FNH (Fig. 10.7) (BARTOLOZZI et al. 1997; GOLLI et al. 1994).

Recently the availability of ultrasound second generation contrast media has permitted the evaluation of the type and the entity of vascularity similar to that observed with dynamic CT or MR. Using this blood pool agent during the arterial phase shows intense enhancement in non-complicated nodules or enhancement in the saved portion of complicated hemorrhagic adenomas. During the portal venous and equilibrium phases non-complicated adenomas may appear as an iso- or slightly hyperechoic mass.

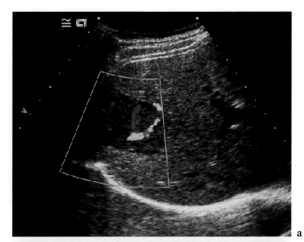

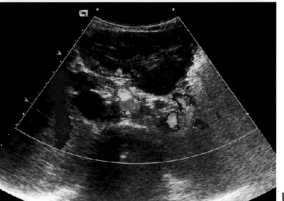

Fig. 10.7a,b. Color scan of hepatocellular adenoma. **a** Color ultrasound examination is able to demonstrate intratumoral vessels and peripheral peritumoral vessels (**b**)

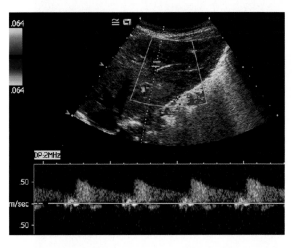

Fig. 10.6. Color Doppler of hepatocellular adenoma. Color Doppler scan reveals the presence of arterial vessels within the lesion with arterial spectrum

10.3.2
Computed Tomography

On multiphasic helical CT, the ability to acquire separate series during the arterial dominant and portal venous dominant phases adds a temporal hemodynamic component to the morphologic depiction of neoplasm. Adenomas consist almost entirely of uniform hepatocytes, with the exception of areas of focal fat, hemorrhage, or calcification. On unenhanced CT scans, fat or hemorrhage can be easily detected,

and the lesion may contain hypodense areas due to the presence of fat within the tumor, or hyperdense ones corresponding to fresh hemorrhage (Figs. 10.8, 10.9). Old hemorrhage is seen as a heterogeneous, hypoattenuating area within the tumor (GRAZIOLI et al. 2001). During dynamic bolus-enhanced CT scanning, non-complicated adenomas may enhance rapidly (about 20–30 s after contrast administration) and appear homogeneously hyperdense compared to the liver. The enhancement usually does not persist in adenomas because of arteriovenous shunting within the lesion (Fig. 10.10). Larger or complicated HA may be more heterogeneous than smaller lesions (Fig. 10.11). However, because adenomas consist of normal hepatocytes and a variable number of Kupffer cells, it is not surprising that most of the adenomas are nearly isoattenuating relative to normal liver on unenhanced, portal venous and delayed phase images (HEIKEN 1998; ROS 1990).

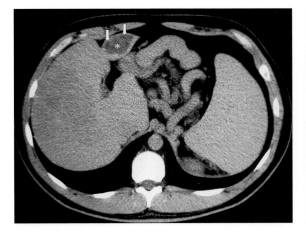

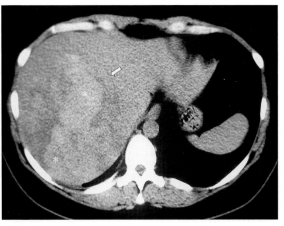

Fig. 10.8. Hepatocellular adenoma: unenhanced CT scan. Unenhanced CT scan shows a heterogeneous hypoattenuating lesion in the left lower lobe of the liver (*asterisk*). The neoplasm contains small, hypodense, peripheral areas related to fat within the tumor (*arrows*)

Fig. 10.9. Complicated hemorrhagic hepatocellular adenoma: unenhanced CT scan. Unenhanced CT scan reveals diffuse intratumoral, fresh hemorrhage characterized by hyperdense intralesion areas (*asterisks*). A peripheral hypodense thin rim represents a fibrous capsule (*arrow*)

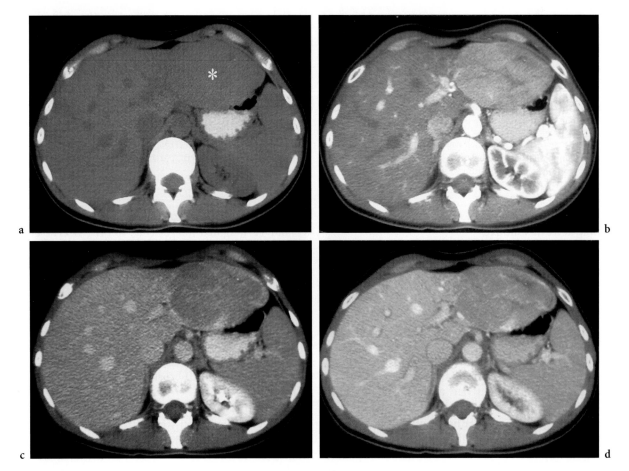

Fig. 10.10a–d. Hepatocellular adenoma: CT evaluation. **a** On precontrast CT scan hepatocellular adenoma (*asterisk*) is isoattenuating to the liver. **b** During the arterial phase after contrast medium administration the nodule shows quite homogeneous enhancement, with a rapid wash-out during the portal venous (**c**) and equilibrium (**d**) phases

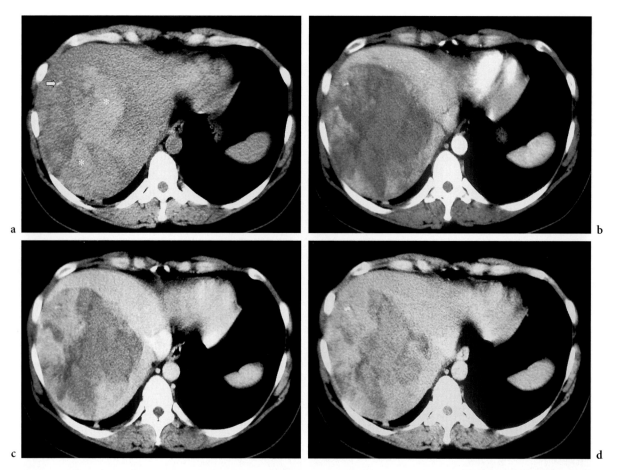

Fig. 10.11a–d. Hepatocellular adenoma: dynamic CT evaluation. **a** On precontrast CT scan the mass appears heterogeneously hyperdense (*asterisks*); a small calcification is visible in the peripheral portion of the tumor (*arrow*). During the dynamic study after contrast medium administration (**b–d**) the lesion shows heterogeneous enhancement, particularly evident during the portal venous and equilibrium phases (**d**)

10.3.3
Magnetic Resonance

On MR images, hepatocellular adenoma can show a variable signal intensity related to tissue components. On T1-weighted images, frequently the lesion is heterogeneous in appearance due to areas of increased signal intensity related to fat, glycogen or recent hemorrhage, and low signal intensity areas corresponding to necrosis or old hemorrhage. Using T1-weighted "out phase" images, adenomas containing fat demonstrate a significant decrease of signal intensity (Fig. 10.12). The neoplasm may appear homogeneously or heterogeneously hyperintense on T2-weighted images, the heterogeneity being mainly due to the presence of hemorrhage and necrosis (Fig. 10.13) (GRAZIOLI et al. 2001; PAULSON et al. 1994). About one-third of adenomas have a peripheral rim, corresponding to a fibrous capsule;

frequently the rim is of low signal intensity on both T1 and T2-weighted images (Fig. 10.14) (ARRIVE et al. 1994).

Dynamic MR imaging, after contrast medium administration, is able to demonstrate the early arterial enhancement that reflects the presence of subcapsular feeding vessels, and a rapid wash-out of the lesion. On portal venous and equilibrium phases hepatic adenoma appears isointense or slightly hyperintense, with focal heterogeneous hypointense areas of necrosis, calcification or fibrosis if present (Fig. 10.15) (CHUNG et al. 1995).

In the delayed liver specific phase after Gd-BOPTA administration, there is usually no substantial uptake of contrast and the lesion is hypointense to the normal liver parenchyma, due to the absence of biliary ducts. This is one of the main features differentiating HA from FNH in the non-complicated form; in fact FNH generally ap-

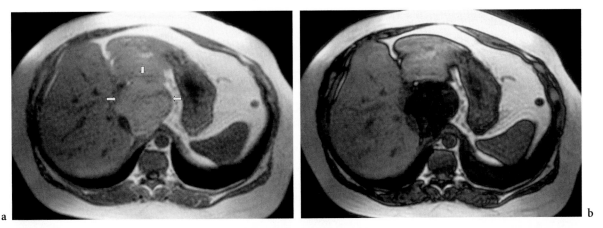

Fig. 10.12a,b. Hepatocellular adenoma: T1-weighted MR evaluation. **a** Unenhanced GRE T1-weighted "in phase" image shows, in segment I of the liver, a homogeneous hyperintense nodule (*arrows*). **b** In an unenhanced T1-weighted "out phase" image, the nodule shows a significant homogeneous signal drop due to the presence of abundant, diffuse fatty infiltration

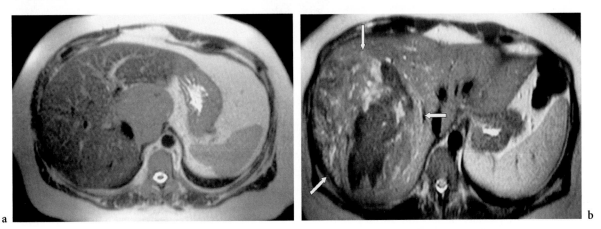

Fig. 10.13a,b. Hepatocellular adenoma: T2-weighted MR evaluation. **a** Same case as in Fig. 10.12. The presence of fatty infiltration determines the homogeneous hyperintensity of the lesion with respect to the surrounding normal liver parenchyma on a HASTE T2-weighted image. **b** Same case as in Fig. 10.3. Cellular composition and intratumoral necrosis and hemorrhage contribute to determining the heterogeneous hyperintensity of the mass on a HASTE T2-weighted image (*arrows*)

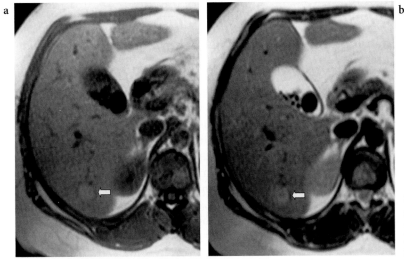

Fig. 10.14a,b. Capsulated hepatic adenoma: MR evaluation. **a** Both T1 and T2 (**b**) weighted images show a peripheral hypointense thin rim representing the fibrous capsule (*arrow*)

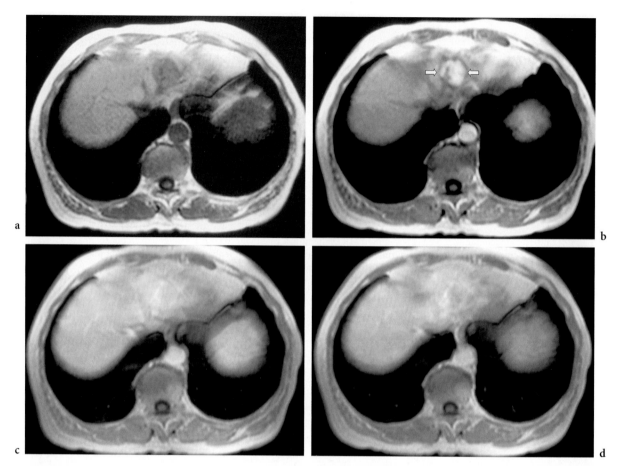

Fig. 10.15a–d. Hepatic adenoma: dynamic MR evaluation. **a** On an unenhanced T1-weighted image the lesion, located in segment II, appears as a well-delimited slightly hypointense nodule. **b** Dynamic MR evaluation after extracellular contrast medium administration shows, during the arterial phase, the early and intense enhancement (*arrows*), and rapid wash-out in the portal (**c**) and equilibrium phases (**d**). In the equilibrium phase a thin hyperintense capsule is also visible

pears isointense or slightly hyperintense to the surrounding parenchyma (GRAZIOLI et al. 2001). Conversely, after Mn-DPDP, hepatic adenoma appears iso- or slightly hyperintense, similarly to FNH, and this contrastographic behavior limits the capability to make a correct differential diagnosis in these primary hepatic nodules (Fig. 10.16) (COFFIN et al. 1999).

Adenomas, in some cases, may take up superparamagnetic iron oxide (SPIO) particles, resulting in decreased signal intensity on DP-T2 or T2*-weighted images, whereas on T1-weighted images the neoplasm usually appears moderately hyperintense. The uptake of SPIO in adenoma is variable, depending on Kupffer's cell content or function, and is usually poorer or heterogeneous compared to that which occurs in the surrounding normal liver parenchyma or in FNH (Fig. 10.17) (VOGL et al. 1996).

10.4
Liver Adenomatosis

Liver adenomatosis (LA) is a distinct clinical entity which can be distinguished from isolated hepatic adenoma by the presence of multiple lesions, usually more than ten nodules. This condition is also characterized by the absence of any correlation with steroid medication, and by involvement in both men and women (GRAZIOLI et al. 2000).

The conditions that may predispose patients to liver adenomatosis are poorly understood, although congenital or acquired abnormalities of the hepatic vasculature, such as portal venous absence, occlusion, portohepatic venous shunts, or vascular tumors may be involved (Fig. 10.18). It was speculated that a focal disturbance of the hepatic blood somehow facilitates the hyperplastic development of this type of lesion (GRAZIOLI et al. 2000; ICHIKAWA et al. 2000).

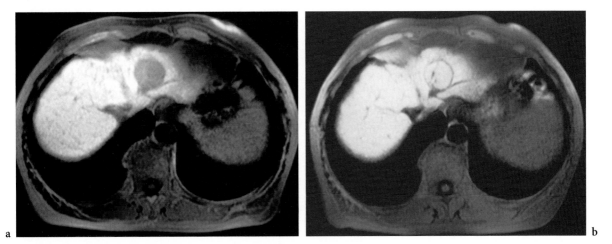

Fig. 10.16a,b. Hepatic adenoma: MR evaluation with Gd-BOPTA and Mn-DPDP. **a** Same case as in Fig. 10.15. On delayed (hepatobiliary phase) GRE T1-weighted fat sat image after Gd-BOPTA administration the lesion appears as a hypointense and homogeneous nodule in comparison with the normal, hyperintense liver parenchyma. **b** Using Mn-DPDP, the lesion demonstrates uptake of the contrast medium and appears isointense to the surrounding normal liver parenchyma

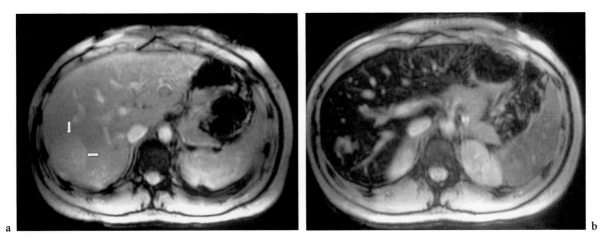

Fig. 10.17a,b. Hepatocellular adenoma: MR evaluation with SPIO. **a** T2*-weighted precontrast image reveals a well-defined, slightly homogeneous hyperintense lesion (*arrows*). **b** On a delayed phase image after SPIO administration, the lesion shows a significant signal drop which reflects the presence of Kupffer's cells

Laboratory analysis has shown an elevation of serum alkaline phosphatase and γ-glutamyltransferase levels (FLEJOU et al. 1985).

Clinically patients with LA can be asymptomatic, can have chronic or acute abdominal pain. The lesions in liver adenomatosis can lead to impaired liver function, and patients are at increased risk for development of hepatocellular carcinoma (HCC); therefore they should be closely monitored with CT or MR imaging as well as with serum α-fetoprotein or other tumor marker examinations (RIBERIO et al. 1998).

The multiple adenomas in liver adenomatosis may have a variety of appearances, but the CT and MR characteristics of individual lesions are similar to those reported for sporadic or solitary adenomas (Fig. 10.19) (GRAZIOLI et al. 2000; ICHIKAWA et al. 2000; PAULSON et al. 1994).

As noted by FLEJOU et al. (1985), liver adenomatosis has features that distinguish it from the more common isolated cases of hepatic adenoma, the latter correlated with hormonal or metabolic disorders. Most steroid-induced or steroid-augmented adenomas are solitary, or at most two or three of these lesions manifest in a patient and typically regress with cessation of exogenous steroid use. Conversely the tumors in patients with liver adenomatosis do not appear to be steroid dependent, and they do not regress with steroid withdrawal or blockage. Most adenomas are

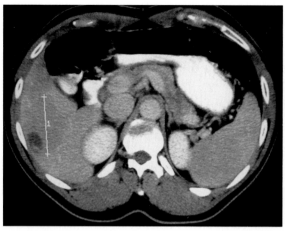
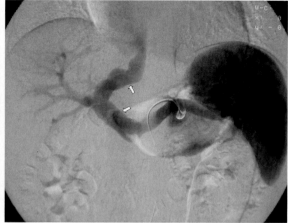

a

b

Fig. 10.18a,b. Hepatocellular adenoma: CT and angiographic examination. **a** CT scan acquired on portal venous phase shows large mass located in the VI segment of the liver (*clippers*). Focal heterogeneous hypodense area represents hepatocellular degeneration. **b** Angiographic scan shows an intrahepatic shunt between the left branch of the portal vein and the intermedius hepatic vein (*arrows*). Right portal venous branches are decreased in size

asymptomatic, unless there is a hemorrhage, which occurs in a minority of patients. The exact frequency of hemorrhage is uncertain, because symptomatic patients are more likely to seek medical attention. Malignant degeneration to HCC has been reported, rarely in adenomas, related to exogenous steroid use or glycogen storage disease. Liver function tests are usually invariably normal (ROOKS et al. 1979). Liver adenomatosis, on the other hand, affects both women and men; liver function abnormalities are almost always present because of the tremendous number of space-occupying tumors.

10.5
Treatment

The hepatic adenoma is the most serious of all hepatic benign neoplasms, because of potential consequences, such as rupture, and dedifferentiation into malignancy. Criteria that guide treatment include the number and size of the nodules, the presence of symptoms, and the surgical risk incurred by the patient (LEESE et al. 1998). Some clinicians have proposed nonsurgical management with cessation of hormone therapy, serial radiologic examination, and screening for elevated α-fetoprotein levels, especially in isolated small adenomas. Conversely, many surgeons have advocated resection of adenomas of larger 5 cm adenomas, due to the recognized risk of complications. Hepatic arterial embolization can be effective for controlling acute hemorrhage in an adenoma (AULT et al. 1996).

In liver adenomatosis, because of the chance of malignant degeneration and hemorrhage, resection of adenomas, or at least of the largest and most vulnerable lesions (such as subcapsular and exophytic lesions), seems to be warranted in many cases, even if some smaller adenomas remain in place. Orthotopic liver transplantation remains a difficult decision, although it is sometimes the last option in progressive forms, or in liver disease impairing socioprofessional day-to-day life in young patients, particularly young women trying to become pregnant. Liver transplantation can be reserved even in patients who have progressive signs or symptoms after partial resection, or in whom HCC is suspected.

10.6
Differential Diagnosis

Another clinical problem concerns the differential diagnosis between patients with hepatic adenoma and patients with different solid, hypervascular hepatic masses.

Focal nodular hyperplasia (FNH), similarly to hepatic adenoma, is a hypervascular and nonencapsulated lesion that occurs predominantly in young women, who probably share a common predisposing factor of hepatic venous abnormality. FNH can be often distinguished from adenoma by the absence of fat, calcification or hemorrhage, and by the presence of a central scar and marked hypervascularity (CHOI and FREENY 1998; ICHIKAWA et al. 2000). Some

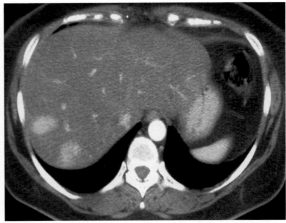

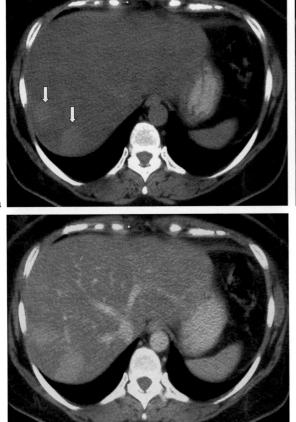

Fig. 10.19a–c. Liver adenomatosis: CT evaluation. **a** On pre-contrast CT scan at least two nodules (*arrows*), slightly hyperdense compared to the normal liver parenchyma, can be detected in the VII and VIII segments. **b** During the arterial phase after contrast medium administration the lesions become homogeneously hyperdense, showing a rapid wash-out in the portal venous phase (**c**)

authors have noted the coexistence of FNH and adenomas both in liver adenomatosis and in cases of sporadic liver adenomas (FRIEDMAN et al. 1984; ICHIKAWA et al. 2000).

Other investigators have reported cases of nodular regenerative hyperplasia demonstrating multiple hypervascular hepatic lesions in young patients without cirrhosis but with underlying vascular abnormalities; nevertheless the nodules are usually multiple, distributed uniformly through the liver and in most cases present a peripheral "ischemic" rim (MOTOORI et al. 1997).

Distinguishing liver adenomatosis from multifocal HCC might be impossible with imaging criteria alone, because HCC lesions are often hypervascular and partially encapsulated and may contain fat (OLIVER et al. 1996). In most cases of diffuse HCC, however, cirrhosis or clinical evidence of chronic liver disease is evident and serum tumor markers are elevated.

Hypervascular liver metastases may share some imaging features with liver adenomatosis. Most patients have a known primary malignancy, such as thyroid or renal carcinoma. Such hepatic metastases almost never contain fat, and the diagnosis is usually easily confirmed by needle biopsy.

References

Arrive L, Flejou JF, Vilgrain V, et al (1994) Hepatic adenoma: MR findings in 51 pathologically proved lesions. Radiology 193:507–512

Ault GT, Wren SM, Ralls PW, et al (1996) Selective management of hepatic adenomas. Am Surg 62:825–829

Bartolozzi C, Lencioni R, Paolicchi A, et al (1997) Differentiation of hepatocellular adenoma and focal nodular hyperplasia of the liver: comparison of power Doppler imaging and conventional color Doppler sonography. Eur Radiol 7:1410–1415

Bianchi L (1993) Glycogen storage disease I and hepatocellular tumors. Eur J Pediatr 152 (Suppl 1):S63–S70

Bluteau O, Jeannot E, Bioulac-Sage P, et al (2002) Bi-allelic inactivation of TCF1 in hepatic adenomas. Nat Genet 32:312–315

Boulahdour H, Cherqui D, Charlotte F, et al (1993) The hot spot hepatobiliary scan in focal nodular hyperplasia. J Nucl Med 34:2105–2110

Chen YW, Jeng YM, Yeh SH, et al (2002) P53 gene and Wnt signaling in benign neoplasms: -catenin mutation in hepatic adenoma but not in focal nodular hyperplasia. Hepatology 36:927–935

Choi CS, Freeny PC (1998) Triphasic helical CT of hepatic focal nodular hyperplasia: incidence of atypical findings. AJR Am J Roentgenol 170:391–395

Chung KY, Mayo-Smith WW, Saini S, et al (1995) Hepatocellular adenoma: MR imaging features with pathologic correlation. AJR Am J Roentgenol 165:303–308

Coffin CM, Diche T, Mahfouz AE, et al (1999) Benign and malignant hepatocellular tumours: evaluation of tumoral enhancement after mangafodipir trisodium injection on MR imaging. Eur Radiol 9:444–449

Flejou JF, Barge J, Menu Y, et al (1985) Liver adenomatosis: an entity distinct from liver adenoma? Gastroenterology 89:1132–1138

Friedman LS, Gang DL, Hedberg SE, et al (1984) Simultaneous occurrence of hepatic adenoma and focal nodular hyperplasia: report of a case and review of the literature. Hepatology 4:536–540

Golli M, Nhieu JTV, Mathieu D, et al (1994) Hepatocellular adenoma: color Doppler US and pathologic correlation. Radiology 190:741–744

Grazioli L, Federle MP, Ichikawa T, et al (2000) Liver adenomatosis: clinical, pathologic, and imaging findings in 15 patients. Radiology 216:395–402

Grazioli L, Federle MP, Brancatelli G, et al (2001) Hepatic adenomas: imaging and pathologic findings. Radiographics 21:877–894

Heiken JP (1998) Liver. In: Lee JKT, Sagal SS, Stanley RJ, et al (eds) Computed body tomography with MRI correlation. Lippincott-Raven, Philadelphia, pp 701–778

Ichikawa T, Federle MP, Grazioli L, et al (2000) Hepatocellular adenoma: multiphasic CT and pathologic findings in 25 patients. Radiology 214:861–868

Ishak K, Anthony P, Sobin L (1994) Histological typing of tumors of the liver. In: WHO International Histological Classification of Tumors, 2nd edn. Springer-Verlag, Berlin

Kawakatsu M, Vilgrain V, Belghiti J, et al (1994) Association of multiple liver cell adenomas with spontaneous intrahepatic portohepatic shunt. Abdom Imaging 19:438–440

Kew MC (1998) Hepatic tumors and cysts. In: Feldman M, Scharschmidt BF, Sleisenger MH (eds) Sleisenger and Fordtran's gastrointestinal and liver disease. WB Saunders, Philadelphia, pp 1364–1387

Labrune P, Trioche P, Duvaltier I, et al (1997) Hepatocellular adenomas in glycogen storaged disease type I and III: a series of 43 patients and review of the literature. J Pediatr Gastroenterol Nutr 24:276–279

Leese T, Farges J, Bismuth H (1998) Liver cell adenomas. Ann Surg 208:558–564

Molina EG, Schiff ER (1999) Benign solid lesion of the liver. In: Schiff ER (ed) Diseases of the liver. Lippincott-Raven, pp 1254–1257

Motoori S, Shinozaki M, Goto N, et al (1997) Case report: congenital absence of the portal vein associated with nodular hyperplasia in the liver. J Gastroenterol Hepatol 12:639–643

Nakasaki H, Tanaka Y, Ohta M, et al (1989) Congenital absence of the portal vein. Ann Surg 210:190–193

Oliver JH, Baron RL, Dod JD, et al (1996) Hepatocellular carcinoma: evaluation with biphasic contrast-enhanced, helical CT. Radiology 199:505–511

Paulson EK, McClellan JS, Washington K, et al (1994) Hepatic adenoma: MR characteristic and correlation with pathologic findings. AJR Am J Roentgenol 163:113–116

Reddy KR, Schiff E (1993) Approach to a liver mass. Semin Liver Dis 13:423–435

Riberio A, Burgart LJ, Nagorney DM et al (1998) Management of liver adenomatosis: results with a conservative surgical approach. Liver Transpl Surg 4:388–398

Rooks JB, Ory HW, Ishak KG, et al (1979) Epidemiology of hepatocellular adenoma: the role of oral contraceptive use. JAMA 242:644–648

Ros PR (1990) Computed tomography-pathologic correlation in hepatic tumors. In: Ferrucci JT, Mathieu DG (eds) Advances in hepatobiliary radiology. CV Mosby, St. Louis, pp 75–108

Rubin R, Lichtenstein G (1993) Hepatic scintigraphy in the evaluation of solitary solid liver masses. J Nucl Med 34:697–705

Soe KL, Soe M, Gluud S (1992) Liver pathology associated with the use of anabolic-androgenic steroids. Liver 12:73–79

Terkivatan T, De Wilt JW, De Man RA, et al (2000) Management of hepatocellular adenoma during pregnancy. Liver 20:186–187

Vogl TJ, Hammerstingl R, Schwarz W, et al (1996) Superparamagnetic iron oxide-enhanced versus gadolinium-enhanced MR imaging for differential diagnosis of focal liver lesions. Radiology 198:881–887

Walness I, Medline A (1982) Role of estrogens as promoters of hepatic neoplasia. Lab Invest 46:313–320

11 Pseudo-Lesions of the Liver

Filipe Caseiro-Alves, Ana Ferreira, and Dider Mathieu

CONTENTS

11.1
Introduction

Liver imaging, currently performed by helical CT and MR, is widely used for the study of focal and diffuse liver disease as well as to obtain angiographic data sets by volumetric 3D reconstructions. The liver, with its dual blood supply, receiving simultaneous arterial (20%) and venous blood (80%), is well suited to cross-sectional imaging, which can provide high intrinsic contrast and temporal resolution, easily depicting the various phases of liver enhancement on dynamic studies performed after the injection of intravenous non-specific, interstitial contrast agents. However, the clear-cut separation of the hepatic phases of liver enhancement routinely achieved by state-of-the-art equipment creates additional problems, mostly related to the presence of perfusion abnormalities resulting in areas of abnormal liver

F. Caseiro-Alves, MD, PhD; A. Ferreira, MD
Department of Radiology, Faculdade de Medicina de Coimbra, Praceta Mota Pinto, 3000 Coimbra, Portugal
D. Mathieu, MD, PhD
Centre de Radiologie, Boulevard de la Republique 1, 13100 Aix en Provence, France

enhancement. In most cases, they are caused by a selective impairment of one of its vascular supplies, either arterial or venous. It is well known that the arterial and portal systems are not independent and may communicate via intrahepatic anastomosis, at the acinus level, using transplexal, transvasal or even transtumoral routes (Fig. 11.1) (Itai and Matsui 1997). Arterioportal shunts can be opened to a further extent in response to a significant portal blood flow reduction or stoppage, which in turn results in a compensatory increase of the arterial flow to the corresponding liver segments. Connections between the intrahepatic vascular systems are not restricted to arterioportal communications but may also occur between the portal vein and the hepatic or systemic veins seen in a variety of conditions such as portal hypertension or in Budd-Chiari syndrome. On other occasions, the liver may be supplied by accessory hepatic arteries such as the inferior diaphragmatic, capsular or hilar arteries (Michels 1966). In the venous counterpart, an accessory network of systemic veins, the so-called "non-portal venous blood" can drain directly into the liver parenchyma as may occur with the parabiliary venous plexus, the cystic veins, the veins of Sappey, or the aberrant drainage of the gastric vein (Itai and Matsui 1999; Matsui et al. 1994). All these feeding vessels may ultimately mimic or conceal focal liver lesions, and thus represent a potential source of interpretation errors. It is therefore important that the radiologist is aware of their true nature, at the same time understanding the basic underlying mechanism of their production.

Besides a pure vascular nature, other focal heterogeneities of the liver parenchyma such as fatty infiltration may be seen on cross-sectional imaging, mimicking focal liver lesions in many cases. Under these circumstances, a multimodality imaging approach may be indispensable to rule out true focal liver lesions. Thus a sound knowledge of the diagnostic capabilities of the various imaging techniques is of the utmost importance to allow a proper choice to be made for the diagnostic workflow of these patients. The present chapter will try to cover the most

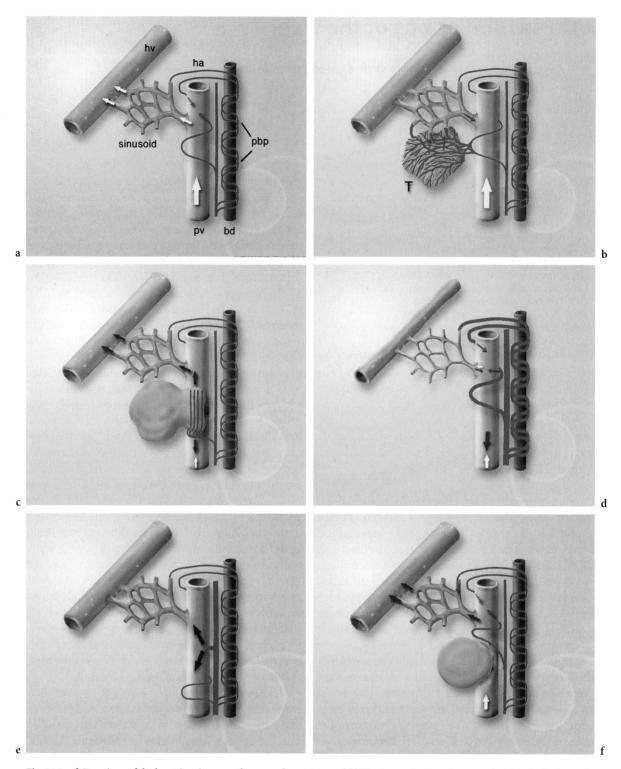

Fig. 11.1a–f. Drawings of the hepatic microvasculature and arterioportal (AP) communications in normal and pathologic conditions. **a** Normal circulation with physiologic AP communications. *ha*, hepatic artery; *hv*, hepatic vein; *pv*, portal vein; *bd*, biliary duct; *pbp*, peribiliary plexus. **b** Tumoral AP shunt via a transtumoral route. *T*, tumor. **c** Tumoral AP shunt via a transvasal (vasa vasorum) route. **d** Cirrhosis with stretching and deformation of hepatic sinusoids causing a compensatory increase of the arterial flow. Note inversion of the direction of the portal vein flow. **e** Iatrogenic AP shunt caused by a fistulous tract after liver biopsy. **f** Portal flow reduction due to extrinsic compression resulting in a compensatory increase of the arterial blood flow. (Courtesy of Yu and Rofsky 2002)

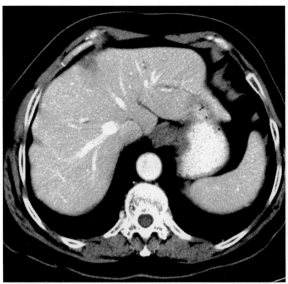
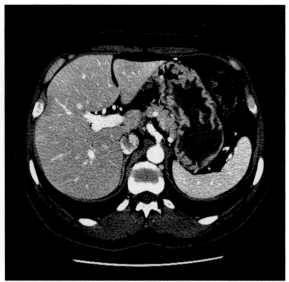

a   b

Fig. 11.2a,b. Pitfalls of liver imaging seen on dynamic multidetector computed Tomography (MDCT) simulating hypodense focal liver lesions due to extrinsic compression caused by diaphragmatic muscle bundles (**a**) and by a rib arch (**b**)

common causes of liver pseudo-lesions seen with cross-sectional imaging, particularly on dynamic helical-CT and MR studies. Several kinds of liver pseudo-lesions have been reported in the literature and they can be broadly divided into three main categories: pitfalls, vascular abnormalities and variants, and focal steatosis.

11.2
Pitfalls

11.2.1
Parenchymal Compression

One of the best known pitfalls, and most commonly seen in the elderly, results from the diaphragmatic compression of liver parenchyma due to uneven contraction of its muscle bundles, creating a hypodense pseudo-nodular area near the dome of the liver, in segments VII and VIII (YOSHIMITSU et al. 2001). The typical location and the observation of the adjacent slices in general readily solve the problem (Fig. 11.2). Another pitfall can be caused by a more medially located rib (in general the seventh to eleventh ribs) that may provoke an extrinsic compression of adjacent parenchyma locally reducing the portal venous flow and mimicking a hypodense focal nodule during the portal phase of liver enhancement. This finding

has been reported to be present in as many as 14% of patients and is most commonly seen in the sub-capsular regions of segments V and VI (YOSHIMITSU et al. 1999).

11.2.2
Unenhanced Vessels

Due to the high temporal resolution achievable nowadays by dynamic studies performed with multislice CT or hypergradient MR, the different phases of liver enhancement can be clearly separated. Since portal and venous vessel enhancement occurs slightly later than arterial enhancement, it may occur at this stage to depict a non-opacified intrahepatic venous vessel. When seen end-on these vascular structures may simulate a hypodense focal nodule, thus mimicking a true focal liver lesion. Besides their typical anatomical distribution, the direct visual comparison with later phases of liver enhancement should be able to rapidly solve the problem and avoid this common pitfall (Fig. 11.3).

11.2.3
Pericaval Fat Collection

Localized fat collections adjacent to the intrahepatic portion of the inferior vena cava have received at-

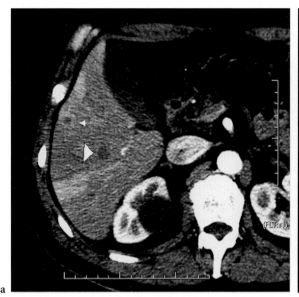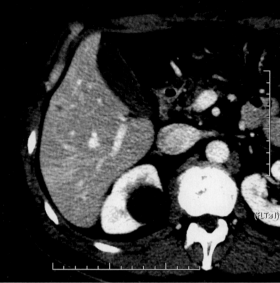

a

b

Fig. 11.3a,b. Dynamic MDCT obtained in a patient with rectal carcinoma during upper abdominal work-up depicting the arterial (**a**) and portal (**b**) phases of liver enhancement. **a** A small 1-centimeter metastasis is depicted showing ring enhancement (*arrow*) as well as two THAD in segments V and VI related to other intrahepatic metastases not shown in the present scans. There is a pseudo-nodular appearance at segment V (*arrowhead*) that could easily mimic a focal malignant deposit. **b** Comparison with the portal phase of liver enhancement clearly shows that the "nodule" corresponds to the unopacified right hepatic vein sliced end-on

tention in recent years because they can be a source of error, mimicking intracaval fat-containing lesions or even lipomatous liver masses (HAN et al. 1997). Although considered an anatomic variation, they are most commonly seen in cases of obesity or chronic liver disease with parenchymal atrophy. The typical location is around the inferior vena cava (IVC) and due to volume averaging effects an intracaval thrombus may even be erroneously diagnosed (Fig. 11.4). In general, observation of the adjacent contiguous slices is enough to solve any diagnostic dilemma, but in doubtful cases a second series of scans obtained at end-expiration can be performed in order to modify the anatomical relationship between the pericaval fat and the vessel itself.

11.3
Vascular Abnormalities and Variants

11.3.1
Portal Venous Inflow Obstruction

Reduction of the portal blood flow to the liver can be due to thrombosis, stricture or compression of the main portal vein or to a more peripheral, intrahepatic compromise. In both cases, on dynamic liver stud-

ies, an area of parenchymal staining on the arterial phase can be seen, reflecting the increased compensatory arterial flow, showing a rapid return to near isodensity on the subsequent portal venous phase of liver enhancement (CHEN et al. 1999). These areas are typically fan-shaped showing a broad peripheral base and may be lobar, segmental, subsegmental or subcapsular in location (Fig. 11.5).

The term "transient hepatic attenuation differences" (THAD) has been coined, a designation that expresses well their transitory nature (ITAI et al. 1987). THAD can obscure or artificially increase the size of a focal liver lesion located within the hyperattenuating fan-shaped area (Fig. 11.6).

It must be stressed that THAD, reflecting a local vascular disturbance, is a rather non-specific imaging feature, since it can be due to other causes than portal flow obstruction such as arteriovenous communications, a subject that will be dealt later in this chapter. In some instances, however, their nature is not apparent and a real intrahepatic vascular mechanism remains to be proved since there may be no associated evidence of a focal liver lesion even on follow-up scans (Fig. 11.7).

Areas of hyperattenuation/hyperintensity of liver enhancement can also be depicted on dynamic CT/MR around inflammatory processes such as liver abscesses or acute cholecystitis artificially increas-

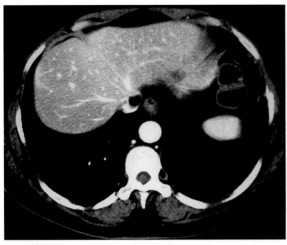
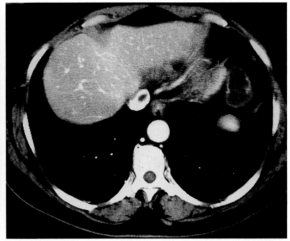

a   b

Fig. 11.4a,b. Helical dynamic CT obtained in a non-cirrhotic patient in end-inspiration and during the portal phase of liver enhancement. There is a small fat collection around the IVC simulating an intracaval thrombus

ing the lesion size (Fig. 11.8). A double mechanism has been pointed out: the local hyperemia related to the inflammatory process itself increases arterial perfusion and the parenchymal compression exerted by the mass further contributes to a locally reduced portal flow (MATHIEU et al. 2001).

Cavernomatous transformation of the portal vein may be another cause for reduction of the portal blood flow to the liver and especially to the most peripheral areas, since the hilar collateral vessels are insufficient to adequately supply the more peripheral liver in contrast to the periportal regions. Dynamic studies may reveal a heterogeneous liver enhancement associated with one or more THAD, reflecting the compensatory increase in the arterial flow (Fig. 11.9).

11.3.2
Hepatic Vein Obstruction

A reduction in the efferent blood flow via the hepatic veins such as seen in Budd-Chiari syndrome causes several liver flow abnormalities which are quite different in the acute and chronic forms of the disease (MATHIEU et al. 1987). In the acute phase, besides obvious liver enlargement, the postsinusoidal obstruction causes a severe reduction in the portal vein flow and a compensatory increase in the arterial flow delivered through the hepatic artery. Since blood flow is not able to perfuse the more peripheral liver areas properly, and since there is a pressure gradient between the arterial vessels and liver veins, functional intrahepatic arterioportal shunts are used that may

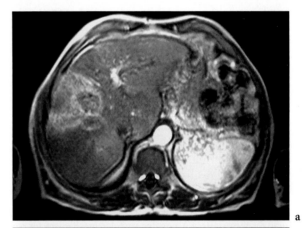

a

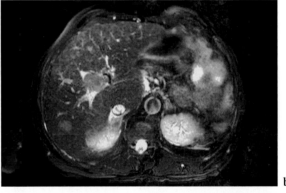

b

Fig. 11.5a,b. MR imaging of a patient with hepatocellular carcinoma and tumor thrombus within the right portal vein. **a** The dynamic liver study obtained at the arterial phase of liver enhancement shows a fan-shaped area of hyperintensity with a broad capsular base corresponding to the THAD in the territory affected by the portal flow interruption. **b** On the T2-weighted fast spin-echo sequence a tumoral portal vein thrombus is depicted causing vessel enlargement

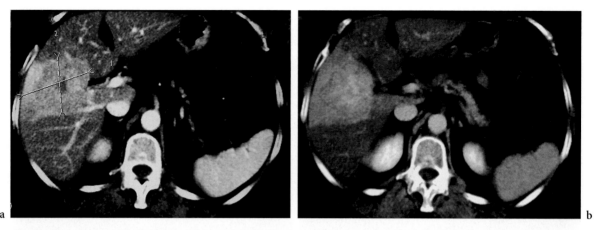

Fig. 11.6a,b. Dynamic helical CT in a patient with hepatic metastasis from lung cancer located at the central liver. **a** Due to its central location with probable portal vein involvement there is a peripheral fan-shaped perfusion abnormality artificially increasing the lesion size. **b** This finding is exacerbated at a later phase of liver enhancement due to the interstitial diffusion of iodinated contrast material within the metastasis

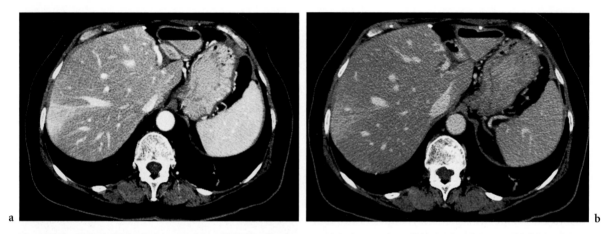

Fig. 11.7a,b. Helical CT depicting a peripheral THAD of unknown origin in a patient with previous history of left liver lobectomy for metastasis. **a** A possible vascular mechanism for the THAD seen on segment VII was presumed since small venous collaterals are seen around the stomach but without discernible portal vein thrombosis or cavernomatous transformation. **b** At a later phase of liver enhancement the THAD returns to near isodensity with the remaining liver. A follow-up CT performed 6 months later did not show any additional abnormalities

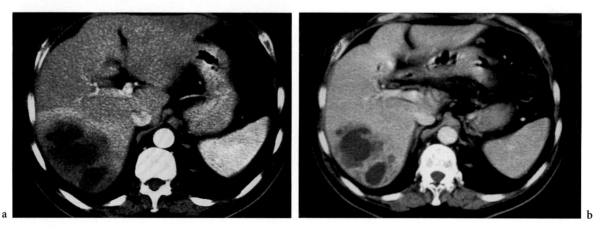

Fig. 11.8a,b. Dynamic CT of liver abscess. **a** There is a peripheral rim of increased attenuation at the late arterial phase of liver enhancement. **b** A later phase of liver enhancement showing return to isodensity

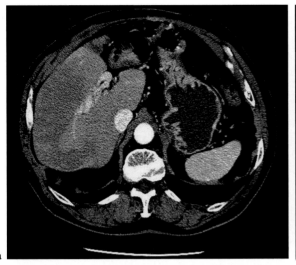
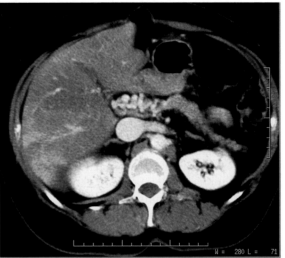

Fig. 11.9a,b. Dynamic multislice helical CT of two cases of portal cavernoma. **a** The collateral hilar vessels show early staining and there is a better perfusion of the central liver displaying enhancement to a higher level compared to the peripheral parenchyma. **b** Another patient showing several peripheral THADs at the right liver lobe

ultimately lead to a complete flow reversal within the portal vein. This phenomenon can be depicted by dynamic CT or MR that will show at the arterial phase of liver enhancement an isolated and vigorous enhancement of the portal vein (Fig. 11.10).

In the later phases of liver enhancement a mottled parenchymal appearance is the net result of the efferent vessel obstruction, causing stasis and distal accumulation of the intravascular contrast material. This imaging finding is, however, not specific to Budd-Chiari syndrome, since it can also be seen in advanced right-sided cardiac failure, explained by the same hemodynamic effects related to the outflow disturbances within the hepatic veins (Fig. 11.11). In the chronic phase of Budd-Chiari disease, the venous obstruction is well established, giving rise to the appearance of typical comma shaped branching vascular structures, corresponding to an intrahepatic network of venous collaterals trying to bypass the obstruction. These abnormal vessels tend to be

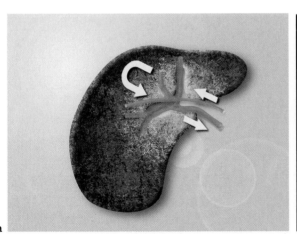
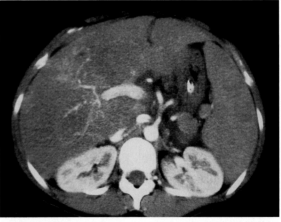

Fig. 11.10a,b. Abnormal liver hemodynamics in the acute phase of Budd-Chiari syndrome. **a** Due to the hepatic venous flow obstruction there is rising pressure in the portal system resulting in reduced intrahepatic portal venous flow and a compensatory increase of the arterial flow. Since there is a normal pressure gradient between the arterial and portal systems, functional AP shunts are used leading to total inversion of the direction of the blood flow within the main portal vein that acts as a draining vein. **b** In the arterial phase of liver enhancement, iodinated blood conveyed by the hepatic artery perfuses the central areas of the liver. Due to the complete flow reversal within the portal vein early and isolated enhancement is observed

more peripherally located and to be most prominent around the caudate lobe due to its separate, autonomous venous drainage.

11.3.3
Intrahepatic Vascular Shunts

Intrahepatic shunts can be divided into tumorous or non-tumorous depending on the underlying cause and into arterioportal, arteriosystemic or portosystemic according to the established vascular connection. Arterioportal shunting (AP shunting) is one of the most common intrahepatic shunts and in general is observed in the context of hepatocellular carcinoma, but it may be iatrogenic and related to prior liver biopsy. Tumoral AP shunting occurs essentially by a transtumoral route, when a direct communication between the feeding arterial vessels of the tumor and the draining portal venules and/or sinusoids is established, resulting in increased arterial flow around the tumor (Fig. 11.1). Since these vascular communications are generally too small, they are below the threshold of detection with cross-sectional imaging, and only the parenchymal perfusion changes are depicted (ITAI and MATSUI 1997; LANE et al. 2000). Imaging findings are thus manifested by a peritumoral THAD whose size depends on the magnitude of the shunt associated with early enhancement of the draining veins (portal or systemic) (Fig. 11.12) (YU and ROFSKY 2002).

Besides the appearance of a THAD and since there is a pressure gradient between the high pressure arterial system and the low pressure portal system, a localized inversion of the portal flow may occur, demonstrated by early enhancement of portal vein branches, during the arterial phase of the dynamic liver study. AP shunts can occur not only with malignant tumors such as hepatocellular carcinoma (HCC) but also with other liver tumors and have been recently demonstrated in association with the so-called "flash-filling" hemangiomas. The underlying mechanism seems to be related to the hyperdynamic status of this benign vascular tumor possessing a large arterial flow, quick enhancement and quick outflow to the draining vein (YU and ROFSKY 2002). In these circumstances flow direction in the draining portal vessel may be inverted (Fig. 11.13).

Apart from tumors and liver biopsy, AP shunts may also be seen in the context of liver cirrhosis due to the parenchymal damage with chronic scarring, ischemia and nodular regeneration, which altogether tend to modify the hepatic flow dynamics (Fig. 11.1d). AP shunts in the cirrhotic patient can be a source of potential confusion with HCC since they may also appear as small arterial enhancing nodules (KIM et al. 1988). The use of MR enhanced with reticuloendothelial superparamagnetic iron oxide agents may be of some use in this regard. In principle, the parenchyma affected by a non-tumorous AP shunt should reveal a signal loss comparable to the normal parenchyma on T2-weighted images, in contrast to the tumoral AP

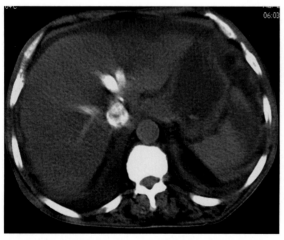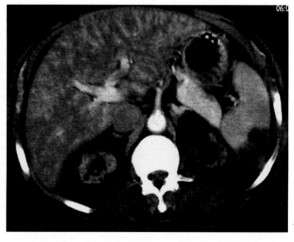

a   b

Fig. 11.11a,b. Dynamic liver MDCT in a patient with severe right-sided cardiac failure and renal insufficiency. **a** Intense reflow of the iodinated contrast agent within the hepatic veins is seen shortly after the i.v. injection in the arm vein, with severe delay of aortic enhancement. **b** Mottled appearance of the liver parenchyma in the later phase of liver enhancement due to stagnation of iodinated contrast material within hepatic sinusoids. There is a hypodense area on the splenic parenchyma corresponding to a local infarction

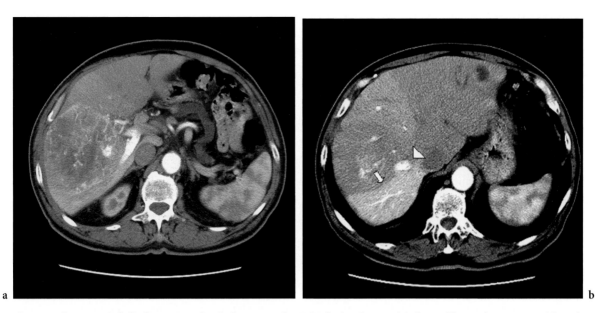

Fig. 11.12a,b. Dynamic helical MDCT study of a hypervascular HCC during the arterial phase of liver enhancement. **a** There is early enhancement of the portal vein consistent with arterioportal shunting. **b** A THAD is also seen in the posterior segments of the right liver lobe (*arrow*). An arteriosystemic fistula was suspected in this case due to the early enhancement of the right hepatic vein (*arrowhead*)

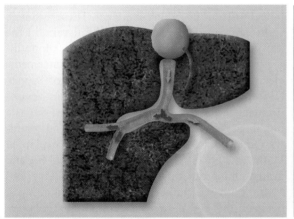

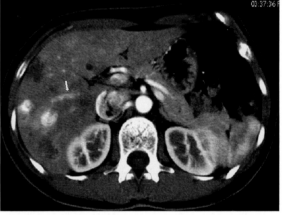

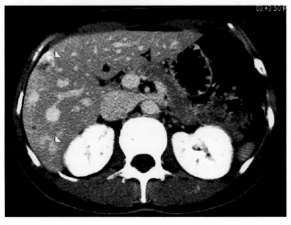

Fig. 11.13a–c. Schematic drawing (**a**) and dynamic CT (**b,c**) of a flash filling hemangioma causing localized inversion of the portal vein flow. The dynamic CT depicts, on the arterial phase of liver enhancement (**b**), two small hypervascular hemangiomas showing early and vigorous enhancement associated with subtle peritumoral enhancement representing perfusion abnormalities. There is concomitant enhancement of a small intrahepatic branch (*arrow*) of the portal vein near one of the hemangiomas leading to localized inversion of the portal blood flow. The right liver lobe also shows two additional hemangiomas (*arrowheads*) that display the usual pattern of enhancement

shunt, which will remain hyperintense, since it is devoid of the Kupffer cells responsible for the contrast media retention (Mori et al. 2000).

Intrahepatic portosystemic venous shunts (IPSVS) consist of the direct communication between the portal vein and the systemic veins and they can also mimic a hypervascular liver lesion. According to Itai et al. (2001), they can be subdivided into internal and external subtypes, depending on whether the portal vein communicates with the hepatic vein (internal type) or with a systemic vein outside the liver (external type). Outside the setting of liver cirrhosis with portal hypertension that may be accompanied by the presence of intra- and extrahepatic portosystemic collateral circulation, IPSVS are seldom seen and a congenital origin has been postulated due to the persistence of an omphalomesenteric venous system with the right horn of the sinus venosus or rupture of a portal vein aneurysm into a hepatic vein (Lane et al. 2000). With the advent of CT and color Doppler, they have been increasingly reported (Itai et al. 2001; Lane et al. 2000). They can be recognized by any cross-sectional imaging method, particularly Doppler sonography, by the demonstration of a direct connection between a dilated segment of the portal vein and the adjacent draining vein (Fig. 11.14). If they attain a large size, hepatic encephalopathy might be induced.

11.3.4
Non-portal Venous Supply to the Liver

In some instances, veins from the digestive organs may not flow into the portal vein trunk, but instead may drain directly into the liver parenchyma. These anatomical variations have been consistently reported, with angiographic demonstration from the splanchnic circulation such as the cystic vein from the gallbladder for segments IV–V, the parabiliary venous system draining the pancreatic head, duodenum and distal stomach for the posterior aspect of segment IV and the aberrant gastric venous drainage from the gastric antrum and pancreatic head to segments I and IV (Fig. 11.15) (Itai and Matsui 1999).

Since parenchymal perfusion to these liver areas does not depend on portal venous blood, they will show lack of enhancement on CT arterial portography, thus mimicking hypodense focal tumors. On intravenous dynamic CT/MR these areas show early enhancement due earlier venous return of less diluted contrast agent when compared with the portal blood flow coming from the intestine and spleen. Since the venous blood supply to these liver areas is subtracted from the normal portal blood flow that carries hormonal substances and other dietary elements, it is not surprising that focal sparing in cases of fatty liver may occur. This imaging finding has been consecutively demonstrated using cross-sectional imaging techniques on the gallbladder bed or in the posterior edge of segment IV (Fig. 11.16). Conversely, focal fatty infiltration can also occur in the hilar region of segment IV, or adjacent to the gallbladder neck. The explanation for this local distribution remains unclear, but when segment IV receives its venous blood supply directly from the pancreas it is exposed to higher levels of insulin, which may act as a promoting factor (Itai and Matsui 1999).

Apart from the vascular variants of the splanchnic circulation other systemic venous shunts can be associated with liver pseudo-lesions, as is the case in superior vena cava obstruction with subsequent development of a collateral thoracic circulation by intermediates of the intercostal veins, the internal mammary, hemiazygos and paravertebral veins. These veins ultimately connect the superior epigastric vein to the portal system via the paraumbilical veins at the round ligament. These systemic veins can end deeply in the umbilical vein, in the left portal vein or can enter the left liver lobe directly around the falciform ligament by intermediates of the paraumbilical inferior veins of Sappey (Hashimoto et al. 2002). This systemic venous drainage to the liver has also been pointed out as a possible explanation for the cases of focal fatty infiltration around the falciform ligament as explained by the low portal blood flow causing local hepatic injury and promoting fatty infiltration (Itai and Matsui 1999). Another rare anastomotic network between the portal and systemic circulations can be seen through the veins of the coronary and falciform ligaments interconnecting the diaphragmatic veins to the portal system.

In cases of superior vena cava obstruction, the recruitment of the collateral circulation can cause a dense focal parenchymal stain in the early phases of liver enhancement around the round ligament, the left portal vein or even in more remote subcapsular areas, corresponding to the early arrival of a considerable amount of minimally diluted contrast agent to these areas of liver parenchyma (Maldjian et al. 1995). The parenchymal staining in these cases can be so intense that it can mimic a true hypervascular neoplasm (Fig. 11.17).

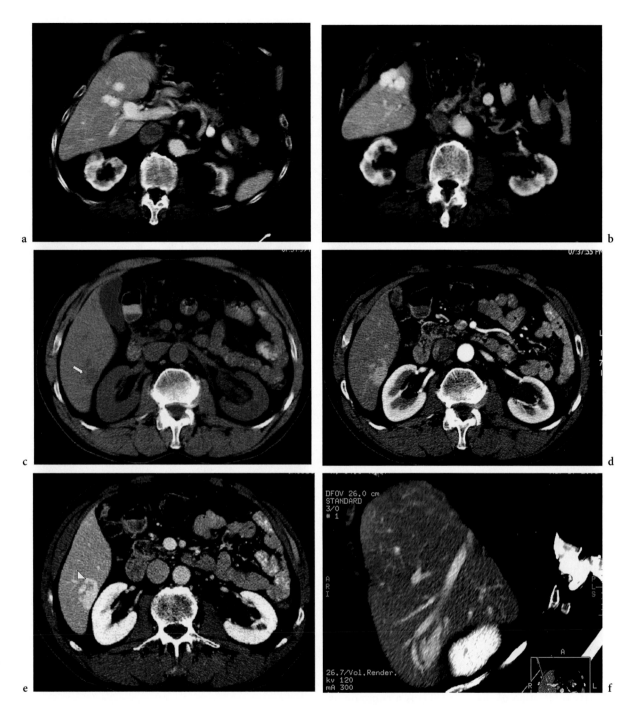

Fig. 11.14a–f. Multislice helical CT of intrahepatic portosystemic venous shunts of the external (**a,b**) and internal subtypes (**c–f**). **a** Portal venous phase of liver enhancement depicting an abnormal vessel adjacent to the portal vein. **b** This venous vessel runs to the periphery of segment V interconnecting with subcapsular systemic veins. **c** Another case showing on plain CT a hypodense nodule on segment VI (*arrow*). **d,e** Arterial and portal phases of dynamic liver study showing progressive enhancement of the "nodule" to the same extent as portal vessels. An abnormal branching structure corresponding to the connecting vein can be seen (*arrowhead*). **f** MIP reconstruction showing the direct connection of the intrahepatic "nodule" with the right hepatic vein

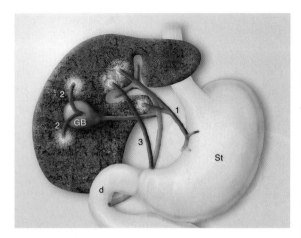

Fig. 11.15. Schematic drawing of non-portal splanchnic perfusion to the liver parenchyma. 1, aberrant gastric vein drainage to segments I and IV; 2, cystic veins to segments IV and V; 3, parabiliary venous system to the posterior aspect of segment IV; GB, gallbladder; ST, stomach; d, duodenum

11.3.5
Steal Phenomena

Another cause of abnormal liver enhancement can be seen in the arterial phase around highly vascularized liver neoplasms. In the dynamic study, the liver around a hypervascular neoplasm can be significantly hypodense compared to the remainder of the normal parenchyma since the iodinated arterial blood flow is strongly diverted to feed the hypervascular liver lesion. This phenomenon may be seen around benign or malignant liver tumors, which are essentially dependent on the amount of arterial vascularization of the hepatic neoplasm (Fig. 11.18). The phenomenon is transitory and in the portal venous phase of liver enhancement it returns to isodensity.

11.4
Focal Fatty Infiltration and Focal Fatty Sparing

Fatty infiltration of the liver (FFI) is a common asymptomatic condition reported to be present in as much as 10% of the adult population and is usually associated with a variety of clinical situations, of which alcoholism, diabetes and obesity are the most common in the developed countries (EL-HASSAN et al. 1992). There are many other reported causes that include inborn metabolic errors, drug toxicity, glucocorticoid therapy, and infections (ALPERS et al. 1993). KAMMEN et al. (2001) described an overall incidence of focal fatty liver in as many as 9% of children and

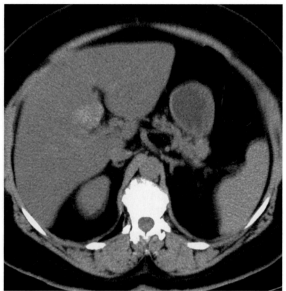

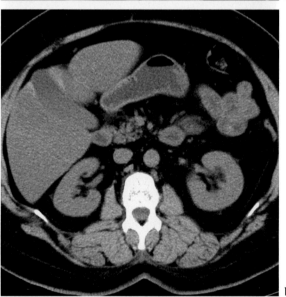

Fig. 11.16a,b. Obese patient with low hepatic attenuation consistent with diffuse steatosis. Areas of focal fatty sparing displaying normal attenuation values are recognized at the posterior aspect of segment IV (**a**) and adjacent to the gallbladder fossa (**b**)

young adults so the disease is not exclusively seen in adult patients. In patients displaying fatty liver infiltration, about 31% may possess focal forms consisting of multiple or solitary nodular foci (EL-HASSAN et al. 1992). Several etiologic explanations have been advanced for the focal cases of liver steatosis. The most commonly accepted theory is related to local disturbances of liver perfusion since the laminar flow of the splenic vein entering the portal vein is not

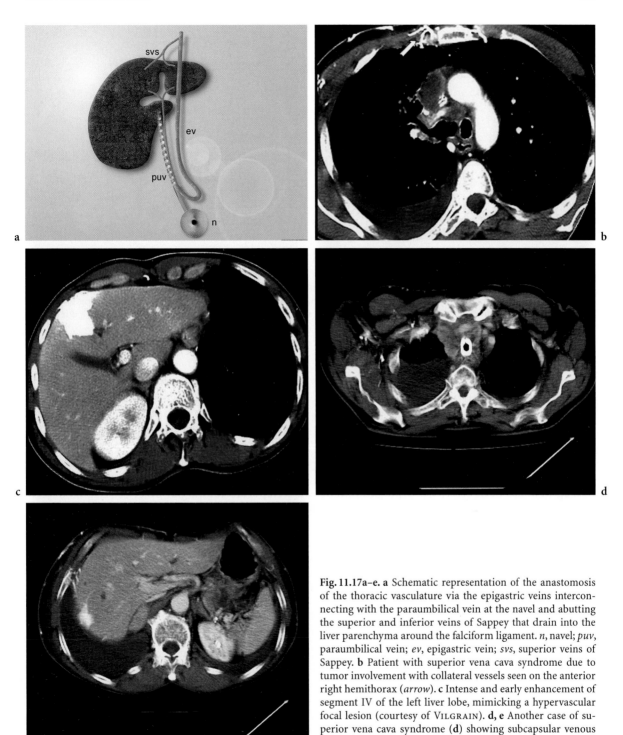

Fig. 11.17a–e. a Schematic representation of the anastomosis of the thoracic vasculature via the epigastric veins interconnecting with the paraumbilical vein at the navel and abutting the superior and inferior veins of Sappey that drain into the liver parenchyma around the falciform ligament. *n*, navel; *puv*, paraumbilical vein; *ev*, epigastric vein; *svs*, superior veins of Sappey. **b** Patient with superior vena cava syndrome due to tumor involvement with collateral vessels seen on the anterior right hemithorax (*arrow*). **c** Intense and early enhancement of segment IV of the left liver lobe, mimicking a hypervascular focal lesion (courtesy of VILGRAIN). **d, e** Another case of superior vena cava syndrome (**d**) showing subcapsular venous collateral vessels at the right liver lobe leading to a hyperdense pseudo-tumoral focal lesion (**e**).

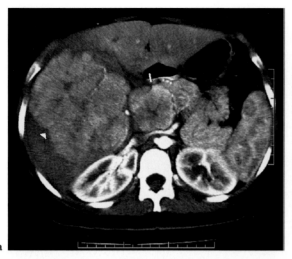
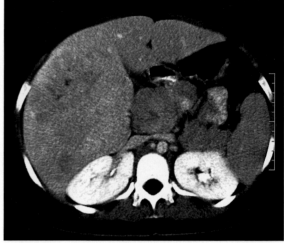

a   b

Fig. 11.18a,b. Dynamic helical CT of a hypervascular liver metastasis from non-functioning malignant neuroendocrine pancreatic tumor. **a** The primary tumor (*arrow*) and the liver metastasis (*arrowhead*) are similarly enhanced during the arterial phase of liver enhancement. The parenchyma around the metastasis is less dense than the normal left liver lobe due to steal phenomena. This finding is transitory and not depicted in the later phases of the dynamic study (**b**)

exposed to hormones and other lipotropic-promoting substances that arise via the superior mesenteric vein, which is preferentially directed towards the right liver lobe (ITAI and MATSUI 1999; ARAI et al. 1988; ARITA et al. 1996; BAKER et al. 1985). Other causes, also of vascular origin, are related to the presence of anatomical variants in liver vasculature, comprising what has been described as the third inflow feeding vessel, which was discussed earlier in this chapter. Since these aberrant vessels carry non-portal, nutrient-poor blood flow towards the liver, one should expect that focal fatty sparing (FFS) should arise instead of FFI. However, for reasons that for the time being are unclear, both kinds of pseudo-lesions can be observed (ITAI and MATSUI 1999; GABATA et al. 1997; TOCHIO et al. 1999). The aberrant vessels tend to perfuse specific liver areas, so abnormalities are confined to expected locations within the parenchyma, following a relatively constant pattern. The areas involved are thus commonly observed near the falciform ligament, the gallbladder, the posterior aspect of segment IV, the anterior aspect of segment I and the subcapsular regions (Fig. 11.16) (ITAI and MATSUI 1999; ARAI et al. 1988).

Since these liver areas do not receive portal blood flow, it is also not surprising that they can be a source for the pseudo-lesions seen on angiographically assisted CT arterial portography, where they are represented by focal non-enhancing areas,

ultimately leading to the high number of false positives reported for this technique (BLUEMKE et al. 1995; PAULSON et al. 1993). Another vascular change that has been implied in the development of focal fatty infiltration relates to liver hypoxia, mainly observed on the more peripheral subcapsular parenchyma. Finally, focal fatty sparing can be caused by arterioportal shunting or other causes that deprive the portal blood flow to the affected areas of the parenchyma, such as compression or occlusion of the portal vein (ARITA et al. 1996). The diagnosis of the diffuse forms of hepatic steatosis is in general straightforward, since it consists of a diffuse increase in liver echogeneity on ultrasound or hypodensity on CT scans, producing no apparent vascular distortion, amputation or mass effect. In contrast to the diffuse forms, however, the diagnosis of the focal forms can be very troublesome since the foci of fatty infiltration are in general too small to be able to produce significant vessel distortion or expectable mass effect. Focal fatty infiltration is a frequent source of liver pseudo-lesions and may mimic other true focal lesions known to be primarily hyperechoic on sonography such as hemangiomas, metastases from digestive tract or endocrine tumors. On CT they can mimic hypodense secondary liver deposits or other primaries such as adenoma and HCC, and problems in the differential diagnosis are exacerbated by the fact that density measurements are not reliable due to an overlap between FFI and true hypodense focal liver lesions.

For many years it has been known that MR is the best way to adequately characterize fat (Thu et al. 1991). Fat causes T1-shortening, so FFI is in general brighter on T1-weighted images, an effect that is more pronounced at lower field strengths, since the T1 relaxation time of fat is directly proportional to the intensity of the static magnetic field. However, T1 hyperintensity is not a specific finding for fat, and other diagnostic possibilities can be proposed, such as hemorrhage, melanin-containing nodules or peliosis (Mathieu et al. 1997). To adequately characterize fat on MR it is mandatory to use some kind of chemical-shift imaging, a technique that explores the difference in resonant frequencies between water and fat, which, at 1.5 T, are separated by 220 Hz. Chemical shift imaging can be done by integrating an additional destructive radiofrequency pulse to the sequence design centered on the resonant frequency of fat. These sequences are known as fat-saturated (fat-sat) and they are able to nullify the signal generated from fatty tissues.

FFI and FFS share, on MR, the same morphological aspects as other imaging modalities, but on MR they tend to appear isointense and virtually undetectable on FATSAT T2-weighted and T1-weighted images, which are helpful features for differentiation from true focal liver lesions (Fig. 11.19). Another approach to characterizing fat is currently performed by the technique of phase cancellation (opposed-phase imaging), which has gained a wide popularity due to its ease of performance and excellent results in the demonstration of the milder forms of FFI (Hood et al. 1999). This technique is based on the different precession velocities of fat and water observed after excitation in the transverse plane and the condition to be observed is that water and fat coexist in the same tissue voxel. At 1.5 T and using a T1-weighted gradient-echo sequence, the signal intensity of water and fat protons is additive every 4.2 ms (in-phase) and subtractive, due to phase cancellation phenomena, in between, that is, adding an extra 2.1 ms to the original TE value. This means that, simply by varying the echo time (TE) of a T1-weighted gradient-echo sequence, the operator can obtain in-phase or opposed-phase images for the tissues under appreciation. State-of-the-art equipment can currently obtain a simultaneous set of images respectively in and out-of-phase in the same single breath-hold period, matching exactly for visual comparison of the pertinent anatomy. The

opposed-phase images are readily recognized due to the presence of a thin black rim delineating the solid organs in contact with intra-abdominal fat due to phase cancellation in areas of abrupt change in signal intensity (Rofsky et al. 1996). This kind of chemical-shift imaging is more effective at higher field strengths, which maximizes the resonant frequency difference between water and fat (Fig. 11.20).

In practical terms, the signal intensity of the liver and/or of any suspected nodule is subject to a direct visual assessment of the signal intensity comparative to the spleen, an organ where signal intensity remains unaltered between the two sets of images. When defining the protocol for the breath-hold GRE in opposed-phase sequence it is usually preferable to choose between the lowest possible TE values, not only to allow an increased number of slices to be acquired, but also to minimize any T2 interference that could lead to confusion, notably with liver signal intensity drop-out, caused, for instance, by a previously unsuspected iron deposition. Despite the exquisite information provided by MR and chemical-shift imaging, the mere characterization of fat may not be enough to allow the straightforward exclusion of liver tumors that may contain fat such as hepatocellular carcinoma, adenoma or, more rarely, angiomyolipoma. Dynamic MR using gadolinium chelates adds additional arguments to the accurate diagnosis of fatty pseudo-lesions against true focal fatty liver masses. In contrast to FFI, hepatocellular carcinoma, adenoma and even angiomyolipomas may be distinguished by their strong enhancement on the arterial phase of the dynamic study, reflecting its hypervascular nature, and also by their expected heterogeneity (Yoshimura et al. 2002). Whenever doubt remains, MR can again provide additional arguments with the use of more sophisticated specific contrast agents targeted to Kupffer cells or hepatocytes, such as iron-oxide particles and mangafodipir. With this approach, a significant uptake of both classes of contrast agent by fatty pseudo-tumors is expected, in contrast to true focal liver lesions, which contain fat components but are devoid of Kupffer cells. As a note of caution it must be emphasized, however, that both a less pronounced and an increased signal drop-out in the areas of FFI compared to normal liver parenchyma have been reported when using iron-oxide enhanced MR, probably reflecting quantitative and/or qualitative alterations of the Kupffer cells inside the areas of FFI (Hirohashi et al. 2000; Lwakatare et al. 2001).

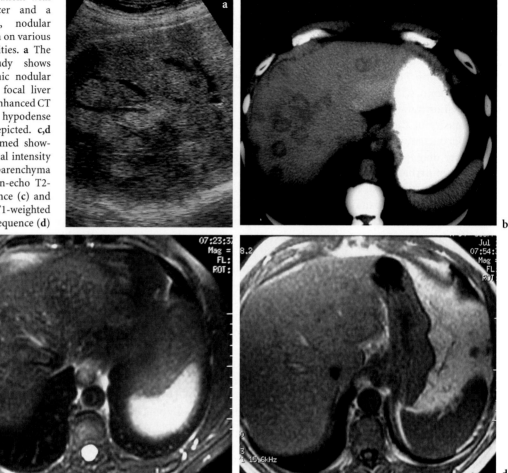

Fig. 11.19a–d. Patient with colorectal cancer and a pseudo-tumoral, nodular form of FFI seen on various imaging modalities. **a** The ultrasound study shows several echogenic nodular foci simulating focal liver lesions. **b** Non-enhanced CT where several hypodense nodules are depicted. **c,d** MR was performed showing normal signal intensity of the liver parenchyma both in the spin-echo T2-weighted sequence (**c**) and in the in-phase T1-weighted gradient-echo sequence (**d**)

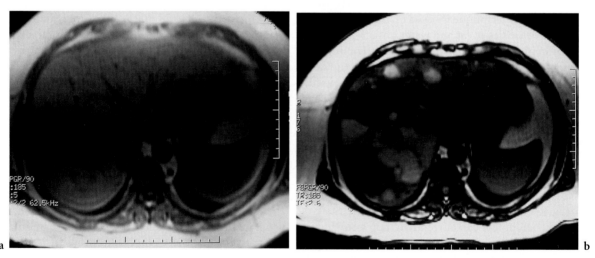

Fig. 11.20a,b. Opposed-phase imaging for MR depiction and characterization of FFI on gradient-echo T1-weighted images is advantageous. **a** In the in-phase image the liver is practically homogeneous, but on opposed-phase imaging (**b**) areas of FFI become hypointense compared to the signal intensity of the spleen. A pseudo-tumoral form of FFS is now apparent corresponding to the nodular areas of liver parenchyma devoid of fatty infiltration

References

Alpers DH, Sabesin SM, White HM (1993) Fatty liver: biochemical and clinical aspects. In: Schiff L, Schiff E (eds) Diseases of the liver, 7th edn. JB Lippincott, Philadelphia

Arai K, Matsui O, Takashima T, et al (1988) Focal spared areas in fatty liver caused by regional decreased portal flow. AJR Am J Roentgenol 151:300–302

Arita T, Matsunaga N, Homma Y, et al (1996) Focally spared area of fatty liver caused by arterioportal shunt. J Comput Assist Tomogr 20:360–362

Baker MK, Wenker JC, Cockerill EM, et al (1985) Focal fatty infiltration of the liver: diagnostic imaging. Radiographics 5:923–929

Bluemke DA, Soyer P, Fishman EK (1995) Non-tumorous low attenuation defects in the liver on helical CT during arterial portography: frequency, location and appearance. AJR Am J Roentgenol 164:1141–1145

Chen WP, Chen JH, Hwang JI, et al (1999) Spectrum of transient hepatic attenuation differences in biphasic helical CT. AJR Am J Roentgenol 172:419–424

el-Hassan AY, Ibrahim EM, al-Mulhim FA, et al (1992) Fatty infiltration of the liver: analysis of prevalence, radiological and clinical features and influence on patient management. Br J Radiol 65:774–778

Gabata T, Matsui O, Kadoya M, et al (1997) Aberrant gastric venous drainage in focal fatty liver of segment IV: demonstration with color Doppler sonography. Radiology 203:461–463

Han BK, Im JG, Jung JW, et al (1997) Pericaval fat collection that mimics thrombosis of the inferior vena cava: demonstration with use of multi-directional reformation CT. Radiology 203:105–108

Hashimoto M, Heianna J, Tate E, et al (2002) Small veins entering the liver. Eur Radiol 12:2000–2005

Hirohashi S, Ueda K, Uchida H, et al (2000) Nondiffuse fatty change of the liver: discerning pseudo-tumor on MR images enhanced with ferumoxides. Initial observations. Radiology 217:415–420

Hood MN, Ho VB, Smirniotopoulos JG (1999) Chemical shift: the artifact and clinical tool revisited. Radiographics 19:357–371

Itai Y, Matsui O (1997) Blood flow and liver imaging. Radiology 202:306–314

Itai Y, Matsui O (1999) "Non-portal" splanchnic venous supply to the liver: abnormal findings on CT, US and MRI. Eur Radiol 9:237–243

Itai Y, Hachiya J, Makita K, et al (1987) Transient hepatic attenuation differences at dynamic computed tomography. J Comput Assist Tomogr 11:461–465

Itai Y, Saida Y, Irie T, et al (2001) Intrahepatic portosystemic venous shunts: spectrum of CT findings in external and internal subtypes. J Comput Assist Tomogr 25:348–354

Kammen BF, Pacharn P, Thoeni RF, et al (2001) Focal fatty infiltration of the liver: analysis of prevalence and CT findings in children and young adults. AJR Am J Roentgenol 177:1035–1039

Kim TK, Choi BI, Chung JW, et al (1988) Nontumorous arterioportal shunt mimicking hypervascular tumor in the cirrhotic liver: two-phase spiral CT findings. Radiology 208:597–603

Lane MJ, Jeffrey B, Katz DS (2000) Spontaneous intrahepatic vascular shunts. AJR Am J Roentgenol 174:125–131

Lwakatare F, Yamashita Y, Nakayama M, et al (2001) SPIO-enhanced MR imaging of focal fatty liver lesions. Abdom Imaging 26:157–160

Maldjian P, Obolevich A, Cho K (1995) Focal enhancement of the liver on CT. A sign of SVC obstruction. J Comput Assist Tomogr 19:316–318

Mathieu D, Vasile N, Menu Y, et al (1987) Budd-Chiari syndrome. Dynamic CT. Radiology 165:409–413

Mathieu D, Paret M, Mahfouz AE (1997) Hyperintense benign liver lesions on spin-echo T1-weighted MR images: pathologic correlations. Abdom Imaging 22:410–417

Mathieu D, Luciani A, Achab A, et al (2001) Hepatic pseudolesions. Gastroenterol Clin Biol 25 (Suppl 4):B158–166

Matsui O, Takahashi S, Kadoya M, et al (1994) Pseudo-lesion in segment IV of the liver at CT during arterial portography: correlation with aberrant gastric venous drainage. Radiology 193:31–36

Michels NA (1966) Newer anatomy of the liver and its variant blood supply and collateral circulation. Am J Surg 112:337–347

Mori K, Yoshioka H, Itai Y, et al (2000) Arterioportal shunts in cirrhotic patients: evaluation of the difference between tumorous and nontumorous arterioportal shunts on MR imaging with superparamagnetic iron oxide. AJR Am J Roentgenol 175:1659–1664

Paulson EK, Baker ME, Spritzer CE, et al (1993) Focal fatty infiltration: a cause of nontumorous defects in the left hepatic lobe during CT arterial portography. J Comput Assist Tomogr 17:590–595

Rofsky NM, Weinreb JC, Ambrosino MM, et al (1996) Comparison between in-phase and opposed-phase T1-weighted breath hold flash sequences for hepatic imaging. J Comput Assist Tomogr 20:230–235

Thu TH, Mathieu D, Nguyen-Than T, et al (1991) Value of MR imaging in evaluating focal fatty infiltration of the liver: preliminary results. Radiographics 11:1003–1012

Tochio H, Kudo M, Okabe Y, et al (1999) Association between a focal spared area in the fatty liver and intrahepatic efferent blood flow from the gallbladder wall: evaluation with color Doppler sonography. AJR Am J Roentgenol 172:1249–1253

Yoshimitsu K, Honda H, Kuroiwa T, et al (1999) Pseudolesion of the liver possibly caused by focal rib compression: analysis based on hemodynamic change. AJR Am J Roentgenol 172:645–649

Yoshimitsu K, Honda H, Kuroiwa T, et al (2001) Unusual hemodynamics and pseudolesions of the noncirrhotic liver at CT. Radiographics 21:S81–S96

Yoshimura H, Murakami T, Kim T, et al (2002) Angiomyolipoma of the liver with least amount of fat component: imaging features of CT, MR, and angiography. Abdom Imaging 27:184–187

Yu JS, Rofsky NM (2002) Magnetic resonance imaging of arterioportal shunts in the liver. Top Magn Reson Imaging 13:165–176

Primary Malignancies in Cirrhotic Liver

12 Clinico-Pathological Features of Hepatocellular Carcinoma

Massimo Colombo and Guido Ronchi

CONTENTS

12.1 Introduction

Hepatocellular carcinoma (HCC) is a major health problem worldwide due to its high incidence (approximately 600,000 new cases in 2000), and severe natural history. Indeed, the incidence and mortality rates associated with this disease significantly overlap worldwide (Parkin et al. 2001). The identification of chronic liver disease as the relevant risk factor for this tumor has made surveillance aimed at early detection of HCC possible and surveillance is now universally recognized to be the practical approach for improving the treatment of HCC patients (Bruix et al. 2001). The few cases (<5%) of HCCs that do not develop with a background of chronic liver disease present late and usually have poor prognosis (Bralet et al. 2000). The understanding of both the natural history and staging of HCC is hampered by the epidemiologic and clinical variability of the tumor. This, in turn, is influenced by the concurrence of multiple co-morbidity factors in the same patient as well as by the presence of multiple distinct cell lines in the liver that may develop into liver cell cancer (Sell 2002).

M. Colombo, MD; G. Ronchi, MD
Department of Gastroenterology and Endocrinology, IRCCS Maggiore Hospital, University of Milan, Via Pace 9, 20122 Milano, Italy

12.2 The Pathological Classification

HCC is classified as nodular, massive or diffuse. The nodular type occurs as a nodule sharply delineated from the surrounding liver. The massive type occupies a large area and infiltrates the neighboring hepatic tissue with satellite nodules. The diffuse type is characterized by the diffuse involvement of the liver (Kojiro 1997). All three forms of HCC occur with a background of chronic liver disease or of an otherwise normal liver. The growth pattern of HCC may be infiltrative, expanding, multinodular and mixed type. Based on histology, the WHO proposed a classification of HCC into trabecular, acinar, compact and scirrhous (Gibson and Sobin 1978). In the trabecular type, tumor cells are arranged in cords of variable cell thickness separated by sinusoids, with minimal or no fibrosis (Fig. 12.1). The acinar (pseudoglandular) type is characterized by cells arranged in gland-like structures, filled with cellular debris, exudates and macrophages (Figs. 12.2, 12.3). The compact type shows tumor cells that are packed in a solid mass with inconspicuous sinusoids (Fig. 12.4). In the scirrhous type, significant fibrous tissue separates cords of tumor cells. Each histological type is

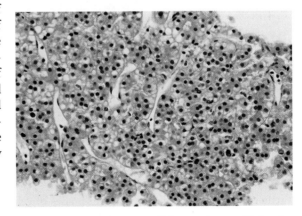

Fig. 12.1. Trabecular hepatocellular carcinoma. Trabecular pattern of well-differentiated neoplastic hepatocytes arranged in plates which are between three and four cells in thickness (×30)

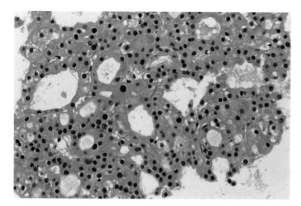

Fig. 12.2. Acinar hepatocellular carcinoma. Prevalence of acinar pattern of well-differentiated hepatocytes arranged in acini with dilated lumen (×30)

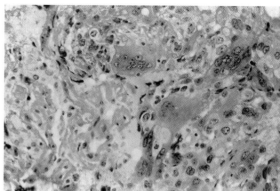

Fig. 12.5. Undifferentiated hepatocellular carcinoma. Pleomorphic liver cells growing in solid pattern with evidence of many syncytial giant cells (×75)

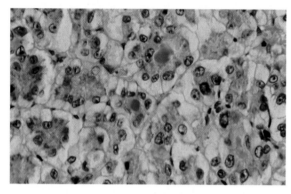

Fig. 12.3. Acinar clear-cell hepatocellular carcinoma. Clear-cell hepatocytes are arranged in glands with lumen filled by biliary plugs (×120)

12.3
Early Detected Tumors

Surveillance of patients with cirrhosis has led to an increasing number of cancers detected early in the form of small nodules that first appear as well-differentiated tumors and proliferate along with gradual dedifferentiation (KOJIRO 1998). A sizable number of tumors arising in cirrhotic livers seem to occur in a multicentric distribution and a certain proportion of them may arise from dysplastic nodules (INTERNATIONAL WORKING PARTY 1995). HCCs ranging from 1–2 cm in size may present with a fibrous capsule and/or fibrous septa in contrast to other indistinct nodular small cancers that have indistinct margins despite such tumors being clearly detected as hypoechoic or hyperechoic focal lesions on ultrasound (US) examination. The latter have been considered carcinoma in situ of the liver due to the absence of invasion into the portal vein branches and intrahepatic metastases (KOJIRO 2002). Minute HCCs of the indistinct nodular type are difficult to differentiate from high grade dysplastic nodules. The majority of small (less than 1.5 cm) HCCs of the indistinct nodular type are not detected as hypervascular tumors by contrast imaging, whereas distinct nodular type tumors almost invariably show hypervascular features during the arterial phase of contrast imaging (KOJIRO 2002). A combination of the lack of fibrotic capsule and reduced number of unpaired arteries per square millimeter in less than 1.5 cm tumors accounts for many false negative diagnoses of HCC with contrast imaging. Since well-differentiated tumors in the early stages proliferate along with the occurrence of gradual dedifferentiation (KOJIRO 1998), more histological grades are seen in tumors greater than 1 cm in size. A "nodule-in-nodule"

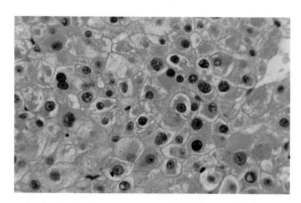

Fig. 12.4. Solid hepatocellular carcinoma. Nodular growth of neoplastic hepatocytes with prominent nucleoli. The cells grow in solid sheets with few vascular channels (×120)

further classified according to different grades of cell differentiation. Well differentiated HCC is a trabecular tumor with two- to three-cell thick cords. The anaplastic tumor usually shows a solid growth pattern, with pleomorphic and giant syncytial cells (Fig. 12.5).

appearance has been documented in less differentiated tumors expanding with a clear boundary within a well-differentiated tumor.

Biopsy examination of 1–2 cm nodules in patients with cirrhosis often implies differential diagnosis between a well-differentiated HCC and a large regenerative nodule. Histological changes seen in a biopsied nodule are best evaluated in comparison with those of control extranodular tissue from the same liver (Table 12.1) (Borzio et al. 1994). Moderately differentiated HCC has a typical trabecular pattern, whereas poorly differentiated HCC may show a trabecular, solid or sarcomatous like pattern.

12.4
Special Types of Tumors

Special types of HCC have distinct histologic patterns and natural history: fibrolamellar carcinoma, clear cell HCC and pedunculated HCC. Fibrolamellar carcinoma is composed of large eosinophilic cells arranged in thin or thick trabeculae that are surrounded by fibrous bounds with lamellar stranding

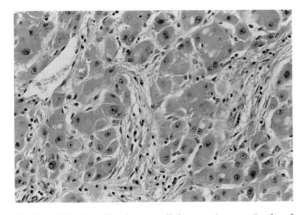

Fig. 12.6. Fibrolamellar hepatocellular carcinoma. Cords of neoplastic liver cells are separated by lamellar fibrous strands (×75)

(Fig. 12.6). The tumor occurs primarily in non-cirrhotic livers of young adults with equal frequency in males and females. In the USA the incidence of this tumor is approximately 1% of all HCCs. Serum α-fetoprotein (AFP) is elevated in a minority of the patients. In half the patients, an abdominal X-ray reveals minute calcifications within the tumor that are uncommon in HCC. The fact that the tumor is sharply demarcated and arises in non-cirrhotic livers

makes fibrolamellar carcinoma more often suitable for resection than the usual HCC (Craig 1997).

12.5
Diagnosis

Both cytohistologic criteria and non-invasive criteria allow diagnosis of HCC (Table 12.2). In patients with chronic liver disease, large tumors are easily diagnosed by combining clinical and radiological procedures. Arterial hypervascularization by triphasic spiral CT or MR of a liver mass identified by abdominal US, is diagnostic for HCC (Bruix et al. 2001). Diagnosis is further confirmed by greater than 400 ng/ml serum levels of AFP. During the arterial phase of spiral CT highly vascularized HCCs appear against a background of relatively unenhanced liver that is primarily contrasted during the late portal vein phase. In patients not fulfilling these diagnostic criteria, the diagnosis of HCC is made by echo-guided aspiration cytology or microhistology (Bruix et al. 2001). The histological diagnosis of HCC is needed in the absence of contraindications and when a definite diagnosis may influence the choice of treatment. The diagnosis of small HCCs (1–2 cm in diameter) identified by chance or during surveillance, may be difficult. In principle, a lesion seen as either a hypoechoic or hyperechoic nodule in the liver of a patient with chronic liver disease should be presumed to be a preneoplastic lesion, like a macroregenerative nodule, or an HCC, and should be investigated accordingly. For tumors of 1–2 cm in diameter the risk of false negative diagnoses with contrast imaging technique could be as high as 50% due to immature arterial vascularization of the nodule (Kojiro 2002). The highest diagnostic accuracy (85%) for these nodules was provided by the combined use of fine needle aspiration cytology plus intranodular and extranodular fine needle microhistology (Table 12.1) (Borzio et al. 1994). Complications in patients subjected to

Table 12.1. Diagnostic accuracy of fine-needle aspiration (A) and biopsy (B) of 36≤2-cm nodules developing in patients with compensated cirrhosis

Liver sampling	Accuracy
Intra- + extranodular A+B	85%
Intranodular A+B	78%
Intra- + extranodular B	67%
Intranodular B	54%
Intranodular A	31%

fine-needle biopsy are hemoperitoneum (<0.5%) and tumor seeding along the needle track (3%–5%) (Takamori et al. 2000; Kim et al. 2000). Recently, 3D image reconstruction techniques by MR was proven to be superior to spiral CT in the diagnosis of HCC nodules of 1–2 cm in size (84% vs 47% detection rates). As expected both imaging techniques failed to recognize tumors of less than 1 cm in diameter (32% vs 10% detection rates) as a consequence of poor arterialization of small nodules (Table 12.3) (Burrel

Table 12.2. Diagnostic criteria for hepatocellular carcinoma as proposed during the Conference of the European Association for the Study of the Liver in Barcelona

- Cytohistologic criteria
- Non-invasive criteria (cirrhotic patients)

  1. Radiological criteria:
     Two coincident imaging techniques[a]
     Focal lesion >2 cm with arterial hypervascularization

  2. Combined criteria:
     One imaging technique associated to AFP
     Focal lesion >2 cm with arterial hypervascularization
     AFP levels >400 ng/ml

[a]Four techniques considered: US, spiral CT, MR and angiography.

Table 12.3. Superiority of magnetic resonance (MR) angiography with respect to helical computerized tomography (CT) for detection of early hepatocellular carcinoma prior to liver transplantation

Tumor size (mm)	Number of tumors	Detected by MR	Detected by CT	pValue
<10	22	7 (22%)	2 (10%)	n.s.
11–20	19	16 (84%)	9 (47%)	p=0.04
>20	6	6 (100%)	6 (100%)	n.s.

et al. 2003). Cases not resolved by imaging or liver biopsy should be followed up with imaging techniques performed at 3-month intervals (enhanced follow-up), until diagnosis is obtained (Fig. 12.7). The differential diagnosis of HCC or fibrolamellar carcinoma includes focal nodular hyperplasia, metastatic carcinomas, neuroendocrine carcinoma and cholangiocarcinoma (Craig 1997).

12.6
Staging

Staging is a crucial variable in treatment outcome since many therapeutic failures have resulted from incorrect patient selection. Tumor dedifferentiation and vascular invasion by tumor cells have constantly emerged as independent predictors of shortened survival in patients undergoing hepatic resection or transplantation for HCC. Although, tumor size and number appear to be clinical surrogates predicting tumor dedifferentiation and vascular invasion, tumor-related criteria like the tumor, node and metastases (TNM) classification do not accurately predict patient survival. The latter is better predicted by criteria combining tumor characteristics, functional status and liver function. Triphasic spiral CT and dynamic MR are currently used for assessing the number, size and vascular invasiveness of the tumor. In the Barcelona Clinic Liver Cancer staging classification the functional status of the patient and the liver status are measured by the Performance Status and Child-Pugh score system, respectively (Llovet et al. 1999). The Barcelona classification comprises four stages that select the best candidates for the best therapies available, i.e. from early tumor stage (Stage

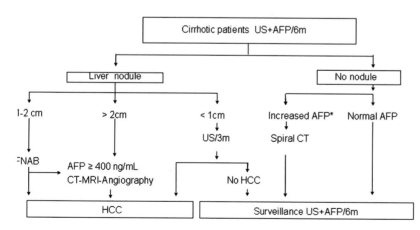

* Serum levels to be defined

Fig. 12.7. Surveillance of patients with compensated cirrhosis as suggested by the Conference of the European Association for the Study of the Liver

A) that includes asymptomatic patients with small tumors suitable for radical therapies to late tumor stage (Stage D) that includes patients with untreatable disease (Table 12.4).

The Cancer of the Liver Italian Program (CLIP) system allocates points for four variables that affect prognosis including Child-Pugh stage, tumor morphologic features (single, multiple or massive tumor), serum AFP level and portal vein thrombosis (Table 12.5) (CLIP 1998). Although this scoring system has been partially validated (CLIP 2000) and is easy to use, the CLIP score has suboptimal sensitivity for tumor invasiveness, since patients with a score of 0 may have from 0% to 50% of their liver replaced by HCC. Since the score is definitively skewed toward more severely affected patients whose disease is not amenable to curative treatment, too many patients with a CLIP score of 0 will not meet currently accepted criteria for surgery or locoregional ablation of the tumor that have been proven to be efficacious in patients in whom there is one tumor node of less than 5 cm in size (BRUIX et al. 2001). In recent years, other staging systems have been proposed including the Chinese University Prognostic Index (LEUNG et al. 2002), the modified TNM (HENDERSON et al. 2003), a French score system (CHEVRET et al. 1999) and a German score system (RABE et al. 2003). Tumor aggressiveness appears to be predicted also by the tissue expression of genetically modified estrogen receptors (VER): VER identified tumors with shorter doubling time and was a negative predictor of survival compared to patients with a HCC expressing wild ER (VILLA et al. 2000). In a comparative study, patient classification based on ER was a better predictor of survival in patients with inoperable HCC compared to CLIP, Barcelona and French staging scores (VILLA et al. 2003). However, one important limitation of the ER score system is its invasive approach to obtain a sample of liver tissue. Since staging scores developed thus far reflect differences in demographic features

Table 12.4. The Barcelona Clinic Liver Cancer Staging Classification of patients with hepatocellular carcinoma

Staging	Performance status	Tumor stage	Child-Pugh
(A) Early	0	Single <5 cm 3 nodes <3 cm	A & B
(B) Intermediate	0	Large/multinodular	A & B
(C) Advanced	1–2	Vascular invasion extrahepatic spread	A & B
(D) End-stage	3–4	Any of the above	C

Table 12.5. Cancer of the Liver Italian Program (CLIP) staging classification of hepatocellular carcinoma

Score	Tumor morphology	Child-Pugh	AFP	Vascular invasion
0	Uninodular <50% of the liver	A	<400 mg/dl	No
1	Multinodular >50% of the liver	B	>400 mg/dl	Yes
2	Massive	C	-	-

of the patients seen locally, expertise and treatment algorithms adopted in different centers, one wonders whether it is worth attempting to reach consensus on a single model for staging HCC. From a clinical point of view, it appears mandatory that prognostication of liver cancer should always incorporate treatment-dependent variables.

12.7
Natural History of the Tumor

The tumor size when HCC is first detected does not predict the course of the disease in all cases. In fact, the median time of doubling volume for a small HCC may range from 1 to 20 months (BARBARA et al. 1992; EBARA et al. 1986; OKAZAKI et al. 1989). The tumor is a clinically indolent disease during the early phases of growth, whereas in the advanced stages it often presents with painful hepatomegaly and/or jaundice. In the majority of patients with compensated cirrhosis undergoing surveillance, HCC is first detected as a single node (Table 12.6). The multinodular pattern of the tumor appears to be more common in patients with multiple etiological factors than in those with a single etiologic factor (BENVEGNÙ et al. 2001; FASANI et al. 1999). Primary and secondary HCCs may be differentiated by matching radiological and histopathological findings on explanted or resected livers only. Distinction between these two conditions bears important clinical implications, since second primary tumors appear to be less aggressive than metastatic tumors and recur less frequently after ablation than the former tumors (KUMADA et al. 1997). The growth pattern of HCC varies greatly from one tumor to another and may have clinical implications, since it influences the choice and outcome of treatments. Slowly expanding tumors (FRANCO et al. 1990) are more commonly seen in Caucasian and Asian pa-

Table 12.6. Prevalence of single, small nodes of hepatocellular carcinoma (HCC) detected during surveillance programs with abdominal ultrasound (US) of patients with compensated cirrhosis

Study	Patients with cirrhosis	US periodicity (months)	HCC × year	Single HCC <5 cm
Oka et al. 1990	140	3	6.5%	82%
Colombo et al. 1991	447	12	3.2%	54%
Cottone et al. 1994	147	6	4.4%	83%
Bolondi et al. 2001	313	6	4.1%	80%

tients than in South African patients who have more fast growing, replacing type tumors (Anthony 1973). Further complicating the assessment of tumor course is that some HCC nodes have constant rates of growth during follow-up, while others either have a declining growth rate in the late phases of follow-up or, after an initial phase of resting, increase in volume exponentially (Ebara et al. 1986; Okazaki et al. 1989). This great diversity of the tumor growth patterns makes the predictive power of the size of the tumor at diagnosis not absolute and explains why prognostication in HCC patients can be more reliably obtained by combining tumor size with liver function.

One controversial issue that bears important clinical implication is the presence of microscopic vessel invasion by the tumor, that is considered direct evidence of intrahepatic metastasis. Although macroscopic venous invasion seen with CT or MR scan is a well-established prognostic indicator and is one of the variables in the pathologic staging of HCC, the clinical significance of microscopic venous invasion in patients with operable HCC, remains unclear. Patients with microscopic venous invasion have higher serum levels of AFP, a larger tumor size and more nodules lacking a fibrous capsule (Tsai et al. 2000). Interestingly, up to 40% of less than 2-cm explanted tumors show microscopic venous invasion, a feature that overestimates the actual risk of tumor recurrence in patients with less than 5-cm tumors undergoing liver transplantation (Mazzaferro et al. 1996). Interestingly, circulating tumor cells have been demonstrated in the blood of 23 of 44 patients with HCC using a cytomorphological approach but only one patient ultimately developed extrahepatic metastases during a 3-year follow-up period (Vona et al. 2004). This clearly suggests that the presence of tumor cells within tu-

mor vessels is not synonymous of tumor metastasis in all cases, thus attenuating the predictive value of this pathological feature.

12.8
Conclusions

The understanding of the natural history of HCC has led to significant improvements in the management of patients with this tumor and made surveillance programs aimed at early diagnosis of HCC, possible. Surveillance programs with abdominal US and serum AFP have been of strategic importance since HCC treatment could only be improved in tumors diagnosed early. Chronic carriers of hepatitis B and patients with cirrhosis are the ideal target population for prospective surveillance (Bruix et al. 2001). Abdominal US is the best tool for surveillance with its greater predictive value for HCC than serum AFP (54% vs 32%) (Colombo et al. 1991; Oka et al. 1994). Since the average volume doubling time of HCC arising in patients with cirrhosis is 6 months, a 6-month interval between surveillance is considered cost-effective by many (Bruix et al. 2001). Although surveillance can identify tumors at an early stage and increase the chances of successful treatment, it is still not clear whether it reduces liver-related mortality in parallel. Ageing of the patient population and deterioration of liver function during surveillance, occurrence of multinodular tumors and limited access to liver transplantation may hamper surveillance program effectiveness. Two non-randomized studies in the Far East (Chen et al. 2002; Yuen et al. 2000) and one in Italy (Bolondi et al. 2001) provided conflicting results in terms of survival when patients with an HCC detected during surveillance were compared to patients with an incidentally diagnosed tumor. However, those studies did not adequately assess patient survival in relation to the significant improvements in management of HCC that have occurred in recent years. The reanalysis of a cohort of 417 HCC-free patients with compensated cirrhosis who had been under prospective surveillance for 148 months, showed a fall in liver-related mortality rates in HCC patients identified between 1997 and 2001. Mortality rates fell from 45% in the first 5-year period (1986–1991) to 37% in the second (1991–1996) and 10% in the third (1997–2001; first vs second not significant, first vs third $p=0.0009$, second vs third $p=0.018$) in parallel with a reduction in yearly mortality of treated patients (34%, 28% and 5%: first vs second not significant, second vs third $p=0.036$; first vs third $p=0.0024$) (SANGIOVANNI et al. 2004). During the last 5-year surveillance period, there was a shift of more patients from surgery towards the less aggressive locoregional ablative techniques, favored by the application of stringent criteria for patient selection to hepatic resection and the limited availability of donated organs for treating HCC with liver transplantation (BRUIX et al. 1996; MAZZAFERRO et al. 1996). Also, fewer patients with a single small tumor were left untreated or missed radical treatment compared to previous periods (46% vs 38% vs 26%), and fewer patients treated with hepatic resection or locoregional ablative therapies died of causes unrelated to cancer (35%, 25%, 0%). The gain in survival of cirrhotic patients developing an HCC during the last 5 years was likely to be the consequence of improved management of the tumor and complications of cirrhosis.

References

Anthony PP (1973) Primary carcinoma of the liver. A study of 282 cases in Ugandan Africans. J Pathol 110:37–48

Barbara L, Benzi G, Gaiani S, et al (1992) Natural history of small untreated hepatocellular carcinoma in cirrhosis: a multivariate analysis of prognostic factors of tumor growth rate and patient survival. Hepatology 16:132–137

Benvegnù L, Noventa F, Bernardinello E, et al (2001) Evidence for an association between the aetiology of cirrhosis and pattern of hepatocellular carcinoma development. Gut 48:110–115

Bolondi L, Sofia S, Siringo S, et al (2001) Surveillance programme of cirrhotic patients for early diagnosis and treatment of hepatocellular carcinoma: a cost effectiveness analysis. Gut 48:251–259

Borzio M, Borzio F, Macchi R, et al (1994) The evaluation of fine-needle procedures for the diagnosis of focal liver lesions in cirrhosis. J Hepatol 20:117–121

Bralet MP, Regimbeau JM, Pineau P, et al (2000) Hepatocellular carcinoma occurring in nonfibrotic liver: epidemiologic and histopathologic analysis of 80 French cases. Hepatology 32:200–204

Bruix J, Castells A, Bosch J, et al (1996) Surgical resection of hepatocellular carcinoma in cirrhotic patients: prognostic value of preoperative portal pressure. Gastroenterology 111:1018–1022

Bruix J, Sherman M, Llovet JM, et al (2001) Clinical management of hepatocellular carcinoma conclusions of the Barcelona-2000 EASL Conference, Barcelona September 15-17, 2000. J Hepatol 35:421–430

Burrel M, Llovet JM, Ayuso C, et al (2003) MRI angiography is superior to helical CT for detection of HCC prior to liver transplantation: an explant correlation. Hepatology 38:1034–1042

Chen TH, Chen CJ, Yen MF, et al (2002) Ultrasound screening and risk factors for death from hepatocellular carcinoma in a high risk group in Taiwan. Int J Cancer 98:257–261

Chevret S, Trinchet JC, Mathieu D, et al (1999) A new prognostic classification for predicting survival in patients with hepatocellular carcinoma. Groupe d'Etude et de Traitement du Carcinome Hepatocellulaire. J Hepatol 31:133–141

CLIP, the Cancer of the Liver Italian Program Investigators (1998) A new prognostic system for hepatocellular carcinoma: A retrospective study of 435 patients. Hepatology 28:751–755

CLIP, the Cancer of the Liver Italian Program (CLIP) Investigators (2000) Prospective validation of the CLIP score: a new prognostic system for patients with cirrhosis and hepatocellular carcinoma. Hepatology 31:840–845

Colombo M, de Franchis R, Del Ninno E, et al (1991) Hepatocellular carcinoma in Italian patients with cirrhosis. N Engl J Med 325:675–680

Craig JR (1997) Fibrolamellar carcinoma: clinical and pathologic features. In: Okuda K, Tabor E (eds) Liver Cancer. Churchill Livingston, New York, pp 255–262

Ebara M, Ohto M, Shinagawa T, et al (1986) Natural history of minute hepatocellular carcinoma smaller than three centimeters complicating cirrhosis. A study in 22 patients. Gastroenterology 90:289–298

Fasani P, Sangiovanni A, De Fazio C, et al (1999) High prevalence of multinodular hepatocellular carcinoma in patients with cirrhosis due to multiple etiological factors. Hepatology 29:1704–1707

Franco D, Capussotti L, Smadja C, et al (1990) Resection of hepatocellular carcinomas. Results in 72 European patients with cirrhosis. Gastroenterology 98:733–738

Gibson JB, Sobin LH (1978) Histological typing of tumours of the liver, biliary tract and pancreas. WHO, Geneva

Henderson JM, Sherman M, Tavill A, et al (2003) AHPBA/AJCC consensus conference on staging of hepatocellular carcinoma: consensus statement. HPB 5:143–250

International Working Party (1995) Terminology of nodular hepatocellular lesions. Hepatology 22:983-993

Kim SH, Lim HK, Lee WJ, et al (2000) Needle tract implantation in hepatocellular carcinoma: frequency and CT finding after biopsy with a 19.5-gauge automated biopsy gun. Abdom Imaging 25:246–250

Kojiro M (1997) Pathology of hepatocellular carcinoma. In:

Okuda K, Tabor E, (eds) Liver Cancer. Churchill Livingston, New York, pp 165–187

Kojiro M (1998) Pathology of early hepatocellular carcinoma: progression from early to advanced. Hepatogastroenterology 45:1203–1205

Kojiro M (2002) The Evolution of pathologic features of hepatocellular carcinoma. In: Zuckerman AJ, Mushahwar IK (eds) Viruses and Liver Cancer. Elsevier, Amsterdam, pp 113–122

Kumada T, Nakano S, Takeda I, et al (1997) Patterns of recurrence after initial treatment in patients with small hepatocellular carcinoma. Hepatology 25:87–92

Leung TW, Tang AM, Zee B, et al (2002) Construction of the Chinese University Prognostic Index for hepatocellular carcinoma and comparison with the TNM staging system, the Okuda staging system, and the Cancer of the Liver Italian Program staging system: a study based on 926 patients. Cancer 94:1760–1769

Llovet JM, Bru C, Bruix J (1999) Prognosis of hepatocellular carcinoma: the BCLC staging classification. Semin Liver Dis 19:329–338

Mazzaferro V, Regalia E, Doci R, et al (1996) Liver transplantation for treatment of small hepatocellular carcinomas in patients with cirrhosis. N Engl J Med 334:693–699

Oka H, Tamori A, Kuroki T, et al (1994) Prospective study of α-fetoprotein in cirrhotic patients monitored for development of hepatocellular carcinoma. Hepatology 19:61–66

Okazaki N, Yoshino M, Yoshida T, et al (1989) Evaluation of the prognosis for small hepatocellular carcinoma based on tumor volume doubling time. A preliminary report. Cancer 63:2207–2210

Parkin DM, Bray F, Ferlay J, et al (2001) Estimating the world cancer burden: Globocan 2000. Int J Cancer 94:153–156

Rabe C, Lenz M, Schmitz V, et al (2003). An independent evaluation of modern prognostic scores in a central European cohort of 120 patients with hepatocellular carcinoma. Eur J Gastroenterol Hepatol 15:1305–1315

Sangiovanni A, Del Ninno E, Fasani P, et al (2004). Increased survival of cirrhotic patients with a hepatocellular carcinoma detected during surveillance. Gastroenterology 126:1005–1014

Sell S (2002) Cellular origin of hepatocellular carcinoma. Sem Cell Develop Biol 13:419–424

Takamori R, Wong LL, Dang C, et al (2000). Needle-tract implantation from hepatocellular cancer: is needle biopsy of the liver always necessary? Liver Transpl 6:67–72

Tsai TJ, Chau GY, Lui WY, et al (2000) Clinical significance of microscopic tumor venous invasion in patients with resectable hepatocellular carcinoma. Surgery 127:603-608

Villa E, Moles A, Ferretti I, et al (2000) Natural history of inoperable hepatocellular carcinoma: estrogen receptors' status in the tumor is the strongest prognostic factor for survival. Hepatology 32:233-238

Villa E, Colantoni A, Camma C, et al (2003) Estrogen receptor classification for hepatocellular carcinoma: comparison with clinical staging systems. J Clin Oncol 21:441–446

Vona G, Estepa L, Beroud C, et al (2004) Impact of cytomorphological detection of circulating tumor cells in patients with liver cancer. Hepatology 39:792–797

Yuen MF, Cheng CC, Lauder IJ, et al (2000) Early detection of hepatocellular carcinoma increases the chance of treatment: Hong Kong experience. Hepatology 31:330–335

13 Diagnosis and Staging of Hepatocellular Carcinoma

Dania Cioni, Riccardo Lencioni, Jacopo Lera, Andrea Conti, Elisa Batini, and Carlo Bartolozzi

CONTENTS

13.1 Introduction

Diagnostic confirmation and careful staging of the cirrhotic patient with hepatocellular carcinoma (HCC) are key aspects for establishing the patient's prognosis and planning an appropriate treatment. For years, the diagnosis of HCC was based mainly on percutaneous biopsy, and accurate tumor staging required invasive procedures, such as angiography or angiographically assisted techniques. Currently, owing to the advances in imaging modalities, a reliable diagnostic assessment can be based in most instances on noninvasive examinations in combination with clinical and laboratory findings (Bruix et al. 2001). HCC, however, shows a variety of imaging features that reflect the variable gross and microscopic characteristics of this malignancy, and imaging evaluation of cirrhotic patients with suspected HCC is a challenging issue, as nonmalignant hepatocellular lesions arising in liver cirrhosis, such as regenerative (RN) and dysplastic nodules (DN), may simulate a small HCC (Bartolozzi and Lencioni 1999). One

of the key pathologic factors for differential diagnosis that is reflected in imaging appearances is the vascular supply to the nodule. Through the progression from RN, to low-grade DN, to high-grade DN, to frank HCC, one sees development of nontriadal arteries, which become the dominant blood supply in overt HCC (Tajima et al. 2002). It is this neovascularity that allows HCC to be diagnosed. It is currently accepted that imaging techniques may confidently establish the diagnosis, without needing biopsy confirmation, in HCCs larger than 2 cm. In lesions ranging from 1 to 2 cm, biopsy can still be recommended, but a negative response can never be used to completely rule out malignancy. While ultrasound (US) is widely accepted as the imaging modality of choice for HCC screening, spiral computed tomography (CT) or dynamic magnetic resonance (MR) imaging are required for intrahepatic staging of the disease. These examinations have replaced invasive procedures, such as angiography and angiographically assisted CT techniques, but remain relatively insensitive for the detection of tiny HCCs and tumor vascular invasion into peripheral portal vein branches (Choi et al. 2001).

13.2 Ultrasound

The use of US as the imaging modality of choice for HCC screening has been widely accepted, as this technique enables a rapid and noninvasive evaluation of liver parenchyma. Nevertheless, a comprehensive US assessment of the liver parenchyma is sometimes impossible because of the patient's body habitus or colonic interposition. In addition, when careful imaging-pathologic correlation was performed, the sensitivity of US in the detection of small HCCs was shown to be much lower than previously estimated (Kim et al. 2001).

New, contrast-specific techniques that display enhancement of microbubble US contrast agents

D. Cioni, MD; R. Lencioni, MD; J. Lera, MD; A. Conti, MD; E. Batini, MD; C. Bartolozzi, MD
Division of Diagnostic and Interventional Radiology, Department of Oncology, Transplants and Advanced Technologies in Medicine, University of Pisa, Via Roma 67, 56126 Pisa, Italy

in gray-scale, improve tumor-to-liver contrast, and seem to increase lesion detection and characterization (EFSUMB STUDY GROUP 2004; LENCIONI et al. 2002a).

Small HCC tumors less than 3 cm usually show a nodular configuration and can be divided into four types: single nodular type, single nodular type with extranodular growth, contiguous multinodular type, and poorly demarcated nodular type (BARTOLOZZI and LENCIONI 1999). On US, small, nodular type HCC typically appears as a round or oval mass lesion, with either hypoechoic or hyperechoic appearance and sharp and smooth boundaries. In contrast, the single nodular type with extranodular growth, the contiguous multinodular type, and the poorly demarcated nodular type show a nodular configuration with an irregular or blurred margin. The hyperechoic pattern of small HCC usually indicates fatty metamorphosis or, less frequently, pseudoglandular arrangement of the cancer cells or peliotic changes of tumor vascular spaces. Small, nodular type HCC is usually indistinguishable from RN or DN.

Advanced HCC tumors are classified into three major types: nodular, expansive type; massive, infiltrative type; and diffuse type (BARTOLOZZI and LENCIONI 1999). The typical nodular, expansive type HCC is a sharply demarcated lesion that may be unifocal or multifocal. Large, nodular type HCC typically shows inhomogeneous internal architecture with components of different echogenicity separated by thin septa (mosaic pattern). Most expansive type HCCs have a well-developed fibrous capsule that shows itself as a peripheral hypoechoic halo. The infiltrative type HCC is characterized by an irregular and indistinct tumor-nontumor boundary. The tumor strands into surrounding tissue, and frequently invades vascular structures, particularly portal vein branches. Infiltrative HCCs may create a massive involvement of the liver, replacing large parts of the parenchyma. The diffuse type is by far the most unusual presentation of HCC. This type is characterized by numerous nodules of small size scattered throughout the liver.

Doppler US techniques have long been used in attempts to evaluate tumor vascularity of HCC. On color or power Doppler US, HCC is usually displayed as a vascular rich lesion containing intratumoral flow signals with an arterial Doppler spectrum (LENCIONI et al. 1996a). A basket pattern, which is a fine blood-flow network surrounding the nodule, or tumor vessels flowing into the lesion and branching within it, are typically observed in large HCC. Doppler interrogation shows a pulsatile Doppler waveform with high frequency shifts and abnormally elevated resistive and pulsatility indexes. Since RNs and DNs usually do not show intratumoral arterial vessels, detection of neovascularity on Doppler US imaging supports the diagnosis of HCC. In small HCCs, however, the sensitivity of Doppler techniques in showing arterial hypervascularity is low, and a pulsatile flow with arterial waveform can be demonstrated in less than 50% of the lesions (LENCIONI et al. 1996a).

The introduction of US contrast agents and, more recently, the development of contrast-specific techniques that display microbubble enhancement in gray-scale have substantially improved the ability of US studies to assess the vascularity of HCCs. These techniques, in fact, optimize contrast and spatial resolution, and offer real-time imaging of contrast enhancement, thus allowing evaluation of tumor microcirculation (EFSUMB STUDY GROUP 2004; LENCIONI et al. 2002a). After intravenous administration of an US contrast agent, HCC typically shows strong intratumoral enhancement in the arterial phase (i.e. within 20–30 s after the start of the injection) followed by an isoechoic or hypoechoic appearance in the portal venous and delayed phases (EFSUMB STUDY GROUP 2004; FRACANZANI et al. 2001; LENCIONI et al. 2002a). In contrast, RNs and DNs usually do not show any early contrast uptake, and resemble the enhancement pattern of liver parenchyma.

In a series in which 72 HCCs ranging from 1.2 to 7.5 cm in greatest dimension were studied with contrast US by using continuous, low mechanical index, real-time scanning after bolus injection of 2.4 ml of a second-generation agent, contrast US studies showed arterial contrast uptake, occurring 11–31 s after the start of the injection, in 61 (92%) of 66 hypervascular HCCs on spiral CT with a sensitivity of 92%, and a specificity of 100% in distinguishing hypervascular HCCs from hypovascular HCCs. Of these 66 hypervascular tumors on spiral CT, arterial contrast uptake was observed in a contrast US study in 44 (92%) HCCs smaller than or equal to 3 cm, in 17 (94%) HCCs larger than 3 cm with no statistical significant difference, in 37 (95%) HCCs which were superficially located, and in 24 (89%) HCCs which were deeply located within the liver parenchyma with no statistical significant difference (Figs. 13.1, 13.2) (LENCIONI et al. 2002b).

In another series, 25 small (3 cm or less) nodular lesions detected by baseline US in 14 pre-transplant cirrhotic patients were examined with contrast-enhanced US, and contrast US findings were correlated lesion-by-lesion with pathology findings. On pathology examination, the 25 lesions were classified as HCC (n=18), high-grade DN (n=3), and low-grade

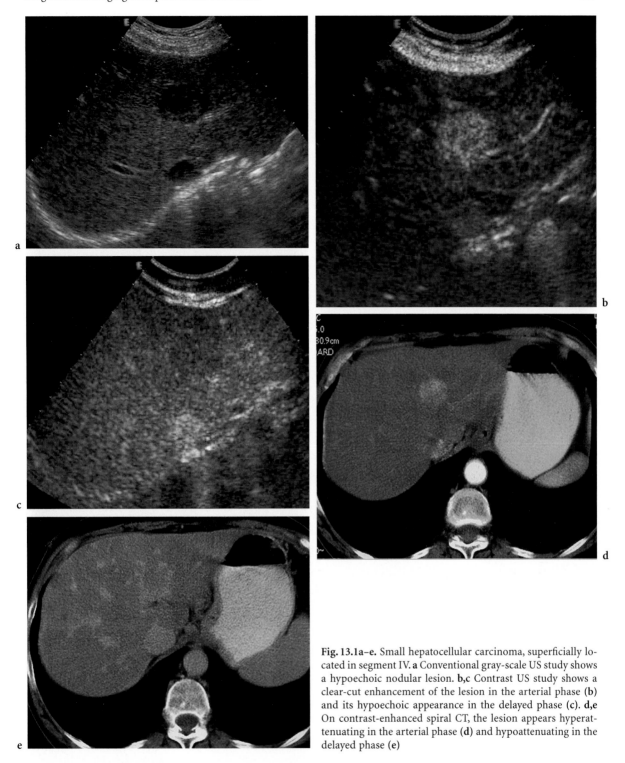

Fig. 13.1a–e. Small hepatocellular carcinoma, superficially located in segment IV. **a** Conventional gray-scale US study shows a hypoechoic nodular lesion. **b,c** Contrast US study shows a clear-cut enhancement of the lesion in the arterial phase (**b**) and its hypoechoic appearance in the delayed phase (**c**). **d,e** On contrast-enhanced spiral CT, the lesion appears hyperattenuating in the arterial phase (**d**) and hypoattenuating in the delayed phase (**e**)

DN (*n*=4). Contrast-enhanced US studies showed arterial contrast uptake in 14 of 18 HCCs and in 1 of 3 HG-DNs. No arterial enhancement was seen on contrast US in 4 of 18 HCCs, 2 of 3 HG-DNs and 4 of 4 LG-DNs. In the delayed phase, 13 of 18 HCCs, 3 of 3 HG-DNs, and 4 of 4 LG-DNs were isoechoic with respect to liver parenchyma. Delayed lesion hypoechogenicity was observed in 5 of 18 HCCs and none of the DNs (Figs. 13.3, 13.4) (LENCIONI et al. 2004a).

Doppler US techniques are useful in evaluating presence and extension of portal vein thrombosis caused by tumor invasion. The peculiar aspect seen in

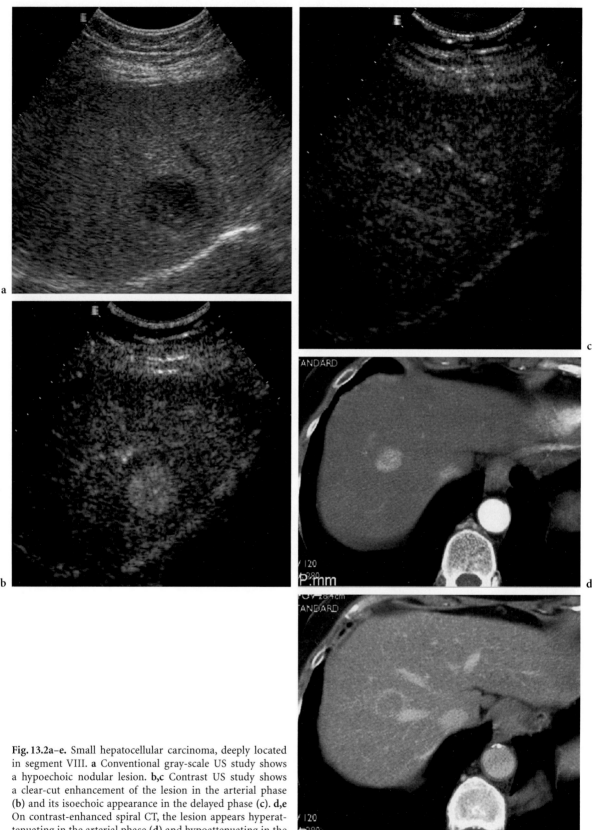

Fig. 13.2a–e. Small hepatocellular carcinoma, deeply located in segment VIII. **a** Conventional gray-scale US study shows a hypoechoic nodular lesion. **b,c** Contrast US study shows a clear-cut enhancement of the lesion in the arterial phase (**b**) and its isoechoic appearance in the delayed phase (**c**). **d,e** On contrast-enhanced spiral CT, the lesion appears hyperattenuating in the arterial phase (**d**) and hypoattenuating in the delayed phase (**e**)

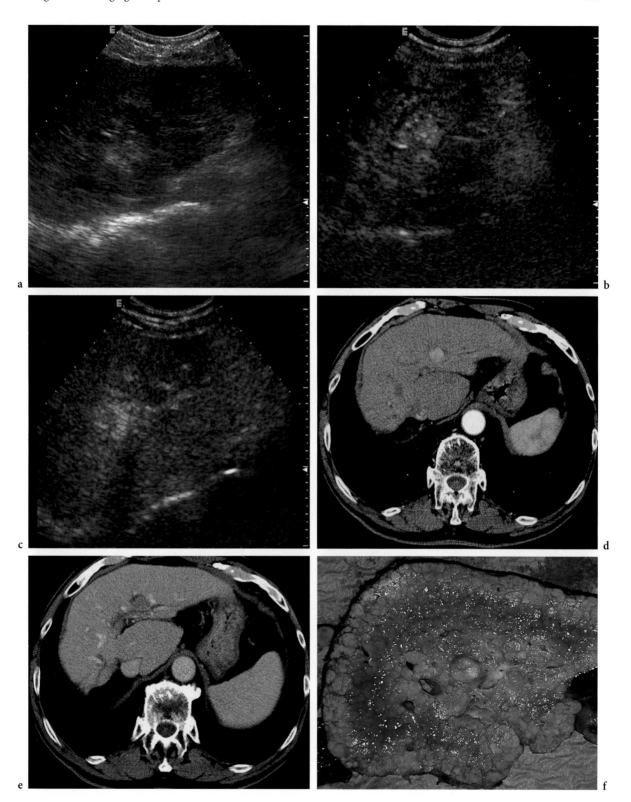

Fig. 13.3a–f. Small hepatocellular carcinoma located in segment IV in a cirrhotic patient, candidate for liver transplantation. **a** Conventional gray-scale US study shows a hypoechoic nodular lesion. **b,c** Contrast US study shows a clear-cut enhancement of the lesion in the arterial phase (**b**) and its hypoechoic appearance in the delayed phase (**c**). **d,e** On contrast-enhanced spiral CT, the lesion appears hyperattenuating in the arterial phase (**d**) and hypoattenuating in the delayed phase (**e**). **f** Pathology examination of the explanted liver confirms the presence of the small hepatocellular carcinoma

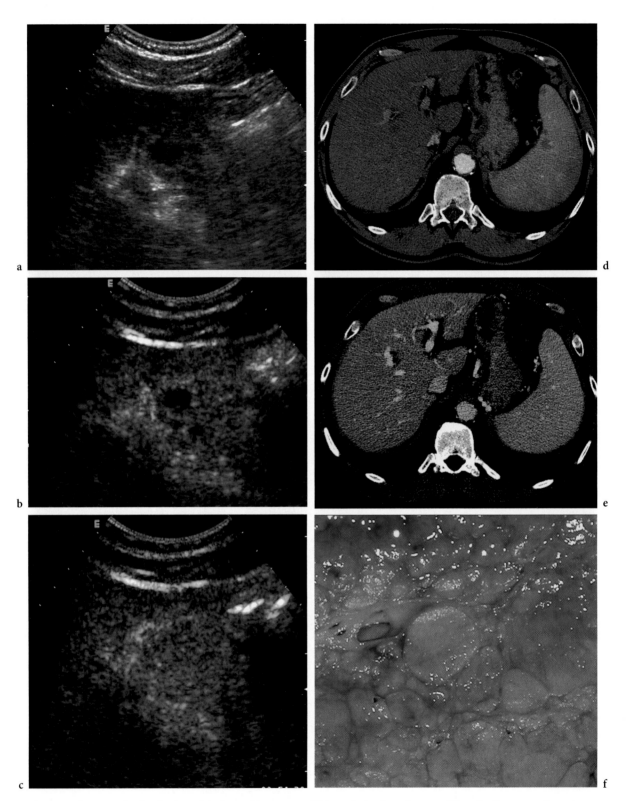

Fig. 13.4a–f. Low-grade dysplastic nodule, located in segment III in a cirrhotic patient, candidate for liver transplantation. **a** Conventional gray-scale US study shows a hypoechoic nodular lesion. **b,c** Contrast US study does not show a clear-cut enhancement of the lesion in the arterial phase (**b**), and the lesions appear isoechoic in the delayed phase (**c**). **d,e** On contrast-enhanced spiral CT, the lesion fails to enhance in the arterial phase (**d**) and appears hypoattenuating in the delayed phase (**e**). **f** Pathology examination of the explanted liver confirms the presence of the low-grade dysplastic nodule

cases of malignant thrombosis is the presence of pulsatile arterial flow within the thrombus (LENCIONI et al. 1995a). This finding is the expression of hypervascular neoplastic tissue growing into the portal vein. The sensitivity of US in detecting the arterial neovascularity within tumor thrombi may be increased by using microbubble contrast agents: enhancement of the thrombus in the arterial phase will indicate malignant thrombosis.

13.3
Computed Tomography

Spiral CT, with the recent introduction of multidetector-row scan technology, currently plays a fundamental role in the diagnosis and staging of HCC (AWAI et al. 2002; KAWATA et al. 2002). The different blood supply to the lesion, in fact, is the most important CT feature that may help differentiate among small hepatocellular lesions that have emerged in a cirrhotic liver (CHOI 2004). Indeed, small, overt HCCs show a typical hypervascular pattern, with clear-cut enhancement in the predominantly arterial phase and rapid wash-out in the portal venous phase (Fig. 13.5) (ICHIKAWA et al. 2002; LAGHI et al. 2003; LEE et al. 2004; MURAKAMI et al. 2001). In contrast, early-stage HCCs, RNs or DNs fail to exhibit this feature and appear isoattenuating or hypoattenuating with respect to surrounding liver parenchyma on CT images (Fig. 13.6) (LENCIONI et al. 1996b). Nevertheless, high-grade DNs may show increased arterial blood supply and be indistinguishable from a small HCC (FREENY et al. 2003).

Small, nodular type HCC tumor is a sharply demarcated lesion that may or may not be encapsulated. The CT detection rate of the capsule is low in small tumors because the capsule is thin and poorly developed. The capsule is seen as a peripheral rim that is hypoattenuating on unenhanced and arterial-phase contrast-enhanced images and hyperattenuating on delayed contrast-enhanced images (Fig. 13.7) (KARAHAN et al. 2003; ROS et al. 1990). The single nodular type with extranodular growth, the contiguous multinodular type, and the poorly demarcated

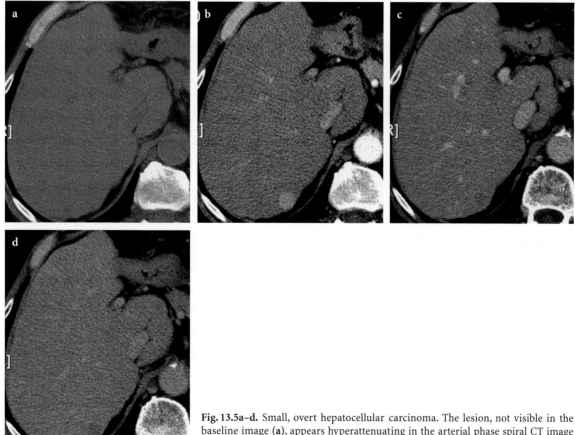

Fig. 13.5a–d. Small, overt hepatocellular carcinoma. The lesion, not visible in the baseline image (**a**), appears hyperattenuating in the arterial phase spiral CT image (**b**) and hypoattenuating in the portal venous (**c**) and delayed phase (**d**) images

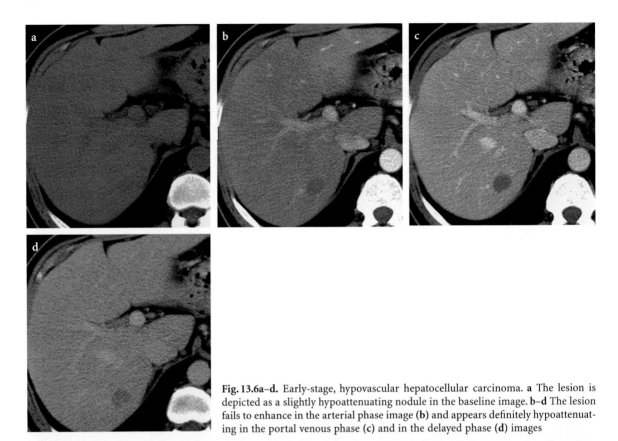

Fig. 13.6a–d. Early-stage, hypovascular hepatocellular carcinoma. **a** The lesion is depicted as a slightly hypoattenuating nodule in the baseline image. **b–d** The lesion fails to enhance in the arterial phase image (**b**) and appears definitely hypoattenuating in the portal venous phase (**c**) and in the delayed phase (**d**) images

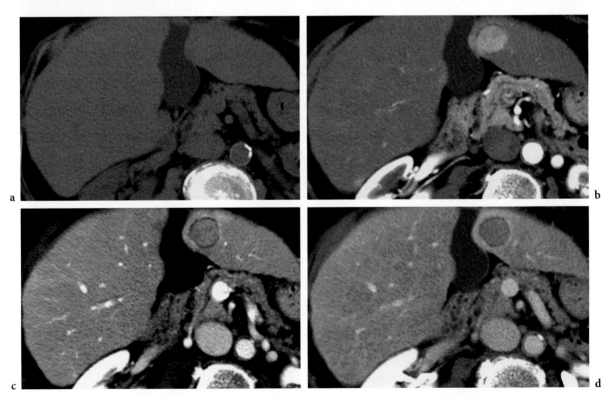

Fig. 13.7a–d. Small, encaspulated hepatocellular carcinoma. **a,b** The lesion, hardly visible in the baseline image (**a**), is well depicted in the arterial phase spiral CT image (**b**). **c,d** In the portal venous (**c**) and delayed phase (**d**) images, a peripheral rim of enhancement corresponding to the capsule is observed

nodular type show a nodular configuration with an irregular or unclear margin on CT images (Fig. 13.8) (MATSUI et al. 1991; UEDA et al. 1995).

Among the advanced HCC tumors, the typical expansive type of HCC is a sharply demarcated lesion that may be unifocal or multifocal. Typical features of expansive type HCC include tumor capsule and internal mosaic architecture. Most expansive HCC lesions have a well-developed fibrous capsule. The fibrous capsule is demonstrated by CT as a hypoattenuating rim which enhances in the delayed phase (KARAHAN et al. 2003; Ros et al. 1990). Internal mosaic architecture is characterized by components separated by thin fibrous septa. The different components may show various attenuation indexes on CT images, particularly if areas of well-differentiated tumor with different degrees of fatty metamorphosis are present. Internal septa show delayed enhancement, similar to that of the fibrous capsule (Fig. 13.9) (YOSHIKAWA et al. 1992). The infiltrative type HCC is characterized by an irregular and indistinct tumor-nontumor boundary. This type is demonstrated as a mainly uneven hypodense area with unclear mar-

gins (Fig. 13.10). The tumor strands into surrounding tissue, and frequently invade vascular structures, particularly portal vein branches. HCC, in fact, has a great propensity for invading and growing into the portal vein, eliciting tumor thrombi. Identification of neoplastic thrombosis of the portal vein is a crucial staging and prognostic factor (CHOI 1995; KARAHAN et al. 2003). Infiltrative HCC may create a massive involvement of the liver, replacing large parts of the parenchyma. The diffuse type is by far the most unusual presentation of HCC. This type is characterized by numerous nodules of small size scattered throughout the liver. The nodules do not fuse with each other and are visualized as diffusely distributed hypodense lesions (Fig. 13.11).

In addition to these morphological features, HCC has a typical tendency to produce small or minute satellite nodules ("daughter" lesions), frequently located in the vicinity of the main tumor. These nodules, representing intrahepatic metastases usually developed via the portal vein branches, show the same CT appearance of the main tumor. Identification of these satellite lesions is of the utmost importance for thera-

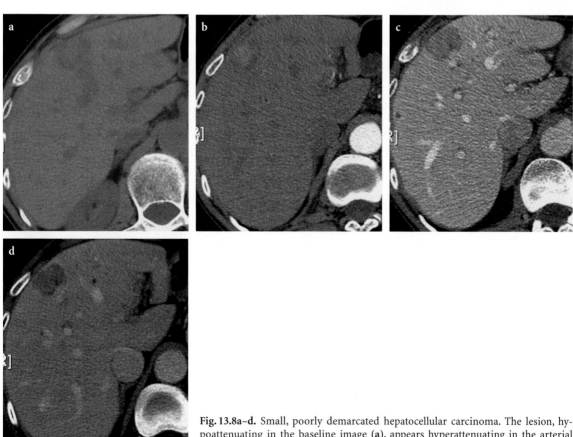

Fig. 13.8a–d. Small, poorly demarcated hepatocellular carcinoma. The lesion, hypoattenuating in the baseline image (a), appears hyperattenuating in the arterial phase image (b) and hypoattenuating in the portal venous (c) and delayed phase (d) images

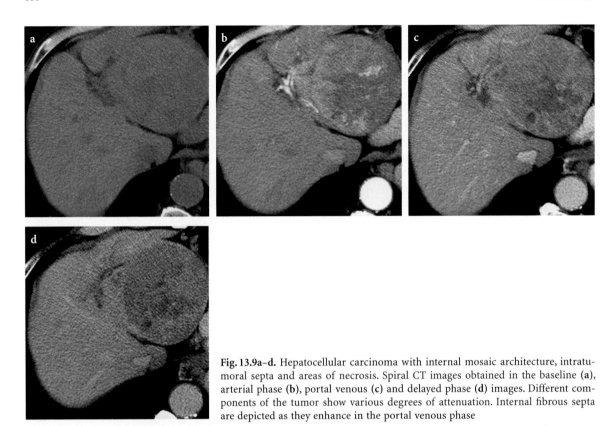

Fig. 13.9a–d. Hepatocellular carcinoma with internal mosaic architecture, intratumoral septa and areas of necrosis. Spiral CT images obtained in the baseline (**a**), arterial phase (**b**), portal venous (**c**) and delayed phase (**d**) images. Different components of the tumor show various degrees of attenuation. Internal fibrous septa are depicted as they enhance in the portal venous phase

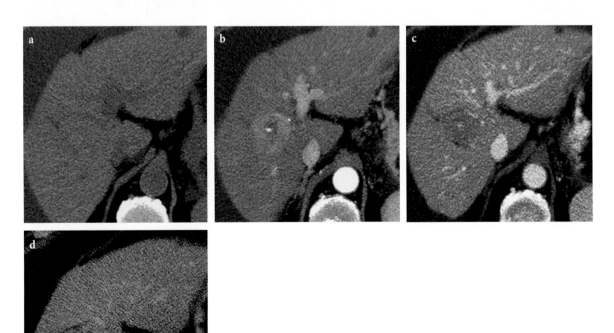

Fig. 13.10a–d. Infiltrative type hepatocellular carcinoma. The lesion is depicted by baseline (**a**), arterial phase (**b**), portal venous phase (**c**) and delayed phase (**d**) images as an uneven area with irregular borders and inhomogeneous enhancement which strands into surrounding tissue

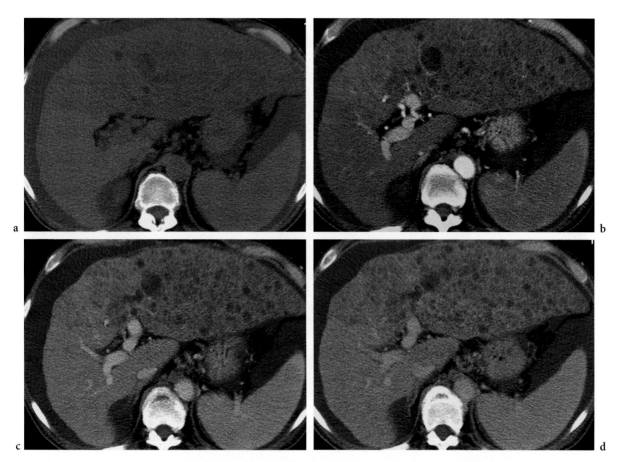

Fig. 13.11a–d. Diffuse type hepatocellular carcinoma. The lesion depicted by baseline (**a**), arterial phase (**b**), portal venous phase (**c**) and delayed phase (**d**) images is characterized by numerous nodules of small size scattered throughout the left liver lobe. The nodules do not fuse with each other and are visualized as diffusely distributed hypoattenuating lesions

peutic planning, and represents one of the most challenging issues in HCC patients (Fig. 13.12) (CHOI et al. 1997). Satellite lesions should be distinguished from multiple small HCC tumors caused by multicentric development. Such a distinction is important since the presence of intrahepatic metastases indicates a more advanced stage and is associated with a worse prognosis. In the case of multicentric development, multiple small tumors may exhibit a different enhancement pattern on CT, reflecting different degrees of tumor differentiation (UEDA et al. 1995).

Unusual histopathologic characteristics of HCC may modify the typical CT appearance of this tumor. These unusual histopathologic characteristics include marked fatty change, massive necrosis, abundant fibrous stroma (sclerosing type HCC), sarcomatous change, copper accumulation, and calcifications (FREENY et al. 1992). When fatty metamorphosis is severe, CT shows usually areas of negative attenuation value within the tumor, allowing the diagnosis of the fat component (Fig. 13.13). When the degree of fatty

deposition differs among internal portions of the tumor, the mosaic architecture can be visualized and the diagnosis of HCC made (YOSHIKAWA et al. 1998). Spontaneous massive necrosis within HCC is shown as a non-enhanced area, similar to other necrotic tumors (Fig. 13.9). HCC with abundant fibrous stroma (sclerosing type HCC) demonstrates hypovascularity on arterial-phase CT images and shows delayed enhancement (YAMASHITA et al. 1993). The same enhancement pattern may be seen in HCC with sarcomatous change, which is a very rare histotype. These CT features are commonly seen in lesions with a rich fibrous component, such as confluent hepatic fibrosis in cirrhotic liver and cholangiocellular carcinoma. Deposition of copper and copper-binding protein in some HCCs has been recognized, resulting in increased attenuation on precontrast CT images (KITAGAUA et al. 1991). The presence of calcifications is uncommon in HCC, being detected in about 0.2–1% of tumors. Calcifications, however, are not rare in fibrolamellar carcinoma and in mixed cholangiocellular-hepatocellular carcinoma.

Fig. 13.12a–d.
Hepatocellular carcinoma
with satellite lesions. The
daughter nodules are
better depicted in the
arterial phase spiral CT
image (**b**) with respect
to the baseline (**a**), portal
venous (**c**) and delayed
phase (**d**) images

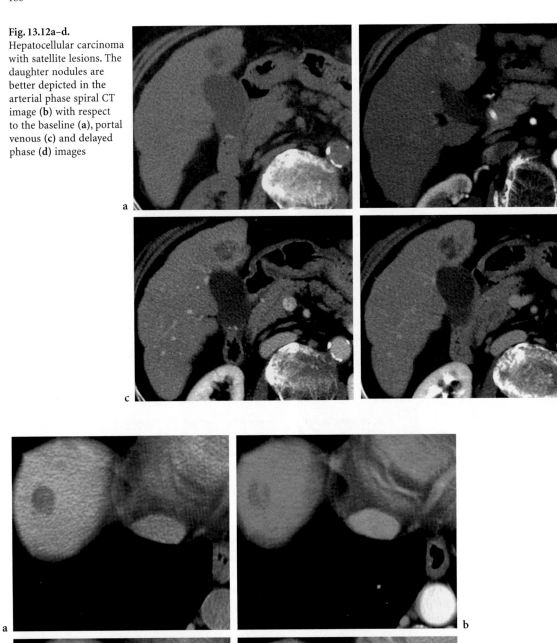

Fig. 13.13a–d. Hepatocellular carcinoma with fatty metamorphosis. Spiral CT images obtained in the baseline (**a**), arterial phase (**b**), portal venous (**c**) and delayed phase (**d**) images. The lesion appears hypoattenuating in the baseline image, shows inhomogeneous enhancement in the arterial phase image and appears hypoattenuating in the portal venous (**c**) and delayed phase (**d**) images, due to intratumoral fatty change

13.4
Magnetic Resonance Imaging

Recent advances in MR imaging include the introduction of high performance gradients, which have made possible the volumetric three-dimensional imaging techniques, as well as the development of liver-specific contrast agents, with a substantial impact on the diagnosis and staging of HCC (KEOGAN and EDELMAN 2001; SEMELKA and HELMBERGER 2001; AUGUI et al. 2002; HUSSAIN et al. 2003; LAISSY et al. 2002; SEMELKA et al. 1999).

If the dynamic study is often the single most important component of an MR examination, much information can be obtained from baseline images. Tumor architecture, grading, stromal component, as well as intracellular content of certain substances, such as fat, glycogen, or metal ions, greatly affect the MR imaging appearance of the lesion on T1-weighted and T2-weighted images (LENCIONI et al. 2004b). The signal intensity may range from hypointensity to isointensity to hyperintensity on T1-weighted images and from isointensity to hyperintensity on T2-weighted images. Hyperintensity on T1-weighted images and isointensity on T2-weighted images are typical features of well-differentiated tumors, while hypointensity on T1-weighted images and hyperintensity on T2-weighted images are usually associated with moderately or poorly differentiated tumors (Figs. 13.14, 13.15) (LENCIONI et al. 2004b). Tumor capsule is usually depicted as a thin rim with hypointense signal intensity on T1-weighted images

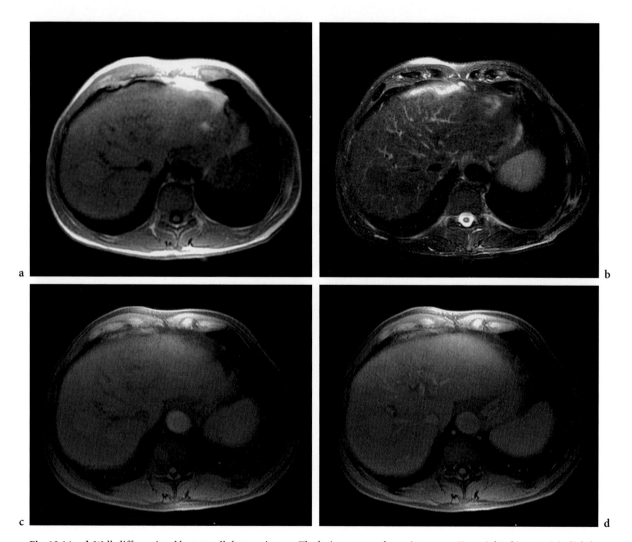

Fig. 13.14a–d. Well-differentiated hepatocellular carcinoma. The lesion appears hyperintense on T1-weighted images (**a**), slightly hypointense on T2-weighted images (**b**), does not show a clear-cut enhancement in the arterial phase (**c**) and appears isointense in the portal venous phase (**d**) on dynamic study

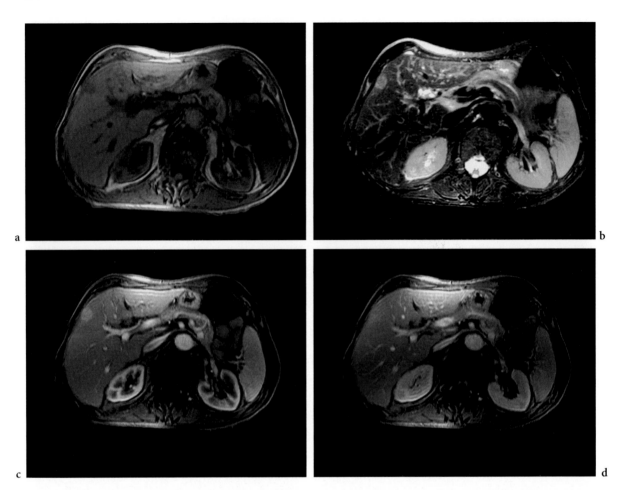

Fig. 13.15a–d. Poorly differentiated hepatocellular carcinoma. The lesion appears hypointense on T1-weighted images (**a**) and hyperintense on T2-weighted images (**b**), showing a clear-cut enhancement in the arterial phase (**c**) and wash-out in the portal venous phase (**d**) on dynamic study

due to its fibrotic composition. T2-weighted images delineate a single ring with hypointense signal intensity or a double ring with inner hypointensity and outer hyperintensity due to a thin fibrous inner zone and an outer zone consisting of compressed small vessels and bile ducts (BARTOLOZZI et al. 2001). In the mosaic pattern, intratumoral, linear-like hypointense areas on T1-weighted images and a nonuniform signal on T2-weighted images are detected due to intratumoral septa and a variety of histopathological findings within the tumorous tissue (BARTOLOZZI et al. 2001). Central necrosis presents itself usually with hypointensity on T1-weighted images, with marked hyperintensity on T2-weighted images in the case of liquefaction (BARTOLOZZI et al. 2001). Stromal (fibrous) component reduces signal intensity on T2-weighted images (BARTOLOZZI et al. 2001). Intracellular accumulation of fat or gly-cogen increases signal intensity on T1-weighted

images (BARTOLOZZI et al. 2001). While the intra-tumoral content of copper usually has limited influence on MR signal intensity of the lesion, iron deposits may greatly reduce signal intensity, especially on T2-weighted images (BARTOLOZZI et al. 2001).

The signal intensity of HCCs may be inhomogeneous, reflecting the presence of areas with different degrees of differentiation. Lesion signal intensity on baseline T1-weighted and T2-weighted images may help differentiate HCCs from RNs or DNs in cirrhosis (LENCIONI et al. 2004b). In fact, benign hepatocellular lesions almost never show hyperintensity on T2-weighted images, while malignant nodules almost never show hypointensity on T2-weighted images. Isointensity on T2-weighted images, however, is a common finding both in DN and well-differentiated HCC and, therefore, considerable overlap exists.

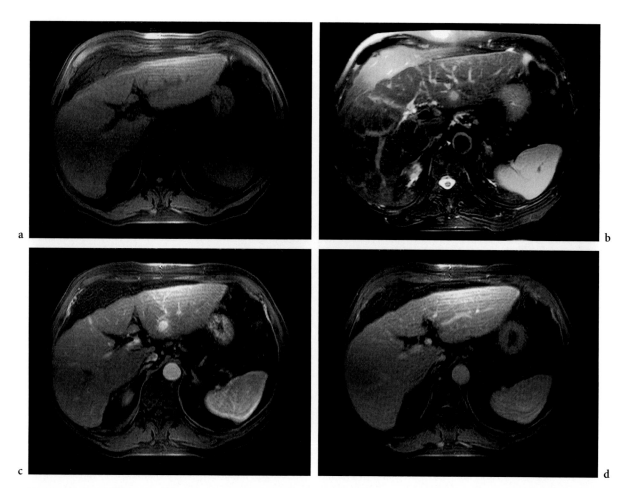

Fig. 13.16a–d. Small hepatocellular carcinoma. The lesion appears hypointense on T1-weighted images (**a**) and hyperintense on T2-weighted images (**b**), showing a clear-cut enhancement in the arterial phase (**c**) and wash-out in the portal venous phase (**d**) on dynamic study

The key pathologic factors for differential diagnosis between HCC and RNs or DNs is reflected in imaging appearances of vascular supply to the lesion, because the HCC neovascularity allows HCC to be diagnosed (Lencioni et al. 1996b). Dynamic MR imaging well demonstrates the hallmark of HCC in the cirrhotic liver, that is, arterial phase enhancement with portal venous phase wash-out (Fig. 13.16) (Eubank et al. 2002; Lencioni et al. 1996b; Noguchi et al. 2002; Noguchi et al. 2003). This feature enables one to distinguish frank HCC from DN, which are not usually hypervascular on arterial phase MR imaging, and enhance homogeneously on portal venous phase imaging, appearing isointense or nearly isointense to surrounding liver tissue (Fig. 13.17). Well-differentiated tumors, however, may not exhibit the typical hypervascularity of overt HCC and show slight progressive enhancement with no peak in the ar-

terial phase (Bartolozzi et al. 2001). Sclerosing HCC can show some delayed enhancement due to the abundant fibrous component (Bartolozzi et al. 2001).

While the dynamic study performed by using gadolinium chelates is currently a key part of the MR imaging examination, liver-specific contrast agents have also been used in attempts to improve the information provided by MR imaging in HCC detection and characterization. It has been shown that some well-differentiated HCCs may show a positive enhancement after the administration of a hepatobiliary contrast agent because of their affinity with normal hepatocytes. In one study, owing to this peculiar feature, early-stage tumors that were missed by spiral CT because of their immature neovascularity were detected (Bartolozzi et al. 2000). However, since uptake of the hepatobiliary contrast agent also occurs in DNs, differential

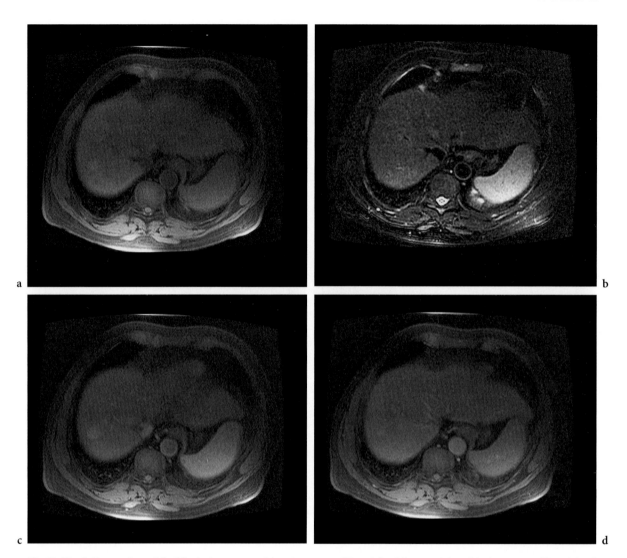

Fig. 13.17a–d. Dyspastic nodule. The lesion appears hyperintense on T1-weighted images (**a**) and isointense on T2-weighted images (**b**), but does not show clear-cut enhancement in the arterial phase (**c**) and appears isointense in the portal venous phase (**d**) on dynamic study

diagnosis among these entities cannot be achieved (Bartolozzi et al. 2000). HCC conspicuity after the administration of RES-specific contrast agents depends on differences in the number of Kupffer cells within the nodule and the surrounding cirrhotic liver (Lim et al. 2001). While moderately or poorly differentiated HCCs containing few or no Kupffer cells show high contrast-to-noise ratio, well-differentiated HCCs (as well as DNs) have a Kupffer cell population that may not significantly differ from that of surrounding parenchyma, which results in a signal-to-noise ratio close to zero and, thus, in

low detectability rates (Figs. 13.18, 13.19) (Lim et al. 2001). Although in one study MR imaging with use of a RES-targeted agent was superior to spiral CT for the detection of HCCs, in a comparative study the sensitivity of RES-targeted-enhanced imaging in detection of small HCCs was inferior to that of gadolinium-enhanced MR (Kang et al. 2003; Pauleit et al. 2002). In addition, the specificity may not improve after the administration of RES-targeted agents because of the false-positive lesions that may be caused by fibrotic changes (Mori et al. 2002)

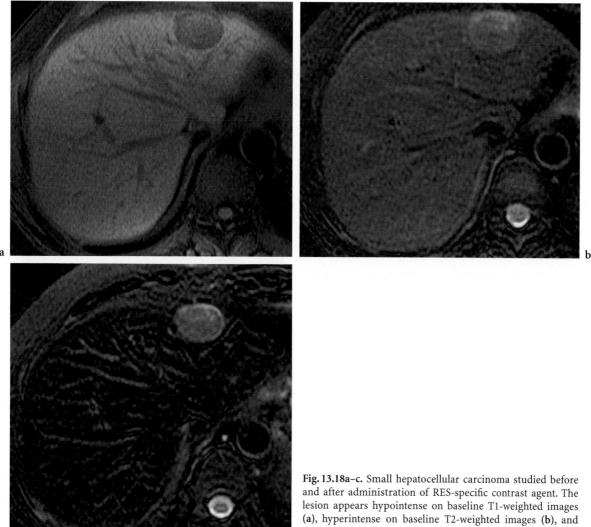

Fig. 13.18a–c. Small hepatocellular carcinoma studied before and after administration of RES-specific contrast agent. The lesion appears hypointense on baseline T1-weighted images (**a**), hyperintense on baseline T2-weighted images (**b**), and hardly hyperintense on T2-weighted images after contrast agent administration (**c**)

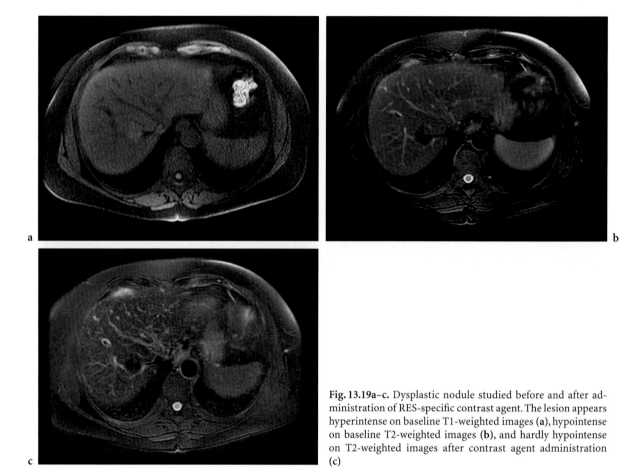

Fig. 13.19a–c. Dysplastic nodule studied before and after administration of RES-specific contrast agent. The lesion appears hyperintense on baseline T1-weighted images (**a**), hypointense on baseline T2-weighted images (**b**), and hardly hypointense on T2-weighted images after contrast agent administration (**c**)

13.5
Angiography and Angiographically Assisted Techniques

Angiography has long been used to diagnose HCC through the demonstration of abnormal arterial tumor vessels and nodular tumor stain. Following the advances in CT and MR imaging, angiography has lost almost any diagnostic role. The sensitivity of angiography in the depiction of small HCCs is inferior to that of spiral CT or dynamic MR imaging. In addition, angiography does not provide accurate anatomic localization of tumors. Angiography can be used in combination with spiral CT to perform CT hepatic arteriography (CTHA), CT arterial portography (CTAP), or Lipiodol CT.

In spiral CTHA, contrast material is injected directly into the proper or common hepatic artery. This technique is based on the fact that all but very few HCCs are fed from the hepatic artery. On spiral CTHA images, HCCs show high-attenuation blushes compared with the surrounding normal liver and stand out against the faintly enhanced normal parenchyma. Spiral CTAP is based on the reverse pathologic substratum with respect to CTHA, that is, on the fact that almost no HCCs are fed by the portal vein. This procedure produces dense enhancement of portal venous blood, so that the arterially supplied HCCs are highlighted as negative defects. However, variations in vascular anatomy, flow-related artifacts (especially perfusion defects in CTAP), and altered hemodynamics due to the associated cirrhosis may significantly change the patterns of enhancement and produce both false-negative and false-positive results (CHOI et al. 2001).

In Lipiodol CT, iodized oil is injected into the hepatic artery through angiographic catheterization. Most of the iodized oil droplets flow into HCCs by virtue of the increased blood supply to the tumor and, once deposited in the tumor, disappear at a far slower rate compared with those deposited in the normal liver tissue. Hence, on CT scans acquired 3-4 weeks later, HCCs appear as highly hyperattenuating areas compared with nontumorous liver tissue. However, when careful imaging-pathologic correlation was performed, the sensitivity of the technique was shown to be lower than previously estimated (BIZOLLON et al. 1998; LENCIONI et al. 1997). Also, findings on Lipiodol spiral CT have limited specificity, as Lipiodol accumulation has been demonstrated in benign lesions, including RN and DN (BIZOLLON et al. 1998).

13.6
Percutaneous Biopsy

Percutaneous biopsy has long been considered the method of choice for diagnosis of HCC. It is routinely performed with local anesthesia and without a hospital stay. US is the preferred imaging modality for guidance, because real-time control allows for a faster procedure time and precise centering of the needle in the target. Percutaneous biopsy can be performed by using either noncutting aspiration needles for cytology examination or cutting needles (Menghini modified needles or Tru-cut needles) for histology examination. The sensitivity of biopsy for the diagnosis of HCC ranges from 75% to 97%, while the specificity approaches 100% in most published series (BARTOLOZZI and LENCIONI 1999; LENCIONI et al. 1995b; LONGCHAMPT et al. 2000). False-negative results may be caused by either sampling mistakes or misinterpretations of a well differentiated tumor such as a DN or RN. Four cytologic features (increased nuclear/cytoplasmic ratio, cellular monomorphism, nuclear crowding, loss of bile duct cells) and four histologic features (increased nuclear/cytoplasmic ratio, decreased Kupffer cells, cellular monomorphism, increased trabeculae thickness) were identified as predictive of HCC in biopsy specimens (LONGCHAMPT et al. 2000). To improve the accuracy of the biopsy, combined cytology and histology sampling is recommended. Performing a double biopsy into the lesion and in normal parenchyma may also improve the accuracy of the technique (BARTOLOZZI and LENCIONI 1999).

Fatal complications following biopsy are extremely rare and almost always related to post-biopsy bleeding. A possible major complication is represented by tumor seeding along the needle track. The risk of seeding depends on several factors, including needle caliber, number of passes, tumor histology, and lesion location. The combination of superficial location and poor tumor differentiation significantly enhances the risk of seeding. Although the true incidence of this event is difficult to establish, in two series in which careful post-biopsy follow-up was performed seeding occurred in 3.5% and 5.1% of cases, respectively (KIM et al. 2000; TAKAMORI et al. 2000).

13.7
Diagnostic Workup

While the detection of a focal lesion in cirrhosis during US follow-up should always raise the suspicion of HCC, it has been shown by pathologic studies that many small nodules detected by US in cirrhotic livers do not correspond to HCC, but rather to non-neoplastic hepatocellular nodules, such as RN or DN. The prevalence of HCC among US-detected nodules is strongly dependent on the size of the lesion: while half of the nodules less than 1 cm in size are not malignant, the large majority of the lesions exceeding 2 cm are true HCC or contain HCC foci (BRUIX et al. 2001). The differential diagnosis between small HCC and RN or DN remains one of the greatest challenges in liver imaging. The diagnostic protocol, therefore, should be structured according to the actual risk of malignancy and the possibility of achieving a reliable diagnosis.

The following workup has been devised by a panel of experts from the European Association for the Study of the Liver, and offers guidelines for the clinical management of suspected HCC lesions (BRUIX et al. 2001). In nodules smaller than 1 cm detected by US in a cirrhotic patient, in view of the high prevalence of nonmalignant lesions and the difficulty of achieving a final diagnosis of HCC, a reasonable protocol is to repeat US every 3 months, until the lesion grows to more than 1 cm, at which point additional diagnostic techniques are applied. It has to be emphasized, however, that the absence of growth during the follow-up period does not rule out the malignant nature of the nodule because even an early-stage HCC may take more than 1 year to increase in size.

When the nodule exceeds 1 cm in size, the lesion is more likely to be HCC and diagnostic confirmation should be pursued. If the nodule does not exceed 2 cm, biopsy of the nodule can be recommended since the imaging techniques do not seem to have sufficient accuracy to distinguish HCC from benign conditions and AFP concentration will usually remain within normal values or be slightly elevated. Pathological confirmation may be best obtained by histology or combined cytology and histology sampling. The presence of an expert pathologist and the use of standardized interpretation criteria are crucial aspects of the technique. Nevertheless, a negative biopsy of a nodule which has emerged in a cirrhotic liver can never be taken as a criterion to rule out malignancy. Hence, lesions in which malignancy is not confirmed should be carefully followed over time and additional diagnostic techniques must be applied in the case of lesion growth.

For nodules above 2 cm, imaging techniques may confidently establish the diagnosis without needing confirmation with a positive biopsy (TORZILLI et al. 1999). Thus, in the setting of liver cirrhosis, HCC can be diagnosed by the coincident findings in at least two techniques (out of US, CT and MR imaging) showing characteristic features in a focal lesion larger than 2 cm. Imaging techniques should evidence arterial hypervascularization, and angiography can be used for this purpose if the others are not available. Ultimately, the decision to request a diagnostic biopsy should take into account the clinical impact of the result, and the balance between the potential risks of biopsy and the risk of invasive treatments in a patient due to a possible false-positive diagnosis based solely on imaging techniques.

The HCC nature of a nodule may also be confirmed by the concomitant detection of an increased α-fetoprotein (AFP) concentration. Published data suggest using values above 400 ng/ml for diagnostic confirmation, but future investigations may prompt a reduction of this limit to lower values, probably in the light of a comparison with values obtained prior to the nodule detection (BRUIX et al. 2001).

13.8
Staging Workup

The indication to perform an accurate assessment of disease extension depends on the clinical need. In patients diagnosed at an advanced stage of disease with no therapeutic options, the results of diagnostic US provide enough information and no other techniques are necessary. In those individuals in whom a treatment decision has to be taken, in contrast, accurate staging is necessary to determine the best treatment method. In these patients, tumor staging should include the assessment of number, size, location, and characteristics of the tumor nodules; tumor vascular invasion; and nodal and extrahepatic metastases.

US is definitely insufficient to define accurately the degree of intrahepatic and extrahepatic tumor spread. US, in fact, has a low detection rate for small intrahepatic metastatic nodules of HCC. When US findings were compared with explanted liver specimens, US lesion detection sensitivity for HCCs and DNs was in the ranges of 33–46% and 0–33%, respectively (KIM et al. 2001; RODE et al. 2001). Also, US is insensitive in the identification of tumor invasion in peripheral portal vein branches.

Spiral CT is a much better technique for staging, as it provides reliable detection of both intrahepatic and extrahepatic spread of the tumor. Dynamic MR imaging may in any case substitute for CT scanning (KIM et al. 2004; SUGIHARA et al. 2003). Spiral CT and dynamic MR imaging provide accurate assessment of the number and size of HCCs, enabling identification of even small intrahepatic metastatic nodules. These tiny tumor deposits, in fact, are usually hypervascular, like the main tumor, and therefore well depicted in arterial phase spiral CT or MR images. Nevertheless, when careful lesion-by-lesion imaging-pathologic correlation was performed in explanted livers, the sensitivity of both spiral CT and MR imaging in the detection of intrahepatic metastatic nodules was shown to be much lower than previously estimated (BHARTIA et al. 2003; BURREL et al. 2003; DE LEDINGHEN et al. 2002; VALLS et al. 2004). In studies in which the results of preoperative spiral CT were correlated with histopathologic results after 3-mm slicing of the explanted liver, the sensitivity of spiral CT was in the range 37–75% for the detection of HCCs, and 39–50% for the detection of DNs (LIM et al. 2000; PETERSON et al. 2000; ZACHERL et al. 2002). With dynamic gadolinium-enhanced MR imaging, lesion-by-lesion analysis revealed a sensitivity of 55–77% in the detection of HCCs and 15–50% for the detection of DNs (KRINSKY et al. 2001; RODE et al. 2001). In a series in which 55 patients with liver cirrhosis and HCC were examined with multidetector spiral CT and then submitted to liver transplantation within 3 months, pathology examinations showed 41 HCCs in 24 of 55 patients, ranging from 0.5 to 5 cm in diameter. Thirty of 41 lesions were detected by CT (lesion sensitivity 73%). Nine of the 11 lesions undetected by CT were smaller than 1 cm. Eight false-positive CT findings were observed (positive predictive value, 79%). Patient sensitivity and specificity in the detection of HCC were 79% (19/24) and 90% (28/31), respectively (Fig. 13.20) (CIONI et al. 2004).

Spiral CT and dynamic MR imaging have, however, substantially restricted the indication for more complex and invasive angiographically assisted CT techniques for the detection of satellite lesions even if they still remain relatively insensitive for the detection of tiny HCCs (Table 13.1).

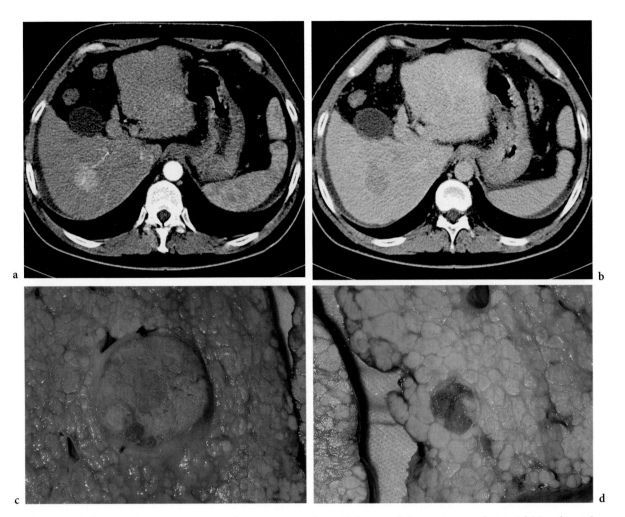

Fig. 13.20a–d. Preoperative CT in a pre-transplant cirrhotic patient with hepatocellular carcinoma. **a,b** Arterial (**a**) and portal venous phases (**b**) images show a typical hypervascular hepatocellular carcinoma located in segment VII. **c,d** On pathology examination of the explanted liver, the lesion is confirmed (**c**), but a second tiny tumor is also depicted (**d**)

Table 13.1. Sensitivity and positive predictive value of gadolinium-enhanced dynamic magnetic resonance imaging (MR) and spiral computed tomography (CT) in the diagnosis of hepatocellular carcinoma (HCC) according to lesion size. All series have pathologic examination of the explanted liver as term of reference. N/P= not performed; N/A= not available

Author year	No. of patients/ No. of lesions	Overall sensitivity	Sensitivity for lesions <1 cm	Sensitivity for lesions 1-2 cm	Sensitivity for lesions >2 cm	Positive predictive value
KRINSKY et al. 2001	71 / 19	MR, 10/19 (53%) CT, N/E	1/3 (33%)	6/12 (50%)	3/4 (75%)	19/34 (56%)
RODE et al. 2001	43 / 13	MR, 10/13 (77%) CT, 7/13 (54%)	MR, 5/7 (71%) CT, 3/7 (43%)	MR, 4/5 (80%) CT, 3/5 (60%)	MR, 1/1 (100%) CT, 1/1 (100%)	MR, N/A CT, N/A
DE LÉDINGHEN et al. 2002	34 / 54	MR, 33/54 (61%) CT, 28/54 (52%)	MR, 2/8 (25%) CT, 2/8 (25%)	MR, 19/34 (56%) CT, 15/34 (44%)	MR, 12/12 (100%) CT, 11/12 (92%)	MR, 33/37 (89%) CT, 28/37 (76%)
BURREl et al. 2002	50 / 76	MR, 58/76 (76%) CT, 43/70 (61%)	MR, 7/22 (32%)[1] CT, 2/19 (10%)	MR, 16/19 (84%)[1] CT, 9/19 (47%)	MR, 6/6 (100%)[1] CT, 6/6 (100%)	MR, 58/64 (90%) CT, 43/49 (87%)
BHARTIA et al. 2003	31 / 32	MR, 25/32 (78%)[2] CT, N/P	3/8 (38%)	12/13 (92%)	10/11 (91%)	25/46 (54%)
TEEFEY et al. 2003	22 / 18	MR, 14/18 (77%) CT, 13/18 (72%)	N/A	N/A	N/A	MR, 14/19 (74%) CT, 13/22 (59%)
VALLS et al. 2004	51 / 85	MR, N/P CT, 67/85 (79%)	N/A	23/28 (61%) 3	44/47 (94%)	67/76 (88%)

[1] Analysis of sensitivity according to lesion size was focused on 47 satellite nodules and did not include 29 main tumors
[2] MR examination protocol included dynamic gadolinium-enhanced, and ferumoxide-enhanced imaging
[3] The subgroup includes lesions smaller than or eqaul to 2 cm

The use of Lipiodol CT, in particular, is no longer recommended because of its invasiveness and limited accuracy (BIZOLLON et al. 1998; LENCIONI et al. 1997).

Vascular invasion by the tumor is a crucial staging factor. Tendency to grow into the portal veins, eliciting tumor thrombi, is a peculiar feature of HCC. Spiral CT and MR imaging allows accurate identification of tumor thrombi in the main portal veins. Tumor thrombi are shown as solid masses in the blood vessels with a marked hypervascularity often seen on arterial-phase images. Arteriovenous shunting may be present within thrombi. The hepatic segment in which the feeding portal vein branch is obstructed demonstrates hyperperfusion abnormality on arterial-phase CT or MR images, as a result of arterial compensation and lack of dilution of the enhanced arterial blood with the unenhanced portal blood. Identification of tumor invasion in peripheral (segmental or subsegmental) portal vein branches, however, is unreliable with both spiral CT and MR imaging.

Lymphatic metastases in HCC are not common. They are seen in no more than 10–15% even in autopsy cases, especially in the hepatic hilar lymph nodes (BARTOLOZZI and LENCIONI 1999). Extrahepatic hematogenous metastases are usually associated with advanced-stage tumors. The lung is the most common site of metastases, followed by the bone and the adrenal gland. CT is valuable for the diagnosis of adenopathies and distant metastatic disease, except for bone metastases. Assessment of tumor spread in selected patients (i.e. candidates for liver transplantation, inclusion in therapeutic trials) may therefore require thin section spiral CT of the chest and bone scintigraphy.

References

Augui J, Vignaux O, Argaud C, et al (2002) Liver: T2-weighted MR imaging with breath-hold fast-recovery optimized fast spin-echo compared with breath-hold half-Fourier and non-breath-hold respiratory-triggered fast spin-echo pulse sequences. Radiology 223:853–859

Awai K, Takada K, Onoshi H, et al (2002) Aortic and hepatic enhancement and tumor-to-liver contrast: analysis of the effect of different concentrations of contrast material at multidetector row helical CT. Radiology 224:757–763

Bartolozzi C, Lencioni R (1999) Liver malignancies. Springer, Berlin Heidelberg New York

Bartolozzi C, Donati F, Cioni D, et al (2000) MnDPDP-enhanced MRI vs dual-phase spiral CT in the detection of hepatocellular carcinoma in cirrhosis. Eur Radiol 10:1697–1702

Bartolozzi C, Cioni D, Donati F, et al (2001) Focal liver lesions: MR imaging-pathologic correlation. Eur Radiol 11:1374–1388

Bhartia B, Ward J, Guthrie JA, et al (2003) Hepatocellular carcinoma in cirrhotic livers: double-contrast thin-section MR imaging with pathologic correlation of explanted tissue. AJR Am J Roentgenol 180:577–584

Bizollon T, Rode A, Bancel B, et al (1998) Diagnostic value and tolerance of Lipiodol-computed tomography for the detection of small hepatocellular carcinoma: correlation with pathologic examination of explanted livers. J Hepatol 28:491–496

Bruix J, Sherman M, Llovet JM, et al (2001) Clinical management of hepatocellular carcinoma. Conclusions of the Barcelona-2000 EASL conference. European Association for the Study of the Liver. J Hepatol 35:421–430

Burrel M, Llovet JM, Ayuso C, et al (2003) MRI angiography is superior to helical CT for detection of HCC prior to liver transplantation: an explant correlation. Hepatology 38:1034–1042

Choi BI (1995) Vascular invasion by hepatocellular carcinoma. Abdom Imaging 20:277–278

Choi BI (2004) The current status of imaging diagnosis of hepatocellular carcinoma. Liver Transpl 10:S20–S25

Choi BI, Lee HJ, Han JK, et al (1997) Detection of hypervascular nodular hepatocellular carcinomas: value of triphasic helical CT compared with iodized-oil CT. AJR Am J Roentgenol 168:219–224

Choi D, Kim SH, Lim JH, et al (2001) Detection of hepatocellular carcinoma: combined T2-weighted and dynamic gadolinium-enhanced MRI versus combined CT during arterial portography and CT hepatic arteriography. J Comput Assist Tomogr 25:777–785

Cioni D, Lencioni R, Crocetti L, et al (2004) Multidetector spiral CT in the detection of hepatocellular carcinoma in transplant cirrhotic patients. Eur Radiol 14 (Suppl 6):18

de Ledinghen V, Laharie D, Lecesne R, et al (2002) Detection of nodules in liver cirrhosis: spiral computed tomography or magnetic resonance imaging? A prospective study of 88 nodules in 34 patients. Eur J Gastroenterol Hepatol 14:159–165

EFSUMB Study Group (2004) Guidelines for the use of contrast agents in ultrasound. Ultrashall Med 25:249–256

Eubank WB, Wherry KL, Maki JH, et al (2002) Preoperative evaluation of patients awaiting liver transplantation: comparison of multiphasic contrast-enhanced 3D magnetic resonance to helical computed tomography examinations. J Magn Reson Imaging 16:565–575

Fracanzani AL, Burdick L, Borzio M, et al (2001) Contrast-enhanced Doppler ultrasonography in the diagnosis of hepatocellular carcinoma and premalignant lesions in patients with cirrhosis. Hepatology 34:1109–1112

Freeny PC, Baron RL, Teefey SA (1992) Hepatocellular carcinoma: reduced frequency of typical findings with dynamic contrast enhanced CT in a non Asian population. Radiology 185:143–148

Freeny PC, Grossholz M, Kaakaji K, et al (2003) Significance of hyperattenuating and contrast-enhancing hepatic nodules detected in the cirrhotic liver during arterial phase helical CT in pre-liver transplant patients: radiologic-histopathologic correlation of explanted livers. Abdom Imaging 28:333–346

Hussain HK, Londy FJ, Francis IR, et al (2003) Hepatic arterial phase MR imaging with automated bolus-detection three-dimensional fast gradient-recalled-echo sequence: comparison with test-bolus method. Radiology 226:558–566

Ichikawa T, Kitamura T, Nakajima H, et al (2002) Hypervascular hepatocellular carcinoma: can double arterial phase imaging with multidetector CT improve tumor depiction in the cirrhotic liver? AJR Am J Roentgenol 179:751–758

Kang BK, Lim JH, Kim SH, et al (2003) Preoperative depiction of hepatocellular carcinoma: ferumoxides-enhanced MR imaging versus triple-phase helical CT. Radiology 226:79–85

Karahan OI, Yikilmaz A, Isin S, et al (2003) Characterization of hepatocellular carcinoma with triphasic CT and correlation with histopathologic findings. Acta Radiol 44:566–571

Kawata S, Murakami T, Kim T, et al (2002) Multidetector CT: Diagnosis impact of slice thickness on detection of hypervascular hepatocellular carcinoma. AJR Am J Roentgenol 179:61–66

Keogan MT, Edelman RR (2001) Technologic advances in abdominal MR imaging. Radiology 220:310–320

Kim SH, Lim HK, Lee WJ, et al (2000) Needle-tract implantation in hepatocellular carcinoma: frequency and CT findings after biopsy with a 19.5-gauge automated biopsy gun. Abdom Imaging 25:246–250

Kim CK, Lim JH, Lee WJ (2001) Detection of hepatocellular carcinomas and dysplastic nodules in cirrhotic liver: accuracy of ultrasonography in transplant patients. J Ultrasound Med 20:99–104

Kim YK, Kim CS, Lee YH, et al (2004) Comparison of superparamagnetic iron oxide-enhanced and gadobenate dimeglumine-enhanced dynamic MRI for detection of small hepatocellular carcinomas. AJR Am J Roentgenol 182:1217–1223

Kitagaua K, Matsui O, Kadoya M, et al (1991) Hepatocellular carcinomas with excessive copper accumulation: CT and MR findings. Radiology 180:623–628

Krinsky GA, Lee VS, Theise ND, et al (2001) Hepatocellular carcinoma and dysplastic nodules in patients with cirrhosis: prospective diagnosis with MR imaging and explantation correlation. Radiology 219:445–454

Laghi A, Iannaccone R, Rossi P, et al (2003) Hepatocellular carcinoma: detection with triple-phase multidetector row helical CT in patients with chronic hepatitis. Radiology 226:543–549

Laissy JP, Trillaud H, Douek P (2002) MR angiography: noninvasive vascular imaging of the abdomen. Abdom Imaging 27:488–506

Lee KHY, O'Malley ME, Haider MA, et al (2004) Triple-phase MDCT of hepatocellular carcinoma. AJR Am J Roentgenol 182:643–649

Lencioni R, Caramella D, Sanguinetti F, et al (1995a) Portal vein thrombosis after percutaneous ethanol injection for hepatocellular carcinoma: value of color Doppler sonography in distinguishing chemical and tumor thrombi. AJR Am J Roentgenol 164:1125–1130

Lencioni R, Caramella D, Bartolozzi C (1995b) Percutaneous biopsy of liver tumors with color Doppler US guidance. Abdom Imaging 20:206–208

Lencioni R, Pinto F, Armillotta N, et al (1996a) Assessment of tumor vascularity in hepatocellular carcinoma: comparison of power Doppler US and color Doppler US. Radiology 201:353–358

Lencioni R, Mascalchi M, Caramella D, et al (1996b) Small hepatocellular carcinoma: differentiation from adenomatous hyperplasia with color Doppler US and dynamic Gd-DTPA-enhanced MR imaging. Abdom Imaging 21:41–48

Lencioni R, Pinto F, Armillotta N, et al (1997) Intrahepatic metastatic nodules of hepatocellular carcinoma detected at lipiodol-CT: imaging-pathologic correlation. Abdom Imaging 22:253–258

Lencioni R, Cioni D, Bartolozzi C (2002a) Tissue harmonic and contrast-specific imaging: back to gray scale in ultrasound. Eur Radiol 12:151–165

Lencioni R, Cioni D, Franchini C, et al (2002b) Assessment of tumor vascularity in hepatocellular carcinoma: value of real-time contrast-enhanced US. Radiology 225(P):247

Lencioni R, Cioni D, Crocetti L, et al (2004a) Small nodules in liver cirrhosis: correlation between contrast-enhanced US and pathologic examination of explanted liver. Eur Radiol 14(Suppl 2):260

Lencioni R, Cioni D, Crocetti L, et al (2004b) Magnetic resonance imaging of liver tumors. J Hepatol 40:162–171

Lim JH, Kim CK, Lee WJ, et al (2000) Detection of hepatocellular carcinomas and dysplastic nodules in cirrhotic livers: accuracy of helical CT in transplant patients. AJR Am J Roentgenol 175:693–698

Lim JH, Choi D, Cho SK, et al (2001) Conspicuity of hepatocellular nodular lesions in cirrhotic livers at ferumoxides-enhanced MR imaging: importance of Kupffer cell number. Radiology 220:669–676

Longchampt E, Patriarche C, Fabre M (2000) Accuracy of cytology vs microbiopsy for the diagnosis of well-differentiated hepatocellular carcinoma and macroregenerative nodule. Definition of standardized criteria from a study of 100 cases. Acta Cytol 44:515–523

Matsui O, Kadoya M, Kameyama T, et al (1991) Benign and malignant nodules in cirrhotic livers: distinction based on blood supply. Radiology 178:493–497

Mori K, Scheidler J, Helmberger T, et al (2002) Detection of malignant hepatic lesions before orthotopic liver transplantation: accuracy of ferumoxides-enhanced MR imaging. AJR Am J Roentgenol 179:1045–1051

Murakami T, Kim T, Katamura M et al (2001) Hypervascular hepatocellular carcinoma: detection with double arterial phase multi-detector row helical CT. Radiology 218:763–767

Noguchi Y, Murakami T, Kim T, et al (2002) Detection of hypervascular hepatocellular carcinoma by dynamic magnetic resonance imaging with double-echo chemical shift in-phase and opposed-phase gradient echo technique: comparison with dynamic helical computed tomography imaging with double arterial phase. J Comput Assist Tomogr 26:981–987

Noguchi Y, Murakami T, Kim T, et al (2003) Detection of hepatocellular carcinoma: comparison of dynamic MR imaging with dynamic double arterial phase helical CT. AJR Am J Roentgenol 180:455–460

Pauleit D, Textor J, Bachmann R, et al (2002) Hepatocellular carcinoma: detection with gadolinium- and ferumoxides-enhanced MR imaging of the liver. Radiology 222:73–80

Peterson MS, Baron RL, Marsh JW Jr, et al (2000) Pretransplantation surveillance for possible hepatocellular carcinoma in patients with cirrhosis: epidemiology and CT-based tumor detection rate in 430 cases with surgical pathologic correlation. Radiology 217:743–749

Rode A, Bancel B, Douek P, et al (2001) Small nodule detection in cirrhotic livers: evaluation with US, spiral CT, and MRI and correlation with pathologic examination of explanted liver. J Comput Assist Tomogr 25:327–336

Ros PR, Murphy BJ, Back JL, et al (1990) Encapsulated hepatocellular carcinoma: radiologic findings and pathological correlation. Gastrointest Radiol 15:233–237

Semelka RC, Helmberger KG (2001) Contrast agents for MR imaging of the liver. Radiology 218:27–38

Semelka RC, Balci NC, Op de Beeck B, et al (1999) Evaluation of a 10-minute comprehensive MR imaging examination of the upper abdomen. Radiology 211:189–195

Sugihara E, Murakami T, Kim T, et al (2003) Detection of hypervascular hepatocellular carcinoma with dynamic magnetic resonance imaging with simultaneously obtained in-phase and opposed-phase echo images. J Comput Assist Tomogr 27:110–116

Tajima T, Honda H, Taguchi K, et al (2002) Sequential hemodynamic change in hepatocellular carcinoma and dysplastic nodules: CT angiography and pathologic correlation. AJR Am J Roentgenol 178:885–897

Takamori R, Wong LL, Dang C, et al (2000) Needle-tract implantation from hepatocellular cancer: is needle biopsy of the liver always necessary? Liver Transpl 6:67–72

Torzilli G, Minagawa M, Takayama T, et al (1999) Accurate preoperative evaluation of liver mass lesions without fine-needle biopsy. Hepatology 30:889–893

Ueda K, Kitigawa K, Kadoya M, et al (1995) Detection of hypervascular hepatocellular carcinoma by using spiral volumetric CT: comparison of US and MR imaging. Abdom Imaging 20:547–554

Valls C, Cos M, Figueras J, et al (2004) Pretransplantation diagnosis and staging of hepatocellular carcinoma in patients with cirrhosis: value of dual-phase helical CT. AJR Am J Roentgenol 182:1011–1017

Yamashita Y, Fan ZM, Yamamoto H, et al (1993) Sclerosing hepatocellular carcinoma: radiologic findings. Abdom Imaging 18:347–351

Yoshikawa J, Matsui O, Kadoya M, et al (1992) Delayed enhancement of fibrotic areas in hepatic masses: CT-pathologic correlation. J Comput Assist Tomogr 16:206–211

Yoshikawa J, Matsui O, Takashima T, et al (1998) Fatty metamorphosis in hepatocellular carcinoma: radiologic features in 10 cases. AJR Am J Roentgenol 151:717–720

Zacherl J, Pokieser P, Wrba F, et al (2002) Accuracy of multiphasic helical computed tomography and intraoperative sonography in patients undergoing orthotopic liver transplantation for hepatoma: what is the truth? Ann Surg 235:528–532

Primary Malignancies in Non-Cirrhotic Liver

14 Clinico-Pathological Classification

Clotilde Della Pina, Erika Rocchi, Andrea Conti, Sara Montagnani, and Laura Crocetti

14.1 Introduction

Primary malignant tumors of the liver can be classified into three groups according to their origins: those derived from the hepatocytes, those arising from the bile-duct epithelium, and those originating from the mesenchymal tissues of the liver. In this chapter, clinico-pathological features of hepatocellular malignancies arising in noncirrhotic liver are discussed, including hepatocellular carcinoma, fibrolamellar carcinoma and hepatoblastoma. Cholangiocellular tumors (cholangiocarcinoma and cystoadenocarcinoma) and tumors that origin from hepatic mesenchymal tissues (epithelial hemangioendothelioma, angiosarcoma and primary hepatic lymphoma) will also be examined.

C. Della Pina, MD; E. Rocchi, MD; A. Conti, MD;
S. Montagnani, MD; L. Crocetti, MD
Division of Diagnostic and Interventional Radiology, Department of Oncology, Transplants and Advanced Technologies in Medicine, University of Pisa, Via Roma 67, 56126 Pisa, Italy

14.2 Hepatocellular Tumors

14.2.1 Hepatocellular Carcinoma

Most cases of hepatocellular carcinoma (HCC) can be attributed to chronic hepatitis B (HBV) and/or C (HCV) (Llovet et al. 2003). However, some cases of HCC are not associated with cirrhosis (Nzeako et al. 1996). Nzeako et al. (1996) estimated that 40% of the HCC seen in North America occurs in noncirrhotic livers; they reported that only 10% of those patients had evidence of viral hepatitis or alcoholism. In a more recent study serologic evidence of hepatitis B or C or history of alcohol intake was present in only 36% of noncirrhotic patients with HCC, the remaining 64% having no evidence of risk factors for cirrhosis or HCC (Brancatelli et al. 2002). These data support the fact that HBV and HCV are associated with carcinogenesis of the HCC arising in noncirrhotic liver, but in most cases the cause of HCC remains uncertain. Recent reports have shown that transplacental transmission of HBV and HBV DNA integration into the cellular genomic DNA during fetal life is a possible explanation of HBV-related HCC in young adults without cirrhosis (Sezaki et al. 2004). The suspicion that oral contraceptives might play a role in the genesis of liver cancer has yet to be confirmed (Smalley et al. 1988).

When the tumor develops in the absence of cirrhosis, the course of the disease is generally turbulent. These patients are younger, generally about 40 years old, and with abnormally elevated serum tumor markers. Patients generally have severe, diffuse abdominal pain; weakness, weight loss, and lack of appetite may also be present. Extrahepatic extension of HCC is common in noncirrhotic patients (Trevisani et al. 1995). Noncirrhotic patients with HCC have a relatively favourable prognosis, with a median survival of 2.7 years and with 25% of patients surviving for at least 5 years after resection (Smalley et al. 1988).

The hepatic mass is commonly a large, lobulated and encapsulated solitary mass; necrosis and hypervascularity are prominent features. Vascular and biliary invasion are common. HCC had been reported as well-differentiated in 15% of patients, moderately differentiated in 82%, and poorly-differentiated in 3% of cases (BRANCATELLI et al. 2002).

14.2.2
Fibrolamellar Carcinoma

Fibrolamellar carcinoma (FLC) is a rare neoplasm of hepatocellular origin, considered as independent entity from HCC (EL-SERAG and DAVILA 2004). FLC occurs predominantly in young people of both sex, usually without preexisting liver disease (CRAIG et al. 1980). FLC does not appear to be related to previous HBV or HCV infection, and is not associated with elevated alpha-fetoprotein levels. Serum unsaturated vitamin B_{12} binding capacity and plasma neurotensin may be used as tumoral markers (KWEE 1989). In most patients signs and symptoms are represented by abdominal pain, hepatomegaly or palpable mass in the abdomen. In a recent study, the survival rates were significantly longer in patients with FLC than HCC: the 5-year relative survival rate was 31% for FLC and 6% for HCC (EL-SERAG and DAVILA 2004).

The neoplasm usually presents as a large, lobulated and solitary mass with a central fibrous scar that may be calcified (ICHIKAWA et al. 1999). Microscopically, FLC is characterized by cords of tumor cells surrounded by abundant avascular fibrous tissue. Fibrotic lamellae often form a central scar and multiple septa which radiate from the centre of the lesion.

14.2.3
Hepatoblastoma

Hepatoblastoma is the most common hepatic neoplasm in the paediatric age, comprising approximately 1% of all paediatric cancers (SCHNATER et al. 2003). The tumor is often detected before 3 years of age, more frequently in males, with a median survival of 1 year (JUNG et al. 2001). The neoplasm is frequently combined with congenital disorders and malformations of other organ such as hemihypertrophy, glycogen storage disease, diaphragmatic and umbilical hernias, and Wilms tumor (LACK et al. 1982; MANN et al. 1990). Presentation is often due to the mass effects accompanied by anorexia, vomiting, fever, and weight loss. The serum α-fetoprotein level

is usually high. Metastases can be found in the abdominal lymph nodes, the lungs, and, less commonly, the brain (BEGEMANN et al. 2004). Recent evidence suggests the possible association between prematurity and hepatoblastoma (FEUSNER and PLASCHKES 2002).

On macroscopic examination, hepatoblastoma is, in most cases, a solid, solitary and lobulated mass. Areas of necrosis and calcification are commonly present. Microscopically it can be classified as an epithelial or mixed (epithelial-mesenchymal) neoplasm. Epithelial hepatoblastoma is composed of fetal or embryonal malignant hepatocytes. Mixed hepatoblastoma has epithelial and mesenchymal component as osteoid material or cartilage. The histologic classification has prognostic implications: the epithelial type, particularly fetal histologic type, is associated with improved survival when compared with other histologic patterns (HAAS et al. 1989).

14.3
Cholangiocellular Tumors

14.3.1
Cholangiocellular Carcinoma

Cholangiocellular carcinoma or cholangiocarcinoma (CCA) is a primary malignancy arising from the bile duct epithelium. The incidence of CCA among primary liver tumors is around 20% of the cases. It generally occurs during the sixth and seventh decades of life (OKUDA et al. 2002). Risk factors are primary sclerosing cholangitis, congenital anomalies of the biliary tree, hepatolithiasis, infection with Clonorchis sinensis, familial polyposis and congenital hepatic fibrosis (ABDEL-RAHIM 2001; BURAK et al. 2004; KIM et al. 2003). Some data point to a potential role for chronic liver disease, hepatitis B and C in development of intrahepatic CCA (SHAIB and EL-SERAG 2004; LIU et al. 2003). Peripheral intrahepatic CCA usually presents with non-specific symptoms, such as anorexia and weight loss, or can be detected as incidental lesion by ultrasound examination (KACZYNSKI et al. 1998). On the other hand perihilar or extrahepatic tumours present signs and symptoms related to the biliary obstruction. In most cases serum α-fetoprotein level is normal whereas a recent study had shown that serum CA 19-9 could be an effective tumor marker (QIN et al. 2004).

According to the site of origin, CCA can be classified into: 1) peripheral CCA, which arises from intrahepatic bile ducts; 2) hilar CCA (Klatskin's tumor), which originates from one of the hepatic ducts or from the bifurcation of both hepatic ducts; 3) classical bile-duct carcinoma from the extrahepatic bile ducts (Nakeeb et al. 1996). However, this classification scheme is controversial because the differentiation between peripheral and hilar forms is sometimes difficult: peripheral CCA can spread into the hepatic hilum, and hilar CCA can infiltrate intrahepatic bile ducts (Yamasaki 2003). The Liver Cancer Study Group of Japan (1997) has proposed a new classification based on macroscopic appearance and growth characteristics. Among all CCA, the peripheral CCA represents 20%, hilar CCA 60% and bile-duct carcinoma 20% of cases.

Macroscopically CCA is a grayish-white, firm and fibrous mass because of its large amount of fibrous stroma. Characteristically this tumor has a large central core of fibrotic tissue, due to the desmoplastic reaction induced by the neoplastic cells. CCA differs from HCC since it is poorly vascularised, and the invasion of the portal tree is an infrequent complication. Hilar and bile-duct CCA grow into the walls of the bile ducts with invasion of the lumen, so obstructive jaundice and dilatation of the biliary tree are early signs. In the bile ducts, CCA presents papillary growth and periductal infiltration. Microscopically CCA represent an adenocarcinoma with its tubular or acinar-glandular structures. The neoplastic cells induce a variable desmoplastic reaction.

14.3.2 Cystoadenocarcinoma

This rare neoplasm is seen predominantly in females in the middle age. It arises from a cystoadenoma or a congenital biliary cyst (Devaney et al. 1994). When present, the symptoms are due to the growing abdominal mass. Most of the lesions are intrahepatic, less than 10% are extrahepatic, arising in the extrahepatic biliary ducts. Connections to the biliary tree may be seen, but are uncommon.

From a macroscopic point of view, cystadenocarcinoma is a large cystic mass containing bile-stained mucus and divided by internal septa. The neoplasm originates from the mucinous-secreting epithelium of the biliary ducts. Microscopically cystoadenocarcinoma shows similar features to those of mucinous cystic tumors of pancreas and ovary. The neoplastic tissue consists in epithelial cells arranged in papillary structures circumscribed by an abundant mesenchymal stroma, that can bear some resemblance to ovarian stroma (Gourley et al. 1992). Biliary cystadenocarcinoma with ovarian stroma is documented only in women developing from a pre-existing biliary cystadenoma and has a good prognosis. In contrast cystadenocarcinoma without ovarian stroma is seen both in men and women and is not associated with a pre-existing cystadenoma (Devaney et al. 1994).

14.4
Mesenchymal Tumors

14.4.1
Angiosarcoma

Angiosarcoma is a very rare neoplasm, but it is the most common hepatic tumor of mesenchymal origin. It displays a predilection for males and generally occurs during the sixth and seventh decade of life. Angiosarcoma has been associated to the exposure to a variety of chemical agents (inorganic arsenic, vynil chloridre) and radiation (radium, thorium oxide [Thorotrast]) (Ito et al. 1988; Kojiro et al. 1985). Association with hemochromatosis, von Reckinghausen's disease, and alcoholic cirrhosis have also been noted (Locker et al. 1979). Primary hepatic angiosarcoma is highly aggressive and, therefore, symptoms and signs are those of a rapidly progressive disease. The patient complains of pain, anemia, fever of unknown origin, weight loss, and abdominal mass (Molina and Hernandez 2003). The median survival after diagnosis is only 6 months (Molina and Hernandez 2003). This tumor metastasize early, particularly to lung and spleen (Buetow et al. 1994).

Macroscopically, angiosarcoma presents often multifocal growth pattern, with nodules ranging from few millimeters to several centimeters. Angiosarcoma may also appear as solitary, not encapsulated, large mass with large cystic areas filled with blood debris. Microscopically the neoplastic tissue is characterised by malignant endothelial cells that line dilated sinusoidal spaces. As the tumor grows, the dilated sinusoids become cavernous cavities with poorly defined borders (Ito et al. 1988).

14.4.2
Epithelioid Haemangioendothelioma

Epithelioid haemangioendothelioma (EHE) is a rare malignant hepatic tumor of vascular origin that occurs generally in young females. This neoplasm has a lower grade of malignancy than angiosarcoma, but is however progressive: overall metastasis rate is 45% with preferential involvement of lungs and bones (LAUFFER et al. 1996). The clinical signs and symptoms of patients with EHE are non-specific; the tumor is usually discovered incidentally, although symptoms like weakness, weight loss, and jaundice can occur. The 5-years survival of 55% for EHE is significantly better than for other hepatic malignancies (LAUFFER et al. 1996).

Macroscopically, EHE presents as multiple nodules or large intrahepatic mass, the latter being the natural evolution of multiple confluent nodules (MILLER et al. 1992). EHE characteristically has a fibrotic hypovascular central area and a peripheral hyperemic rim. At the outer edge of these tumors there is often a narrow avascular zone where hepatic sinusoids and small vessels are infiltrated by advancing tumor (MILLER et al. 1992). The hepatic capsule overlying an EHE is frequently retracted inward, probably due to fibrosis induced by the tumor. The neoplastic tissue is composed of epithelioid cells that proliferate into the sinusoids and central hepatic veins.

14.4.3
Lymphoma

Lymphoma is considered to be a primary neoplasm of the liver when the tumor is limited to hepatic parenchyma. Primary lymphoma of the liver is extremely rare, and is more common among immunocompromised patients. It typically occurs during the fifth decade of life and has a male predominance (AVLONITIS and LINOS 1999; HARRIS et al. 1987; SISKIN et al. 1995). Some studies have highlighted the association between hepatic lymphoma, arising in the post-transplant time or in patients with AIDS, and the infection with Epstein-Barr virus (NALESNIK et al. 1988). It has also been suggested that HCV plays a role in the pathogenesis of lymphoma (BRONOWICKI et al. 2003; KIM et al. 2000). Abdominal pain or discomfort, weight loss and fever are the most frequent presenting symptoms (AVLONITIS and LINOS 1999; RYAN et al. 1988). Serum tumor markers are usually normal but serum lactic dehydrogenase activity may be increased (SCOAZEC et al. 1991). Follow-up studies show that hepatic lymphoma had a relatively favorable prognosis when early detection of the disease was possible (OHSAWA et al. 1992; SCOAZEC et al. 1991).

Macroscopically, the liver may be occupied by solitary mass, multiple masses or a diffuse lesion without nodule formation (OHSAWA et al. 1992). Hodgkin's disease occurs more often as miliary lesions than masses. According to the WF classification, most cases of primary lymphoma of the liver are of intermediate or high grade. Diffuse large cell lymphoma is the most commonly encountered histological subtype and most of cases are B-cell lymphoma. In both Hodgkin and non-Hodgkin's lymphoma, initial involvement is seen in the portal areas, because here the majority of the lymphatic tissue of the liver is found.

References

Abdel-Rahim AY (2001) Parasitic infections and hepatic neoplasia. Dig Dis 19:288-291

Avlonitis VS, Linos D (1999) Primary hepatic lymphoma: a review. Eur J Surg 165:725-729

Begemann M, Trippett TM, Lis E, et al (2004) Brain metastases in hepatoblastoma. Pediatr Neurol 30:295-297

Brancatelli G, Federle MP, Grazioli L, et al (2002) Hepatocellular carcinoma in noncirrhotic liver: CT, clinical, and pathologic findings in 39 U.S. residents. Radiology 222:89-94

Bronowicki JP, Bineau C, Feugier P, et al (2003) Primary lymphoma of the liver: clinical-pathological features and relationship with HCV infection in French patients. Hepatology 37:781-787

Buetow PC, Buck JL, Ros PR, et al (1994) Malignant vascular tumors of the liver: radiologic-pathologic correlation. Radiographics 14:153-1 66

Burak K, Angulo P, Pasha TM, et al (2004) Incidence and risk factors for cholangiocarcinoma in primary sclerosing cholangitis. Am J Gastroenterol 99:523-526

Craig JR, Peters RL, Edmondson HA, et al (1980) Fibrolamellar carcinoma of the liver: a tumor of adolescents and young adults with distinctive clinico-pathologic features. Cancer 46:372-379

Dean PJ, Haggitt RC, O'Hara CJ (1985) Malignant epithelioid hemangioendothelioma of the liver in young women: relationship to oral contraceptive use. Am J Surg Pathol 9:695-704

Devaney K, Goodman ZD, Ishak KG (1994) Hepatobiliary cystadenoma and cystadenocarcinoma. A light microscopic and immunohistochemical study of 70 patients. Am J Surg Pathol 18:1078-1091

El-Serag HB, Davila JA (2004) Is fibrolamellar carcinoma different from hepatocellular carcinoma? A US population-based study. Hepatology 39:798-803

Feusner J, Plaschkes J (2002) Hepatoblastoma and low birth weight: a trend or chance observation? Med Pediatr Oncol 39:508-509

Gourley WK, Kumar D, Bouton MS, et al (1992) Cystadenoma and cystadenocarcinoma with mesenchymal stroma of the liver. Immunohistochemical analysis. Arch Pathol Lab Med 116:1047-1050

Haas JE, Muczynski KA, Krailo M, et al (1989) Histopathology and prognosis in childhood hepatoblastoma and hepatocarcinoma. Cancer 64:1082-1095

Harris KM, Schwartz ML, Slasky BS, et al (1987) Post-transplantation cyclosporine-induced lymphoproliferative disorders: clinical and radiologic manifestations. Radiology 162:697-700

Ichikawa T, Federle MP, Grazioli L, et al (1999) Fibrolamellar hepatocellular carcinoma: imaging and pathologic findings in 31 recent cases. Radiology 213:352-361

Ishak KG, Sesterhenn IA, Goodman ZD, et al (1984) Epithelioid hemangioendothelioma of the liver: a clinicopathologic and follow-up study of 32 cases. Hum Pathol 15:839-852

Ito Y, Kojiro M, Nakashima T, et al (1988) Pathomorphologic characteristics of 102 cases of Thorotrast-related hepatocellular carcinoma, cholangiocarcinoma, and hepatic angiosarcoma. Cancer 62:1153-1162

Jung SE, Kim KH, Kim MY, et al (2001) Clinical characteristics and prognosis of patients with hepatoblastoma. World J Surg 25:126-130

Kaczynski J, Hansson G, Wallerstedt S (1998) Incidence, etiologic aspects and clinicopatholgic features in intrahepatic cholangiocarcinoma. A study of 51 cases from a low-endemicity area. Acta Oncol 37:77-83

Kelleher MB, Iwatsuki S, Sheahan DG (1989) Epithelioid hemangioendothelioma of the liver. Clinicopathological correlation of 10 cases treated by orthotopic liver transplantation. Am J Surg Pathol 13:999-1008

Kim JH, Kim HY, Kang I, et al (2000) A case of primary hepatic lymphoma with hepatitis C liver cirrhosis. Am J Gastroenterol 95:2377-2380

Kim YT, Byun JS, Kim J, et al (2003) Factors predicting concurrent cholangiocarcinomas associated with hepatolithiasis. Hepatogastroenterology 50:8-12

Kojiro M, Nakashima T, Ito Y, et al (1985) Thorium dioxide-related angiosarcoma of the liver. Pathomorphic study of 29 autopsy cases. Arch Pathol Lab Med 109:853-857

Kwee HG (1989) Fibrolamellar hepatocellular carcinoma. Am Fam Physician 40:175-177

Lack EE, Neave C, Vawter GF (1982) Hepatoblastoma. A clinical and pathologic study of 54 cases. Am J Surg Pathol 6:693-705

Lauffer JM, Zimmermann A, Krahenbuhl L, et al (1996) Epithelioid hemangioendothelioma of the liver. A rare hepatic tumor. Cancer 78:2318-2327

Liu XF, Zou SQ, Qin FZ (2003) Pathogenesis of cholangiocarcinoma in the porta hepatic and infection of hepatitis virus. Hepatobiliary Pancreat Dis Int 2:285-289

Liver Cancer Study Group of Japan (1997) Intrahepatic cholangiocarcinoma, macroscopic typing. In: Okamoto E (ed) Classification of primary liver cancer. Kanehara, Tokyo, pp 6-7

Llovet JM, Borroughs A, Bruix J (2003) Hepatocellular carcinoma. Lancet 362:1907-1917

Locker GY, Doroshow JH, Swelling LA, et al (1979) The clinical features of hepatic angiosarcoma: a report of four cases and a review of the English literature. Medicine 58:48-63

Mann JR, Kasthuri N, Raafat F (1990) Malignant hepatic tumours in children: incidence, clinical features and aetiology. Paediatr Perinat Epidemiol 4:276-289

Miller WJ, Dood GD III, Federle MP, et al (1992) Epithelioid hemangioendothelioma of the liver: imaging findings with pathologic correlation. AJR Am J Roentgenol 159:53-57

Molina E, Hernandez A (2003) Clinical manifestations of primary hepatic angiosarcoma. Dig Dis Sci 48:677-682

Nakeeb A, Pitt HA, Sohn TA, et al (1996) Cholangiocarcinoma. A spectrum of intrahepatic, perihilar, and distal tumors. Ann Surg 224:463-473

Nalesnik MA, Jatfe R, Starzl TE, et al (1988) The pathology of posttransplant lymphoproliferative disorders occurring in the setting of cyclosporine A-prednisone immunosuppression. Am J Pathol 133:173-192

Nzeako UC, Goodman ZD, Ishak KG (1996) Hepatocellular carcinoma in cirrhotic and noncirrhotic livers. A clinico-histopathologic study of 804 North American patients. Am J Clin Pathol 105:65-75

Ohsawa M, Aozasa K, Horiuchi K, et al (1992) Malignant lymphoma of the liver. Report of five cases and review of the literature. Dig Dis Sci 37:1105-1109

Okuda K, Nakanuma Y, Miyazaki M (2002) Cholangiocarcinoma: recent progress. Part 1: epidemiology and etiology. J Gastroenterol Hepatol 17:1049-1055

Qin XL, Wang ZR, Shi JS, et al (2004) Utility of serum CA 19-9 in diagnosis of cholangiocarcinoma: in comparison with CEA. World J Gastroenterol 10:427-432

Radin DR, Craig JR, Colletti PM, et al (1988) Hepatic epithelioid hemangioendothelioma. Radiology 169:145-148

Ryan J, Straus DJ, Lange C, et al (1988) Primary lymphoma of the liver. Cancer 61:370-375

Sanders LM, Botet JF, Straus DJ, et al (1989) CT of primary lymphoma of the liver. AJR Am J Roentgenol 152:973-976

Schnater JM, Kohler SE, Lamers WH, et al (2003) Where do we stand with hepatoblastoma? A review. Cancer 98:668-678

Scoazec JY, Degott C, Brousse N, et al (1991) Non-Hodgkin's lymphoma presenting as a primary tumor of the liver: presentation, diagnosis and outcome in eight patients. Hepatology 13:870-875

Sezaki H, Kobayashi M, Hosaka T (2004) Hepatocellular carcinoma in noncirrhotic young adult patients with chronic hepatitis B viral infection. J Gastroenterol 39:550-556

Shaib Y, El-Serag HB (2004) The epidemiology of cholangiocarcinoma. Semin Liver Dis 24:115-125

Siskin GP, Haller JO, Miller S, et al (1995) AIDS-related lymphoma: radiologic features in pediatric patients. Radiology 196:63-66

Smalley SR, Moertel CG, Hilton JF, et al (1988) Hepatoma in the noncirrhotic liver. Cancer 62:1414-1424

Trevisani F, D'Intino PE, Caraceni P, et al (1995) Etiologic factors and clinical presentation of hepatocellular carcinoma. Differences between cirrhotic and noncirrhotic Italian patients. Cancer 75:2220-2232

Weiss SW, Enzinger FM (1982) Epithelioid hemangioendothelioma: a vascular tumor often mistaken for a carcinoma. Cancer 50:970-981

Yamasaki S (2003) Intrahepatic cholangiocarcinoma: macroscopic type and stage classification. J Hepatobiliary Pancreat Surg 10:288-291

15 Hepatocellular and Fibrolamellar Carcinoma

Giuseppe Brancatelli, Michael P. Federle, Valérie Vilgrain, Luigi Grazioli, Massimo Midiri and Roberto Lagalla

CONTENTS

15.1
Hepatocellular Carcinoma

15.1.1
Epidemiologic and Clinical Features

Hepatocellular carcinoma is one of the most common malignant neoplasm world-wide, with an estimated incidence of more than 500,000 new cases per year (Llovet et al. 2003). Hepatocellular carcinoma usually occurs in patients with long standing cirrhosis induced by hepatitis B or C viral infections or protracted alcohol intake. In cirrhotic liver, hepatocellular carcinoma is the result of the evolution of regenerative nodules into dysplastic nodules, with different degree of atypia, and finally into overt hepatocellular carcinoma (Arakawa et al. 1986). However,

G. Brancatelli, MD; M. Midiri, MD; R. Lagalla, MD
Department of Radiology, Policlinico Universitario, Via del Vespro 127, 90127 Palermo, Italy
M. P. Federle, MD
Department of Radiology, Abdominal Imaging Offices, University of Pittsburgh Medical Center, Room 4660, CHP, MT, 200 Lothrop Street, Pittsburgh, PA 15213, USA
V. Vilgrain, MD
Department of Radiology, Hospital Beaujon, Avenue Du General Leclerc 100, 92118 Clichy, France
L. Grazioli, MD
Department of Radiology, University of Brescia, Spedali Civili di Brescia, Piazzale Spedali Civili 1, 25023 Brescia, Italy

20%–40% of cases of hepatocellular carcinoma are not associated with cirrhosis (Nzeako et al. 1996).

Mechanism of hepatocarcinogenesis in patients without cirrhosis are not fully understood. In some cases, virus B and C exert directly their carcinogenic effect (Trevisani et al. 1995). In a series of 39 patients, serologic evidence of hepatitis B or C or history of alcohol intake was present in 15 cases (38%) (Brancatelli et al. 2002). These data support the fact that HBV and HCV viral proteins have direct oncogenic role on hepatocellular carcinoma arising in non-cirrhotic liver. In other cases, hepatocellular carcinoma is the result of the malignant transformation of hepatocellular adenoma (Ferrell 1993). However, in many patients with hepatocellular carcinoma developing in non-cirrhotic liver, etiology is unknown (Brancatelli et al. 2002). Recent reports have shown that non-alcoholic steatohepatitis is a risk factor for the development of hepatocellular carcinoma (Bugianesi et al. 2002).

Hepatocellular carcinoma in non-cirrhotic liver is more common in males (65%) than females (Brancatelli et al. 2002). Patients with hepatocellular carcinoma arising in non-cirrhotic liver usually are in their sixties (Brancatelli et al. 2002; Winston et al. 1999). Patients are typically symptomatic, and abdominal pain is by far the most common symptom, being present in half of patients (Brancatelli et al. 2002). Otherwise, hepatocellular carcinoma presents with fever, weight loss, hepatomegaly or ascites. The average level of serum α-fetoprotein is usually very high (more than 18,000) (Brancatelli et al. 2002). Complications are spontaneous rupture and massive hemoperitoneum. Due to its large size, treatment is either resection or intraarterial chemotherapy.

15.1.2
Histopathologic Features

Many studies on hepatocellular carcinoma arising in non-cirrhotic liver did not provide detailed enough data in terms of the fibrotic degree of the non-neoplastic part of the liver. The term "non-cirrhotic" liver ranges from no fibrosis to incomplete cirrhosis, encompassing all the intermediate steps as portal fibrosis, portal and periportal fibrosis, septa and bridging fibrosis and incomplete cirrhosis. Hepatocellular carcinoma in non-fibrotic liver is far less common than hepatocellular carcinoma in fibrotic liver. In a series of 39 patients, only two livers were interpreted as non-fibrotic (Brancatelli et al. 2002). Tumor can present as a solitary mass, as a predominant mass with satellite nodules, or as a multifocal or diffuse mass, and frequently shows necrosis and hemorrhage due to lack of stroma. Vascular and biliary invasion are common. Calcifications and fat can be observed in 10% of cases. Regarding the hepatocellular carcinomas, they are reported as well-differentiated in 15% of patients, moderately differentiated in 82% of patients, and poorly-differentiated in 3% of patients (Brancatelli et al. 2002). Microscopically, hepatocytes may show a trabecular, acinar or pseudoglandular pattern. Cells are pleomorphic or anaplastic, and cytoplasm can show increased fat and glycogen.

15.1.3
Imaging Features

Hepatocellular carcinoma in non-cirrhotic liver is usually large, with a mean diameter of 12.4 cm (Figs. 15.1–15.3). It presents usually as a solitary or dominant mass with smaller satellite lesions, while in a few cases it presents as multiple masses without a dominant lesion. The dominant mass or largest cluster of hepatocellular carcinoma can be found either in the right or left lobe, with no predominance. At ultrasonography, hepatocellular carcinoma shows mixed echogenicity due to tumor necrosis and hypervascularity. Hypoechoic appearance is usually due to solid tumor, while hyperechoic appearance can be due to fatty metamorphosis. In those encapsulated hepatocellular carcinomas, the capsule can be seen at ultrasound as a thin hypoechoic band. At CT and MR imaging, the tumor margins can either be well- or ill-defined, and the surface is usually lobulated. A tumor capsule is noted in only half of patients. Calcification are present within tumors in one every four patients,

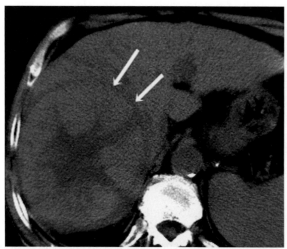

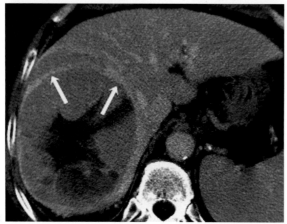

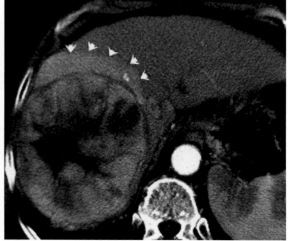

Fig. 15.1a–c. Hepatocellular carcinoma in non-cirrhotic liver in an 80-year-old man. **a** Non-enhanced transverse CT scan demonstrates a large, encapsulated mass (*arrows*) in the right lobe, with an hypoattenuating necrotic center. **b** Hepatic arterial contrast-enhanced transverse CT scan shows heterogeneous enhancement of the tumor. The central hypoattenuating area does not enhance. The portion of the non-tumorous liver adjacent to the lesion (*arrowheads*) is homogeneously hyperattenuating to normal liver due to thrombosis of a branch of the right portal vein (not shown) and hyperarterialization. **c** Portal venous contrast-enhanced transverse CT scan demonstrates that both the lesion and the adjacent area of hyperarterialization are hypoattenuating to the normal parenchyma. The capsule (*arrows*) is now best seen, due to contrast retention

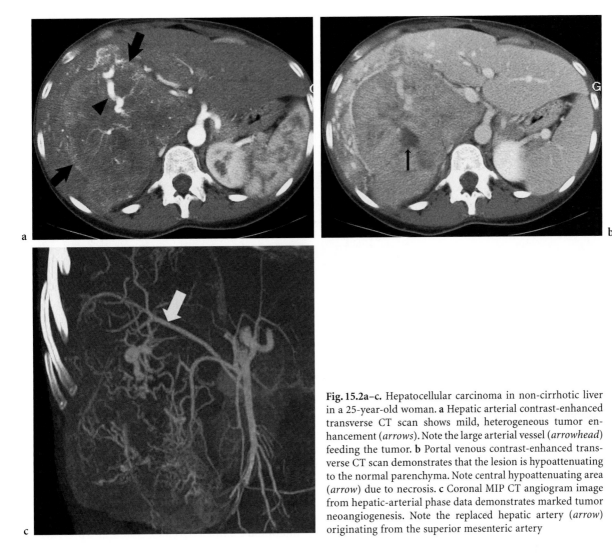

Fig. 15.2a–c. Hepatocellular carcinoma in non-cirrhotic liver in a 25-year-old woman. **a** Hepatic arterial contrast-enhanced transverse CT scan shows mild, heterogeneous tumor enhancement (*arrows*). Note the large arterial vessel (*arrowhead*) feeding the tumor. **b** Portal venous contrast-enhanced transverse CT scan demonstrates that the lesion is hypoattenuating to the normal parenchyma. Note central hypoattenuating area (*arrow*) due to necrosis. **c** Coronal MIP CT angiogram image from hepatic-arterial phase data demonstrates marked tumor neoangiogenesis. Note the replaced hepatic artery (*arrow*) originating from the superior mesenteric artery

and are most of the times peripheral. Calcifications are better seen with CT than with MR imaging. Necrotic non-enhancing portions of tumor are present virtually in all of cases (Fig. 15.1). Hyperattenuating/ hyperintense areas compatible with hemorrhage can be found within tumors. Low-attenuating areas compatible with a fat component are unusually seen. Dilated intrahepatic bile ducts can be observed, indicative of hepatocellular carcinoma obstruction of more central ducts. Tumor thrombus or encasement of either the portal or hepatic veins is seen in some cases. Upper abdominal lymphadenopathy is noted in a minority of patients. On nonenhanced CT/MR images, the typical hepatocellular carcinoma is predominantly hypoattenuating/hypointense to liver. On hepatic arterial phase CT/MR images, the tumor

is heterogeneously hyperattenuating/hyperintense. Occasionally, wedge-shaped areas of increased density on hepatic arterial phase are observed, and are due to perfusion abnormalities (increased arterial flow) due to portal vein occlusion by tumor thrombus (Fig. 15.1). On portal venous phase CT/MR, hepatocellular carcinoma shows decreased attenuating/ intensity with heterogeneous areas of contrast accumulation (Figs. 15.1–15.3) (BRANCATELLI et al. 2002; WINSTON et al. 1999). On delayed phase, the tumor is hypoattenuating/hypointense to adjacent nontumorous liver. Angiography shows an hypervascular tumor with mixed neovascularity and arteriovenous shunting. A large hepatic artery is noted, as well as vascular invasion. The "thread and streak sign" is due to tumor thrombus in portal vein. Hepatobiliary

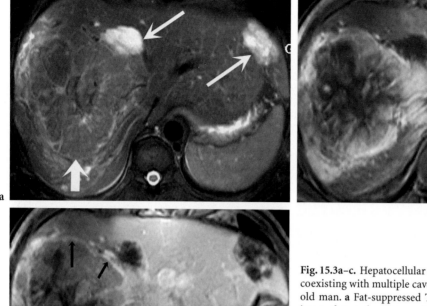

Fig. 15.3a–c. Hepatocellular carcinoma in non-cirrhotic liver coexisting with multiple cavernous hemangioma in a 45-year-old man. **a** Fat-suppressed T2-weighted turbo spin-echo MR image shows a large tumor (*short thick arrow*) in the right lobe of the liver that is slightly hyperintense to the surrounding non-tumorous parenchyma. Two hemangiomas (*long thin arrows*) with signal intensity as strong as that of the cerebrospinal fluid are seen adjacent to the tumor and in the left lobe in a subcapsular location. **b** Gadolinium-enhanced T1-weighted gradient-echo MR image obtained during arterial-phase shows strong intensity of the hepatocellular carcinoma, except for a central area that is hypointense due to necrosis. Hemangiomas show initial nodular peripheral enhancement. **c** Gadolinium-enhanced T1-weighted gradient-echo MR image obtained during portal-phase shows hypointensity of the hepatocellular carcinoma, and enhancement of the surrounding capsule (*arrows*). Hemangiomas show progressive nodular centripetal filling

scans show uptake in 50% of lesions. At technetium sulfur colloid, hepatocellular carcinoma shows heterogeneous uptake. At gallium scan, hepatocellular carcinoma shows uptake in 90% of cases.

15.2
Fibrolamellar Hepatocellular Carcinoma

15.2.1
Epidemiologic and Clinical Features

Fibrolamellar hepatocellular carcinoma has distinct features in comparison to hepatocellular carcinoma. It accounts for only 1%–9% of all cases of hepatocellular carcinoma, but for as many as 40% of those in patients 32 years of age or younger (CRAIG et al. 1980). It arises in non-cirrhotic liver in the majority of cases (90%), and the typical patient has an average age of 28 years, with no sex predilection. No specific risk factors have been identified for the development of fibrolamellar hepatocellular carcinoma. Signs and symptoms are initially non-specific, and represented by pain, abdominal distention, hepatomegaly or palpable mass in the abdomen. Jaundice can occasionally be present if the tumor invades the biliary tract. Rarely, fibrolamellar hepatocellular carcinoma can present with metastatic disease, fever, gynecomastia or portal, hepatic, or inferior vena cava thrombosis. The tumor is associated with an elevated plasma level of vitamin B_{12}, while levels of α-fetoprotein are typically normal, being mildly increased in 10% of cases (<200 ng/l). Rarely, a marked increase in α-fetoprotein levels is seen, similar to conventional hepatocellular carcinoma (10,000 ng/l). Prognosis in patients with fibrolamellar hepatocellular carcinoma is better than for patients with typical hepatocellular carcinoma. The tumor is resectable in half of patients, although it tends to recur. Treatment consists of surgical resection of the mass and the associated regional lymph nodes. Liver transplantation has been performed in those cases in whom hepatectomy was not possible. In inoperable cases, chemotherapy is administered. Patients with fibrolamellar hepatocel-lular carcinoma have a survival rate of 34% at 5 years, and the rate rises to 63% if the tumor has been completely resected (BERMAN et al. 1980).

15.2.2
Histopathologic Features

Fibrolamellar hepatocellular carcinoma is usually a solitary, lobulated, non-encapsulated well-circumscribed mass with a prominent central, stellate scar (ICHIKAWA et al. 1999). It is found more commonly in the left lobe, and at cut section it presents as a large (mean 13 cm), firm, bile-stained, tan-yellow or brown mass with streaks of fibrous tissue. It may sometimes show large necrotic or cystic areas and hemorrhage. Fibrolamellar hepatocellular carcinoma are typically slow-growing. No specific risk factors are known for the occurrence of fibrolamellar hepatocellular carcinoma, therefore there is usually no cirrhosis or hepa-

titis in the underlying liver. Punctuate calcifications located within the scar are observed in 68% of cases. Microscopically, the mass consists of cords and trabeculae of large polygonal neoplastic cells containing large nuclei with prominent nucleoli and intranuclear cytoplasmic pseudo-inclusions, eosinophilic hyaline globules, pale bodies. Cells are divided into nodules by a dense, avascular collagenous stroma composed of lamellae that form multiple fibrous septa which radiate from the central scar.

15.2.3
Imaging Features

At ultrasonography, fibrolamellar hepatocellular carcinoma usually present as a large, solitary, well-defined and lobulated mass, with variable echotexture. The central scar is usually hyperechoic.

CT demonstrates typically a solitary mass with well-defined, lobulated margins (Figs. 15.4–15.6).

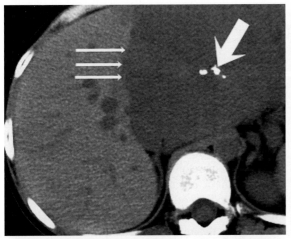

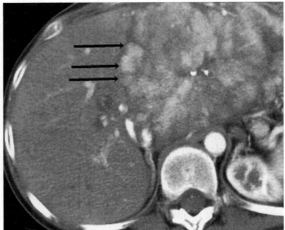

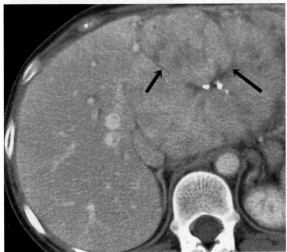

Fig. 15.4a–c. Fibrolamellar hepatocellular carcinoma in the left lobe in a 21-year-old woman. **a** Non-enhanced transverse CT scan shows a large mass (*long thin arrows*) replacing the left lobe of the liver, hypoattenuating to the non-neoplastic parenchyma, with central calcifications (*short thick arrow*). **b** Hepatic arterial contrast-enhanced transverse CT scan demonstrates moderate, heterogeneous enhancement within the tumor (*arrows*), with a central hypoattenuating scar. **c** Portal venous contrast-enhanced transverse CT scan shows isoattenuation of the tumor. Note septa (*arrows*) radiating from the center to the periphery

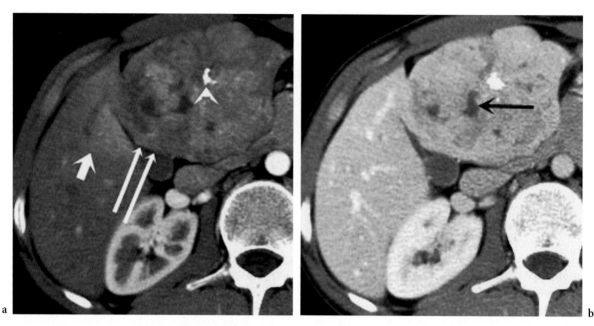

a   b

Fig. 15.5a,b. Fibrolamellar hepatocellular carcinoma in the left lobe in a 22-year-old man. **a** Hepatic arterial contrast-enhanced transverse CT scan shows a heterogeneous hypervascular tumor (*long thin arrows*) with a central calcification (*arrowhead*). The scattered hypoattenuating foci represent areas of necrosis. The adjacent non-tumorous liver enhances to an abnormal degree (*short thick arrow*), due to increased arterial flow and decreased portal venous flow. **b** Portal venous contrast-enhanced transverse CT scan shows the heterogeneous tumor, with hypoattenuating necrotic areas (*arrow*). Compression of a branch of the portal vein, responsible for the segmental increased arterial flow, was seen on an adjacent image (not shown)

A usually incomplete tumor capsule surrounds the mass in 35% of cases, and small calcifications are seen in the center of the tumor in 68% of cases. Cyst-like or necrotic areas are noted in 65% of cases, while fat is never observed. On non-enhanced CT images, the tumor is heterogeneous and hypoattenuating to adjacent normal liver. On hepatic-arterial phase, the tumor is usually heterogeneously and strongly hyperattenuating to liver. On portal venous phase, the tumor is iso- to hypoattenuating to liver, while on delayed-phase imaging the tumor is usually hypoattenuating. A stellate, central scar is noted at CT in 71% of cases, with radial septal bands extending toward the periphery of the tumor. The central scar and septa are hypoattenuating on unenhanced, arterial and portal venous phase, while they can become hyperattenuating to liver on delayed-phase. Lymphadenopathy is noted in 65% of cases, involving most commonly the hepatic hilum. Malignant features that are occasionally observed are biliary invasion or lung metastases.

At magnetic resonance imaging, the tumor is hypointense to liver on T1-weighted images, and hyperintense on T2-weighted images. In the arterial phase of imaging the tumor is usually markedly heterogeneous and hyperintense. The tumor becomes hypointense on both portal venous and delayed phase. Calcifications can be suspected as hypointense spots on both T1-weighted and T2-weighted images. Cyst-

Fig. 15.6a–f. Fibrolamellar hepatocellular carcinoma in the right lobe in a 21-year-old woman. **a** Non-enhanced transverse CT scan shows a large hypoattenuating mass (*short arrows*) in the right hepatic lobe. A calcification (*long arrows*) is noted within the center of the tumor. **b** Hepatic arterial contrast-enhanced transverse CT scan demonstrates heterogeneous tumor enhancement (*arrows*). An enlarged lymph node (LN) is seen at hilum. **c** Delayed contrast-enhanced transverse CT scan. The lesion becomes hypoattenuating to the surrounding liver. Septa (*arrows*) radiating from the center to the periphery are better seen on this phase of enhancement. **d** Fat-suppressed T2-weighted turbo spin-echo MR image shows the mass as of slightly higher intensity compared to the surrounding liver parenchyma. The central scar (*arrowhead*) is hypointense. The peripheral hyperintense foci (*arrow*) represent areas of necrosis. **e** Gadolinium-enhanced T1-weighted gradient-echo MR image obtained during arterial-phase shows marked hypervascularity of the tumor, central scar, fibrous septa and a non-enhancing capsule (*arrows*) that surrounds most of the lesion. **f** Gadolinium-enhanced T1-weighted gradient-echo MR image obtained during portal-phase shows isointensity of the tumor to the normal surrounding liver. A peripheral portion of the tumor that was of high signal intensity on T2-weighted imaging is noted as of low-signal intensity (*arrow*) on this sequence

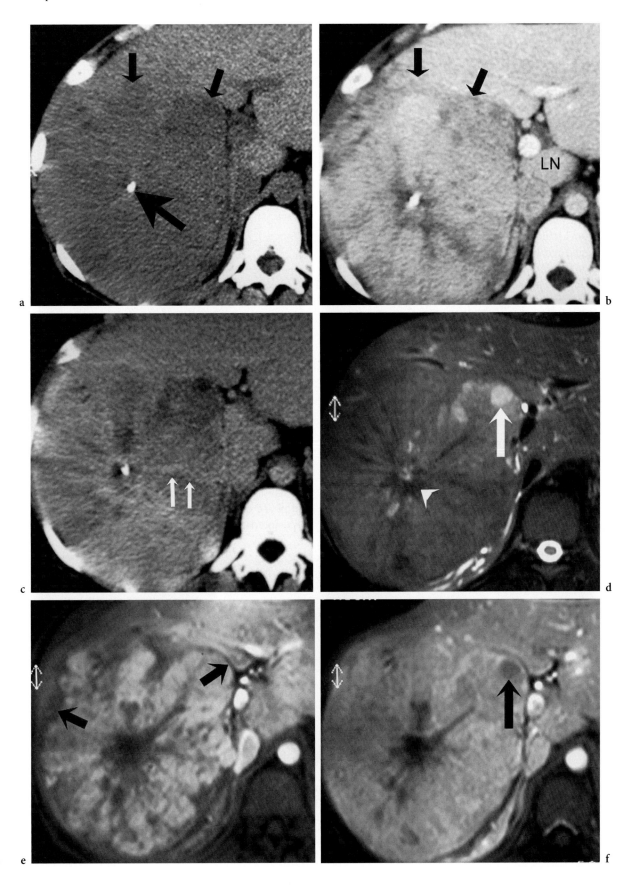

like or necrotic areas appear as hypointense on T1-weighted and markedly hyperintense on T2-weighted images. The central scar and septa are hypointense on both T1-weighted and T2-weighted images, and can show partial enhancement on delayed phase. Rarely, however, the scar may show hyperintensity on T2-weighted imaging, rendering difficult the differential diagnosis with focal nodular hyperplasia.

At angiography, fibrolamellar hepatocellular carcinoma is usually seen as a hypervascular mass with enlarged feeding arteries and dense tumor blush. No arteriovenous or arterioportal shunts are usually noted. Fibrous septa are seen as multiple serpiginous hypovascular areas, while central scar is avascular. At tagged red blood cell scan, fibrolamellar hepatocellular carcinoma shows early uptake and late defect. At Tc-99m-labeled sulfur colloid examination, if solitary, the mass is seen as a single photopenic defect, if multifocal as multiple defects. It is however difficult to differentiate fibrolamellar hepatocellular carcinoma from hepatocellular carcinoma or metastases with nuclear medicine alone.

15.3
Differential Diagnosis

Table 15.1 shows the main distinguishing features between hepatocellular carcinoma arising in non-cirrhotic liver and fibrolamellar hepatocellular carcinoma. Both hepatocellular carcinoma in non-

Table 15.1. Epidemiological, clinical, pathologic and imaging features of hepatocellular carcinoma arising in non-cirrhotic liver and fibrolamellar hepatocellular carcinoma

	Fibrolamellar hepatocellular carcinoma	Hepatocellular carcinoma
Sex	M=F	M>F
Average age	28	61
Lobe	Left in 65%	Right in 54%
Calcifications	68%	28%
Location of calcifications	Central in 95%	Peripheral
Surface	Lobulated	Lobulated
Capsule	35%	51%
Size	13 cm	12.4 cm
Lymphadenopathy	65%	21%
Fat	~0%	10%

cirrhotic liver and fibrolamellar hepatocellular carcinoma have to be differentiated from focal nodular hyperplasia, because both are seen in young individuals with no history of cirrhosis and both have a central scar or an area of reduced contrast-enhancement in the center of the lesion. Focal nodular hyperplasia usually has a smaller diameter (mean 5 cm), and calcifications are extremely rare. Focal nodular hyperplasia is isointense or isoattenuating to liver on non-enhanced, portal venous and delayed-phase CT and MR imaging, while it is strongly and homogeneously hyperattenuating/hyperintense on the arterial phase of imaging (Fig. 15.7). The scar is usually hyperintense on T2-weighted images, and this is the

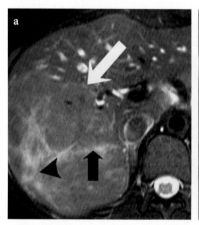
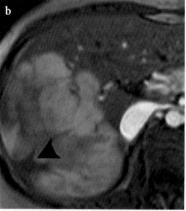
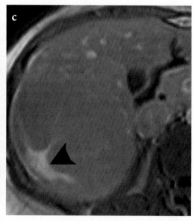

Fig. 15.7. a Fat-suppressed T2-weighted turbo spin-echo MR image shows a large tumor (*white arrow*) in the right lobe of the liver that is slightly hyperintense to the surrounding non-tumorous parenchyma, with a central, large hyperintense scar (*arrowhead*) and septa (*black arrow*). **b** Gadolinium-enhanced T1-weighted gradient-echo MR image obtained during arterial-phase shows strong enhancement of the lesion. The central area (*arrowhead*) does not show enhancement. **c** Delayed-phase (5 min) gadolinium-enhanced T1-weighted gradient-echo MR image shows isointensity of the focal nodular hyperplasia lesion and hyperintensity (*arrowhead*) of the central scar. Strong enhancement and homogeneity of the tumor and scar hyperintensity are the key to correct diagnosis

most valuable feature to differentiate focal nodular hyperplasia from fibrolamellar hepatocellular carcinoma, which usually exhibits a hypointense scar on T2-weighted images.

References

Arakawa M, Kage M, Sugihara S, et al (1986) Emergence of malignant lesions within an adenomatous hyperplastic nodule in a cirrhotic liver. Gastroenterology 91:198–208

Berman MM, Libbey NP, Foster LH (1980) Hepatocellular carcinoma: polygonal cell type with fibrous stroma-an atypical variant with a favorable prognosis. Cancer 46:1448–1455

Brancatelli G, Federle MP, Grazioli L, et al (2002) Hepatocellular carcinoma in noncirrhotic liver: CT, clinical, and pathologic findings in 39 U.S. residents. Radiology 222:89–94

Bugianesi E, Leone N, Vanni E, et al (2002) Expanding the natural history of nonalcoholic steatohepatitis: from cryptogenic cirrhosis to hepatocellular carcinoma. Gastroenterology 123:134–140

Craig JR, Peters RL, Edmondson HA, et al (1980) Fibrolamellar carcinoma of the liver: a tumor of adolescents and young adults with distinctive clinico-pathologic features. Cancer 46:372–379

Ferrell L (1993) Hepatocellular carcinoma arising in a focus of multilobular adenoma. A case report. Am J Surg Pathol 17:525–529

Ichikawa T, Federle MP, Grazioli L, et al (1999) Fibrolamellar hepatocellular carcinoma: imaging and pathologic findings in 31 recent cases. Radiology 213:352–361

Llovet JM, Borroughs A, Bruix J (2003) Hepatocellular carcinoma. Lancet 362:1907–1917

Nzeako UC, Goodman ZD, Ishak KG (1996) Hepatocellular carcinoma in cirrhotic and noncirrhotic livers. A clinico-histopathologic study of 804 North American patients. Am J Clin Pathol 105:65–75

Trevisani F, D'Intino PE, Caraceni P, et al (1995) Etiologic factors and clinical presentation of hepatocellular carcinoma. Differences between cirrhotic and noncirrhotic Italian patients. Cancer 75:2220–2232

Winston CB, Schwartz LH, Fong Y, et al (1999) Hepatocellular carcinoma: MR imaging findings in cirrhotic livers and noncirrhotic livers. Radiology 210:75–79

16 Cholangiocellular Carcinoma

Sylvain Terraz and Christoph D. Becker

CONTENTS

S. Terraz, MD; C. D. Becker, MD
Division of Diagnostic and Interventional Radiology, Geneva
University Hospital, 24, Rue Micheli du Crest, 1211 Geneva 14,
Switzerland

16.1 Introduction

16.1.1 Epidemiology

Cholangiocellular carcinoma or cholangiocarcinoma (CCA) is a malignant tumour arising from bile duct epithelium and is the second most common primary liver cancer world-wide. In Caucasians, the relative frequency of CCA among histologically confirmed primary liver cancers is 19%–25%. Epidemiological studies have demonstrated increasing mortality rates and a nearly twofold increase of CCA in the past 20 years. CCA is mainly a disease of the elderly, with peak prevalence during the seventh decade of life and a slight male predilection, although most patients with risk factors often develop this neoplasm at a younger age (Okuda et al. 2002).

Primary sclerosing cholangitis (PSC), with or without ulcerative colitis, is the commonest known predisposing condition to the development of CCA in Western countries, with a lifetime risk of 5%–15%. If chronic inflammatory processes of the biliary tract were sustained for a long period of time, they would cause the multiple chromosomal changes necessary to trigger the development of cholangiocarcinogenesis. The etiological factors that influence the regional epidemiology are liver fluke infection and hepatolithiasis. Two species of liver fluke, Clonorchis sinensis (clonorchiasis) and Opisthorchis viverrini (opisthorchiasis) that are endemic in South Eastern Asia and the Far East, are known to be associated with CCA. Besides the fluke, some chemical carcinogens that are present in local food may be involved as cofactors. The presence of a parasite in the bile duct mechanically damages tissues, resulting in chronic cholangitis (recurrent pyogenic cholangitis), and increased cell proliferation. Chronic hepatolithiasis (intrahepatic gallstones) is very uncommon in Western countries, but is endemic in some parts of the Far East. It was suggested that bacterial infection and bile stasis cause stenoses and dilatation of the duct, which further facilitates stone formation, persistent cholangitis, and eventually an increased risk of malignant transformation. An excessive risk of CCA was demonstrated with Thorotrast (thorium dioxide), a radiological agent no longer licensed for use, and smoking in association with PSC, but no relationship was found with organic solvent, alcohol intake or oral contraceptive use. Others predisposing factors for CCA include Caroli's disease with a lifetime risk of 7%, familial polyposis and congenital hepatic fibrosis. On rare occasions, CCA can develop from benign tumours, like biliary papilloma and adenoma, or from choledochal cysts with a 10%–30% risk of malignancy. Recent evidence now suggests a possible etiological role of hepatitis C virus (HCV) infection in CCA. Hepatocytes and cholangiocytes share the same precursor cell, called the oval cell. It is possible that oval cells are infected with HCV and develop into cholangiocytes with acquisition of certain genetic changes associated with carcinogenesis.

16.1.2
Clinical Features

CCA usually presents after the disease is advanced with non-specific symptoms. This is particularly true with more peripheral intrahepatic or perihilar tumours obstructing one duct, which often produce systemic manifestations of malignancy, such as malaise, fatigue, anorexia and weight loss, or vague gastrointestinal symptoms and ill-defined upper abdominal discomfort. Most common presenting clinical features of perihilar or extrahepatic tumours are those of biliary obstruction: jaundice, pale stool, dark urine and intractable pruritus. Some cases are detected incidentally by elevated serum alkaline phosphatase and bilirubin levels, or ultrasonography (US) performed for other indications. Right upper quadrant pain, fever, and rigors suggest cholangitis, which is an unusual clinical presentation.

16.2
Pathology

CCA may arise from any portion of the bile duct epithelium, that is, from the terminal ductules to the papilla of Vater, as well as at the peribiliary glands. Most of these ductal tumours are adenocarcinomas (95% of cases), but various other histological types

are seen at microscopy, such as mucinous, squamous, adenosquamous and cystadenocarcinoma. It is often impossible to histologically distinguish CCA from other adenocarcinomas that have metastasized to the liver.

In the surgical literature, CCA is usually classified as either intrahepatic or extrahepatic, and intrahepatic CCA is further classified as either peripheral tumour that arises distal to second-order bile duct branches, or hilar tumour (Klatskin's tumour) that arises from one of the hepatic ducts or the bifurcation of both hepatic ducts. This last entity is classified as intrahepatic, even though the right and left hepatic ducts join outside the liver anatomically. These three types of CCA, peripheral (20%–25%), hilar (50%–60%) and extrahepatic (20%–25%), are traditionally regarded as distinct disease entities from a clinical, therapeutic, and radiological point of view. However, this classification scheme is controversial. Differentiation between peripheral and hilar forms is difficult, since peripheral CCA can spread continuously into the hepatic hilum, whereas hilar CCA often shows continuous infiltration to the intrahepatic bile ducts. In addition, the distinction between hilar CCA and extrahepatic CCA is not clearly defined.

The Liver Cancer Study Group of Japan (1997) has proposed a new classification based on macroscopic appearance and growth characteristics, which divides intrahepatic CCA into mass-forming, periductal-infiltrating, and intraductal-growing types. Because some authors have reported that two growth patterns could coexist in the same patient, the combined type was defined. The prognosis for mass-forming and periductal-infiltrating CCA is generally unfavourable, whereas the prognosis for intraductal-growing CCA is much better after surgical resection. The different biologic behaviour of the tumours seem to be caused by their various locations and their size at the time of diagnosis. Further molecular or biochemical investigations are needed to support the "field theory", which states that all CCAs are biologically the same tumour originating from the same biliary epithelium.

16.2.1
Mass-Forming Type

Mass-forming CCA is the most common type of peripheral CCA. This neoplasm arises from the mucosa of a branch of the bile ducts in the peripheral or hilar area of the liver, invades and penetrates the bile duct wall, spreads between hepatocyte plates, expands via the hepatic sinusoidal spaces and grows three-dimensionally. Similar to hepatocellular carcinoma (HCC), tumour cells have a propensity to invade small adjacent portal branches in the form of venous tumoral thrombi. As the primary mass and satellite nodules within portal veins grow, they fuse together and form a large mass, up to 15 cm in diameter. On gross specimens, the tumour is firm and whitish grey because of its large amount of fibrous stroma and central necrosis may be present. The margin is usually wavy or lobulated but sharply circumscribed.

16.2.2
Periductal-Infiltrating Type

Periductal-infiltrating CCA is the most common type of hilar CCA. Arising from the mucosa of the intrahepatic or extrahepatic bile ducts, the tumour invades the wall and penetrates to the serosa. In contrast to mass-forming CCA, infiltrating CCA tends to spread along the bile duct wall via the nerve and perineural tissue of Glisson's capsule toward the porta hepatis. Thus, the tumour grows longitudinally and extends along the axis of the bile duct. Macroscopically, this neoplasm appears as elongated, spiculated or branch-like, with a firm, grey-white, annular thickening of the bile duct walls that measure up to 1 cm. Irregular narrowing of the involved bile ducts eventually results in obstruction of the lumen. The tumoral extension varies, ranging from 0.5 to 6 cm in length, sometimes involving all the extrahepatic ducts and extending proximally as far as the intrahepatic ducts. Associated tumour formation may occur outside the bile ducts in the liver parenchyma.

16.2.3
Intraductal-Growing Type

Intraductal-growing CCA, accounting for 8%–18% of reported cases, is a low-grade papillary adenocarcinoma, consisting of innumerable frond-like infoldings of proliferated columnar epithelial cells and slender fibrovascular cores. The neoplastic cells are confined within the mucosal layer, spread superficially without invading the submucosal layer. Since the intraluminal papillary projections grow to a certain size, the tumour becomes friable and may slough spontaneously from the wall of the bile ducts. Sometimes, the detached tumour forms implants in the lumen of the adjacent bile ducts, resulting in multiple tumours, so-called papillomatosis. The sloughed and floating tumoral debris may partially occlude the bile flow or drain through the orifice of the papilla of Vater. The tumours are usually small, sessile or polypoid but sometimes a large mass occludes an aneurysmally dilated bile duct. The biliary tree may be dilated diffusely, in a lobar or segmental fashion, because of obstruction by a tumour, by sloughed debris or by excessive mucin. When an intraductal CCA produces a large amount of mucus, it is considered as a variant and is labelled intraductal papillary mucinous tumour (IPMT) of the bile ducts. Some IMPT of the bile ducts may occasionally impede the flow of bile, resulting in obstructive jaundice. This tumour bears a striking similarity to IPMT of the pancreas, in terms of histopathology and pathophysiology.

16.3
Imaging Findings

16.3.1
Peripheral Cholangiocarcinoma

Since mass-forming CCA is the most common type of peripheral CCA, its most common appearance on cross-sectional imaging is a single, predominantly homogeneous mass with well-defined irregular borders and with a distinct right lobe predilection. Its size is usually large because early symptoms are rarely present. Satellite nodules are frequent and vary in size. Capsular retraction is relatively frequent as a result of subjacent lobar atrophy by chronic compression of portal venous and biliary systems. The bile ducts peripheral to the tumour are usually focally dilated because of obstruction by the tumour. Periductal-infiltrating peripheral CCA is often difficult to detect by imaging. Early findings include diffuse architectural changes of a hepatic segment or lobe with discrete and focal bile ducts dilatation. In the later stage, the tumour may invade the hepatic parenchyma and hilum.

16.3.1.1
Ultrasonography

Mass-forming intrahepatic CCA manifests as a solitary mass in liver parenchyma with a nodular pattern. Increasing tumour echogenicity together with increasing tumour size is a well-documented finding (WIBULPOLPRASERT and DHIENSIRI 1992).

Nodules less than 3 cm tend to be hypoechoic or isoechoic, whereas lesions greater than 3 cm are predominantly hyperechoic. When multiple lesions are present, the larger mass shows higher echogenicity compared to the daughter nodules. A peripheral hypoechoic area, so-called halo sign, is observed in 1/3 of cases. These US findings did not differ from those found in cases of metastases from extrahepatic adenocarcinomas, which have also histological similarities. Sometimes, the central portion of the tumour may appear hypoechoic, due to the presence of necrosis, or markedly hyperechoic with acoustic shadowing, due to the presence of calcifications. Because of the peripheral location of the mass, bile duct obstruction is not often seen and, when present, it is a helpful sign for the differential diagnosis with HCC. Owing to its hypovascular nature, CCA shows scanty signals on power Doppler US, which also helps to differentiate it from the typically hypervascular HCC.

Recently, new echo-enhancing agents have been developed to improve detection and characterisation of liver nodules. The marked increase in the echogenicity of the liver parenchyma greatly improves the contrast between liver and non-hepatocytic components such as portal triads and liver masses. The use of galactose microaggregates with a small admixture of palmitic acid (Levovist, Schering, Berlin, Germany) intravenously and coded phase inversion harmonic US imaging provides detailed information about tumour vascularity. Progressive peripheral enhancement was observed in CCA nodules (Furuse et al. 2003). New contrast-specific imaging techniques combined with a second-generation agent, which contained sulphur hexafluoride (Sonovue, Bracco, Milan, Italy), can display microbubble enhancement in grey-scale, thus maximising contrast and spatial resolution and enabling the analysis of the microcirculation of focal hepatic lesions. These techniques offer high sensitivity either to microbubble movement at low mechanical index (MI) or to microbubble collapse at high MI and related to microbubble concentration. Hypovascular tumours such as nodular CCA appear as black spots in the hepatic arterial and portal venous phase, with a progressive peripheral enhancement and concentric filling in the delayed phases (Lencioni et al. 2002). Currently available US contrast media have not so far enabled to distinguish reliably between CCA and adenocarcinoma metastases.

16.3.1.2
Computed Tomography

Unenhanced computed tomography (CT) scan shows a predominantly hypodense mass, either solitary or with several satellite nodules. Calcifications may be seen in the central portion of the lesions, especially in mucin-secreting CCA. The most common pattern of mass-forming CCA on contrast-enhanced CT is a mild, incomplete and thin, rim-like or thick, band-like contrast enhancement around the periphery of the main tumour on scans obtained at hepatic arterial phase and as gradual centripetal enhancement on subsequent phases (Fig. 16.1a) (Kim et al. 1997). The distinctive intratumoral appearance of peripheral cholangiocarcinoma on two-phase spiral CT scans is a markedly hypodense mass mixed with stippled and slightly hyperdense foci during both the hepatic arterial and portal venous phase. The hypodense part corresponds to diffuse and microcystic changes of necrotic material and the slightly hyperdense areas in

---

Fig. 16.1a–f. Peripheral mass-forming cholangiocarcinoma in a 59-year-old man with weight loss and epigastric pain. **a** Arterial-phase CT scan shows a large, heterogeneous and hypodense mass with lobulated margins and satellite nodules in the IV–VIII liver segments. The contrast enhancement around the tumour is thin, irregular, incomplete and rim-like. **b** Equilibrium phase CT scan shows concentric filling of contrast material, thus making the whole tumour slightly denser than surrounding liver parenchyma. Central low density areas correspond to microcystic alterations of necrosis. **c** Coronal image from a PET study after intravenous injection of 218 MBq of [18]FDG. The liver mass demonstrates a marked increased activity with mean SUV between 3.5 and 6.1 within this area. Furthermore, there is a hot spot at the right lung apex (*arrow*), probably corresponding to a lung metastasis. **d** Unenhanced axial T1-weighted GRE image (TR/TE/flip angle: 106/4 ms/80°) shows the extensive lesion with a homogeneous low signal and well-defined borders. **e** Axial T2-weighted FSE image (TR/TE/flip angle: 586/80 ms/90°) reveals a heterogeneous and predominantly hyperintense tumour with areas of lower or higher signal intensity, depending on the fibrous content or degree of necrosis respectively. **f** Axial T2*-weighted GRE SENSE image (TR/TE/flip angle: 220/18 ms/25°) after intravenous injection of 1.4 ml of ferucarbotran (Resovist, Schering, Berlin, Germany). This technique shows a diffuse signal drop in the normal liver parenchyma. The tumour appears as a homogenously bright lesion with margins that are more clearly depicted. Furthermore, the daughter nodules around the primary mass and in the left hepatic lobe become more conspicuous, allowing a better delineation of tumour extension. After core biopsy, histopathology revealed an undifferentiated mass-forming cholangiocellular carcinoma. Since the tumour had been staged T4 Nx M1, the patient was treated by Gemzar-oxaliplatin chemotherapy

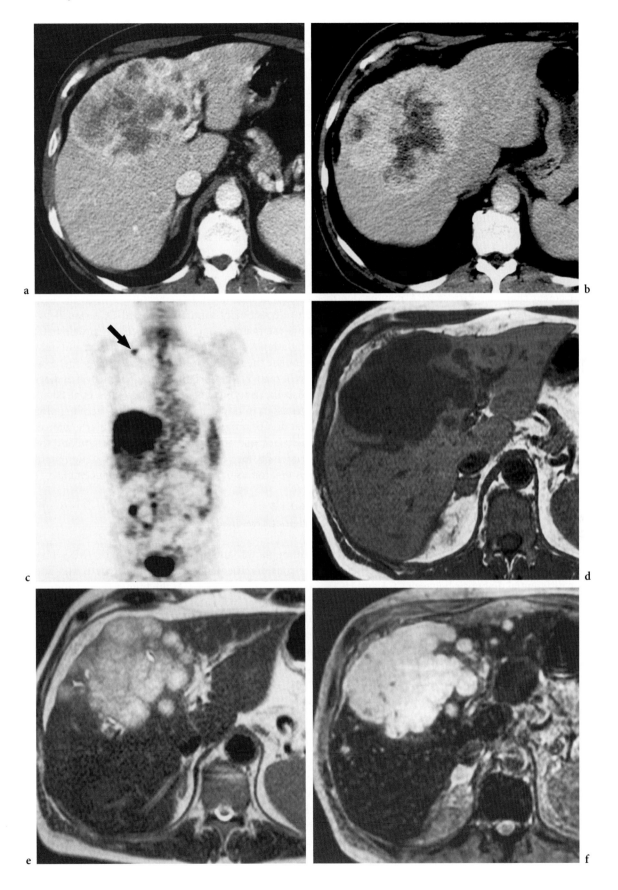

the mass may be consistent with mucinous substances (Ros et al. 1988). CT findings of daughter nodules are similar of those of the primary mass. In the vast majority, tumour shows a greater enhancement than the surrounding liver parenchyma on post-equilibrium-phase (Fig. 16.1b) (LACOMIS et al. 1997). Delayed imaging is of great diagnostic importance, since some CCA nodules are only depicted on delayed phase images, sometimes more than 30 min after contrast administration. Delayed imaging is also useful in differentiating intrahepatic CCA nodules from dilated bile ducts or fatty infiltration of the liver, and better defining their margins. In addition, although not necessary for diagnosis, delayed enhancement can be helpful as a target for CT-guided biopsy. These findings are explained by slow diffusion into the interstitial spaces of the tumour. It has also been suggested that the delayed enhancement characteristics of CCA may be due to contrast material retention within the fibrous stroma of these tumours. Besides fibrosis, other factors affect the delayed enhancement, like distribution of fibrosis, tumour grading and tumour differentiation: for instance, better differentiated tumours are more likely to show delayed contrast material retention than poorly differentiated ones (LACOMIS et al. 1997).

The contrast enhancement pattern of CCA differs from that of HCC or other hypervascular tumours, which typically show a single, early peak of enhancement followed by a rapid decrease in tumour attenuation, so-called washout (LOYER et al. 1999). Sclerosing and fibrolamellar HCC are distinctly different entities in clinicopathologic features, but both have abundant fibrous stroma. Therefore, both types of HCC show hypervascularity and prolonged enhancement on imaging studies. Other criteria are helpful for the differential diagnosis between CCA and HCC, which represent the two most common primary liver cancers. Most CCA occur in non-cirrhotic livers, may show intratumoral calcifications but no intratumoral fat, do not have a pseudocapsule, are not associated with arterioportal shunting and frequently cause bile ducts dilatation. Extension trough the liver capsule and invasion of organs adjacent to the liver is common in intrahepatic CCA, but rare in HCC, which is more expansive than infiltrative. Interestingly, the invasion of vascular structures around the liver is rare in peripheral CCA. Cholangiohepatocellular carcinoma (combined HCC and CCA) is a rare primary liver cancer that contains unequivocal elements of both neoplasms. CT findings of the HCC-component-dominant type resemble those of HCC, whereas CT findings of CCA-component-dominant type mimic those of cholangiocarcinoma. In exceptional cases,

concomitant but distinct CCA and HCC may emerge in the same cirrhotic patient and HCV infection would be probably their common pathogen.

Hypovascular metastases, especially from adenocarcinoma of the gastrointestinal tract, may have a similar pattern to that of mass-forming CCA and the differential diagnosis can be very difficult. Suggestive features for the diagnosis of intrahepatic CCA are unknown primary tumour, a relatively large single tumour at discovery, few satellites nodules rather than multiple scattered nodules, and other additional findings such as segmentary or subsegmentary bile duct dilatation, and retraction of liver capsule. Some primary malignant tumours (i.e. embryonal sarcoma, neuroendocrine carcinoma) or mesenchymal metastases (i.e. metastatic leiomyosarcoma) that rarely occur in the liver, may appear as a thick-walled, bulky mass that contains a large necrotic area in the liver and occasionally mimic peripheral CCA. Small hypodense hemangiomas are particularly problematic in patients with underlying malignancy and may simulate the satellite lesions of CCA or liver metastases. If present, the "bright-dot" sign is helpful in diagnosis these atypical hemangiomas (JANG et al. 2003). It consists in tiny enhancing dots in the hemangioma that do not progress to the classic globular enhancement because of the small size of the lesion and the propensity for very slow fill-in. However, a number of hemangiomas have no discernible enhancement.

16.3.1.3
Magnetic Resonance

Although CT and magnetic resonance (MR) may be considered equally effective in the detection and correct diagnosis of CCA, the higher tissue contrast resolution of magnetic resonance imaging facilitates the detection and evaluation of hepatic parenchymal changes peripheral to the tumour (ZHANG et al. 1999). The MR imaging appearance of peripheral CCA is invariably that of a homogenous hypointense mass on T1-weighted images with a peripheral hyperintense rim on T2-weighted images (Fig. 16.1d). Since internal desmoplastic changes are intermingled with various degrees of fibrosis, coagulative necrosis, and mucinous material, signal intensity of the centre of the tumour on T2-weighted images is extremely variable (Fig. 16.1e) (MAETANI et al. 2001). With respect to the central portion of the tumour, the stronger the fibrotic change, the lower the signal intensity on T2-weighted images. Although a central scar is not pathognomonic, this finding that reflects severe fibrosis appears to be a characteristic marker of intrahepatic CCA. Central areas with high signal intensity or with mixed high and low signal intensity on T2-weighted images, correspond to necrosis and cell debris with various amount of fibrosis respectively. Mucinous CCA is one of the histological subtypes of CCA and can be extremely hypointense on T1-weighted images and homogeneously hyperintense on T2-weighted images, due to large amount of mucinous lakes within the tumour.

Differentiating intrahepatic CCA from metastatic adenocarcinomas is difficult, since these secondary hepatic tumours also exhibit necrosis and show sometimes hypointense areas. Dynamic MR imaging studies may provide additional information because intratumoral fibrous stroma displays marked delayed or prolonged enhancement on the delayed phase of contrast-enhanced T1-weighted imaging and necrosis have been known to show no enhancement. Some authors emphasised the importance of "ultra-delayed" images, obtained 1–4 h after the administration of gadolinium chelates in order to investigate the different tissue components present in hepatic tumours. Typically, CCA revealed minimal or moderate initial rim enhancement, followed by progressive and concentric incomplete filling with contrast material. This characteristic enhancement pattern of central scar is similar of those seen in focal nodular hyperplasia. Small CCA (2–4 cm) may enhance homogeneously and simulate an HCC. Nevertheless, CCA do not show early phase hypervascularity and ancillary findings similar to those of CT imaging may help to differentiate both tumours. Although some studies have stressed that the portal and hepatic veins are not commonly invaded and make this a differentiating point from HCC, most authors believe the portal vein is commonly involved with tumour and emphasise the role of MR imaging in this field. Rarely, atypical hemangiomas with regressive changes, such as thrombosis, haemorrhage or hyalinisation, may show T2 signal intensity that is similar to that of CCA. Conversely, peripheral CCA may show progressive, centripetal and prolonged contrast-enhancement that may mimic peripheral globular enhancement of typical hemangioma. Interpretation should be based on the combination of two or more imaging characteristics (JANG et al. 2003).

Recently, diffusion-weighted MR sequences has been proposed for the characterisation of focal hepatic lesions by using single-shot echo-planar imaging (EPI) technique with diffusion gradients in three directions and with different b values (TAOULI et al. 2003). There is a significant difference between apparent diffusion coefficient (ADC) of cyst, heman-gioma and benign hepatocellular nodules (mean ADC 2.45x10-3 mm2/s) and ADC of HCC and metastases (mean ADC 1.08x10-3 mm2/s). Thus, diffusion-weighted MR imaging can potentially be useful for the differentiation between benign and malignant hepatic lesions.

16.3.1.4
Liver-Specific MR Contrast Agents

A variety of liver contrast agents have been developed for contrast-enhanced MR imaging of the liver, which are designed to overcome the limitations of extracellular low molecular gadolinium chelates. The two main classes of liver-specific contrast agents are the superparamagnetic iron oxide (SPIO) with uptake via the reticuloendothelial system (RES) mainly into the liver and spleen, and the hepatobiliary contrast agents with uptake into hepatocytes followed by variable biliary excretion.

As a negative contrast material, the particles of SPIO are taken up by the hepatosplenic Kupffer's cells, leading to a significant decrease of signal intensity of normal liver parenchyma on T2*-weighted images and remarkable improvement for detection of neoplastic focal lesion, which lack Kupffer's cells. SPIO particles may be slowly injected as ferumoxides diluted solution (Endorem, Guerbet, Roissy, France) or administered as direct bolus injection of undiluted ferucarbotran (Resovist, Schering, Berlin, Germany). SPIO-enhanced MR imaging can significantly improve the visualisation of intrahepatic CCA and the evaluation of the tumour margins, in a manner previously shown for colon metastases (Fig. 16.1f) (BRAGA et al. 2001). For CCA, the contrast-to-noise ratio is increased of about 90% compared to unenhanced imaging, similar to colorectal metastases. Therefore, SPIO are useful for defining the extent and location of intrahepatic CCA and are recommended prior to surgical exploration when CT shows a potentially resectable tumour. Benign hepatocellular lesions, such as focal nodular hyperplasia or liver cirrhotic nodules, are easily characterised by SPIO particles, with a significant signal intensity reduction in the lesions. HCC shows variable signal decrease on T2*-weighted images compared to surrounding liver, according to tumour differentiation. In addition, the degree of fibrosis of the underlying cirrhosis may decrease the tumour-to-liver contrast.

Mangafodipir trisodium, known as Mn-DPDP (Teslascan, Amersham Health, Oslo, Norway), is a paramagnetic complex that is metabolised following i.v. administration. After intracellular uptake of released Mn2+, T1 relaxivity of liver tissue is three times greater than that of gadolinium. Post-contrast imaging may start as soon as 20 min after the start of the infusion (5 mmol/kg), but longer time intervals are possible because of a plateau-like enhancement. Mn-DPDP enhances the performance of MR for classification of focal liver lesions as either hepatocellular or non-hepatocellular and benign or malignant (OUDKERK et al. 2002). Since CCA do not contain hepatocytes, they do not take up Mn-DPDP and typically demonstrate no central enhancement. Thus, lesion conspicuity is significantly increased after contrast administration. Occasionally, a peripheral rim or a wedge-shaped area of increased enhancement of the surrounding liver tissue may be found on early (20 min) and delayed (4–24 h) imaging, probably due to compression of surrounding parenchyma or functional biliary obstruction with subsequent retention of contrast agent. These findings are very similar to liver metastases. Other non-hepatocellular liver lesions, such as hemangiomas and cysts, do not take up the contrast agent either, but they rarely show peripheral rim enhancement and differentiation is primarily based on T2-weighted sequences. HCC tends to show a considerable variability in Mn-DPDP uptake: well-differentiated HCC may show significant contrast uptake, whereas poorly differentiated HCC tends to show only minimal or no enhancement.

Gadobenate dimeglumine or Gd-BOPTA (MultiHance, Bracco, Milan, Italy) differs from other gadolinium chelates in that it distributes not only to the extracellular fluid space, but is selectively taken up by functioning hepatocytes and excreted into the bile. Gd-BOPTA can be used for rapid dynamic imaging of the liver following bolus injection (50 mmol/kg) in the same way in which other non-liver-specific contrast materials are used, improving visualisation of hypervascular lesions. The liver parenchyma enhancement obtained with Gd-BOPTA between 40 and 120 min post-injection is equivalent to that achieved with purely liver-specific contrast media. Hence, Gd-BOPTA also significantly increases detection rate of hypovascular lesions (PETERSEIN et al. 2000). Typically, primary CCA nodules and liver metastases are obscured by the parenchyma or slightly hypointense on the hepatic arterial and portal venous phase images. In the equilibrium phase, these lesions are again detectable presenting with a hypointense rim surrounding them, known as peripheral washout sign. This sign is highly specific for non-hepatocellular malignant nodules. This observation is due to a

washout of contrast medium in the peripheral vital parts of the tumour, whereas the contrast medium in the more central parts demonstrates a delayed uptake, most likely because of its diffusion. In the delayed scans, an increase of the signal intensity of normal liver parenchyma is visible. Therefore, a higher contrast between normal liver tissue and the neoplasms is observed.

Gadoxetic acid or Gd-EOB-DTPA (Primovist, Schering, Berlin, Germany) is a paramagnetic contrast agent with hepatocellular uptake via the anionic-transporter protein. In human plasma, Gd-EOB-DTPA exhibits a higher T1-relaxivity than that of other gadolinium chelates. Dynamic imaging can start immediately after bolus injection (25 mmol/kg) and accumulation phase imaging can be performed at 20 min post-injection. Liver metastases and CCA show highest enhancement 90–120 s following i.v. injection of Gd-EOB-DTPA and then showed lower enhancement than normal liver after 3 min post-contrast (HUPPERTZ et al. 2004). A prolonged enhancement of hemangiomas compared to normal liver up to 10 min post-contrast was observed, differentiating them from metastases and CCA. HCC demonstrated an enhancement similar to liver parenchyma during the initial distribution phase and on delayed scans and thus were harder to detect on post-contrast images than on pre-contrast images. Additional information for differential diagnosis was achieved using Gd-EOB-DTPA-enhanced dynamic and static MR imaging for the characterisation of malignant and benign liver lesions and classification according to lesion type.

16.3.1.5
Cholangiography and Angiography

Direct cholangiography is indicated in patients with peripheral CCA only in rare situations, i.e. to detect contralateral bile duct involvement. The mass and its satellites give the intrahepatic ducts an encased or scalloped appearance. The smooth, variable length stricture affects adjacent ducts within the same hepatic territory. This appearance is usually not mistaken for the peripherally invading Klatskin's tumour, but care is required not to interpret these findings as primary sclerosing cholangitis (PSC).

Angiographically, peripheral CCA is predominantly hypovascular, with thin dysplastic vessels corresponding to neovascularity and fibrous transformation of the tumour (SOYER et al. 1995a). Intrahepatic CCA are purely hypervascular in 30% of cases, but shows no arteriovenous fistulas, as seen commonly in large HCC. Encasement of hepatic arteries and other major vessels is essentially due to sclerosis resulting from the tumour.

16.3.2
Hilar Cholangiocarcinoma

Most hilar CCA are of the periductal-infiltrating type, and it is therefore difficult or impossible to depict the tumour mass on imaging studies and to distinguish between a carcinoma arising from the hepatic bifurcation and a mass-forming peripheral CCA that secondarily obliterates the hilar area. The lesion may also represent infiltrating intrahepatic CCA that involves the hepatic hilum by intraductal spreading and the hepatic parenchyma by direct invasion.

16.3.2.1
Ultrasonography

Dilatation of the intrahepatic bile ducts is the most frequently seen US abnormality in patients with infiltrating CCA. Klatskin's tumours classically manifest as segmental dilatation and non-union of the right and left ducts at the porta hepatis. These findings may be the first and only clues to the presence of this pathologic condition. Dilated intrahepatic ducts with a normal-calibre extrahepatic duct are also suggestive of Klatskin's tumour. Characterisation of a CCA requires meticulous evaluation of the point of calibre alteration or ductal occlusion. If the level of obstruction is segmental, this scrutiny should include all the segmental ducts. Periductal-infiltrating CCA is the most common subtype at the hilus but is the most difficult to appreciate at US. In some patients, infiltrating CCA may appear as an obvious small central mass with associated mural thickening. More often, however, isoechoic infiltration of the periductal soft tissue and liver may produce a mass effect that may be inferred from the distance that separates the dilated segmental ducts (HANN et al. 1997). Subtle alterations in liver echogenicity and pressure effects on adjacent vascular structures, especially the portal vein, may also be helpful. On occasion, focal irregularity of the ducts may be used to suggest the US diagnosis as well as to establish the extent of tumour extension. Tissue harmonic imaging proved to be superior to conventional US in the examination of the biliary ductal system (ORTEGA et al. 2001). Imaging improvements include better sharpness of the duct walls, a clearer bile duct lumen, improved detection of intraluminal and juxtaluminal masses and reduc-

tion of side lobe artefacts. Second-generation US contrast agents also improve the contrast resolution of the modality and therefore its sensitivity for tumour detection (KHALILI et al. 2003). Further mass extent or satellite nodules not visualised on the baseline image are depicted on Levovist-enhanced US as small invasive foci following the ducts into the liver.

Although its appearance at CT is usually obvious, lobar atrophy is often more difficult to detect on real-time US. When lobar atrophy is present, US scans demonstrate crowded, dilated ducts within the atrophic lobe. The dilated ducts will often reach unusually close to the surface of the involved atrophic segment. The constellation of these three findings (dilated ducts, ductal crowding, lobar atrophy) is strongly suggestive of CCA, although long-standing biliary obstruction from surgical trauma or focal biliary obstruction from other causes may produce similar findings. In addition to these features, differences in lobar echogenicity may also reflect either ischemic or fatty changes.

Besides ductal involvement, vascular invasion and lymphadenopathy will influence the resectability of hilar CCA. The portal vein is more frequently involved (41%–63% of cases) and easier to evaluate with US than hepatic artery, which may be invaded, encased, or obliterated by the tumour. These findings are often better appreciated at grey-scale US, which provides higher resolution than its colour Doppler counterpart. Conversely, a vessel within a tumour may be detected only from its colour signal. Alteration in the calibre of the vessel with findings of waveform alterations and focal velocity increases at spectral Doppler US is suggestive of direct involvement of the vessel wall. Detection of lymphadenopathy in the hepatoduodenal ligaments and the peripancreatic region is sensitive but not specific because not all large nodes may contain tumour tissue. A flat lymph node with preservation of the echogenic hilar stripe is more likely of reactive inflammatory origin than are nodes that are round and hypoechoic.

16.3.2.2
Computed Tomography

Hilar CCA typically results in focal thickening of the bile duct walls with subsequent obstruction and pre-stenotic bile duct dilatation, although exophytic growth may also occur. CT is more sensitive than US in detecting an obstructive ductal lesion, showing an abnormality in 69%–90% of cases (TILLICH et al. 1998). In periductal-infiltrating hilar CCA, irregular and ill-defined thickening of the ductal wall can be seen in contrast-enhanced CT, which is often hypoattenuating relative to the liver parenchyma in the portal venous phase and hyperattenuating in the delayed phase (Fig. 16.2a). Lobar hepatic atrophy with marked dilatation and crowding of bile ducts is easily seen on CT scans in approximately 1/4 of patients with hilar CCA.

When using multislice CT (MSCT) technology, dilated bile ducts and the level of obstruction may be visualised by three-dimensional CT cholangiography with minimum intensity projection (minIP). Some authors have proposed this technique as an alternative of MRCP or cholangiography (PARK et al. 2001). CT cholangiography after slow infusion or oral administration of biliary excreted contrast agents has been used in the early 1990s. This method is time-consuming and is of limited value in patients with advanced bile duct obstruction and renal failure. These drawbacks prevented widespread use of this technique. A detailed representation of vascular structures allows a good depiction of invasion of the hepatic arteries and portal venous branches.

The hepatoduodenal ligament is commonly invaded in advanced Klatskin's tumour, appearing as dense masses in hypoattenuating tissue of the ligament. Lymphatic metastases most commonly involve the portocaval, the superior and posterior pancreaticoduodenal lymph nodes. Retroperitoneal lymphadenopathy, peritoneal spread, and proximal intestinal obstruction occur in advanced stages of hilar CCA. Both CT and US tend to understage hilar CCA, as local tumour extension along the bile ducts, peritoneal spread, and metastases in normal sized lymph nodes may not be appreciated.

Mirizzi syndrome is an uncommon cause of extrahepatic bile duct obstruction due to an impacted stone in the cystic duct that creates extrinsic compression of the common hepatic duct. The inflammatory component of this syndrome may be infiltrative or mass-like at the hilum and suggest CCA. Even, identification of a hyperattenuating stone on unenhanced images cannot always ascertain benign disease, since both entities may coexist (BECKER et al. 1984). Gallbladder carcinoma with contiguous spread to the bile ducts at the porta hepatis is often indistinguishable from CCA. The epicentre of this tumour is the gallbladder rather than the hilum and it is usually associated with gallbladder wall thickening and enhancement. Complications of biliary stone disease such as inflammatory strictures after stone passage or due to bacterial cholangitis are conditions in which the differential diagnosis can also cause difficulties.

16.3.2.3
Magnetic Resonance

On cross-sectional MR imaging, a periductal-infiltrating CCA appears as an ill-defined circumferential or nodular tumour with hypointense or occasionally isointense signal to liver on T1-weighted images and moderately hyperintense signal on T2-weighted images (Fig. 16.2b) (GUTHRIE et al. 1996). The central scar of the mass-forming type is an unusual feature of

---

Fig. 16.2a–f. Hilar periductal-infiltrating cholangiocarcinoma in a 62-year-old woman with progressive jaundice and mild abdominal discomfort. Initial ultrasound showed diffuse dilatation of the intrahepatic bile ducts with a normal-calibre extrahepatic duct and non-union of the right and left ducts at the porta hepatis. Right branch of portal vein was invisible. **a** Portal-phase CT scan confirms the diffuse dilatation of both intrahepatic bile ducts and reveals infiltration of the hilum by an ill-defined mass that is heterogeneously enhanced by contrast (*arrow*). Right branch of portal vein is completely obstructed by this lesion. **b** Unenhanced axial T1-weighted SE image (TR/TE/flip angle: 186/19 ms/90°) shows an irregular hypointense mass that extends proximally along intrahepatic bile ducts from hepatic hilum. **c** Axial T1-weighted fat-suppressed GRE image (TR/TE/flip angle: 102/6 ms/80°) 120 s after intravenous injection of 6.1 mmol of Gd-DTPA (Magnevist, Schering, Berlin, Germany). The tumour exhibits a strong and homogenous enhancement and its margins are better delineated. Dilated intrahepatic bile ducts are easily differentiated from intrahepatic vessels. In this case, the right branch of hepatic artery is encased within the tumour (*arrow*). Digital subtraction angiography (not shown) demonstrated a slightly irregular vessel at this level, confirming arterial invasion. **d** Coronal breath-hold single-shot FSE T2-weighted MR cholangiography (TR/TE/flip angle: 1800/350/90°) with 3D-MIP reconstruction. Bile duct confluence is obliterated, with upstream bilateral extension to the confluence of segmental branches. According to Bismuth-Corlette classification, it is a type IV biliary obstruction. **e** Double oblique axial 3D-MIP reconstruction oriented along the course of the left hepatic duct and perpendicular to the course of the right hepatic duct allows a better visualisation of bile ducts anatomy and a better assessment of common bile duct, and right and left hepatic ducts involvement. *CBD*, common bile duct. **f** Gadolinium-enhanced T1-weighted 3D-GRE sequence (TR/TE/flip angle: 6/2/60°) with coronal oblique MIP reconstruction of portal system. This image nicely depicts the extrinsic occlusion of the right portal branch, with tapering of its proximal part (*arrow*). Distal portal vessels on the right side and left portal branch are patent. The tumour was confirmed histologically after brush cytology. Since the malignant biliary obstruction was classified as type IV, the palliative treatment consisted in placement of three metallic stents (one in the left segmental branches confluence, one in the anterior sector confluence and one in the posterior sector confluence), in order to prevent tumour overgrowth

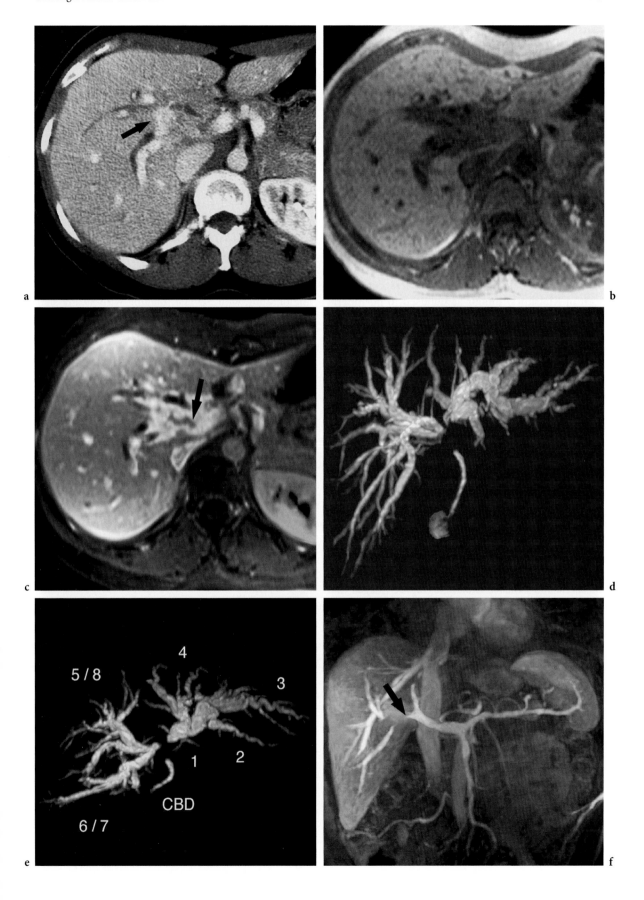

Klatskin's tumour. Hilar CCA does not show a unique enhancement pattern. The majority are hypovascular compared with adjacent liver parenchyma, showing a heterogeneous enhancement that gradually increases on delayed images. This pattern is consistent with the fibrous nature of the tumour. Circumferential tumours may cause minimally increased duct wall thickness and are most clearly shown as moderate periductal enhancement on gadolinium-enhanced fat-suppressed gradient echo images (Fig. 16.2c) (WORAWATTANAKUL et al. 1998). Since appreciable duct wall enhancement has been demonstrated in normal subjects previously, isolated duct wall enhancement may not be a predictor of tumour involvement. A small percentage of infiltrating CCA are hypervascular but without immediate diffuse enhancement. Satellite nodules are less commonly seen in Klatskin's tumour as opposed to peripheral CCA. Invasion of adjacent liver parenchyma and assessment of the atrophy-hypertrophy complex are important in determining tumour non-resectability. Cross-sectional MR images can detect a mass that frequently grows beyond the duct and invades the adjacent liver parenchyma. Morphologic alterations of the liver may also be evaluated by this imaging modality. Lymphadenopathy in the porta hepatis or in the coeliomesenteric and retroperitoneal spaces are more clearly defined on gadolinium-enhanced fat-suppressed gradient echo images.

Over the past decade, projectional MR cholangiopancreatography (MRCP), used in conjunction with MR imaging, has been introduced to evaluate the extent of tumours in the bile ducts. MRCP, with respiratory-gated 3D fast spin echo (FSE) or breath-hold single-shot FSE T2-weighted sequences, can produce excellent non-invasive cholangiographic images that depict hilar obstruction and subsequent dilatation of upstream bile ducts (BECKER et al. 1997). Further, this technique permits visualisation of the ductal irregularity and narrowing characteristic of hilar CCA and the intraluminal tumour extent (SCHWARTZ et al. 2003). The morphology of a bile duct stricture detectable on the images closely reflects the gross anatomic changes occurring along the biliary duct walls. A periductal-infiltrating cancer may be seen either as a stretch of narrowed lumen with a sclerosed appearance, or as an annular stricture. The mass-forming type tends to produce complete obstruction with protuberant-shaped end morphology of the bile duct, whereas the intraductal-growing type appears as an intraluminal filling defect, usually larger than 1 cm. MRCP accurately assesses the level of bile duct involvement with proximal and distal extension of the disease, according to the Bismuth-Corlette classification, although underestimation or overestimation may occur (Fig. 16.2d) (BISMUTH et al. 1992). Double oblique axial thin MIP slices oriented along the course of the left hepatic duct and perpendicular to the course of the right hepatic duct allows interactive 3D post-processing to depict even small bile duct stenosis (Fig. 16.2e). It is an advantage of MRCP over direct cholangiography that an undrained bile duct cephalad to the stenosis can be visualised without injection of contrast medium.

Although hilar CCA has a propensity to compress hepatic vessels (50%–82% of cases), frank vascular invasion is rare. Compression of central portal branches is most frequent, as these have thinner walls than hepatic arteries. Until recently, assessment of resectability in CCA usually required the use of digital subtraction angiography (DSA) to determine vessel involvement. MR angiography, with 3D fast imaging with steady-state precession (FISP) technique, is comparable to DSA in the evaluation of the portal vasculature invasion in patients with cholangiocarcinoma (LEE et al. 2003). For this purpose, dynamic imaging in the coronal oblique plane is particularly useful for distinguishing vessels from bile ducts and for showing the relation of the lesion to the portal veins, because the whole portal veins are typically seen on one or two sections, hilar lesions are more easily localised, and the coronal anatomy is similar to that seen at surgery (Fig. 16.2f). Contrast-enhanced 3D FISP MR angiography has the potential to also substitute DSA in the preoperative evaluation of hepatic arterial invasion, even though DSA has a greater specificity.

16.3.2.4
Cholangiography and Angiography

The role of cholangiography is twofold: first, to help make the diagnosis in difficult cases of Klatskin's tumour where no mass was defined in cross-sectional imaging, and, second, to determine the extent of disease, especially if contralateral involvement exists (SOYER et al. 1995b). Unlike ERCP, percutaneous cholangiography delineates the morphology of hilar CCA in almost all cases. However, the majority of hilar CCA are adequately diagnosed and staged by non-invasive procedures, such as MRCP or CT cholangiography. The cholangiographic appearance of Klatskin's tumour is variable but mainly appears as a ductal narrowing or obstruction of the right and left and common hepatic ducts. As it extends beyond 3 cm, intrahepatic tumours invade the liver. The contour of the stenosed duct may be smooth or moderately irregular. The strictures tend to branch and may extend into the secondary order biliary radicles. Isolation of segments of bile ducts is common in advanced disease. Cholangiography often underestimates the extent of submucosal spread of CCA. Furthermore, hilar CCA should be differentiated cholangiographically from malignant extrinsic strictures and benign intrinsic strictures. Lymphadenopathy and extrahepatic metastases compress and displace rather than invade the extrahepatic ducts. Benign strictures almost invariably occur after cholecystectomy or distal gastric surgery, are short, and cause symmetric narrowing of the common hepatic bile duct. Rarely, lymphoma or sarcoidosis of the bile ducts are indistinguishable from CCA.

Angiography does not depict hilar CCA directly but can show stenosis or occlusion of the hilar or intrahepatic portions of the portal vein or hepatic artery. Nowadays, venous invasion can be accurately demonstrated by contrast-enhanced multiphasic CT or dynamic MR imaging, but angiography still remains the gold standard technique to exclude arterial involvement.

16.3.3
Intraductal Cholangiocarcinoma

Even though mass-forming intrahepatic CCA and periductal-infiltrating hilar CCA and their imaging findings have been exhaustively discussed in the literature, intraductal-growing CCA has been less commonly described. On cholangiographic imaging (MRCP, PTC or ERCP), the bile ducts proximal to the tumour are dilated, the degree of dilatation depending on the degree of obstruction. The intraductal CCAs is depicted as polypoid filling defects or irregularities of the bile duct wall. Usually the tumour is small and flat, but occasionally it is large enough to be visualised on cross-sectional examinations. The mass is confined within the bile ducts, and thus the thickened wall of the bile duct remains invariably intact. Intraductal-growing CCA tends to spread superficially along the lumen for a variable length and sometimes implants along the inner surface of the bile ducts, creating multiple discrete tumours.

16.3.3.1
Ultrasonography

On US, intraductal-growing CCA presents with focal, segmental or diffuse bile duct dilatation with single or multiple papillary intraductal masses or without visible tumour. An intraductal mass appears as a well-defined, polypoid or sessile, echogenic nodule filling the lumen of one or more bile ducts (ROBLEDO et al. 1996). Sometimes, a polypoid tumour causes expansion of the adjacent bile duct and its frond-like surface excrescences are well depicted. Colour Doppler may reveal some faint signals within the tumour.

Biliary stasis secondary to a stricture from PSC may predispose to bile salt deposition and resultant formation of non-shadowing stones and sludge, which may be virtually indistinguishable from intraductal CCA. These oval and avascular intraductal masses often become impacted within the common bile duct, which restricts their mobility. Occasionally, hemobilia secondary to hepatobiliary interventions or blunt trauma will form an intraluminal cast. Although these conditions are mimicking intraductal tumour, the patient's recent medical history and lack of mass effect are usually diagnostic.

16.3.3.2
Computed Tomography

Characteristic features of intraductal peripheral CCA at CT include segmental or lobar dilatation of the intrahepatic bile ducts with higher attenuation than that of bile. An obstructing mass is occasionally seen as a spontaneously hypodense lesion relative to the liver parenchyma, when it is larger than 1 cm. On contrast-enhanced CT, it appears as an enhancing soft-tissue intraductal mass (YOON et al. 2000). Because the intraductal-growing tumour does not penetrate the bile duct wall, its outer margin is relatively clear on CT. The tumour may not be depicted when it is small and isodense to the adjacent hepatic parenchyma or when the complex orientation of the dilated bile ducts obscures the presence of the mass.

Intraductal CCA at the hilum also manifests as an intraductal soft-tissue mass but is associated with more diffuse bile duct dilatation. At this location, the tumours are frequently multiple or disseminated within the biliary system and involve both the intrahepatic and extrahepatic bile ducts. Therefore, the true extent of this superficially spreading tumour is difficult to determine. HCC occasionally invades and grows within the bile duct. This tumour appears at imaging as a polypoid mass expanding the bile duct and therefore is difficult to differentiate from intraductal-growing CCA.

16.3.3.3
Magnetic Resonance

Few studies described the appearance of intraductal-growing CCA at MR imaging. The intraductal tumour is depicted as a cast-like or sessile mass (Fig. 16.3). MRCP shows intraluminal filling defect usually larger than 1 cm or irregularity of the bile duct wall (Fig. 16.3a). The bile ducts of the involved hepatic segment or hepatic lobe are dilated. Papillary CCA is frequently multifocal and spreads superficially along the mucosa, often with intervening normal mucosa between papillary lesions. The ability of MRCP to detect minute mucosal changes and small polypoid lesions is limited, and thus tumour size and span of involvement in the biliary tree are underestimated. Some intraductal CCA produce large amounts of mucin, which may result in overestimation of the tumour.

16.3.3.4
Cholangiography

Although the description of the three pathological types of CCA appears straightforward, at times the cholangiographic differentiation may be difficult, especially between focal stenosis of infiltrating type and papillary lesions of intraductal type. On PTC or ERCP, the involved biliary tree is dilated because of partial obstruction, and filling defects appear because of intraductal tumours. When intraductal CCA is small, there may be fine irregularities, with a velvety or serrated contour, along the bile ducts, representing the papillary surface of the tumour protruding into the duct lumen. However, when the polypoid lesion grows into the bile duct lumen, there is slow progress toward the near-total obstruction of the lumen. In this case, the contrast medium is only able to outline the rounded surface interface, causing a meniscus and making difficult to recognise the exact origin of the mass.

16.3.3.5
Intraductal Papillary Mucinous Tumour of the Bile Ducts

Severe dilatation of the intrahepatic and extrahepatic ducts is the hallmark of IPMT of the bile ducts on US, CT, and MRCP (Yoon et al. 2000). Both proximal and distal bile ducts to the tumour are dilated because mucin may obstruct the papilla of Vater. On cross-sectional imaging, the tumour may appear as a small mass. Mucin is echo-free on US, water-attenuating on CT, hypointense on T1-weighted images and hyperintense on T2-weighted images, and therefore is not visible within the bile juice. Cholangiographic techniques (PTC or ERCP) can show large or small, elongated or amorphous filling defects caused by mu-

cin in the dilated bile ducts. Some intrahepatic IPMT may produce cystic dilatation of the bile ducts that harbour multiple, fungating, intraductal papillary tumours that may calcify. Some of the involved bile ducts dilate cystically, whereas others dilate diffusely and proportionally. If superimposed infection occurs, imaging findings may mimic a liver abscess (Jin et al. 2002). Endoscopy may show mucin protruding from the orifice of the duodenal papilla.

16.3.4
Cholangiocarcinoma and Primary Sclerosing Cholangitis

Clearly, the diagnosis of CCA complicating PSC remains a difficult challenge and no approach to detection has proven optimally effective. Furthermore, uncertainty as to the presence of tumour can arise because the imaging findings in PSC may mimic those of CCA. Often a combination of clinical, laboratory, and imaging tests is used to monitor patients with primary sclerosing cholangitis.

Clinically, CCA is suspected when a patient has rapid clinical deterioration in association with a rapid rise in serum markers of cholestasis. Since up to 70% are Klatskin's tumours located at the hilum, cholangiography has traditionally been used to diagnose and follow up patients with PSC for the progression of disease and the development of CCA. Unfortunately, there is no cholangiographic feature specific for CCA. This shortcoming originates primarily from the difficulty in distinguishing benign dominant strictures of PSC from malignant strictures caused by CCA. In several studies, endoscopic brushing cytology of dominant bile duct strictures was shown to have limited sensitivity (30%–85%) and tumour markers were found to have low specificity. Therefore, it is impossible to exclude CCA on the basis of a negative brush biopsy result.

Cross-sectional imaging modalities such as CT and MR imaging can assist in the work-up of suspected CCA by demonstrating extraductal abnormalities. In fact, CT and MR imaging significantly outperform cholangiography in term of sensitivity and specificity (Campbell et al. 2001). Because most CCA have a fibrous centre, they demonstrate delayed accumulation and washout of contrast material, thus producing hyperdense or hyperintense lesions at delayed contrast-enhanced imaging. State of the art CT, with optimised contrast material administration and including delayed imaging, is able to directly depict tumoral masses, particularly those

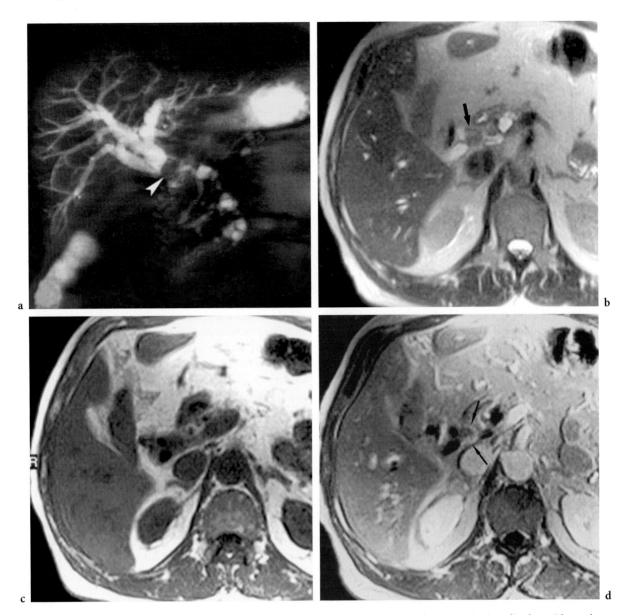

Fig. 16.3a–d. Hilar intraductal-growing cholangiocarcinoma in a 63-year-old man with progressive jaundice but without abdominal symptoms. Initial ultrasound showed diffuse dilatation of the intrahepatic bile ducts with a normal-calibre extrahepatic duct. **a** Coronal breath-hold single-shot FSE T2-weighted MR cholangiography (TR/TE/flip angle: 10000/247/90°) with coronal oblique MIP reconstruction. MRCP also demonstrates diffuse dilatation of intrahepatic bile ducts proximal to a round, faintly irregular intraluminal defect (*arrowhead*) at the origin of the common bile duct. **b** Axial T2-weighted breath-hold single-shot FSE image (TR/TE/flip angle: 80/18000 ms/90°). The 10-mm large intraluminal defect at the bile duct confluence (*arrow*) presents a heterogeneously moderate high signal intensity compared to liver parenchyma, suggesting the soft-tissue nature of this pathological process. **c** Unenhanced axial T1-weighted GRE image (TR/TE/flip angle: 86/4.5 ms/80°) shows a moderate low signal intensity lesion, with slightly hyperintense and thickened duct wall. **d** Axial T1-weighted GRE image (TR/TE/flip angle: 86/4.5 ms/80°) 90 s after intravenous injection of 8.5 mmol of Gd-DTPA (Magnevist, Schering, Berlin, Germany). The intraductal lesion is slightly enhanced by contrast medium and the common bile duct wall shows a marked contrast enhancement (*small arrows*). Surgery revealed a moderately differentiated intraductal papillary cholangiocarcinoma with minimal wall invasion (pT2 N0 M0)

arising within or invading the liver parenchyma, or thickened bile duct wall. Because of its increased contrast resolution, dynamic contrast-enhanced MR imaging has been shown to be more sensitive than CT for the diagnosis and staging of CCA (Vitellas et al. 2000). Periportal changes manifest as low signal intensity on T1-weighted images and high signal intensity on T2-weighted images. Such changes are suggestive of CCA if their extent is greater than 1.5 cm and they enhance after administration of gadolinium contrast material. In addition, MRCP may provide more information than conventional cholangiography about the proximal extent of disease, thereby allowing a more accurate assessment of resectability.

Positron emission tomography (PET) is another non-invasive imaging approach to detecting early CCA in patients with PSC (Keiding et al. 1998). 18Fluoro-2-deoxy-D-glucose (18FDG) is a glucose analogue and a positron-emitting radiolabeled tracer that accumulates in various malignant tumours because of their high glucose metabolic rates. After intravenous injection of 18FDG, CCA masses appear as hot spots on PET scanning of the liver. Preliminary observations suggest that the net metabolic clearance of 18FDG of these tumours is significantly greater than reference liver tissues in the same patients.

16.3.5
Cholangiocarcinoma and Choledochal Cyst

The incidence of malignancy in choledochal cysts is reported at between 10%–30%. The pathogenesis of CCA in choledochal cysts may be caused by the carcinogenic effect of pancreatic reflux. This complication is especially encountered with the most common type I cysts of the Todani classification, which consists in cystic, focal or fusiform dilatation of common bile duct. On the other hand, type III cysts rarely undergo malignant changes.

Most CCA that arise in patients with are papillary. At imaging, they are depicted as either a polypoid mass or an irregularly thickened wall. MRCP represents the current gold standard in the imaging of choledochal cysts and their complications, since it is superior than CT at detecting and defining lesions and as good as cholangiography, without the potential complications of invasive technique (Kim et al. 2000). Also, MRCP may not be as sensitive a tool in paediatric cases as it is in adults, where US has a pre-eminent role.

16.4
Treatment

The management of patients with CCA requires a high degree of expertise in diagnostic imaging techniques, as well as interventional radiological and surgical skills. Early diagnosis and accurate staging is the key to reaching the correct decision regarding the resectability of the tumour. The decision whether the tumour is resectable is based on the imaging information and the result of any biopsies taken.

16.4.1
Surgery

The best chance of cure is offered by complete surgical resection with negative margins and restoration of biliary-enteric continuity. Resectability criteria are based on tumour extension, vascular involvement, distant metastases, the presence of coexistent liver disease or dysfunction, portal hypertension and the general condition of the patient. CCA is resectable if vascular and biliary ductal involvement is limited to one lobe of the liver, if there is no extrahepatic disease, and the patient is fit for surgery. In patients in whom the proportion of the liver to be resected is substantial, it may be useful to carry out preliminary embolisation of the appropriate branch of the portal vein, in order to induce compensatory hypertrophy of the residual lobe, which minimises the risk of postoperative liver failure. In case of doubt, surgical exploration can be performed, in order to determine the chance of resectability.

16.4.2
Palliative and Adjuvant Treatments

Unfortunately, in many cases, imaging delineates an advanced tumour, requiring non-surgical palliative treatment, usually by means of endoscopic or percutaneous radiological techniques. The benefit of external-beam radiotherapy or intra-arterial local chemotherapy is uncertain. Intraluminal 192Ir brachytherapy may restrict tumour spread but to date there is no evidence that it provides any advantage compared with external-beam irradiation. Photodynamic therapy is a safe, minimally invasive palliative therapy, which may be effective in reducing malignant stenosis, leading to a significant longer survival and improved quality of life in patients with hilar CCA. Unresectable or recurrent peripheral CCA may be treated by means of percutaneous radiofrequency thermoablation. Even if there are few reports in the literature, we may reasonably recommend inclusion criteria that are similar to metastases of extrahepatic adenocarcinoma. Patients without known extrahepatic malignancy and with lesions smaller than 5 cm may be good candidates for this type of treatment.

16.4.3
Percutaneous Transhepatic Management

The palliative treatment of malignant hilar biliary obstruction is strongly dependent on individual expertise, but many authors favour the percutaneous approach over the endoscopic approach because the percutaneous technique provides better demonstration of the proximal extent of the tumour, allows easier placement of drainage catheters and avoids the risk of septicaemia due to a failed attempt at endoscopic stent insertion. Moreover, in the presence of multiple duct obstruction, the percutaneous route enables to drain individual branches by means of US guidance and fluoroscopy-directed puncture. If percutaneous transhepatic cholangiography (PTC) demonstrates proximal biliary obstruction, it is desirable that drainage is carried out in order to prevent cholangitis and sepsis (SHERMAN 2001). Unlike ERCP, PTC does not contaminate the bile ducts with enteric flora. Except for patients with acute cholangitis, in whom emergency drainage is mandatory, preoperative biliary drainage is not indicated in lower bile duct obstruction.

16.4.3.1
Biliary Endoprostheses Placement

Metallic endoprostheses offer a better long-term patency than plastic devices (WAGNER et al. 1993). Plastic devices should be used in preference to metallic endoprostheses only when a definitive diagnosis of malignancy has not been made, since metallic endoprostheses cannot be removed. Metallic stents can be inserted in a single-stage procedure in most patients, minimising hospital stay and reducing the associated costs. The proximal end of the stent should be placed in a peripheral intrahepatic duct, in order to minimise the risk of occlusion by tumour overgrowth. Ensuring that the stent extends through the sphincter of Oddi minimises the risk of late non-obstructive cholangitis and reduces post-procedural

morbidity (HATZIDAKIS et al. 2001). In patients with hilar tumours obstructing both the left and right hepatic ducts, bilateral or even triple stent insertion is usually indicated (Fig. 16.4). Parallel deployment of two stents should be achieved by using two separate punctures to gain access to each lobe.

The majority of metallic endoprostheses used are self-expandable devices, such as the Wallstent (Boston Scientific, Watertown, United States), the Zilver stent (Cook, Bloomington, United States) or nitinol stent (Cordis, Waterloo, Belgium). Balloon-expandable stents are infrequently used in the biliary system, because their relatively high rigidity hamper their deployment along a curve. Covered metallic stents offer no significant improvement in patency in comparison with uncovered stents, because overgrowth remains a problem (KANASAKI et al. 2000). On the other hand, peripheral stent placement (in order to minimise occlusion by tumour overgrowth) may lead to inadvertent occlusion of intrahepatic side branches. The possible future role of impregnated stents has yet to be determined.

16.4.3.2
Results of Palliative Treatment by Endoprosthesis

Metallic stents can be inserted successfully in up to 100% of patients. Survival after metallic stent placement has been reported as ranging between 93 and 420 days, depending on patient population, tumour location and stage (COWLING and ADAM 2001). In bifurcation tumours, the longest survival rate has been observed in patients in whom both lobes have been drained. The shortest survival rate has been observed in those with cholangiographic opacification of both lobes but drainage of only one lobe. The 12-month patency of metallic endoprostheses is 46% for hilar and 89% for non-hilar obstructions, with an overall 12-month survival of 35% (BECKER et al. 1993). Stent occlusion is usually caused by tumour overgrowth (2.4%–16%) and less frequently by tumour ingrowth (2.4%–7%). Stent occlusion due to encrustation of bile is uncommon, because of the large stent diameter. This condition may cause jaundice and cholangitis, and should be managed by insertion of a new endoprosthesis to relieve the obstruction. The re-intervention rate is 18%–19.2% after a mean period of 5.9 months (SHERMAN 2001; COWLING and ADAM 2001).

Complications of percutaneous treatment include cholangitis (5%–6.5%), haemorrhage (2%), bile leakage (2%), abscess and catheter dislodgement (COWLING and ADAM 2001; RIEBER and BRAMBS

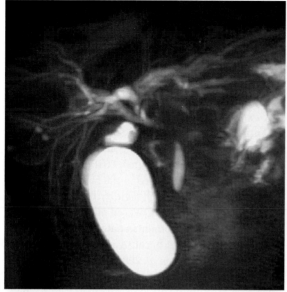
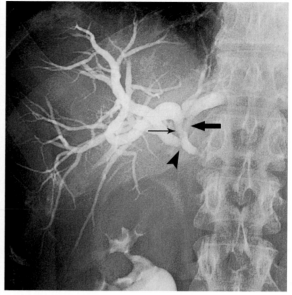

a

b

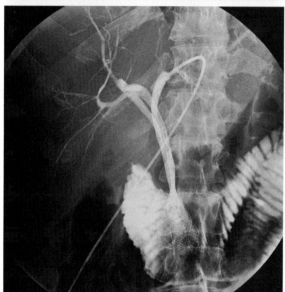

c

Fig. 16.4a–c. Palliative biliary drainage by triple metallic endoprosthesis of a hilar periductal-infiltrating cholangiocarcinoma in a 49-year-old woman with brutal right upper quadrant abdominal pain and vomiting. Initial ultrasound showed diffuse dilatation of intrahepatic bile ducts but without visible mass or wall thickening. **a** Coronal breath-hold single-shot FSE T2-weighted MR cholangiography (TR/TE/flip angle: 8000/247/90°) with coronal oblique MIP reconstruction. MRCP shows a stricture of the common bile duct with a diffuse dilatation of proximal bile ducts. A biliary trifurcation is present, with a separate confluence of V and VIII segments. Because radiological staging did not demonstrate any sign of vascular invasion or extrahepatic dissemination, the patient underwent an exploratory laparotomy, which revealed an invasion of the hepatic ducts, gallbladder and second part of duodenum. Surgical biopsies demonstrated a poorly differentiated periductal-infiltrating cholangiocarcinoma. Due to unresectability, the patient was then treated by palliative biliary stenting. **b** Percutaneous transhepatic cholangiogram obtained before stenting confirms an occlusion of the main bile duct without passage of contrast media distally. At the trifurcation level, left hepatic duct (*arrow*) and, to a lesser extent, confluence of biliary branches V and VIII (*small arrow*), present intraluminal filling defects. Moreover, there is a notch at the inferior aspect of right hepatic duct (*arrowhead*). Therefore, this biliary obstruction may be classified as type IV, according to Bismuth-Corlette classification, as confirmed by surgical exploration. **c** Positioning of three metallic endoprostheses leads to bile duct decompression. Catheter drainage was maintained in the left stent for 24 h to keep control on early reobstruction or haemorrhage

1997). Minor complications are seen in 10%–23% of cases, while the incidence of major complications ranges from 2.3% to 20.8%. Most complications are related to the transhepatic puncture rather than the stent placement (RIEBER and BRAMBS 1997). Aggressive guidewire and catheter manipulations, as well as vigorous filling of multiple undrained segments with contrast medium during cholangiography, can cause cholangitis and septicaemia, especially if stent insertion is unsuccessful. Stent-related complications include malpositioning, migration, inadequate expansion, failure of release of the stent and rarely duodenal erosion when the stent protrudes into the bowel. The 30-day mortality is 6-39%, depending on the patient's general condition, the tumour stage and the therapeutic method used, whereas the procedure-related mortality ranges between 0.8 and 3.4% (COWLING and ADAM 2001).

References

Becker CD, Hassler H, Terrier F (1984) Preoperative diagnosis of the Mirizzi syndrome: limitations of sonography and computed tomography. AJR Am J Roentgenol 143:591–596

Becker CD, Glaettli A, Maibach R, et al (1993) Percutaneous palliation of malignant obstructive jaundice with the Wallstent endoprosthesis: follow-up and reintervention in patients with hilar and non-hilar obstruction. J Vasc Interv Radiol 4:597–604

Becker CD, Grossholz M, Becker M, et al (1997) Choledocholithiasis and bile duct stenosis: diagnostic accuracy of MR cholangiopancreatography. Radiology 205:523–530

Bismuth H, Nakache R, Diamond T (1992) Management strategies in resection for hilar cholangiocarcinoma. Ann Surg 215:31–38

Braga HJ, Imam K, Bluemke DA (2001) MR imaging of intrahepatic cholangiocarcinoma: use of ferumoxides for lesion localization and extension. AJR Am J Roentgenol 177:111–114

Campbell WL, Peterson MS, Federle MP, et al (2001) Using CT and cholangiography to diagnose biliary tract carcinoma complicating primary sclerosing cholangitis. AJR Am J Roentgenol 177:1095-1100

Cowling MG, Adam A (2001) Internal stenting in malignant biliary obstruction. World J Surg 25:355–361

Furuse J, Nagase M, Ishii H et al (2003) Contrast enhancement patterns of hepatic tumours during the vascular phase using coded harmonic imaging and Levovist to differentiate hepatocellular carcinoma from other focal lesions. Br J Radiol 76:385–392

Guthrie JA, Ward J, Robinson PJ (1996) Hilar cholangiocarcinoma: T2-weighted spin-echo and gadolinium enhanced FLASH MR imaging. Radiology 201:347–351

Hann L, Greatrex K, Bach A et al (1997) Cholangiocarcinoma at the hepatic hilus: sonographic findings. AJR Am J Roentgenol 168:985–989

Hatzidakis AA, Tsetis D, Chrysou E, et al (2001) Nitinol stents for palliative treatment of malignant obstructive jaundice. Should we stent the sphincter of Oddi in every case? Cardiovasc Interv Radiol 24:245–248

Huppertz A, Balzer T, Blakeborough A, et al (2004) Improved detection of focal liver lesions at MR imaging: multicenter comparison of gadoxetic acid-enhanced MR images with intraoperative findings. Radiology 230:266–275

Jang HJ, Kim TK, Lim HK, et al (2003) Hepatic hemangioma: atypical appearances on CT, MR imaging and sonography. AJR Am J Roentgenol 180:135–141

Jin GY, Lee JM, Yu HC, et al (2002) Intraductal papillary cholangiocarcinoma with aneurysmal dilatation: a case of the mimicking abscess. Hepatogastroenterology 49:1523–1525

Kanasaki S, Furukawa A, Kane T, et al (2000) Polyurethane-covered Nitinol Strecker stents as primary palliative treatment of malignant biliary obstruction. Cardiovasc Interv Radiol 23:114–120

Keiding S, Hansen SB, Rasmussen HH, et al (1998) Detection of cholangiocarcinoma in primary sclerosing cholangitis by positron emission tomography. Hepatology 28:700–706

Khalili K, Metser U, Wilson SR (2003) Hilar biliary obstruction: preliminary results with Levovist-enhanced sonography. AJR Am J Roentgenol 180:687–693

Kim TK, Choi BI, Han JK, et al (1997) Peripheral cholangiocarcinoma of the liver: two-phase helical CT findings. Radiology 204:539–543

Kim SH, Lim JH, Yoon HK, et al (2000) Choledochal cyst: comparison of MR and conventional cholangiography. Clin Radiol 55:378–383

Lacomis JM, Baron RL, Oliver JH, et al (1997) Cholangiocarcinoma: delayed CT contrast enhancement patterns. Radiology 203:98–104

Lee MG, Park KB, Shin YM, et al (2003) Preoperative evaluation of hilar cholangiocarcinoma with contrast-enhanced three-dimensional fast imaging with steady-state precession magnetic resonance angiography: comparison with intra-arterial digital subtraction angiography. World J Surg 27:278–283

Lencioni R, Cioni D, Crocetti L, et al (2002) Ultrasound imaging of focal liver lesions with a second-generation contrast agent. Acad Radiol 9 [Suppl 2]:371–374

Liver Cancer Study Group of Japan (1997) Intrahepatic cholangiocarcinoma, macroscopic typing. In: Okamoto E (ed) Classification of primary liver cancer. Kanehara, Tokyo, pp 6–7

Loyer EM, Chin H, Dubrow RA, et al (1999) Hepatocellular carcinoma and intrahepatic peripheral cholangiocarcinoma: enhancement patterns with quadruple phase helical CT. A comparative study. Radiology 212:866–875

Maetani Y, Itoh K, Watanabe C, et al (2001) MR imaging of intrahepatic cholangiocarcinoma with pathologic correlation. AJR Am J Roentgenol 176:1499–1507

Okuda K, Nakanuma Y, Miyazaki M (2002) Cholangiocarcinoma: recent progress. Part 1: epidemiology and etiology. J Gastroenterol Hepatol 17:1049–1055

Ortega D, Burns PN, Simpson DH, et al (2001) Tissue harmonic imaging: is it a benefit for bile duct sonography? AJR Am J Roentgenol 176:653–659

Oudkerk M, Torres CG, Song B, et al (2002) Characterization of liver lesions with mangafodipir trisodium-enhanced MR imaging: multicenter study comparing MR and dual-phase spiral CT. Radiology 223:517–524

Park SJ, Han JK, Kim TK, et al (2001) Three-dimensional spiral CT cholangiography with minimum intensity projection in patients with suspected obstructive biliary disease: comparison with percutaneous transhepatic cholangiography. Abdom Imaging 26:281–286

Petersein J, Spinazzi A, Giovagnoni A, et al (2000) Focal liver lesions: evaluation of the efficacy of gadobenate dimeglumine in MR imaging. A multicenter phase III clinical study. Radiology 215:727–736

Rieber A, Brambs HJ (1997) Metallic stents in malignant biliary obstruction. Cardiovasc Interv Radiol 20:43–49

Robledo R, Muro A, Prieto ML (1996) Extrahepatic bile duct carcinoma: US characteristics and accuracy in demonstration of tumors. Radiology 198:869–873

Ros PR, Buck JL, Goodman ZD, et al (1988) Intrahepatic cholangiocarcinoma: radiologic-pathologic correlation. Radiology 167:689–693

Schwartz LH, Lefkowitz RA, Panicek DM, et al (2003) Breath-hold magnetic resonance cholangiopancreatography in the evaluation of malignant pancreaticobiliary obstruction. J Comput Assist Tomogr 27:307–314

Sherman S (2001) Current status of endoscopic pancreaticobiliary interventions. J Vasc Interv Radiol 12:140–155

Soyer P, Bluemke DA, Reichle R, et al (1995a) Imaging of intrahepatic cholangiocarcinoma: 1. Peripheral cholangiocarcinoma. AJR Am J Roentgenol 165:1427–1431

Soyer P, Bluemke DA, Reichle R, et al. (1995b) Imaging of intrahepatic cholangiocarcinoma: 2. Hilar cholangiocarcinoma. AJR Am J Roentgenol 165:1433–1436

Taouli B, Vilgrain V, Dumont E, et al (2003) Evaluation of liver diffusion isotropy and characterization of focal hepatic lesions with two single-shot echo-planar MR imaging sequences: prospective study in 66 patients. Radiology 226:71–78

Tillich M, Mischinger HJ, Preisegger KH, et al (1998) Multiphasic helical CT in diagnosis and staging of hilar cholangiocarcinoma. AJR Am J Roentgenol 171:651–658

Vitellas KM, Keogan MT, Freed KS, et al (2000) Radiologic manifestations of sclerosing cholangitis with emphasis on MR cholangiopancreatography. Radiographics 20:959–975

Wagner HJ, Knyrim K, Vakil N, et al (1993) Plastic endoprostheses versus metal stents in the palliative treatment of malignant hilar biliary obstruction: a prospective randomized trial. Endoscopy 25:213–218

Wibulpolprasert B, Dhiensiri T (1992) Peripheral cholangiocarcinoma: sonographic evaluation. J Clin Ultrasound 20:303–314

Worawattanakul S, Semelka RC, Noone TC, et al (1998) Cholangiocarcinoma: spectrum of appearances on MR images using current techniques. Magn Reson Imaging 16:993–1003.

Yoon KH, Han HK, Kim CG, et al (2000) Malignant papillary neoplasms of intrahepatic bile ducts: CT and histopathologic features. AJR Am J Roentgenol 175:1135–1139

Zhang Y, Uchida M, Abe T, et al (1999) Intrahepatic peripheral cholangiocarcinoma: comparison of dynamic CT and dynamic MRI. J Comput Assist Tomogr 23:670–677

17 Other Primary Malignant Tumors

Renate M. Hammerstingl, Wolfram V. Schwarz, and Thomas J. Vogl

CONTENTS

17.1
Introduction

Primary hepatic malignant neoplasms may develop from hepatocytes, bile duct epithelium, endothelial cells, or lymphoid cells. Most primary malignant hepatic neoplasms are epithelial in origin, such as hepatocellular carcinoma and cholangiocarcinoma. Mesenchymal tumors such as angiosarcoma and epithelioid hemangio-endothelioma, and other sarcoma and lymphomas are rare and represent a minority of primary hepatic neoplasms (Table 17.1).

This chapter will review rare primary malignant neoplasms such as hepatoblastoma, arising from hepatocytes; cystoadenocarcinoma, arising from biliary cells; angiosarcoma and other sarcomas as well as epithelioid hemangioendothelioma, arising from mesenchymal tissue; and finally primary lymphoma, arising from lymphomatous tissue.

Table 17.1. Histologic classification of primary malignant liver lesions

Epithelial tumors	
Hepatocellular	Hepatocellular carcinoma
	Fibrolamellar carcinoma
	Hepatoblastoma
Cholangiocellular	Cholangiocellular carcinoma
	Cystadenocarcinoma
Mesenchymal tumors	
Vascular tumors	Angiosarcoma
	Hemangiosarcoma
	Epithelioid hemangioendothelioma
	Leiomyosarcoma
	Fibrosarcoma
	Embryonal sarcoma
	Fibrous histiocytoma
	Lymphoma (Hodgkin's disease)
	Lymphoma (non-Hodgkin's disease)

R. M. Hammerstingl, MD; W. V. Schwarz, MD;
T. J.Vogl, MD
Department of Diagnostic and Interventional Radiology, University Hospital Frankfurt, Theodor-Stern-Kai 7, 60590 Frankfurt am Main, Germany

17.2
Hepatoblastoma

17.2.1
Incidence and Clinical Presentation

Hepatoblastoma is the most common symptomatic liver tumor occurring in children under the age of 5 years with a peak age of 3 years. Although it may be present at birth or develop in adolescents and young adults, this tumor has a peak incidence between 18 and 24 months of age. Males are more frequently affected. Recent evidence suggests that an extremely low weight at birth is associated with the occurrence of hepatoblastoma. Although diffuse and multifocal forms have been reported, it most commonly presents as a well circumscribed single mass (TSUCHIDA et al. 1990).

The epithelial type in the presence of hepatocyte predominance has a better prognosis than the other forms. Tumors due to embryonal epithelial cells carry a poorer prognosis.

17.2.2
Pathologic Findings

Hepatoblastoma has been considered a tumor of embryonal origin histopathologically different from HCC in childhood. Epithelial hepatoblastoma consists of fetal and embryonal malignant hepatocytes. A mixed hepatoblastoma presents both a hepatocyte and a mesenchymal component consisting of primitive mesenchymal tissue, osteoid material and cartilage. Amorphous calcifications are seen in about 30% of cases.

Grossly hepatoblastoma is usually a large, well-circumscribed solitary mass that has a nodular or lobulated surface. Twenty percent of cases are multifocal.

Microscopically, it consists of epithelial cells, malignant hepatocytes and tissues of mesenchymal origin (MILLER et al. 1992). Areas of calcification and extramedullary hematopoiesis are often present.

17.2.3
Imaging Findings

Hepatoblastoma needs to be differentiated from hemangioendothelioma, which occurs in the same age group (DACHMAN et al. 1983).

17.2.3.1
Ultrasound

Hepatoblastoma presents as a mass with heterogeneous echogenicity (DACHMAN et al. 1987). The association of the high Doppler frequency shift with neovascularity may prove to be useful in the evaluation of these masses (BATES et al. 1990). In contrast to hepatoblastoma, the great majority of hemangioendotheliomas (differential diagnosis) are hypoechoic.

17.2.3.2
Computed Tomography

On unenhanced CT the tumor appears as a homogeneous hypodense mass with or without calcifications which shows septal and peripheral enhancement. Delayed scanning may show greater enhancement (DACHMAN et al. 1987).

17.2.3.3
MR Imaging

On MR the tumor appears as a heterogeneous isointense or hypointense mass on T1-weighted unenhanced images. The presence of a fibrotic component determines hypointensity of the signal in the mixed type. Intermediate intensity with hypointense septations is seen on T2-weighted images. During the arterial phase of dynamic Gd-enhanced imaging, the lesion becomes heterogeneously hyperintense, except for the fibrotic and necrotic areas. On portal venous and equilibrium phases, the tumor rapidly appears isointense and subsequently hypointense. A stromal component increases in signal intensity. On delayed Gd-enhanced imaging the tumor is usually heterogeneously hypointense or isointense.

17.3
Cystadenocarcinoma

17.3.1
Incidence and Clinical Presentation

Biliary cystadenoma and biliary cystadenocarcinoma are rare neoplasms of the liver and comprise less than 5% of intrahepatic cysts of biliary origin (ISHAK et al. 1977). Cystadenocarcinoma develops mostly in hepatic cystadenoma. Most of the reported cases are in middle-aged women (DEVANEY et al. 1994). Clinical symptoms are abdominal pain, mass, and intermittent jaundice. Right upper quadrant abdominal pain, occasionally irradiating to the scapula, is the chief finding in 60% of patients at presentation (EDMONSON 1976).

17.3.2
Pathologic Findings

Most of the cystic lesions are intrahepatic; less than 10% are extrahepatic involving the extrahepatic biliary tree. Connections to the biliary tree may be seen, but are uncommon.

Macroscopically the lesions are usually multilocular and large. They frequently contain mucoid fluid. Large papillary masses as well as solid areas of gray-white tumor may occur in a thickened wall. The cyst is bloody in one-third of the cases.

Microscopically, a variety of epithelia, including columnar, stratum cuboid, and purely squamous epithelium, is seen. Most cases have invasive tubulo-papillary epithelial components. Areas of preexisting benign cystadenoma are found in about one-third of cases, suggesting that benign lesions may evolve into malignant ones.

Biliary cystadenocarcinoma are subdivided pathologically into two subtypes:
- First of all biliary cystadenocarcinoma with ovarian stroma, containing a typical band of closely bound spindle cells below the epithelium. This type is documented only in women developing from a preexisting biliary cystadenoma.
- Second biliary cystadenocarcinoma without ovarian stroma. This type is seen both in men and women and is not associated with a preexisting cystadenoma. Grossly, these tumors are typically large with variable amounts of internal septation and nodularity. There is variable composition of the cystic fluids contained in the locular compartments of the mass (BUETOW et al. 1995). The loculi may contain bilious, hemorrhagic, mucinous, or clear fluid. Calcification within the septa or wall is rarely seen.

Cystadenocarcinoma with ovarian stroma has a good prognosis, whereas cystadenocarcinoma without ovarian stroma results in death in more than 50% of patients (DEVANEY et al. 1994).

17.3.3
Imaging Findings

The pathologic features of the lesion have been shown to correlate with the imaging features on ultrasound,

CT, and MR imaging. Features such as nodularity and thickened septation are associated with biliary cystadenocarcinoma, the lack of nodularity with cystadenoma. However, there are no consistent morphologic or imaging features that would consistently distinguish neoplasms with ovarian-like stroma from those without it (BUETOW et al. 1995). On all imaging studies, it may be difficult to distinguish biliary cystadenoma and cystadenocarcinoma from other multilocular cystic lesions that occur in the liver, such as abscesses and echinococcal cysts. Correlation with clinical presentation and clinical history, however, should be helpful in this regard (AGILDERE et al. 1991).

17.3.3.1
Ultrasound

On ultrasound, cystadenocarcinoma appears mostly as a multilocular cystic mass. Associated nodularity is observed in half of the patients (BUETOW et al. 1995). The fluid-filled spaces may be either anechoic or hypoechoic.

17.3.3.2
Computed Tomography

On the CT scan, these tumors are predominantly hypodense due to their multilocular cystic nature. Nodular areas are evident as focal regions of soft tissue attenuation. After intravenous contrast, enhancement of the wall and septa is depicted (STOUPIS et al. 1994). The presence of thick, nodular septations and papillary excrescences favors the diagnosis of cystadenocarcinoma.

17.3.3.3
MR Imaging

MR descriptions of biliary cystadenocarcinoma are limited (CHEN et al. 1998; CHOI et al. 1989; STOUPIS et al. 1994). Biliary cystadenocarcinomas are of varied signal intensities on T1- and T2-weighted images depending on the type of fluid present within the locules of these tumors. The degree of internal septations and nodularity within the cyst wall varies.

In T1-weighted sequences there may be increased signal intensity internally if there is proteinaceous or hemorrhagic fluid within the multilocular cystic tumor. On T2-weighted images, biliary cystadenocarcinomas are of predominantly high signal-intensity due to their cystic components. Lower signal-intensity is noted in the walls and the septations of these tumors due to hemorrhage. Due to enhancement of the septa and wall, gadolinium-enhanced imaging should facilitate depiction of the internal architecture.

17.4
Angiosarcoma

17.4.1
Incidence and Clinical Presentation

Although angiosarcoma is a rare hepatic malignancy and accounts for less than 2% of all primary liver neoplasms, it is the most common mesenchymal malignancy in the liver in adults. Primary hepatic angiosarcoma is occurring more frequently than fibrosarcoma, malignant fibrous histiocytoma and leiomyosarcoma (BUETOW et al. 1997).

This tumor originates from the endothelial cells. In 40% of cases, angiosarcomas are associated with one of several toxins including Thorotrast, vinyl chloride, and arsenic ingestion. More rarely, angiosarcomas have been related to radiation and hemochromatosis. Association with hemochromatosis, von Recklinghausen's disease, and alcoholic cirrhosis has also been noted (LOCKER et al. 1979). This tumor occurs predominantly in men between the 6th and 7th decades of life. Angiosarcomas are aggressive malignancies that occur in the adult population, carrying a median survival of 6 months (MOLINA and HERNANDEZ 2003). Clinical symptoms include pain, anemia, fever of unknown origin, weight loss, abdominal mass, and hemoperitoneum (ALMOGY et al. 2004). At the time of diagnosis, most patients have distant metastases, most often to lung or spleen. Tumor markers are negative.

17.4.2
Pathologic Findings

Grossly, angiosarcoma is an unencapsulated multinodular lesion. Angiosarcoma may also diffusely involve the liver in a micronodular form. Mixed types might also be present. Rarely, a solitary mass can be identified (CRAIG et al. 1989). The tumors are predominantly located at the surface of the liver. They are nodular, ill defined, and may contain thrombosis or necrosis. When angiosarcoma appears as a solitary, large mass, it frequently contains large cystic areas filled with blood (ITO et al. 1988).

Microscopically, hepatic angiosarcomas are composed of malignant vascular cells that may form poorly organized vessels, which are variable in size from cavernous to capillary, trying to form sinusoids. The tumor is characterized by dilated sinusoids with hypertrophic or necrotic hepatocytes that leave vascular channels lined with malignant cells. Endothelial lining cells are seen to have increased in number, become enlarged and have large hyperchromatic nuclei. Tumor cells tend to grow along preformed vascular channels, particularly the sinusoid, and may form solid nodules or cavitary spaces (ITO et al. 1988).

17.4.3
Imaging Findings

All presentations are observed from a solitary liver mass to multiple disseminated intrahepatic lesions associated with splenic tumors. Because the origins of hepatic angiosarcoma and hepatic angioma are similar, specific diagnosis of these entities is difficult on imaging but almost always possible. Acute onset of the disease, exposure to chemical carcinogens, and a rapid increase in tumor size are highly suggestive of hepatic angiosarcomas and should allow live biopsy to be avoided (Table 17.2) (GOODMAN 1984).

Table 17.2. Angiosarcoma

Pathologic findings
   Foci of malignant vascular cells
   Grows along vascular spaces
   Displaces Thorotrast granules peripherally
   Appearance: – Multinodular (70%)
                – Solitary
                – Thorotrast
                   Peripherally displaced
                   Reticulated surface fibrosis

Clinical findings
   Most common sarcoma of the liver
   Male predominance: M>F (4:1)
   Non-specific symptoms
   Risk factors:
         Exposure: Thorotrast (10%), vinyl chloride, arsenic
                    Hemochromatosis
                    Neurofibromatosis

Imaging findings
   Multilocular masses with disseminated appearance,
   cystic areas

17.4.3.1
Ultrasound

The echogenicity of angiosarcoma is variable depending on the presence or absence of intralesional hemorrhage and the age of hemorrhage as well as necrosis. If the angiosarcoma is Thorotrast related, foci of increased echoes representing Thorotrast accumulations are noted throughout the liver. Multiple color signals are detected on color coded ultrasound (Fig. 17.1).

17.4.3.2
Computed Tomography

On unenhanced CT scan, angiosarcomas have a non-specific low-attenuation appearance. However, hyperdense areas are sometimes observed within the lesions due to hemorrhage or in non-tumorous liver due to Thorotrast deposit. Thorotrast accumulates as well in lymph nodes and spleen. In cases where remote hemorrhage occurred, necrotic or cystic areas may be noted within the angiosarcoma (Fig. 17.2). In the case of rupture of hepatic angiosarcoma, the diagnosis is ascertained by demonstrating free intraperitoneal fluid and a focal

high-density area adjacent to the tumor consistent with acute clot (MAHONY et al. 1982).

Due to its vascular nature, marked enhancement of angiosarcoma is noted on contrast-enhanced CT. Angiosarcoma may mimic hepatic angioma with progressive spreading enhancement and puddling of contrast material in different portions of the tumor, or it may be heterogeneous. In most described cases, the lesions become isodense on postcontrast images (ITAI and TERAOKA 1989).

Angiosarcomas have been reported to mimic hemangiomas on CT due to their centripetal pattern of enhancement (ITAI and TERAOKA 1989; MAHONY et al. 1982). However, a report of six angiosarcomas studied with spiral CT notes that none of the findings of angiosarcoma could be confused with the typical findings of hepatic hemangioma. In this study, angiosarcoma was multifocal in all patients and showed variable enhancement patterns. In only one patient who had multiple angiosarcomas did a single focus of angiosarcoma simulate hemangioma; all other tumors in this patient showed no imaging features similar to those of hemangioma (PETERSON et al. 2000).

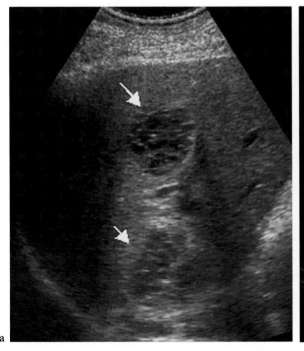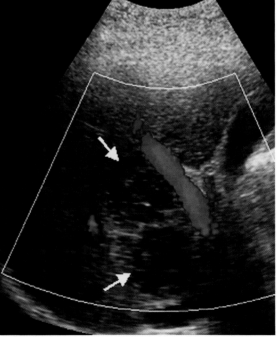

a   b

Fig. 17.1a,b. Angiosarcoma. Ultrasound findings. **a** Documentation of two hypoechoic lesions (*arrows*) in the liver with cystic areas and dorsal increased signal in B-mode imaging. **b** Color coded imaging refers to central non-vascular lesions (*arrows*) with hypervascularity in the periphery of the lesions and feeding vessels

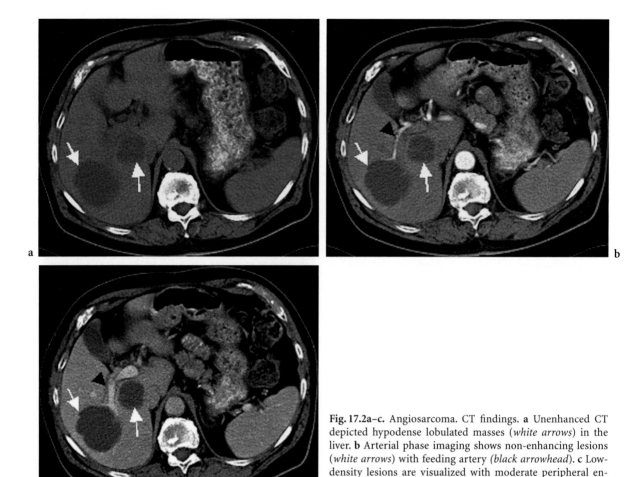

Fig. 17.2a–c. Angiosarcoma. CT findings. **a** Unenhanced CT depicted hypodense lobulated masses (*white arrows*) in the liver. **b** Arterial phase imaging shows non-enhancing lesions (*white arrows*) with feeding artery (*black arrowhead*). **c** Low-density lesions are visualized with moderate peripheral enhancement (*white arrows*) and feeding vessels (*black arrowhead*) in venous phase imaging

17.4.3.3
MR Imaging

The signal intensity on T1-weighted images may be hypointense with areas of hyperintensity related to hemorrhage (Figs. 17.3, 17.4). On T2-weighted images, angiosarcoma should be of increased signal intensity. After intravenous administration of gadolinium, peripheral intense enhancement similar to that seen with intravenous iodinated contrast occurs (Fig. 17.4) (BARTOLOZZI et al. 2001).

The signal intensity features of angiosarcoma are similar to those that may be seen in hemangioma. Both tumors contain abundant blood-filled vascular spaces. However, the peripheral enhancement of angiosarcomas is not of the dense, discontinuous, and globular nature that is typically seen in cases of hemangioma (MARTI-BONMATI et al. 1993).

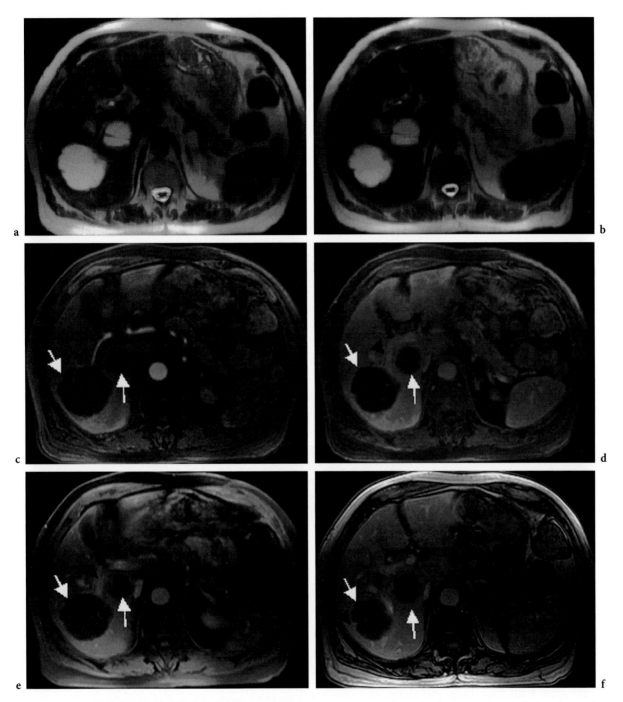

Fig. 17.3a–f. Angiosarcoma. MR findings. **a,b** T2-weighted HASTE imaging confirms the diagnosis of cystic lesions (*arrows*) with hyperintense signal unenhanced (**a**) and no change of signal postcontrast with Ferucarbotran-enhanced (**b**) delayed scans. **c,d** Dynamic gadolinium-enhanced T1-weighted imaging in arterial (**c**) and venous (**d**) phase depicts the non-vascular lesions (*arrows*) with peripheral enhancement as well as the feeding vessels (*black arrowhead*). Delayed static imaging using a fat saturated protocol (**e**) as well as an out-of-phase T1-weighted sequence (**f**) shows an enhanced rim (*black arrowhead*) and vessels near the lesions

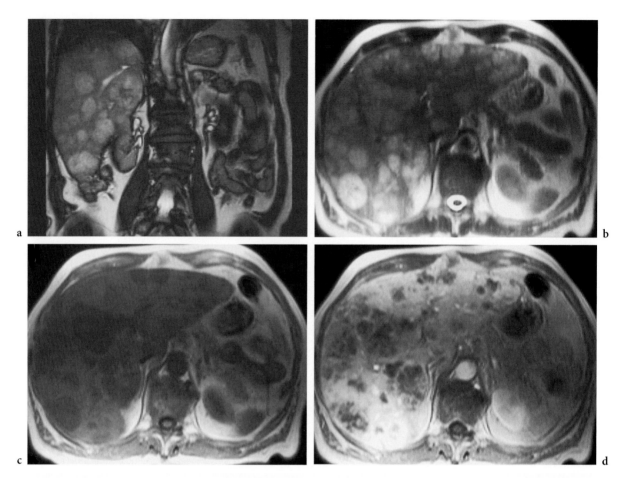

Fig. 17.4a–d. Angiosarcoma. MR findings. **a,b** Coronal and transverse T2-weighted imaging documents well-marginated multiple hyperintense lesions in the liver (true-FISP imaging (**a**) and T2-HASTE (**b**) unenhanced). **c** Lesions appear hypointense on T1-weighted unenhanced imaging. **d** On delayed Gd-enhanced imaging, lesions are hypervascular with predominantly peripheral and inhomogeneous enhancement as well as delayed retention of the contrast medium

17.5
Epithelioid Hemangioendothelioma

17.5.1
Incidence and Clinical Presentation

Epithelioid hemangioendothelioma (EHE) is a rare primary malignant neoplasm of vascular origin that may arise from liver, lung, soft tissue, or bone in adults (Table 17.3). This tumor should not be confused with infantile hemangioendothelioma, which occurs in children who usually are aged 6 months or younger. The tumor has a variable clinical course between that of benign endothelial tumors and malignant angiosarcomas (Weiss et al. 1986). Unlike most primary malignant tumors, two-thirds of patients are middle-aged women. Patients usually present with abdominal pain, weakness, anorexia, jaundice, and hepatosplenomegaly (Ishak et al. 1984). Rare mani-

festations include hemoperitoneum and Budd-Chiari syndrome (Hamm et al. 1994). The most common laboratory abnormality is in serum alkaline phosphatase levels. Tumor markers are negative. No risk factors of a specific cause of hepatic EHE are known (Radin et al. 1988; Weiss et al. 1982). However, oral contraceptive use and a possible linkage to vinyl chlo-

Table 17.3. Epithelioid hemangioendothelioma

Pathologic findings
        Female predominance: F>M (2:1)
        Middle age
        Association with OC or vinyl chloride

Clinical findings
        Non-specific symptoms or asymptomatic (20%)

Imaging findings
        Slow, peripheral, subcapsular growth
        Hypertrophy of uninvolved liver

ride exposure have been suggested (SHIN et al. 1991). The prognosis of patients with EHE is considerably better than that for angiosarcoma, but survival may vary from several months to 2 or 3 decades. Treatment depends on the intrahepatic extent and involvement of other organs. When possible, liver transplantation is the treatment of choice.

17.5.2
Pathologic Findings

Two major manifestations of EHE are multiple, nodular lesions, and large masses. It is speculated that the smaller, multiple, nodular lesions coalesce to form large, conglomerate masses, the uninvolved portions undergoing hypertrophy. They grow usually in the periphery of the liver, owing to the extension of the tumor through the tributaries of the portal and hepatic veins. These solid tumors characteristically have a dense fibrotic hypovascular central core and a peripheral hyperemic rim. Retraction of the adjacent liver capsule may occur, likely as a result of lesion-related fibrosis. This is an unusual feature in malignant lesions of the liver, and is suggestive of EHE (KELLEHER et al. 1989).

Microscopically, EHE is a solid tumor composed of epithelioid-appearing endothelial cells. There are dendritic spindle cells and epithelioid round cells within an abundant matrix of myxoid and fibrous stroma. Neoplastic cells invade and eventually obliterate the sinusoids, terminal hepatic veins, and portal veins. Approximately 30% of patients may demonstrate progressive sclerosis and eventual classification (KELLEHER et al. 1989). The demonstration of cells containing factor VIII-related antigen confirms the endothelial origin of the tumor.

17.5.3
Imaging Findings

Imaging findings using CT or MR are similar. Changes in hepatic contours are more often observed in diffuse lesions than in nodular lesions. These changes include capsular retraction, which is always centered over a peripheral mass and is suggestive of EHE. But it is not a specific finding and could be encountered in other malignant tumors, such as hepatocellular carcinoma (HCC) and cholangiocellular carcinoma (CCC). Moreover a compensatory enlargement may be seen, usually in the left lobe or the caudate lobe in patients with predominant lesions located in the right lobe. In addition, tumor invasion in the portal branches, obliteration of hepatic veins, and signs of portal hypertension are visualized.

Summing up, the following imaging findings are highly characteristic for EHE: predominant distribution at the periphery of the liver, intratumorous calcifications, changes of liver contour with capsular retraction and compensatory hypertrophy of the normal liver, invasion of portal and hepatic veins, tumors composed of concentric zones, and changes of nodular lesions to large coalescent masses (VAN BEERS et al. 1992).

17.5.3.1
Ultrasound

EHE usually presents as multiple peripheral hypoechoic masses. Hyperechoic and mixed hypo-hyperechoic appearances, however, have also been described. The hyperechoic masses may have a peripheral hypoechoic rim. There is no correlation between sonographic pattern and the size of the lesions. In diffuse lesions hyperechoic foci correspond to calcification (MILLER et al. 1992).

17.5.3.2
Computed Tomography

Unenhanced CT presents multiple, round or oval lesions of low attenuation. Intralesional calcifications have occasionally been described (FURUI et al. 1989).

Due to the vascular nature of EHE contrast-enhanced series are better in depiction. A peripheral tumor enhancement is noted surrounding the central low-attenuation fibrous core. A thin hypodense rim may be seen surrounding the enhanced periphery of the EHE, correlating with the avascular rim seen on pathology (Fig. 17.5).

Retraction of the overlying capsule probably due to lesion-related fibrosis is demonstrated in several cases, although this finding has been seen with other malignant liver tumors (SOYER et al. 1994).

Marked enhancement of the lesions is demonstrated on delayed imaging with isoattenuation compared to surrounding liver parenchyma. Incomplete filling of the lesions may be seen on delayed images in tumors with a high content of fibrosis.

In diffuse lesions, unenhanced CT shows large and diffuse areas of overall low attenuation. The vascularity of diffuse lesions is moderate, but delayed fill-in of contrast medium is consistent with fibrosis.

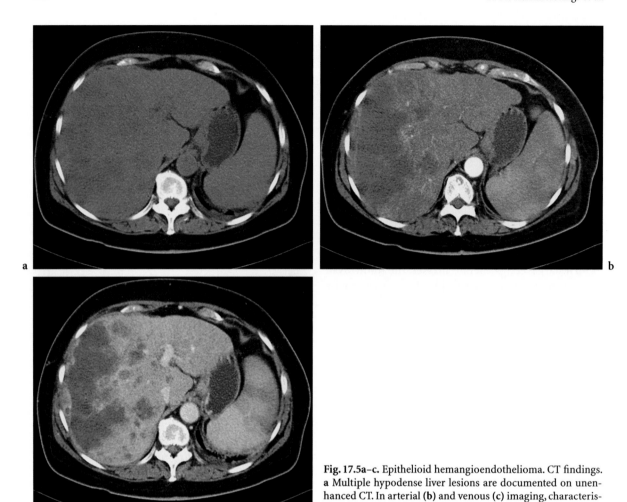

Fig. 17.5a–c. Epithelioid hemangioendothelioma. CT findings.
a Multiple hypodense liver lesions are documented on unenhanced CT. In arterial (**b**) and venous (**c**) imaging, characteristic peripheral distribution and enhancement are noted

17.5.3.3
MR Imaging

Concentric alteration in signal intensity, corresponding to the regions of different histology, are seen on both T1- and T1-weighted images.

The appearance of EHE on T1-weighted images is variable, demonstrating a hypointense lesion, a lesion of low signal intensity with a thin peripheral dark rim, or a isointense tumor with centrally thin dark areas. T2-weighted images show a heterogeneous high signal intensity. The center of the lesion may contain one or several concentric zones of various intensity. These areas are related to connective tissue admixed with calcifications or coagulation necrosis (BARTOLOZZI et al. 2001). The subcapsular nodules demonstrate a high signal intensity but not as intense as the characterizing one of hepatic hemangioma (RADIN et al. 1988). The hyperintense peripheral rim corresponds to viable tumor, the hypointense peripheral rim to the peripheral avascular zone (Fig. 17.6).

Contrast-enhanced series delineate a layered appearance with a central hypointense area, inner hyperintensity, and outer non-enhancing rim. EHE shows peripheral and delayed central enhancement (MILLER et al. 1992).

17.6
Other Sarcomas

17.6.1
Incidence and Clinical Presentation

With the exception of angiosarcomas, sarcomas of the liver are rare tumors. Other sarcomas of the liver include leiomyosarcoma, malignant fibrous histiocy-

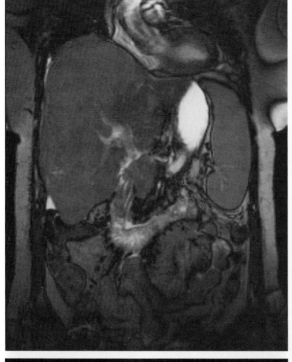

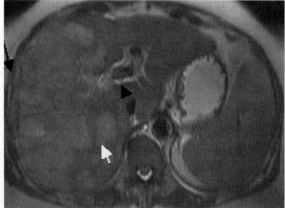

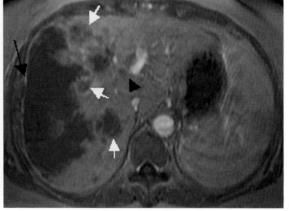

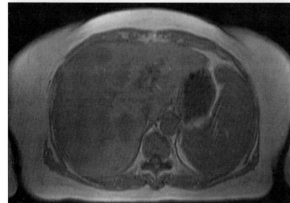

Fig. 17.6a–d. Epithelioid hemangioendothelioma. MR findings. **a** Coronal true FISP imaging refers to multiple moderate hyperintense lesions. **b** In a T2-weighted unenhanced HASTE sequence a retraction of the liver capsule (*black arrow*) as well as portal infiltration (*black arrowhead*) and relatively low-hyperintense multiple lesions (*white arrow*) are depicted. **c** Diffuse hypointense masses are seen on T1-weighted imaging. **d** On delayed Gd-enhanced scans, rim enhancement (*white arrows*), retraction of the liver (*black arrow*), and portal invasion (*black arrowhead*) are excellently documented

toma, and fibrosarcoma. Leiomyosarcoma is the most common (Ishak 1987).

In a recent review of the literature there were 54 cases of primary hepatic leiomyosarcoma: the male-to-female ratio was 25:26; the mean age at diagnosis was 54 years (Gates et al. 1995). Malignant fibrous histiocytomas have become increasingly common since the 1960s and 1970s, when it was introduced as a separate pathologic entity and subsequently popularized. These lesions demonstrate no significant sex predilection and usually occur in patients between 40 and 60 years of age. It is the most common soft tissue sarcoma found in adults.

Fibrosarcoma is a malignant tumor of soft tissue derived from collagen-producing fibroblasts.

17.6.2
Pathologic Findings

These tumors consist of malignant sarcomatous cells corresponding to the respective criteria used for each entity (Enzinger and Weiss 1983).

Grossly, these lesions present as large solitary masses on the background of a normal non-cirrhotic liver. There are variable amounts of internal hemorrhage and necrosis.

Leiomyosarcomas are bulky solid tumors with polylobulated margins and contain areas of hemorrhage. They originate from mesenchymal elements of the liver and are composed of large spindle cells of smooth muscle.

Fibrous histiocytoma is a malignant tumor composed of histiocytes and of macrophages. It is generally regarded as arising from primitive mesenchymal cells that demonstrate partial histiocytic and fibroblastic differentiation.

Fibrosarcoma is composed of cells and fibers derived from fibroblasts, which produce collagen but otherwise lack cellular differentiation. It is grossly grayish white, invades locally and metastases hematogenously.

17.6.3
Imaging Findings

17.6.3.1
Ultrasound

Sonography demonstrates a large mass, with a variable echo pattern depending on the degrees of internal hemorrhage and necrosis (Fig. 17.7). Lesions appear as well-defined masses (BAUR et al. 1993).

17.6.3.2
Computed Tomography

Similarly on CT scan both leiomyosarcomas and malignant fibrous histiocytoma have a similar appearance. A large non-calcified, hypodense, homogeneous mass is depicted, which exhibits heterogeneous peripheral enhancement after contrast medium administration. Non-enhancement corresponds to sites of necrosis with cystic and hemorrhagic spaces. Despite large tumors portal and hepatic veins are not involved in most cases (PINSON et al. 1994).

17.6.3.3
MR Imaging

MR imaging demonstrates a signal intensity that is variable on T1- and T2-weighted images (Fig. 17.8); more frequently they appear as hypointense masses both on T1- and T2-weighted images. Enhancement of the viable portions of the tumor is usually seen peripherally (Fig. 17.9).

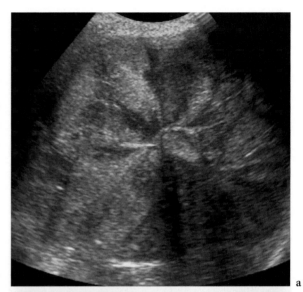

a

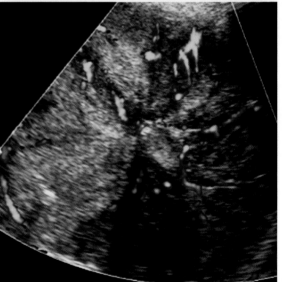

b

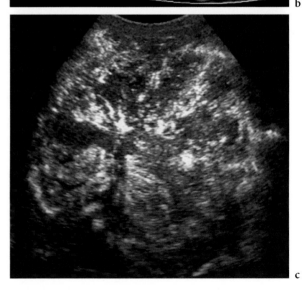

c

Fig. 17.7a–c. Sarcoma. Ultrasound findings. Inhomogeneous lesion of the liver due to clear-cell type of sarcoma revealing mixed echoic pattern using B-mode (**a**) imaging. Color coded (**b**) and contrast-enhanced ultrasound (post-Sonovue intravenously) in the venous phase (**c**) document vascular parts of the large tumor

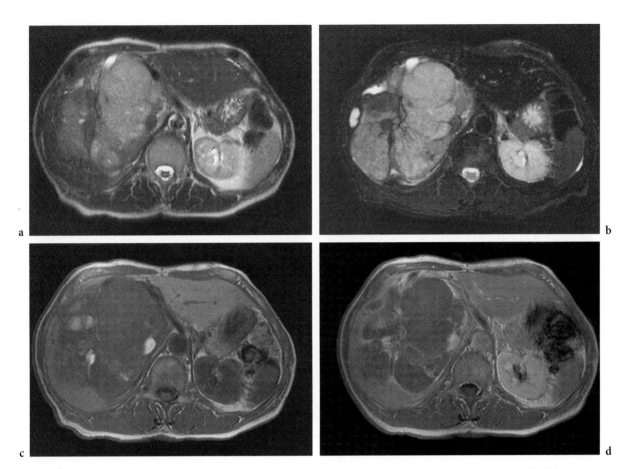

Fig. 17.8a–d. Sarcoma. MR findings. **a,b** Using unenhanced (**a**) and Ferucarbotran-enhanced (**b**) T2-weighted HASTE imaging, a hyperintense inhomogeneous tumor in the right liver lobe with compression of the surrounding vessels is seen. There is no enhancement of superparamagnetic iron oxide contrast agents (SPIO) in delayed Ferucarbotran-enhanced imaging. **c** T1-weighted unenhanced scan shows a mass with mixed signal. **d** Hypervascular areas are demonstrated with inhomogeneous enhancement in a delayed gadolinium-enhanced protocol

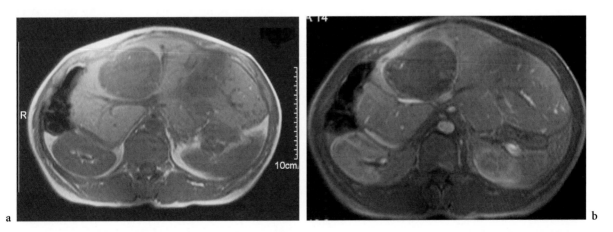

Fig. 17.9a,b. Sarcoma. MR findings. Secondary non-calcified infiltration of the liver due to rectal sarcoma reveals hypointense signal using T1-weighted unenhanced imaging (**a**) and peripheral enhancement post-gadolinium administration (**b**). Inhomogeneous inner structure of the lesion is depicted with several hyperintense areas

17.7
Lymphoma

17.7.1
Incidence and Clinical Presentation

Primary hepatic lymphoma is a rare disease and arises in the liver without nodal or other extrahepatic spread.

These tumors occur more commonly in white middle-aged men. Organ transplant recipients, patients with pharmacologic immunosuppression and AIDS patients have an increased risk of developing primary hepatic lymphoma (BACCHI et al. 1996). Primary hepatic lymphoma may be of either T-cell or B-cell origin, with the large cell lymphocytic type being the most frequently histologic pattern. A strong association has been identified between post-transplant lymphoproliferative disorders and Epstein-Barr virus. Up to 80% of patients with post-transplant lymphoproliferative disorders are infected with the virus at the time of lymphoma diagnosis (NALESNIK et al. 1988). Moreover, a correlation of the presence of Epstein-Barr virus and the appearance of lymphoma in AIDS patients has been reported (BACCHI et al. 1996).

Secondary lymphomatous hepatic involvement is quite common, 60% in Hodgkin's disease and 50% in non-Hodgkin's disease (BECHTOLD et al. 1985). Non-Hodgkin's lymphoma in HIV-positive people is 60 times more common than in the general population. AIDS-related lymphomas are highly aggressive tumors with poorly differentiated histological subtypes associated with a poor prognosis. Patients are typically first seen with advanced stages of the disease.

17.7.2
Pathologic Findings

Grossly, the appearance of primary hepatic lymphoma is variable. There is a large solitary mass with central fibrosis or necrosis. Moreover, multiple smaller nodular lesions are depicted. Furthermore diffuse forms of hepatic lymphoma are seen, documenting hepatomegaly without discrete lesions.

Hodgkin's disease and non-Hodgkin's lymphoma occur more often as miliary lesions than masses (SHIRKHODA et al. 1990).

Microscopically, liver parenchyma involvement occurs early in the disease. With time, small nodules

from a few millimeters to several centimeters in size develop.

In Hodgkin's disease, a Reed-Sternberg variant type of cell is accepted as evidence for liver involvement. Typically these cells are rarely identified in biopsy specimens (JAFFE 1987). In non-Hodgkin's disease, the lymphocytic form tends to be miliary, whereas the large cells or histiocytic varieties are nodular masses (RYAN et al. 1988). In both Hodgkin's and non-Hodgkin's lymphoma initial involvement is seen in the portal areas, because this is where the majority of the lymphatic tissue of the liver is found.

17.7.3
Imaging Findings

Primary lymphoma of the liver usually occurs as a single mass, less often as multiple lesions. It is uncommon for secondary hepatic lymphoma to present with focal masses.

17.7.3.1
Ultrasound

The sonographic pattern of hepatic lymphoma varies from hypoechogenic to highly echogenic (Fig. 17.10). The large mass or multinodular form of lymphoma is seen as one or more hypoechoic masses with regular margins, which is excellently visualized using ultrasound (RIZZI et al. 2001). Echogenic or cystic masses are seen much less frequently. The diffuse form is uncommon and may not be detectable or may result in diffuse hypoechoic or heterogeneous altered echogenicity of the liver (SHIRKHODA et al. 1990).

17.7.3.2
Computed Tomography

While focal primary lymphoma of the liver is more frequently identified by CT due to depiction of a solitary large mass, the typical secondary diffuse lymphomatous involvement is beyond the resolution for CT detection even after contrast injection (SANDERS et al. 1989).

Focal lymphomas are hypodense, homogeneous, and sharply marginated on unenhanced CT scan and do not enhance significantly due their hypovascularity following the administration of contrast (Fig. 17.11). A thin enhancing rim may be depicted

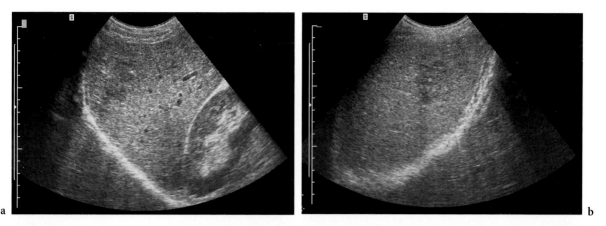

Fig. 17.10a,b. Lymphoma due to Hodgkin's disease. Ultrasound findings. On ultrasound, the tumoral form of the lymphoma appears as an inhomogeneous, hypoechoic mass in B-mode imaging

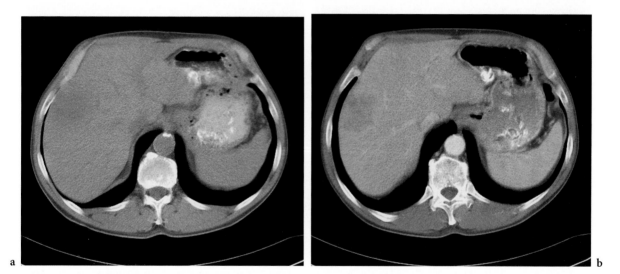

Fig. 17.11a,b. Lymphoma due to Hodgkin's disease. CT findings. **a** On unenhanced scan the lesion is seen as a relatively homogeneous mass. **b** On venous phase imaging lymphoma is depicted as a large well-defined mass with higher attenuation in the periphery of the lesion due to compressed normal liver parenchyma

in some cases (Fig. 17.12) (MAHER et al. 2001; RIZZI et al. 2001). Intratumoral unenhancing hypodense areas suggesting necrosis are not an infrequent finding in focal hepatic lymphomas. Diffuse primary hepatic lymphoma results in a diffusely decreased attenuation of the liver indistinguishable from fatty infiltration of the liver (VINNICOMBE and REZNEK 2003). BECHTOLD et al. (1985) have observed delayed enhancement in a case of primary hepatic lymphoma on CT. It has been shown that infiltration with histologically proven areas of abundant stroma and coagulation necrosis exhibits delayed enhancement on CT.

17.7.3.3
MR Imaging

MR imaging findings are non-specific for lymphoma. On MR images focal lymphomas are hypointense on T1-weighted images and hyperintense on T2-weighted images due to their rich cellularity (BARTOLOZZI et al. 2001; WEISSLEDER et al. 1988). Lymphomas may have a variable signal intensity on T2-weighted images in some cases: they are moderately high in signal intensity compared to surrounding liver parenchyma, whereas some are mildly hypointense to mildly hyperintense. The homogeneity of the tumor is de-

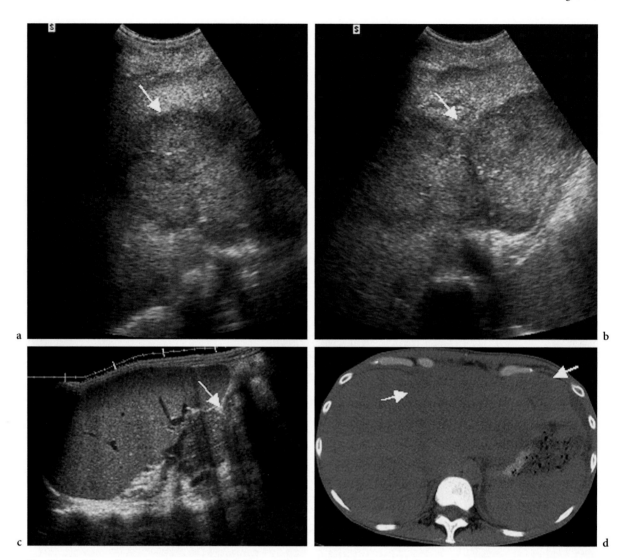

Fig. 17.12a–d. Lymphoma due to non-Hodgkin's disease. Ultrasound and CT findings. **a,b** B-mode ultrasound documents a large hypoechoic lesion (*arrow*) with inhomogeneous inner architecture. **c** Using panorama imaging normal liver parenchyma of the right liver lobe and lymphoma comprising almost the complete left liver lobe (*arrow*) is visualized. **d** Unenhanced CT scan documents a low attenuation mass (*arrows*)

pendent on the presence of necrosis, hemorrhage or fibrosis (ABBAS et al. 1991; NYMAN et al. 1987). A hypointense capsule (T1-weighted images) may be present in some cases (NYMAN et al. 1987).

Lymphomas with relatively low signal on T2-weighted images remain hypointense during the entire dynamic study after the administration of gadolinium-chelates, due to their poor vascularity (Figs. 17.13, 17.14) (FUKUYA et al. 1993).

In cases of relatively high signal in T2-weighted images early post-gadolinium scans present an intense enhancement which constantly increases over time. In addition, there is a centripetal filling-in phenomenon, resulting in an almost total opacification of the tumor in 30 min (KELEKIS et al. 1997). A transient ill-defined perilesional enhancement on immediate post-gadolinium GRE images can be observed independently from signal in T2-weighted images.

In diffuse infiltration due to lymphoma, there is no significant difference in signal intensity of the normal and diffuse lymphomatous liver.

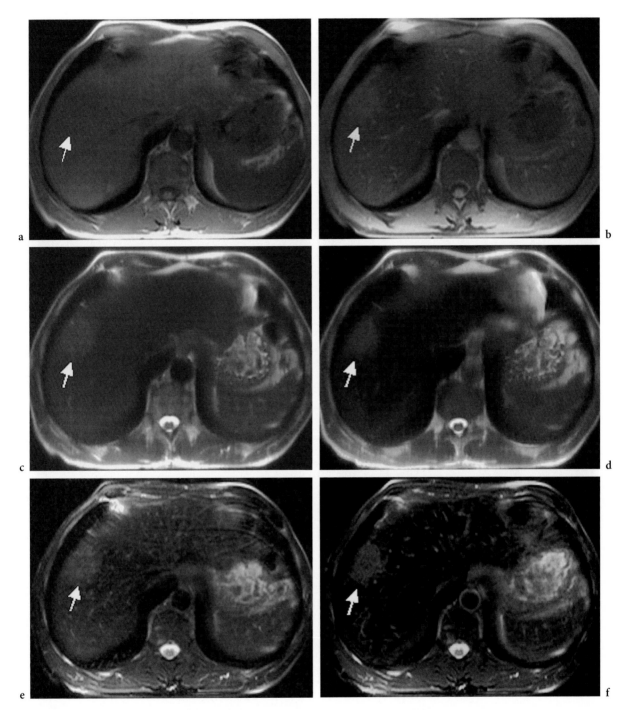

Fig. 17.13a–f. Lymphoma due to Hodgkin's disease. MR findings. **a** T1-weighted unenhanced imaging shows a hypointense well-defined mass (*arrow*). **b** Post-Ferucarbotran moderately hyperintense signal of the lesion (*arrow*) and uptake in the periphery due to compressed normal liver parenchyma is seen. Postcontrast the lesion is hyperintense due to darkening of normal liver parenchyma. **c** A moderately hyperintense lesion (*arrow*) is depicted on T2-weighted unenhanced HASTE imaging. **d** Post-Ferucarbotran there is no evidence of uptake of the lymphoma itself (*arrow*). **e** Using an unenhanced fat-saturated T2-weighted protocol, contrast of lesion (*arrow*) to liver is increased. **f** Visualization of the lymphoma (*arrow*) is best post-Ferucarbotran

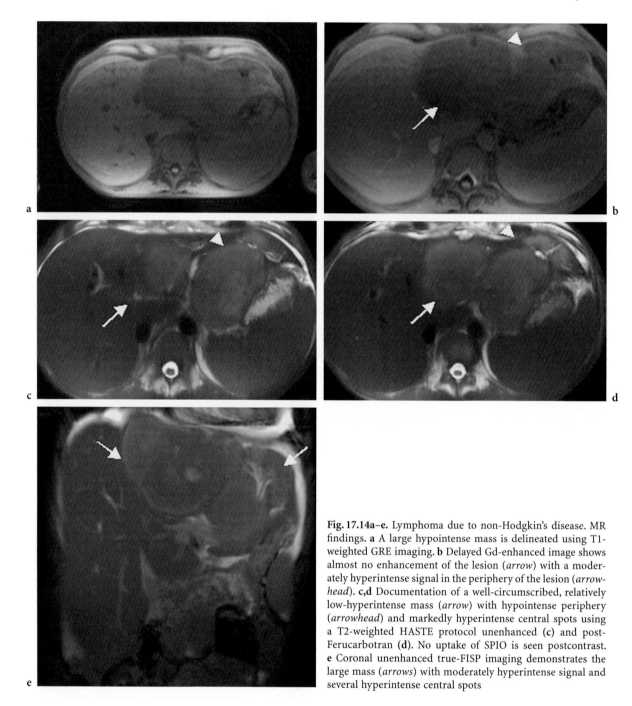

Fig. 17.14a–e. Lymphoma due to non-Hodgkin's disease. MR findings. **a** A large hypointense mass is delineated using T1-weighted GRE imaging. **b** Delayed Gd-enhanced image shows almost no enhancement of the lesion (*arrow*) with a moderately hyperintense signal in the periphery of the lesion (*arrowhead*). **c,d** Documentation of a well-circumscribed, relatively low-hyperintense mass (*arrow*) with hypointense periphery (*arrowhead*) and markedly hyperintense central spots using a T2-weighted HASTE protocol unenhanced (**c**) and post-Ferucarbotran (**d**). No uptake of SPIO is seen postcontrast. **e** Coronal unenhanced true-FISP imaging demonstrates the large mass (*arrows*) with moderately hyperintense signal and several hyperintense central spots

References

Abbas YA, Kressel HY, Wehrli FW, et al (1991) Differential diagnosis of hepatic neoplasms: spin echo versus gadolinium-diethylenetriaminepentaacetate-enhanced gradient echo imaging. Magn Reson Q 7:275–292

Agildere AM, Haliloglu M, Akhan O (1991) Biliary cystadenoma and cystadenocarcinoma. AJR Am J Roentgenol 156:1113

Almogy G, Lieberman S, Gips M, et al (2004) Clinical outcomes of surgical resections for primary liver sarcoma in adults: results from a single centre. Eur J Surg Oncol 30:421–427

Bacchi CE, Bacchi MM, Rabenhorst SH, et al (1996) AIDS-related lymphoma in Brazil. Histopathology, immunophenotype, and association with Epstein-Barr virus. Am J Clin Pathol 105:230–237

Bartolozzi C, Cioni D, Donati F, et al (2001) Focal liver lesions: MR imaging-pathologic correlation. Eur Radiol 11:1374–1388

Bates SM, Keller MS, Ramos IM, et al (1990) Hepatoblastoma: detection of tumor vascularity with duplex Doppler US. Radiology 176:505–507

Baur M, Potzi R, Lochs H, et al (1993) Primary leiomyosarcoma of the liver. Z Gastroenterol 31:20–23

Bechtold RE, Karstaedt N, Wolfman NT, et al (1985) Prolonged hepatic enhancement on computed tomography in a case of hepatic lymphoma. J Comput Assist Tomogr 9:186–189

Buetow PC, Buck JL, Ros PR, et al (1994) Malignant vascular tumors of the liver: radiologic-pathologic correlation. Radiographics 14:153–166

Buetow PC, Buck JL, Pantongrag-Brown L, et al (1995) Biliary cystadenoma and cystadenocarcinoma: clinical-imaging-pathologic correlations with emphasis on the importance of ovarian stroma. Radiology 196:805–810

Buetow PC, Buck JL, Pantongrag-Brown L, et al (1997) Undifferentiated (embryonal) sarcoma of the liver: pathologic basis of imaging findings in 28 cases. Radiology 203:779–783

Chen MF, Jan YY, Chen TC (1998) Clinical studies of mucin-producing cholangiocellular carcinoma: a study of 22 histopathology-proven cases. Ann Surg 227:63–69

Choi BI, Lim JH, Han MC, et al (1989) Biliary cystadenoma and cystadenocarcinoma: CT and sonographic findings. Radiology 171:57–61

Craig JR, Peters RL, Edmondson HA (1989) Tumors of the liver and intrahepatic bile ducts. In: Atlas of tumor pathology, 2nd series, Fascicle 26. Armed Forces Institute of Pathology, Washington DC

Dachman AH, Lichtenstein JE, Friedman AC, et al (1983) Infantile hemangioendothelioma of the liver: a radiologic-pathologic-clinical correlation. AJR Am J Roentgenol 140:1091–1096

Dachman AH, Parker RL, Ros PR, et al (1987) Hepatoblastoma: a radiologic-pathologic correlation in 50 cases. Radiology 164:15–19

Devaney K, Goodman ZD, Ishak KG (1994) Hepatobiliary cystadenoma and cystadenocarcinoma. A light microscopic and immunohistochemical study of 70 patients. Am J Surg Pathol 18:1078–1091

Edmonson HA (1976) Benign epithelial tumors and tumor-like lesions of the liver. In: Okuda K, Peters RL (eds) Hepatocellular carcinoma. Wiley, New York, pp 309–330

Enzinger FM, Weiss SW (1983) Soft-tissue tumors. Mosby Year-Book, St. Louis

Fukuya T, Honda H, Murata S, et al (1993) MRI of primary lymphoma of the liver. J Comput Assist Tomogr 17:596–568

Furui S, Itai Y, Ohtomo K, et al (1989) Hepatic epithelioid hemangioendothelioma: report of five cases. Radiology 171:63–68

Gates LK Jr, Cameron AJ, Nagorney DM, et al (1995) Primary leiomyosarcoma of the liver mimicking liver abscess. Am J Gastroenterol 90:649–652

Goodman ZD (1984) Histologic diagnosis of hepatic tumors. Ann Clin Lab Sci 14:169–178

Hamm B, Thoeni RF, Gould RG, et al (1994) Focal liver lesions: characterization with nonenhanced and dynamic contrast material-enhanced MR imaging. Radiology 190:417–423

Ishak KG (1987) Malignant mesenchymal tumors of the liver. In: Okuda K, Ishak KG (eds) Neoplasms of the liver. Springer, New York, pp 121–156

Ishak KG, Willis GW, Cummins SD, et al (1977) Biliary cystadenoma and cystadenocarcinoma: report of 14 cases and review of the literature. Cancer 39:322–338

Ishak KG, Sesterhenn IA, Goodman ZD, et al (1984) Epithelioid hemangioendothelioma of the liver: a clinicopathologic and follow-up study of 32 cases. Hum Pathol 15:839–852

Itai Y, Teraoka T (1989) Angiosarcoma of the liver mimicking cavernous hemangioma on dynamic CT. J Comput Assist Tomogr 13:910–912

Ito Y, Kojiro M, Nakashima T, et al (1988) Pathomorphologic characteristics of 102 cases of Thorotrast-related hepatocellular carcinoma, cholangiocarcinoma, and hepatic angiosarcoma. Cancer 62:1153–1162

Jaffe ES (1987) Malignant lymphoma: pathology of hepatic involvement. Semin Liver Dis 7:257–268

Kelekis NL, Semelka RC, Siegelman ES, et al (1997) Focal hepatic lymphoma: magnetic resonance demonstration using current techniques including gadolinium enhancement. Magn Reson Imaging 15:625–636

Kelleher MB, Iwatsuki S, Sheahan DG (1989) Epithelioid hemangioendothelioma of the liver. Clinicopathological correlation of 10 cases treated by orthotopic liver transplantation. Am J Surg Pathol 13:999–1008

Locker GY, Doroshow JH, Zwelling LA, et al (1979) The clinical features of hepatic angiosarcoma: a report of four cases and a review of the English literature. Medicine (Baltimore) 58:48–64

Maher MM, McDermott SR, Fenlon HM, et al (2001) Imaging of primary non-Hodgkin's lymphoma of the liver. Clin Radiol 56:295–301

Mahony B, Jeffrey RB, Federle MP (1982) Spontaneous rupture of hepatic and splenic angiosarcoma demonstrated by CT. AJR Am J Roentgenol 138:965–966

Marti-Bonmati L, Ferrer D, Menor F, et al (1993) Hepatic mesenchymal sarcoma: MRI findings. Abdom Imaging 18:176–179

Miller WJ, Dodd GD 3rd, Federle MP, et al (1992) Epithelioid hemangioendothelioma of the liver: imaging findings with pathologic correlation. AJR Am J Roentgenol 159:53–57

Molina E, Hernandez A (2003) Clinical manifestations of primary hepatic angiosarcoma. Dig Dis Sci 48:677–682

Nalesnik MA, Jatfe R, Starzl TE (1988) The diagnosis and treatment of posttransplant lymphoproliferative disorders. Curr Probl Surg 25:367–472

Nyman R, Rhen S, Ericsson A, et al (1987) An attempt to characterize malignant lymphoma in spleen, liver and lymph nodes with magnetic resonance imaging. Acta Radiol 28:527–533

Pinson CW, Lopez RR, Ivancev K, et al (1994) Resection of primary hepatic malignant fibrous histiocytoma, fibrosarcoma, and leiomyosarcoma. South Med J 87:384–391

Radin DR, Craig JR, Colletti PM, et al (1988) Hepatic epithelioid hemangioendothelioma. Radiology 169:145–148

Peterson MS, Baron RL, Rankin SC (2000) Hepatic angiosarcoma: findings on multiphasic contrast-enhanced helical CT do not mimic hepatic hemangioma. AJR Am J Roentgenol 175:165–170

Rizzi EB, Schinina V, Cristofaro M, et al (2001) Non-Hodgkin's lymphoma of the liver in patients with AIDS: sonographic, CT, and MRI findings. J Clin Ultrasound 29:125–129

Ryan J, Straus DJ, Lange C, et al (1988) Primary lymphoma of the liver. Cancer 61:370–375

Sanders LM, Botet JF, Straus DJ, et al (1989) CT of primary lymphoma of the liver. AJR Am J Roentgenol 152:973–976

Shin MS, Carpenter JT Jr, Ho KJ (1991) Epithelioid hemangioendothelioma: CT manifestations and possible linkage to vinyl chloride exposure. J Comput Assist Tomogr 15:505–507

Shirkhoda A, Ros PR, Farah J, et al (1990) Lymphoma of the solid abdominal viscera. Radiol Clin North Am 28:785–799

Soyer P, Bluemke DA, Vissuzaine C, et al (1994) CT of hepatic tumors: prevalence and specificity of retraction of the adjacent liver capsule. AJR Am J Roentgenol 162:1119–1122

Stoupis C, Ros PR, Dolson DJ (1994) Recurrent biliary cystadenoma: MR imaging appearance. J Magn Reson Imaging 4:99–101

Tsuchida Y, Bastos JC, Honna T, et al (1990) Treatment of disseminated hepatoblastoma involving bilateral lobes. J Pediatr Surg 25:1253–1255

van Beers B, Roche A, Mathieu D, et al (1992) Epithelioid hemangioendothelioma of the liver: MR and CT findings. J Comput Assist Tomogr 16:420–424

Vinnicombe SJ, Reznek RH (2003) Computerised tomography in the staging of Hodgkin's disease and non-Hodgkin's lymphoma. Eur J Nucl Med Mol Imaging 30 (Suppl 1): S42–S55

Weiss SW, Enzinger FM (1982) Epithelioid hemangioendothelioma: a vascular tumor often mistaken for a carcinoma. Cancer 50:970–981

Weiss SW, Ishak KG, Dail DH, et al (1986) Epithelioid hemangioendothelioma and related lesions. Semin Diagn Pathol 3:259–287

Weissleder R, Stark DD, Elizondo G, et al (1988) MRI of hepatic lymphoma. Magn Reson Imaging 6:675–681

Hepatic Metastases

18 Sonography of Liver Metastases

Thomas Albrecht

CONTENTS

18.1 Introduction

Both benign and malignant focal liver lesions are extremely common and imaging the liver for focal lesions especially in cancer patients is one of the most frequent tasks in everyday radiological practice.

The most common malignancy of the liver is metastases from other organs: 25–50% patients with a known non-haematological malignancy have liver metastases at the time of diagnosis with decreasing frequency in colon, gastric, pancreatic, breast and lung cancer (EDMUNSON and CRAIG 1987).

The prevalence of solid benign liver tumours has been reported to be more than 20% in autopsy series and in patients with malignancy 25–50% of lesions under 2 cm in size are benign (KARHUNEN 1986; EDMUNSON and CRAIG 1987; JONES et al. 1992;

T. ALBRECHT, MD
Department of Radiology and Nuclear Medicine, Campus Benjamin Franklin, Charité, Universitätsmedizin Berlin, Hindenburgdamm 30, 12200 Berlin, Germany

KREFT et al. 2001). The most frequent benign lesion is haemangioma with a prevalence of 7–21%, followed by focal nodular hyperplasia (FNH), which has a prevalence of up to 3% (KARHUNEN 1986; ISHAK and RABIN 1975; WANLESS et al. 1989). Adenomas are much rarer than FNH (by a factor of approximately 50) and they occur usually in female patients with a history of sexual hormone medication. Other rare benign lesions are pyogenic, parasitic or fungal abscesses. Areas of focal fatty change or focal fatty sparing are very common; they do not represent true lesions but may appear as pseudo-tumours on ultrasound and are thus easily confused with real tumours such as metastases. They are particularly common in patients undergoing chemotherapy.

From the above it is obvious that liver imaging of cancer patients requires an imaging modality that is not only highly sensitive in detection but also provides reliable characterisation of lesions and thus allows differentiation of malignant from benign tumours. Accurate and timely detection of hepatic metastases is very important because of the far-reaching therapeutic and prognostic implications. Especially through the recent improvements in liver resection and local ablation of metastases from colorectal carcinoma, liver imaging has become more demanding. Accurate assessment of number, size and segmental location of metastases is required to identify patients suitable for surgical or interventional therapy, for treatment planning and for follow-up imaging under chemotherapy.

In the past, ultrasound (US) had an important but somewhat limited role in liver imaging of cancer patients. Although commonly the first and most widespread modality used, its detection rate was inferior to that of CT and MR and its ability to differentiate metastases from other focal liver lesions is often limited. With the advent of US contrast agents and new contrast-specific imaging techniques in the last few years, contrast-enhanced ultrasound (CEUS) has become a powerful tool, which has dramatically changed the role of US for liver imaging in cancer patients.

18.2
Examination Technique

The liver is best scanned using a curved array or sector probe with a centre frequency ranging from 2 to 5 MHz. Higher frequency linear array transducers may be employed to image superficial parts of the liver surface in deep inspiration. The left lobe is optimally imaged from a subxiphoid approach with the patient supine. The right lobe is best imaged either subcostally or intercostally. Intercostal scanning should be performed with the patient in the supine position either during quiet respiration or breath-hold on expiration. Using this approach the superior aspects of the liver and subphrenic area can be imaged. Imaging in a plane parallel to the long axis of the intercostal space minimises rib shadowing and by angling the probe anteriorly and posteriorly, liver coverage is maximised from a given intercostal space. The subcostal approach is best performed with the patient in the left lateral decubitus position in deep inspiration allowing insonation of the majority of the right lobe including the dome. Each lobe of the liver should be imaged in at least two orthogonal planes using multiple sweeps covering the entire organ.

The real-time nature of US makes it ideally suited for accurate and safe biopsy of focal lesions, as respiratory motion can be imaged directly during the needle passage and accounted for interactively. Also, US is commonly used for guidance of percutaneous thermal ablation of metastases.

18.2.1
Doppler Techniques

When using colour Doppler the settings must be optimised to achieve the greatest sensitivity to allow the detection of low flow. In practice this means increasing the colour gain to a level just below that which noise or flash artefacts appear. Also the colour box should be made as small as allowable to increase sensitivity and the wall filter and pulse repetition frequency (PRF) should be low. However, if the flow is too high for these settings the wall filter and PRF need to be increased to reduce flash artefact due to motion. The left lobe is particularly susceptible to flash artefacts from cardiac motion. Liver malignancies require a neovascular supply to grow. Conventional colour and spectral Doppler are often limited in their ability to image the vascularity in the majority of metastases since the signals are

too low. This may be improved with the use of power Doppler and contrast agents. Hypovascular metastases typically only show a faint rim of peripheral vessels or no vessels at all (Fig. 18.1). Some benign lesions, such as FNH, exhibit characteristic spoke-wheel arterial vascularity, which aids differential diagnosis (Fig. 18.1).

18.2.2
Tissue Harmonic Imaging

Tissue harmonic imaging (THI) is a grey-scale technique that uses information from harmonic signals (multiples of the insonating frequency) generated by non-linear propagation of a sound wave as it passes through tissue. The transmitted sound wave consists of a series of sine wave oscillations which cause alternate tissue compression and relaxation. Since the velocity of sound propagation is greater in compressed tissue compared to relaxed tissue and since the velocities vary slightly between different tissue materials, harmonics are produced due to these variations in propagation. Whilst conventional US transmits and receives at the same frequency, in THI a low frequency is used and usually the second harmonic signal is received by separating it from the fundamental echoes using filters or phase inversion technology. Since the harmonic signals are generated in the tissue, artefacts from the body wall, side-lobes and scatter are minimised so improving signal to noise ratio. The shorter wavelengths of the harmonic frequency also improve axial resolution. This technique is particularly well suited to imaging "technically difficult" patients.

THI improves spatial and contrast resolution of B-mode US in the majority of cases and the conspicuity of focal liver lesions is often improved. However, the detection rate of focal lesions is only slightly improved. THI should be part of every state-of-the-art sonogram of the liver and abdomen.

18.2.3
Intraoperative Ultrasound

Intraoperative US (IOUS) provides highly accurate information to the surgeon influencing operative management. One prospective study on the impact of IOUS on planned resection of primary or secondary liver malignancies demonstrated a decisive influence on surgical management in almost 50% of

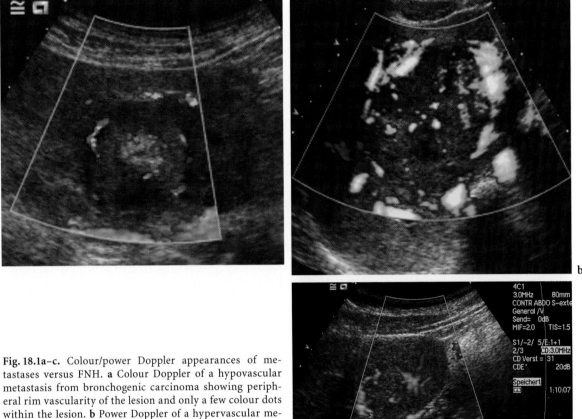

Fig. 18.1a–c. Colour/power Doppler appearances of metastases versus FNH. **a** Colour Doppler of a hypovascular metastasis from bronchogenic carcinoma showing peripheral rim vascularity of the lesion and only a few colour dots within the lesion. **b** Power Doppler of a hypervascular metastasis from malignant melanoma shows stronger rim enhancement and multiple small vessels almost evenly distributed throughout the lesion. **c** Power Doppler of FNH shows the characteristic "spoke-wheel pattern" of a central feeding artery branching and radiating centrifugally towards the periphery of the lesion

cases (CLARKE et al. 1889). In more recent studies the surgical plan was changed after IOUS in 18% of patients with metastatic colorectal carcinoma and additional information of therapeutic relevance was achieved in 15% of patients with gastrointestinal tumours compared to preoperative staging (CONLON et al. 2003; HUNERBEIN et al. 2001).

IOUS detects 10–15% more metastases than CT arterial portography and 19–32% more than SPIO-enhanced MR (BLUEMKE et al. 2000; SCHULTZ et al. 1999; SOYER et al. 1992; WARD et al. 1999). It is able accurately to detect cysts down to 1–3 mm and solid focal lesions of 3–5 mm in size. With a sensitivity of 98% and a specificity of 95%, IOUS is generally considered the gold standard for detecting liver lesions (SCHMIDT et al. 2000). It is used to evaluate the extent of malignant liver disease and to plan resections by assessing the relation of a tumour to large vessels (and thus the segmental borders). Intraoperative

biopsy of small lesions and tumour ablation can be guided by IOUS.

Interpretation of IOUS includes the sonographic information combined with intraoperative inspection and palpation. Surgical mobilisation of the liver with dissection of the falciform ligament is of great help, as it provides easy access to all parts of the organ. Complete visualisation of the liver including its posterior aspect requires insonation from the anterior, lateral and posterior approach. The examination usually takes 10–15 min.

Since the barriers of skin, gas and subcutaneous tissue encountered with US imaging are not present with IOUS, higher transducer frequencies can be used compared to conventional abdominal US, providing better image resolution (Fig. 18.2a). For the liver 7 MHz is the frequency of choice. Probe design also needs to be considered with use of side-fire probes facilitating scanning in tight spaces such as

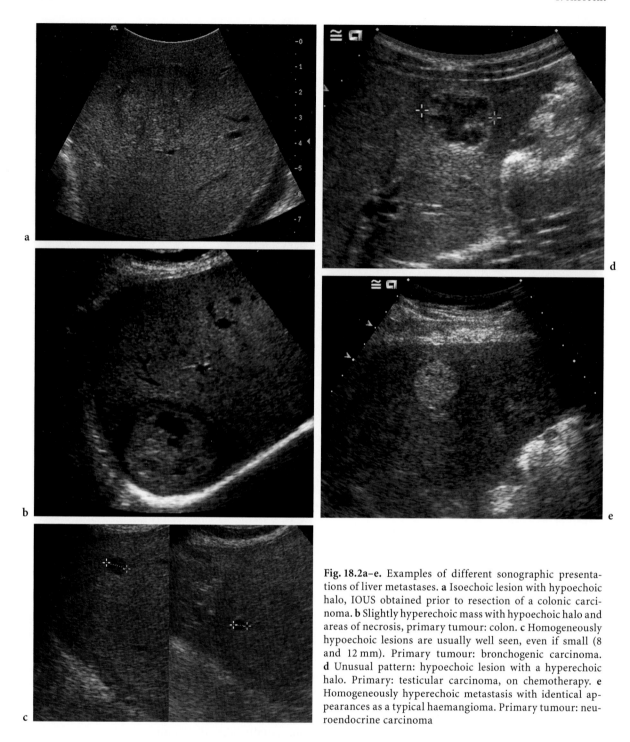

Fig. 18.2a–e. Examples of different sonographic presentations of liver metastases. **a** Isoechoic lesion with hypoechoic halo, IOUS obtained prior to resection of a colonic carcinoma. **b** Slightly hyperechoic mass with hypoechoic halo and areas of necrosis, primary tumour: colon. **c** Homogeneously hypoechoic lesions are usually well seen, even if small (8 and 12 mm). Primary tumour: bronchogenic carcinoma. **d** Unusual pattern: hypoechoic lesion with a hyperechoic halo. Primary: testicular carcinoma, on chemotherapy. **e** Homogeneously hyperechoic metastasis with identical appearances as a typical haemangioma. Primary tumour: neuroendocrine carcinoma

between the ribcage and lateral liver margin as well as the dome, which are difficult to image using end-fire designs.

Transducers should have spectral and colour Doppler to assess tumour vascularisation and vascular invasion, which is especially important in HCC. Sonographic probes may also be incorporated into laparoscopes, allowing the detection of deeper occult lesions undetectable by routine laparoscopy.

Usually IOUS is performed without the use of contrast agents. Reasons are the already high detection rate and, until recently, the fact that contrast-specific imaging modes were not available for intra-operative probes. This has recently been rectified as such probes with contrast capabilities are now becoming available. Early results show that sensitivity and specificity of IOUS are further improved by the use of contrast agents.

18.2.4
Ultrasound Contrast Agents

Unlike all other imaging modalities, US has lacked effective contrast agents until comparatively recently. This was rectified with the introduction of gas microbubble agents, which have had a remarkable impact on liver sonography. Two such agents are currently available for clinical use in Europe: Levovist (Schering AG, Berlin, Germany) and SonoVue (Bracco SPA, Milan, Italy).

Microbubbles are less than 10 µm in diameter and are safe and effective echo enhancers. They are blood pool agents and do not diffuse into the extravascular fluid compartment. When given intravenously microbubbles produce marked signal augmentation on insonation for several minutes, in grey scale and Doppler, with up to 25 dB enhancement in echo strength. In addition to the vascular phase some agents exhibit a delayed liver-specific phase.

Imaging of microbubbles requires highly sensitive contrast-specific imaging techniques. These techniques exploit the non-linear microbubble response which occurs when bubbles interact with US. Contrast-specific imaging techniques use the principles of Doppler (i.e. agent detection imaging, ADI), phase modulation (i.e. phase or pulse inversion mode, PIM), amplitude modulation or a combination of the latter two (contrast pulse sequencing, CPS). There has been rapid development and improvement of such techniques by the manufacturers in the last few years. Detailed explanation of contrast-specific imaging modes is beyond the scope of this chapter and the interested reader is referred to the specialised literature (HOPE SIMPSON and BURNS 1999; ALBRECHT et al. 2000; CHOMAS et al. 2002).

The interactions of microbubbles with US waves are complex. The bubble response is strongly dependent on the acoustic power (amplitude) of the insonating signal, which is indicated on the US scanner as the mechanical index (MI). When a microbubble is exposed to an oscillating acoustic signal, it undergoes alternate expansion and contraction (resonance). At very low acoustic power (MI <approx. 0.05) these alternate expansions and contractions are equal and symmetrical (linear behaviour) and the frequency of the scattered signal is unaltered.

As the acoustic power increases (MI> approx. 0.05), more complex non-linear interactions occur: the expansion and contraction phases become unequal because the microbubbles resist compression more strongly than expansion. This non-linear resonant behaviour is associated with the production of harmonic signals at multiples (or fractions) of the insonating frequency and can be imaged with contrast specific imaging techniques such as phase or pulse inversion mode (PIM). At still higher powers (MI approx. 0.3–1.9), although still within accepted limits for diagnostic imaging, highly non-linear behaviour is associated with microbubble disruption. This disruptive phase can be imaged in several ways, using specially adapted Doppler-based colour overlay modes (ADI) or on grey scale, i.e. with PIM.

High MI imaging is best performed with Levovist. It provides strong non-linear signals from disrupting microbubbles seen on colour modes (ADI) or B-mode (PIM). The disadvantage of this technique is the highly transient nature of the signals, which persist only for a few frames after insonation of an individual area. To exploit the enhancement for clinical use, special scanning techniques such as rapid sweeping through the liver to image undestroyed bubbles with each new frame or intermittent imaging have to be employed.

Conversely, more recent low MI imaging, which is performed with SonoVue, can be performed in real time without substantial bubble destruction. This allows a lesion to be imaged continuously during its vascular phase as well as comprehensive surveying of the liver in multiple planes. Low MI imaging is now preferred in most instances.

During the vascular phase, the dynamic enhancement pattern and the vascular morphology of a lesion are assessed. Additionally some agents have a delayed liver-specific phase where the bubbles accumulate in normal liver parenchyma 2–5 min after injection after the vascular enhancement has faded, analogous to liver-specific contrast agents used in MR (LEEN et al. 2000). This late phase is particularly useful for detection of metastases as they show as non-enhancing defects. Characterisation is also improved as the great majority of benign lesions show contrast uptake in the delayed phase. Microbubble agents known to exhibit liver-specific behaviour are Levovist and Sonavist (Schering AG, Berlin, Germany), Sonazoid (NC100100; Amersham Medical, Amersham, UK) and BR14 (Bracco SPA, Milan, Italy). SonoVue (Bracco SPA) is less liver specific but also shows some degree of hepatic accumulation for approximately 5 min after injection, which can be exploited in a similar way. In the late phase the bubbles are stationary or extremely slow moving, as shown by the absence of conventional Doppler signals. The mechanism of hepatic accumulation is not completely understood. Possible explanations are mediation by the reticuloendothelial system or pooling and endothelial adherence in the liver sinusoids. For some agents (Sonavist and Sonazoid), Kupffer cell uptake has been demonstrated.

18.3
Appearances of Liver Metastases

18.3.1
Unenhanced Ultrasound

The ability of ultrasound to detect a focal lesion depends on a number of factors: size, location, echogenicity and mass effect. Thus detection depends on a combination of spatial resolution and liver-to-lesion contrast: strongly hyper- or hypoechoic lesions are easily detected even when small (Fig. 18.2). Fatty infiltration of the liver aids detection of hypoechoic lesions, since liver-to-lesion contrast is increased. Conversely, isoechoic masses are often missed and require a larger size for detection. Mass effect is important for the detection of isoechoic lesions. It manifests as deviation or invasion of the intrahepatic vasculature and/or bulges of the liver contour.

The echo patterns of metastases are numerous, but some patterns are said to be commonly associated with certain primary tumours (Table 18.1) (Fig. 18.2). US appearances of metastases may vary within a given patient as well as over time and especially following chemotherapy. Most metastases are round with well-defined margins. Hypoechoic metastases are more common (approximately 65%) than hyper- or isoechoic. A hypoechoic halo surrounding the lesions is seen in 40%; it is usually associated with iso- or hyperechoic metastases (HOHMANN et al. 2003). The cause of the halo is controversial. It is not pathognomonic of metastases as it may also be seen in HCC, focal lymphoma, fungal abscess and adenoma and, less commonly, in FNH and haemangioma.

In summary, there are no pathognomonic B-mode features and the differentiation of a single metastasis from other lesions is usually not possible without the use of contrast agents. In a patient with a known primary malignancy, any focal liver lesion seen on unenhanced US must be regarded

as suspicious of metastasis until proven otherwise. However, many lesions (25–50% of lesions ≤2 cm) will eventually prove to be benign, once contrast enhanced US, other imaging tests or biopsy is used to further characterise the lesion (JONES et al. 1992; KREFT et al. 2001).

Doppler typically shows no or some peripheral vascularity in hypovascular metastases, while hypervascular deposits may show vessels throughout the lesion (Fig. 18.1). Use of Doppler can be useful to differentiate metastases from FNH and focal fatty change/infiltration: large FNH (≥approx. 4 cm) often shows a typical "spoke-wheel" arterial pattern, often within a central scar (Fig. 18.1); focal fatty change/sparing shows no abnormal vascularity and normal hepatic vessels crossing the lesion with no deviation.

Multiple lesions in a patient with a known primary malignancy are highly suggestive of metastases. Multiple metastases may show as several individual lesions or as diffuse infiltration, producing the "moth eaten" appearance of a heterogeneous liver combined with definite or questionable individual lesions (Fig. 18.3). Multiple (fungal) abscesses are

Table 18.1. Common sonographic patterns of metastatic liver disease

1. Echogenic
   Colon carcinoma
   Neuroendocrine tumours, i.e. carcinoid, pancreatic islet cell tumours
   Renal cell carcinoma
   Choriocarcinoma
   Multifocal hepatocellular carcinoma

2. Echopoor
   Breast cancer
   Lung cancer
   Lymphoma
   Pancreas

3. Target pattern ("halo")
   Most common lung cancer
   May occur in many others

4. Calcified metastases
   Common; mucinous adenocarcinoma: colon, ovary, stomach, breast (treated)
   Rare; osteosarcoma, chondrosarcoma

5. Cystic
   Ovary, pancreas, colon cancer
   Sarcomas-necrosis
   Squamous cell

6. Infiltrative
   Breast, lung cancer
   Melanoma
   Multifocal hepatocellular carcinoma

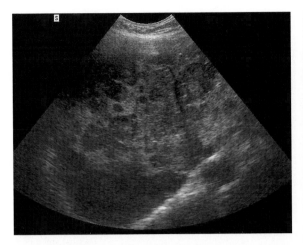

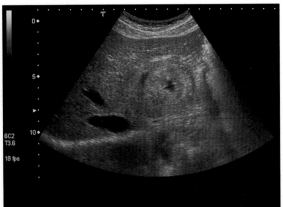
a

Fig. 18.3. Multiple/diffuse metastases giving the "moth-eaten" appearance

the most important differential diagnosis of multiple lesions in patients on chemotherapy; their appearances can be identical to those of metastases.

18.3.2
Contrast Enhanced Ultrasound

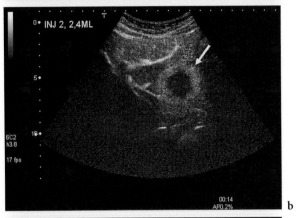
b

Metastases show characteristic dynamic features in all three phases after contrast injection (Figs. 18.4–18.6). In the arterial phase the appearances are twofold: hypovascular metastases show

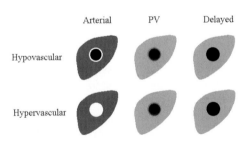

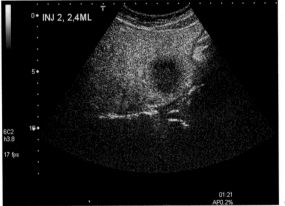
c

Fig. 18.4. Schematic display of the dynamic enhancement of hypo- and hypervascular metastases postcontrast injection during the arterial, portal venous and delayed phase

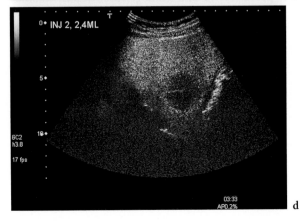
d

Fig. 18.5a–d. Dynamic features of a "hypovascular" hepatic metastasis from a breast primary after contrast injection (SonoVue). **a** Slightly hyperechoic lesion with hypoechoic halo and small central necrosis on unenhanced US. **b** In the arterial phase the lesion displays strong peripheral rim enhancement (*arrow*). **c** Portal venous phase imaging shows fading of the rim. **d** In the delayed phase, the lesion shows as a hypoechoic enhancement defect

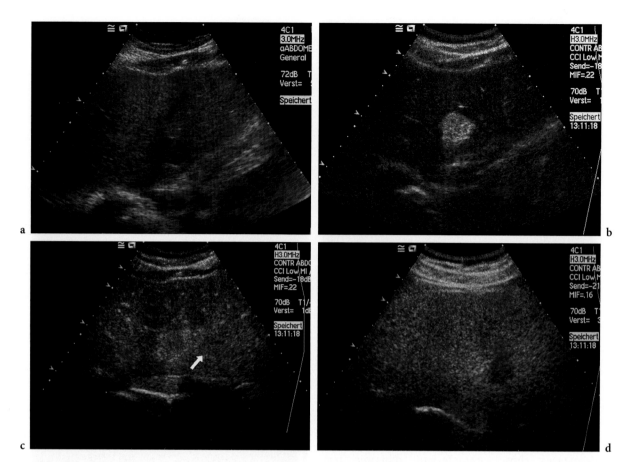

Fig. 18.6a–d. Dynamic features of a "hypervascular" metastasis from a thyroid carcinoma after contrast injection (SonoVue).
a Conventional grey-scale image shows a hypoechoic lesion. **b** During the arterial phase 20 s post injection the lesion enhances homogeneously while there is almost no contrast uptake by the liver parenchyma. **c** Portal venous phase image (43 s post injection) shows enhancement of normal liver and some contrast washout from the lesion (*arrow*) so that the lesion is isoechoic at this point. **d** Delayed phase image (4–5 min post injection) with persistent enhancement of the normal liver and almost complete contrast wash-out from the metastasis

as hyporeflective lesions usually with a typical rim enhancement of varying size, while hypervascular metastatic deposits show as brightly enhancing hyperreflective and homogeneous lesions, sometimes with non-enhancing necrotic areas. At the beginning of the portal venous phase, the (rim) enhancement fades and the entire lesion becomes increasingly hyporeflective. In the delayed phase both hypo- and hypervascular metastases invariably show as dark enhancement defects while the enhancement persists in normal liver parenchyma; this is independent of the contrast agent and imaging technique used (HOHMANN et al. 2003). During the delayed phase metastases are usually particularly well defined often with sharp, "punched out" borders. Both portal venous and delayed phase imaging markedly increase the contrast between the enhancing normal liver and the non-enhancing metastases and thus improve detection, especially of small lesions below 1 cm in diameter and of lesions that are isoechoic on baseline (Figs. 18.7, 18.8).

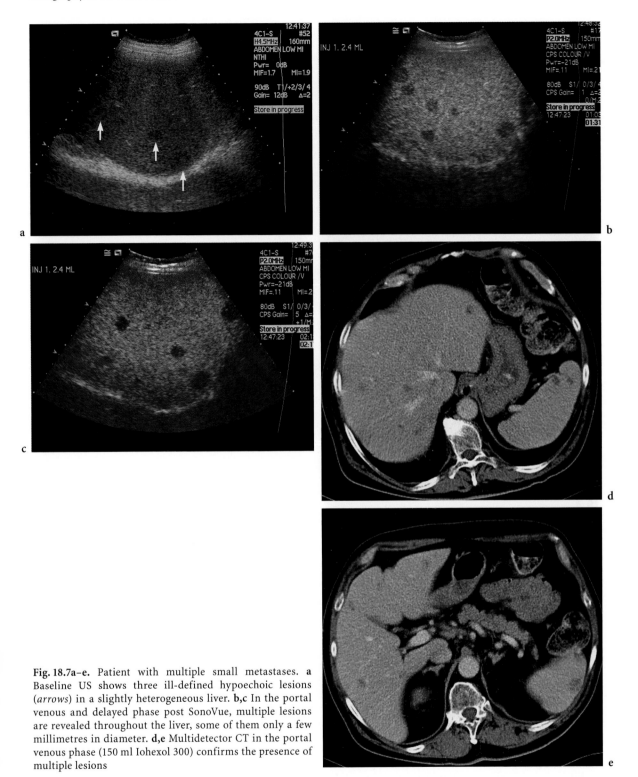

Fig. 18.7a–e. Patient with multiple small metastases. **a** Baseline US shows three ill-defined hypoechoic lesions (*arrows*) in a slightly heterogeneous liver. **b,c** In the portal venous and delayed phase post SonoVue, multiple lesions are revealed throughout the liver, some of them only a few millimetres in diameter. **d,e** Multidetector CT in the portal venous phase (150 ml Iohexol 300) confirms the presence of multiple lesions

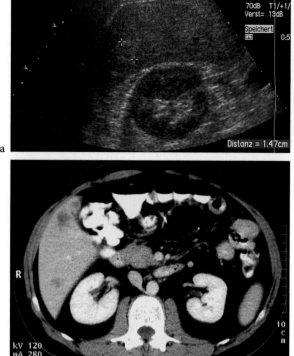

Fig. 18.8a–c. Patient with colorectal carcinoma. **a** Baseline US shows a nearly isoechoic lesion in segment VI measuring 1.5 cm. **b** In the delayed phase post SonoVue (2–5 min) the metastasis appears as a typical enhancement defect and is much more visible. A second metastasis of 2 cm size is now detected in segment V. **c** Spiral CT examination in portal venous phase (150 ml Iohexol 300) confirms the presence of the two metastases

18.4
Differential Diagnosis on Contrast Enhanced Ultrasound

As discussed above, solid benign liver lesions are very common. It is therefore of the utmost importance to differentiate these from metastases in cancer patients. Unenhanced US is usually not able reliably to differentiate metastases from other lesions. Conversely, the use of contrast agents achieves this goal in most cases, since all common solid benign liver lesions have characteristic dynamic imaging features on contrast-enhanced US and their diagnosis is thus usually unproblematic. Most of these features are analogous to those on dynamic CT and MR.

Haemangiomas show a characteristic peripheral nodular arterial phase enhancement followed by gradual centripetal in-filling during the later phases (Fig. 18.9). The filling may be partial or complete. The speed of filling is size dependent: while small haemangiomas often fill within less than a minute, large lesions may take 5 min or more. Many large haemangiomas will not fill completely, and approximately 5–10% of smaller haemangiomas will show only minor peripheral filling. This can lead to confusion with metastases.

FNH appear as lesions with homogeneous enhancement in the arterial phase. In about 50% of FNH this is preceded by a typical spoke-wheel arterial pattern with centrifugal filling early in the arterial phase, lasting for a few seconds (Fig. 18.10). In some cases the feeding artery is also seen. In the subsequent phases the lesions show a similar degree of enhancement as the normal liver, due to the liver-like tissue that the lesion consists of. A non-enhancing central scar is frequently seen in the delayed phase (Fig. 18.10). Delayed phase imaging is particularly useful for FNH as they invariable show as isoechoic or hyperechoic lesions, often with a non-enhancing central scar that was previously invisible. They can thus not be confused with metastases. Not unusually, especially small FNH may become completely occult in the delayed phase due to their liver-like contrast behaviour.

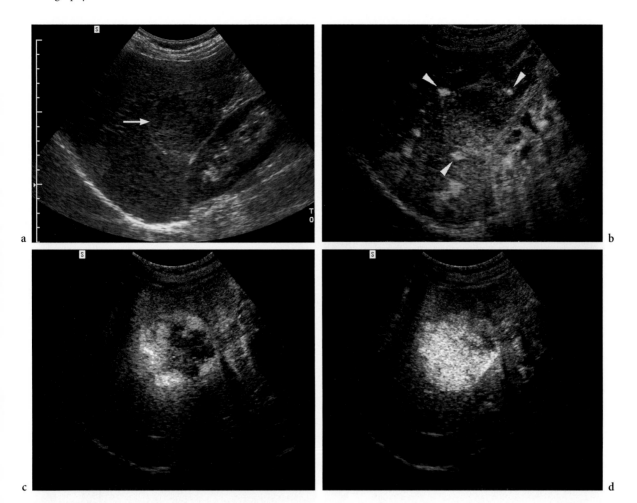

Fig. 18.9a–d. Dynamic enhancement of an haemangioma using Sonazoid. **a** Atypical baseline appearances: isoechoic lesion (*arrow*) indicative of metastases in a patient with colon carcinoma. **b** Arterial phase with peripheral nodular enhancement (*arrowheads*). **c** Partial centripetal fill-in in the portal venous phase (45 s post injection). **d** Complete filling of the haemangioma in the delayed phase (3–5 min post injection)

Focal fatty change and focal fatty sparing show the same contrast behaviour as normal liver parenchyma in all phases, since they contain no abnormal vessels and essentially consist of normal parenchyma. Again, these lesions usually "disappear" after contrast injection (Fig. 18.11).

Liver abscesses are rare; they may, however, be confused with metastases since they also show a rim enhancement in the arterial phase and produce enhancement defects in the later phases. An important differential diagnostic clue is the complete absence of vessels and enhancement in the central liquid portion of an abscess, while even hypovascular metastases will display some weak but visible central enhancement due to small vessels, provided they are not necrotic.

18.5
Detection of Hepatic Metastases with Ultrasound

The accuracy of unenhanced US in the assessment of hepatic metastases is lower than that of contrast-enhanced CT and MR. In series with a true gold standard, its sensitivity ranges between 50% and 76% (Table 18.2) (CLARKE et al. 1989; OHLSSON et al. 1993; WERNECKE et al. 1991). Problems encountered with US are its operator-dependent nature (making it difficult to use for follow-up staging), the sometimes difficult access to subdiaphragmatic areas of segments IVa and VIII and poor liver-to-lesion contrast of isoechoic lesions, especially in small metastases. For lesions smaller than 1 cm, the false-

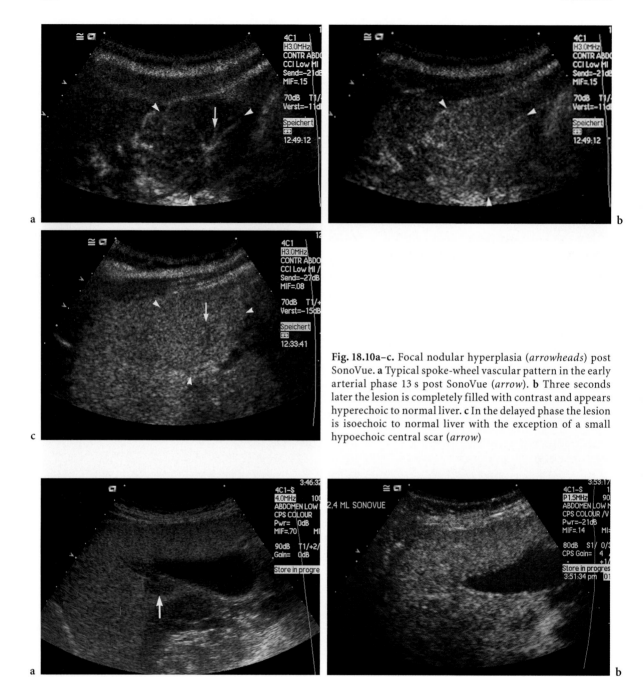

Fig. 18.10a–c. Focal nodular hyperplasia (*arrowheads*) post SonoVue. **a** Typical spoke-wheel vascular pattern in the early arterial phase 13 s post SonoVue (*arrow*). **b** Three seconds later the lesion is completely filled with contrast and appears hyperechoic to normal liver. **c** In the delayed phase the lesion is isoechoic to normal liver with the exception of a small hypoechoic central scar (*arrow*)

Fig. 18.11a,b. Focal fatty sparing near the gallbladder in a patient with pharyngeal carcinoma. **a** Unenhanced US shows a round hypoechoic lesion suggestive of a metastasis (*arrow*). **b** Homogeneous enhancement of the lesion in the delayed phase post SonoVue. The lesion is iso-enhancing compared to normal liver; it has "disappeared"

negative rate is as high as 80% (WERNECKE et al. 1991). The false-positive rate of US is in the order of 5–10% on a by patient basis and considerably higher on a by lesion basis.

As with other imaging modalities, the use of contrast agents improves the ability of US to detect liver metastases substantially. As described above, metas-

tases are seen as non-enhancing defects in an otherwise homogeneously enhancing liver in the portal venous and particularly in the delayed phase after contrast injection. Liver-specific agents are particularly useful for detecting otherwise invisible and often very small (<1 cm) metastases. This improves the sensitivity of US considerably to levels as high

Table 18.2. Performance of conventional US in detection of hepatic metastases (studies with true gold standard only)

Author, year	N (patients)	N (metastases)	Sensitivity	False positives	Gold standard
CLARKE et al. 1989	54	167	76%	?	IOUS
WERNECKE et al. 1991	75	74	53%	0%	IOUS
OHLSSON et al. 1993	71	?	50%	7%	Surgical exploration + follow-up
Own results 2002	35	83	70%	7%	IOUS(± resection)

as 90% when using a combination of other imaging modalities as the standard of reference (ALBRECHT et al. 2001; ALBRECHT et al. 2003a; ALBRECHT et al. 2003b). The detection rate of CEUS is comparable to that of dual phase spiral CT. Specificity is also improved, since benign lesions show late phase enhancement similar to normal liver, independent of their arterial behaviour, and they are thus usually not confused with metastases.

al. 2000). However, some of these results have proven difficult to reproduce by other workers.

Hepatic transit time analysis using a US contrast agent has recently been described as an alternative to DPI measurements. It is also capable of showing hepatic arterialisation by shortening of the transit time (ALBRECHT et al. 1999). Transit time measurements are much less operator dependent than DPI measurements. Whether the technique is able to detect "occult" hepatic metastases remains to be seen.

18.6
Detection of "Occult" Metastases with Functional Imaging

In an effort to further improve the sensitivity of US in the detection of metastases, functional techniques have been applied. One such method is the Doppler perfusion index (DPI), which is based on the fact that arterialisation of the liver's blood supply occurs in metastatic disease at a very early stage before the lesions become visible on any imaging modality including IOUS. The cause of this is unclear; it is likely to be due to some mediator excreted by the metastases.

Spectral Doppler measurements of hepatic arterial and portal venous blood flows are used for calculation of the DPI, i.e. ratio of hepatic arterial flow to total liver flow. In normal subjects the DPI is 0.25 (the hepatic artery contributes <25% of total liver blood flow), but this increases in arterialisation due to metastases. An excellent correlation between raised DPI and overt metastatic disease has been documented in colon and gastric cancer. In colon cancer patients with no overt liver malignancy, a raised DPI preoperatively correlated strongly with a shorter disease free survival and development of overt liver metastases within 5 years postoperatively, indicative of occult disease at presentation (LEEN et

References

Albrecht T, Blomley MJ, Cosgrove DO, et al (1999) Non-invasive diagnosis of hepatic cirrhosis by transit-time analysis of an ultrasound contrast agent. Lancet 353:1579–1583

Albrecht T, Hoffmann CW, Schettler S, et al (2000) B-mode enhancement at phase-inversion US with air-based microbubble contrast agent: initial experience in humans. Radiology 216:273–278

Albrecht T, Hoffmann CW, Schmitz SA, et al (2001) Phase-inversion sonography during the liver-specific late phase of contrast enhancement: improved detection of liver metastases. AJR Am J Roentgenol 176:1191–1198

Albrecht T, Oldenburg A, Hohmann J, et al (2003a) Imaging of liver metastases with contrast-specific low-MI real-time ultrasound and SonoVue. Eur Radiol 13(Suppl 3): N79–86

Albrecht T, Blomley MJ, Burns PN, et al (2003b) Improved detection of hepatic metastases with pulse-inversion US during the liver-specific phase of SHU 508A: multi-center study. Radiology 227:361–370

Bluemke DA, Paulson EK, Choti MA, et al (2000) Detection of hepatic lesions in candidates for surgery: comparison of ferumoxides-enhanced MR imaging and dual-phase helical CT. AJR Am J Roentgenol 175:1653–1658

Chomas J, Dayton P, May D, et al (2002) Nondestructive subharmonic imaging. IEEE Trans Ultrason Ferroelectr Freq Control 49:883–892

Clarke MP, Kane RA, Steele G Jr, et al (1989) Prospective comparison of preoperative imaging and intraoperative ultrasonography in the detection of liver tumors. Surgery 106:849–855

Conlon R, Jacobs M, Dasgupta D, et al (2003) The value of intraoperative ultrasound during hepatic resection compared with improved preoperative magnetic resonance imaging. Eur J Ultrasound 16:211–216

Edmunson H, Craig J (1987) Neoplasms of the liver. In: Schiff L (ed) Diseases of the liver, 8th edn. Lippincott, Philadelphia, p 1109

Hohmann J, Skrok J, Puls R, et al (2003) Characterization of focal liver lesions with contrast-enhanced low MI real time ultrasound and SonoVue. Rofo Fortschr Geb Rontgenstr Neuen Bildgeb Verfahr 175:835–843

Hope Simpson D, Burns PN (1999) Pulse inversion Doppler: a new method for detecting nonlinear echoes from microbubble contrast agents. IEEE Trans Ultrason Ferroelec Freq Contr 46:372–382

Hunerbein M, Rau B, Hohenberger P, et al (2001) Value of laparoscopic ultrasound for staging of gastrointestinal tumors. Chirurg 72:914–919

Ishak KG, Rabin L (1975) Benign tumors of the liver. Med Clin North Am 59:995–1013

Jones EC, Chezmar JL, Nelson RC, et al (1992) The frequency and significance of small (less than or equal to 15 mm) hepatic lesions detected by CT. AJR Am J Roentgenol 158:535–539

Karhunen PJ (1986) Benign hepatic tumours and tumour like conditions in men. J Clin Pathol 39:183–188

Kreft B, Pauleit D, Bachmann R, et al (2001) Häufigkeit und Bedeutung von kleinen fokalen Leberläsionen. Rofo Fortschr Geb Rontgenstr Neuen Bildgeb Verfahr 173:424–429

Leen E, Goldberg JA, Angerson WJ, et al (2000) Potential role of Doppler perfusion index in selection of patients with colorectal cancer for adjuvant chemotherapy. Lancet 355:34–37

Ohlsson B, Tranberg KG, Lundstedt C, et al (1993) Detection of hepatic metastases in colorectal cancer: a prospective study of laboratory and imaging methods. Eur J Surg 159:275–281

Schmidt J, Strotzer M, Fraunhofer S, et al (2000) Intraoperative ultrasonography versus helical computed tomography and computed tomography with arterioportography in diagnosing colorectal liver metastases: lesion-by-lesion analysis. World J Surg 24:43–48

Schultz JF, Bell JD, Goldstein RM, et al (1999) Hepatic tumor imaging using iron oxide MRI: comparison with computed tomography, clinical impact, and cost analysis. Ann Surg Oncol 6:691–698

Soyer P, Levesque M, Elias D, et al (1992) Detection of liver metastases from colorectal cancer: comparison of intraoperative US and CT during arterial portography. Radiology 183:541–544

Wanless IR, Albrecht S, Bilbao J, et al (1989) Multiple focal nodular hyperplasia of the liver associated with vascular malformations of various organs and neoplasia of the brain: a new syndrome. Mod Pathol 2:456–462

Ward J, Naik KS, Guthrie JA, et al (1999) Hepatic lesion detection: comparison of MR imaging after the administration of superparamagnetic iron oxide with dual-phase CT by using alternative-free response receiver operating characteristic analysis. Radiology 210:459–466

Wernecke K, Rummeny E, Bongartz G, et al (1991) Detection of hepatic masses in patients with carcinoma: comparative sensitivities of sonography, CT, and MR imaging. AJR Am J Roentgenol 157:731–739

19 Imaging Features of Hepatic Metastases: CT and MR

Christiane Kulinna and Wolfgang Schima

CONTENTS

19.1
Introduction

Metastatic disease in the liver represents one of the most common problems in oncology. The liver provides a fertile soil for metastases, especially due to its dual blood supply from the systemic and splanchnic system. The liver is second only to regional lymph nodes as a site of metastatic disease (Sugarbaker 1993; Bartolozzi et al. 2001). Metastatic disease is unknown, because most figures are based on autopsy series that reflect the end stage of a disease process, but between 30% and 70%, depending on the primary tumor of patients who die of cancer, have liver metastases on autopsy (Pickren et al. 1982).

C. Kulinna, MD; W. Schima, MD
Department of Radiology, Medical University of Vienna, AKH Vienna, Waehringer Guertel 18–20, 1090 Vienna, Austria

The early detection of liver metastases is of paramount importance in patients suffering from liver malignancies. In most malignancies, the presence of liver metastases indicates non-resectability of the primary tumor for oncologic reasons. In these patients, chemotherapy may be sought. On the other hand colorectal cancer is the prototype of malignant disease, in which the presence of limited metastatic disease does not preclude surgery. Exact knowledge of number, localization and size of metastases is crucial to determine resectability. Thus, the imaging technique used to evaluate the liver must achieve accurate depiction and characterization of both focal and diffuse processes. Additionally, they should provide information on segmental and vascular anatomy to facilitate treatment planning (Funke et al. 2001).

Although less expensive imaging methods, such as sonography, are widely available, patients with equivocal findings at sonography are often referred for definitive evaluation with computed tomography (CT) or magnetic resonance imaging (MR). Indications for liver CT imaging include differentiation of benign liver lesions, i.e. simple cysts, hemangiomas, adenomas, or focal nodular hyperplasia (FNH) from malignant lesions, such as metastasis, hepatocellular carcinoma (HCC), or cholangiocarcinoma. MR imaging is frequently used as a problem solving modality and many patients are referred for MR imaging for the evaluation of lesions considered indeterminate on other imaging modalities (Mueller et al. 2003).

In this chapter, current multi-detector CT (MDCT) and MR imaging protocols including the use of different liver-specific MR contrast agents will be discussed. The CT and MR imaging features of different hepatic metastases and pitfalls will be presented. The role of MDCT and MR in the assessment of patients with extrahepatic malignancies prone to metastasize into the liver and in the preoperative evaluation of surgical candidates will be highlighted.

19.2
Technical Considerations

19.2.1
MDCT

Helical CT is the most commonly used imaging modality for both detection and characterization of hepatic metastases. Single-row detector helical CT (SDCT) has a slow scanning speed (0.8–1 s per rotation) and acquires only one section of CT data with each rotation of the X-ray tube. The whole liver scanning using SDCT only takes 20–25 s. It is recognized that the liver has a dual blood supply, the duration of the virtual hepatic arterial phase equals the interval from the beginning of the contrast inflow into the liver from arteries to the beginning of the contrast inflow from the portal vein. It is so short that it is impossible to cover the whole liver with SDCT during the real hepatic arterial phase (Sun and Tang 2003; Ernst et al. 1999; Guo et al. 2003; Llado et al. 2000; Yamasaki et al. 2002; Yamashita et al. 1995).

With the advent of four-row detector scanners in 1998 coverage of the liver within one breath-hold of 12–14 s became feasible, thus decreasing the likelihood of motion artifacts during scanning. Current MDCT scanners feature up to 16 parallel rows of X-ray detectors that operate simultaneously at a collimation of 0.5–0.75 mm (Ohnesorge et al. 1999). Tube cooling has been improved and tube rotation time has decreased to 0.5 s or, with the newest generation of 16-row detector CT, to 0.4–0.43 s. Therefore, the upper abdomen from the diaphragm to the pelvis can be covered with submillimeter collimation within one breath hold. Image reformatting in any plane is possible without a loss of diagnostic image quality due to MDCT examination of the liver with nearly isotropic data sets. This is the prerequisite for the optimal assessment of very small liver lesions in all planes. The speed of MDCT can either be used to reduce the time to cover a given volume, or to use narrower beam collimation to increase the resolution of details along the z-axis and to reduce volume averaging.

So MDCT with 16-slice scanners needs no longer be restricted to special applications but is indeed ready for routine scanning. The reduced scan time with reduced motion artifacts facilitates the examinations of non-cooperative patients and improves axial resolution which enables for high quality 3D visualization.

19.2.2
MR

MR imaging is commonly used as the definitive imaging modality for the detection and characterization of liver lesions. T1- and T2-weighted sequences still remain the basic requirement for lesion detection and characterization in liver. Key factors that influence the diagnostic quality of MR are relative T1 and T2 relaxation times of lesion and normal parenchyma, pulse sequences and presence of artifacts. The first two factors can be influenced by proper sequence selection and use of appropriate contrast agents. The third factor depends on the technical equipment and the available software options (Bartolozzi et al. 2000). The use of high field strength MR scanners (≥ 1.0 T) is preferable, and phased-array torso coils for signal reception are now standard for all vendors. This improvement of hardware during the last years has made it possible to use breath hold sequences. The standard MR imaging protocol should always include unenhanced T1- and T2-weighted and contrast-enhanced pulse sequences. Newer scanners offer the advantage of rapid scanning with fast/ultrafast spoiled T1-weighted gradient-echo (GRE) sequences like FLASH sequences. In liver MR imaging always a set of T1-weighted in-phase and opposed phase GRE images is acquired to assess the parenchyma for the presence of diffuse or focal fatty infiltration. For T2-weighted images the turbo-spin echo (TSE; synonym: fast spin echo, FSE) with fat-suppression are preferred. For detection of focal lesions a time-to-echo (TE) of approximately 80–100 ms is chosen. In addition, a heavily T2-weighted pulse sequence with a TE of approximately 160–180 ms aids in differentiation between solid (metastases, HCC, etc.) and non-solid lesions (hemangiomas, cysts, etc.) (Ito et al. 1997; Schima et al. 1997). In general, the slice thickness should not exceed 8 mm (with minimal gap). With state-of-the-art T1-weighted 3D-GRE pulse sequences an effective slice thickness of 2–3 mm can be achieved. The standard matrix used is 256×256, but with high power gradients a spatial resolution of 256×512 is feasible.

19.3
Contrast Enhancement

Using contrast agents can increase the detection and improve the characterization of focal liver lesions.

19.3.1
MDCT

For optimal lesion detection a good contrast-to-noise ratio is essential since detection of these lesions depends mainly on contrast resolution. The contrast depends on the CT attenuation of the focal lesion but also on the liver parenchyma. Fatty infiltration of the liver can result in decreased attenuation of the liver and lesion can become imperceptible or even appear hyperattenuating relative to the surrounding parenchyma. In single slice CT, injection of either 2 ml/kg body weight of contrast medium or a fixed volume of 120–150 ml of contrast medium (at 300 mgI/ml), corresponding to a total iodine load of 36–45 g per patient is necessary to achieve adequate liver enhancement (KOPKA et al. 1995; KOPKA et al. 1996; SILVERMAN et al. 1995a). With the introduction of MDCT the total iodine load or the contrast volume could not be reduced, because maximum enhancement of liver parenchyma is provided by the total iodine load, largely independent of examination time (ENGEROFF et al. 2001; FOLEY et al. 2000; SILVERMAN et al. 1995a). However, recent studies found that higher iodine concentrations (400 mgI/ml) with constant total iodine load have a positive impact on abdominal enhancement during arterial phase. Recent studies demonstrated improved detection of hypervascular HCC in the arterial phase with MDCT, if a higher contrast material concentration is used (AWAI et al. 2002). However, the concentration has no influence on the enhancement during the portal venous phase of abdominal MDCT, which is more important for detection of liver metastases of most primary tumors (ENGEROFF et al. 2001).

It has become even more important to time scan acquisition appropriately regarding contrast material injection due to the shortened scan time of MDCT (KULINNA et al. 2001). Missing the arterial phase with MDCT before maximum of arterial liver enhancement is reached is one of the risks of high-speed MDCT scanning. Thus, optimization of scan timing has to be demanded. To obtain optimal enhancement of the liver during the arterial phase a compact bolus of contrast material with a steep upslope and a high injection rate must be used (BADER et al. 2000). In recent years experienced authors recommended at least 3–6 ml/s injection rates to achieve a sufficient conspicuity of hypervascular lesions enhanced in the arterial-dominant phase (ICHIKAWA et al. 2002; KIM et al. 1998a; TUBLIN et al. 1999). At our institution an injection rate of 5–8 ml/

s is preferred in order to optimize liver tumor imaging and depiction of the hepatic vasculature.

Although quadruple-phasic contrast-enhanced MDCT protocols have been advocated, most authors prefer two or maximum three different contrast-enhanced phases, depending on the indication, i.e. three-phasic protocols evaluation of suspected of HCC (LOYER et al. 1999). Whether an unenhanced scan is still of value, is under discussion (KOPKA et al. 2000; OLIVER et al. 1997). No or only limited role of unenhanced scan were found for the evaluation of hypervascular or hypovascular hepatic metastases (PATTEN et al. 1993; PAULSON et al. 1998; SHEAFOR et al. 1999; SICA et al. 2000). However, OLIVER et al. (1998) found that 28% of all hepatic metastases were seen only on the unenhanced scan. At our institution, unenhanced scan is performed in baseline studies, because the differentiation between cysts and small hypovascular metastases and a delineation of calcifications and hemorrhage is improved (Fig. 19.1).

The first contrast-enhanced scan should be a hepatic arterial phase scan. With MDCT two arterial phases can be performed: the early arterial phase starts when the contrast agent reaches the liver via the hepatic artery, followed by the late arterial phase, when there is beginning inflow of contrast-enhanced portal vein blood.

The earlier scan shows no or minimal admixture of enhanced portal venous blood, which is optimal for CT arteriography, but provides only minimal enhancement of liver tumors. The late arterial phase, with portal venous inflow, improves the hypervascular metastases detection. If a fixed delay is used, arterial phase images are obtained 25 s after start of injection of 150 ml contrast medium (300 mgI/ml) with a high flow rate (4–8 ml/s) for single slice and four-row scanners. With 16-row scanners, the delay can be increased to 30 s. However, the strong variability of contrast material transit time strongly advocates the use of automatic bolus triggering for individualization of delay time. If an automatic bolus triggering device (Care Bolus, SmartPrep, etc.) is used, the scanning then should started 12–15 s after a threshold of 100 HU is reached in the aorta. In this late arterial phase inflow of contrast-enhanced blood via the portal vein can already be observed, but there is still excellent opacification of the hepatic arterial system. Enhancement of hypervascular lesions usually peaks in this phase, which gives the best conspicuity of small hypervascular metastases (Fig. 19.2a). It has been recommended to perform double arterial phase scanning in patients with suspected HCC, but for detection of metastases a single (late) arterial phase scan is sufficient. The portal venous phase (PVP) is reached when contrast enhancement via the portal vein becomes dominant. The PVP begins with a 60–70 s delay after beginning of contrast injection. This is the most important phase for detection of hypovascular metastases (FREDERICK et al. 1997; SHEAFOR et al. 1999; VAN LEEUWEN et al. 1996). However, in this phase, many hypervascular metastases and the hyperattenuating rim around some hypovascular lesions will be isoattenuating to the liver parenchyma (Fig. 19.2b).

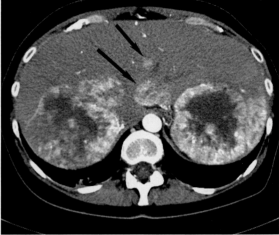

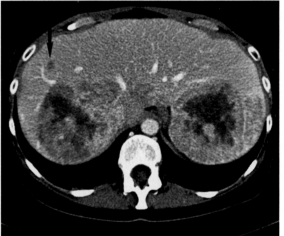

Fig. 19.2a,b. Hypervascular metastases of a glucagonoma. a Small hypervascular lesions are well seen in arterial phase (*arrows*). b The lesions are not or faintly visible on portal venous phase, but another hypovascular lesion is now visible, which was not visible in arterial phase (*arrow*)

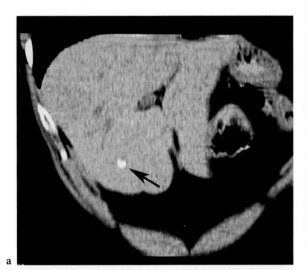

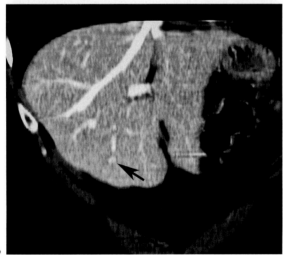

Fig. 19.1a,b. Detection of calcified metastases after chemotherapy: unenhanced scan versus contrast-enhanced scan. a Coronal MPR of unenhanced scan shows two calcified lesions in a patient with colon cancer (*arrow*). b On the portal-venous phase image the two lesions can not be differentiated from adjacent vessels (*arrow*). At surgery vital metastases were found

19.3.2
MR

The diagnostic effectiveness of the resulting MR examination is dependent on the type of contrast agent used, the way and dose in which the agent is administered, and the timing of scans (BARTOLOZZI et al. 2000). According to their biodistribution they can be categorized into three groups:

1. Extracellular contrast agents: non-specific gadolinium chelates
2. Reticuloendothelial system (RES) targeted agents: iron oxide particles
3. Hepatobiliary agents: manganese and gadolinium chelates

These agents can be classified as positive and negative contrast materials, based on their predominant T1 or T2 contrast effect. In general the extracellular and hepatobiliary agents are positive contrast, which means that they cause T1 shortening resulting in increased signal intensity of the liver. The negative contrast agents (RES agents) cause T2 shortening with a decreased signal intensity of the liver (HARISINGHANI et al. 2001).

19.3.2.1
Non-specific Gadolinium Chelates

The liver and liver-lesion enhancement patterns obtained with non-specific gadolinium chelates (extracellular contrast agents) are identical and equivalent to those of iodinated contrast agents currently used in CT. Many non-specific gadolinium chelates are licensed for use in body imaging at the standard dose of 0.1 mmol/kg b.w., including gadopentetate dimeglumine (Schering, Berlin, Germany), Gd-DTPA-BMA (Amersham Health, Oslo, Norway), Gd-DOTA (Guerbet, Aulnay-sous-Bois, France), Gadoteridol (Bracco, Milan, Italy). After i.v. bolus injection they show a brief vascular enhancement, followed by a rapid distribution to the extracellular space and excretion by the kidneys by glomerular filtration. Gadolinium chelates shorten both T1 and T2 relaxation times. The former is used for clinical purposes and results in increase in signal intensity of vascularized lesions on T1-weighted images. Dynamic T1-weighted gradient echo sequences in the arterial (20–30 s post injection), portal venous (60–80 s post injection) and equilibrium phase (3–5 min post injection) are used. Fat suppression should be added to at least one of the post gadolinium spoiled GRE sequences.

Hypervascular metastases exhibit an early, brief and pronounced signal enhancement in the arterial phase, which fades rapidly in the later phases. These lesions appear hyperintense in the arterial phase, but other hypervascular lesions like HCC, adenoma and FNH may show similar pattern. Hypovascular metastases exhibit a delayed contrast enhancement, which means they appear hypointense in the arterial phase. A maximal lesion-to-liver contrast is reached in the PVP. The equilibrium phase is still important, because it can be used for lesion differentiation (i.e. hemangioma versus metastasis). Hemangiomas show persistent enhancement during the equilibrium phase, whereas most metastases appear iso- or hypointense compared to liver parenchyma (Fig. 19.3).

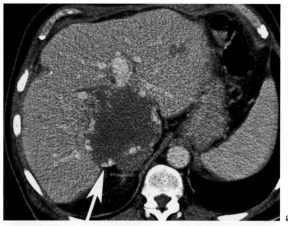

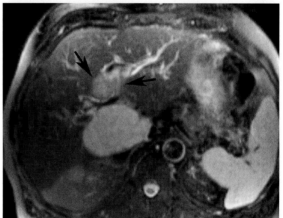

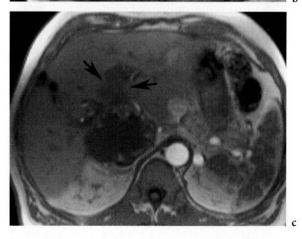

Fig. 19.3a–c. Pre-existing giant hemangioma: difficulty in detection of satellite metastasis. a MDCT shows a large hemangioma centered in the caudate lobe of the liver (arrow). b Follow-up MR 1 year later shows the T2-weighted very hyperintense hemangioma. There is an adjacent tumor anterior to it, which is not as bright (arrows). c Dynamic gadolinium-enhanced T1-weighted GRE image in the arterial phase shows typical peripheral nodular enhancement of the hemangioma. The adjacent lesion shows distinctly different contrast uptake: it is hypovascular (arrows). The anterior "collision tumor" was only seen in retrospect and was subsequently proved to be metastasis of colorectal cancer

19.3.2.2
Reticuloendothelial Agents

All reticuloendothelial agents are iron oxide-based contrast agents (SPIO). They are predominantly phagocytosed by the Kupffer cells in the liver (and in the spleen) and cause local field inhomogeneities, which result in shortened T2 relaxation times and decreased signal intensity of the target tissue. Thus they are called negative contrast agents. Currently, two SPIO agents (Endorem, ferumoxide, Guerbet; Resovist, SHU 555A, Schering) are available on the market. After SPIO administration, the liver parenchyma containing Kupffer cells shows a marked reduction in signal intensity on T2-weighted and T2*-weighted images, whereas liver metastases, containing no Kupffer cells, remain unaffected. Thus, due to the decreased signal intensity of normal liver parenchyma and no signal loss of liver metastases, they appear hyperintense on T2-weighted images postcontrast compared to precontrast MR images (Fig. 19.4). Improved lesion resolution from suppression of peritumoral edema makes these agents useful in preoperative evaluation of hepatic metastases from primary colorectal cancer (HAHN and SAINI 1998). RES-agents are also useful in differentiation metastases from focal liver lesions with phagocytic elements (FNH, adenomas, well-differentiated HCC) that result in RES-agent uptake and show a decreased signal intensity in T2-weighted images. A drop in signal intensity >40% from pre- to postcontrast T2-weighted images suggest a benign lesion (HAHN and SAINI 1998). Well-differentiated HCC have less uptake of RES-agents compared to benign lesions (REIMER and TOMBACH 1998; POECKLER-SCHOENIGER et al. 1999). Current investigations examine the value of dynamic T1-weighted images after ferumoxide administration.

19.3.2.3
Hepatobiliary Agents

Hepatobiliary agents represent a heterogeneous group of paramagnetic molecules of which a fraction is taken up by hepatocytes and excreted in the bile. These agents are designed for greater hepatobiliary uptake and excretion than conventional MR contrast agents. Mangafodipir trisodium, which belongs to this group (Teslascan, Amersham Health), is not specific to hepatocytes, but it is also taken up by the pancreas. The liver takes up free manganese and it acts as an intracellular paramagnetic agent that cause marked shortening of the T1-relaxation time (HARISINGHANI et al. 2001). Focal non-hepatocellular lesions (i.e. metastases) do not enhance post contrast, whereas the parenchyma shows increased signal intensity on T1-weighted images, resulting in improved lesion conspicuity (Fig. 19.5) (AICHER et al. 1993; BERNARDINO et al. 1992; SLATER et al. 1996). Very rarely, metastases from neuroendocrine tumors may show enhancement (WANG et al. 1998). Well differentiated lesions of hepatocellular origin (FNH, adenomas, well-differentiated HCC) show uptake of manganese and late enhancement on T1-weighted images (Fig. 19.6) (RUMMENY et al. 1997).

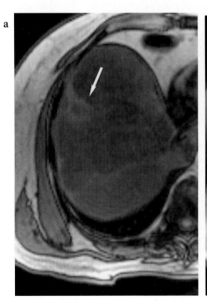 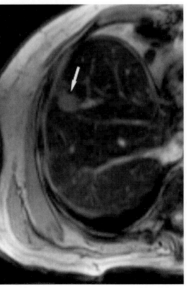

Fig. 19.4a,b. Improvement of lesion detection with iron-oxide based contrast-agent (SHU 555A; Resovist). **a** Unenhanced T2-weighted image with only faint visible lesion (*arrow*). **b** Resovist-enhanced T2-weigthed image shows typical hyperintense appearance of metastases on dark background liver (*arrow*)

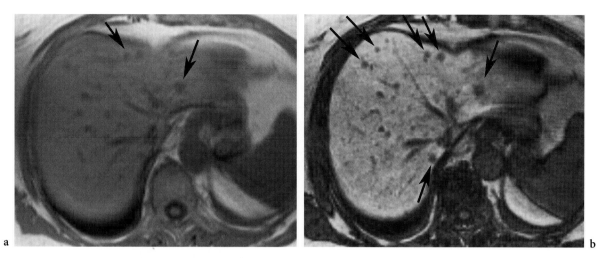

Fig. 19.5a,b. Improvement of lesion detection with liver-specific agent in a patient with breast cancer. **a** Unenhanced T1-weighted GRE image shows three small metastases (*arrows*). **b** Mangafodipir(Teslascan)-enhanced MR demonstrates multiple metastases throughout the liver (*arrows*)

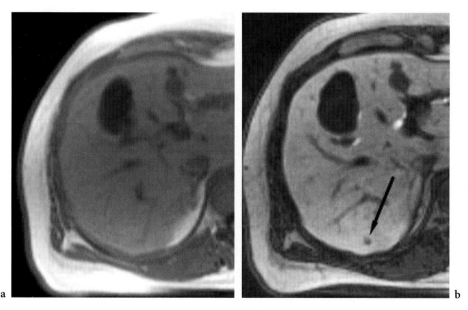

Fig. 19.6a,b. Detection of small metastases: Mangafodipir-enhanced vs gadolinium-enhanced MR. **a** Gadolinium-enhanced image shows three lesions in segment III/IVa of the liver. **b** Mangafodipir-enhanced T1-weighted image shows an additional small lesion (*black arrow*)

Liver-specific gadolinium chelates like Gd-BOPTA (Multihance®, Bracco) and Gd-EOB-DTPA (Primovist, Schering) are selective hepatic agents, because they carry a lipophilic ligand. After injection these agents show biphasic liver enhancement with a rapid rise in T1 signal intensity within the first 5 min post injection (p.i.) like that seen with non-specific extracellular gadolinium agents. Then hepatic signal intensity continues to rise for 20–60 min, reaching a plateau that persists for 2 h, because of hepatobiliary uptake and retention, so static imaging is feasible. However, this results in increasing contrast between liver and non-hepatocellular tumors, but may be problematic in the presence of diffuse liver disease (SIMON et al. 2003).

19.4
Scan Protocol MDCT

For the scan protocol as it is used in our hospital, see Table 19.1.

19.5
Imaging Features at CT/MR

Hepatic metastases generally presenting the histologic type of the primary neoplasm. In patient's setting with suspicion of metastases four questions are important:
1. Does the liver contains focal lesions?
2. Number and localization of lesions
3. Characterization of lesions
4. If metastases are suspected, are they treatable by resection or interventional therapy?

In clinical practice these questions should be answered in the context of the clinical history of the patient and the diagnostic modality. Many modali-

ties are available, but MDCT and MR are most reliable radiological modalities.

19.5.1
Presence of Liver Metastases on Plain MR Images

The majority of liver metastases have a higher cellular and interstitial water content of tumor tissue compared to normal liver parenchyma. Therefore, the mean T1 relaxation time of solid lesions is 1004 ± 234 ms vs 547 ± 80 ms for liver parenchyma, which renders metastases hypointense on nonenhanced T1-weighted images. The mean T2 relaxation time of solid masses is 80 ± 18 ms vs 51 ± 11 ms for liver parenchyma, which results in moderate tumor hyperintensity of metastases (GOLDBERG et al. 1993). Most lesions have irregular margins and show inhomogeneous pattern.

Some pathologic conditions can modify the signal intensity of the metastases. Whenever liquefactive necrosis or edema is present within the metastases, the signal intensity further increases on

Table 19.1. MSCT protocol for liver tumor imaging, 16-row scanner, used at the Department of Radiology, Medical University of Vienna. Unenhanced scan only used in case of HCC; delayed scan only used in case of CCC

Manufacturer	Siemens Sensation 16			
Detector Channels	16			
	Pre	ADP	PVP	Delayed
Collimation (mm)	16×1.5	16×1.5	16×1.5	16×1.5
Feed/rotation	30	30	30	30
Rotation time (s)	0.5			
KV	120			
mAs	120			
Matrix size	512×512			
Scan direction	Craniocaudal			
Slice thickness (mm)	3	2[a]+3	2[a]+3	2[a]+3
Reconstruction interval (mm)	2	1+2	1+2	1+2
Contrast material	150 ml			
Flow rate	5 ml/s			
Scan delay	Bolus tracking +12 s	Interscan delay 30 s	5 min	

ADP, arterial-dominant phase; PVP, portal-venous phase.
[a] Thin slices (2 mm) are used for MPR.

T2-weighted images. On the other hand, the signal intensity on T2-weighted images is decreased, if co-agulation necrosis (after tumor ablation therapy), fibrous matrix, or calcifications are present within metastases. Signal intensity of T1-weighted images is increased when subacute intralesional hemor-rhage with methemoglobin is present or other para-magnetic substances like melanin (seen in metas-tases from melanoma, multiple myeloma) appear within the metastases (KELEKIS et al. 1996; KOKUBO et al. 1988; MAHFOUZ et al. 1996). Depending on their histological type liver metastases may exhibit specific signs on unenhanced MR images: 15%–20% of the hepatic metastases show a central increase in signal intensity on T2-weighted images with a lower signal intensity outer ring, which is called "target" sign (WITTENBERG et al. 1988). It indicates a central hyperintense area of liquefactive necrosis, water content or hemorrhage. On T1-weighted images this feature may present as a central decrease in signal intensity. This finding is not seen in hemangiomas or cysts. Other helpful characteristics to differ ma-lignant necrotic tumors from hemangiomas or cysts are irregular internal morphology, mural nodules, a solid tissue rim or an indistinct interface with adja-cent liver parenchyma.

Approximately 20% of all metastases and 50% of colorectal metastases display a bright "halo" surround-ing a less intense nodule on T2-weighted images, cre-ated by a central area of hypointense fibrosis or necro-sis and a hyperintense rim of viable tumor cells rather than peritumoral edema (SIMON et al. 2003). The peri-tumoral edema may occur if the tumor causes vascular or biliary obstruction (BARTOLOZZI et al. 2001). This finding is usually not seen on T1-weighted images. Peripheral halos can also appear in HCC but have not been reported in benign non-inflammatory lesions.

Another characteristic feature of solid metastases is that they display a considerable signal intensity drop on heavily T2-weighted images using dual- or multiecho T2-weighted pulse sequences (Fig. 19.7). Cysts or hemangiomas show a relative signal in-

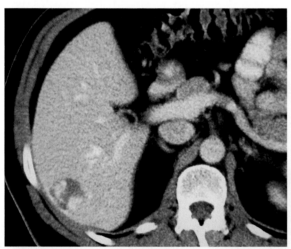

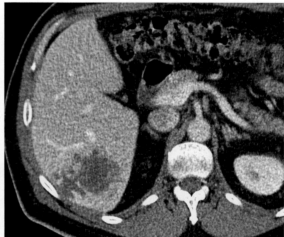

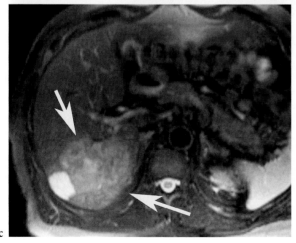

a

b

c

Fig. 19.7a–c. Hemangioma or metastasis: characterization with MR. **a** MDCT in the portal-venous phase shows a typi-cal hemangioma in a patient with colon cancer. Follow-up was recommended. **b** Follow-up portal-venous phase MDCT shows interval growth of a large lesion with change of con-trast enhancement characteristics, indicative of a metasta-sis. **c** T2-weighted fat-suppressed TSE MR image reveals the truth. There is a large moderately hyperintense metastasis (*arrows*) growing next to and compressing a small, T2-weighted very bright hemangioma

tensity increase with increasing TE on T2-weighted images. Only cystic or mucinous metastases may exhibit the same hyperintensity on heavily T2-weighted images (SIMON et al. 2003).

19.5.2
Vascularity of Hepatic Metastases in MDCT and MR

The vascularity of hepatic metastases determines their behavior after i.v. injection of extracellular CT or MR contrast medium. In contrast to the liver parenchyma, hepatic metastases get their blood supply almost exclusively by the hepatic artery. Only small metastases with a diameter of less then 1.5 cm may be found to have residual portal venous blood supply. Contrast enhancement therefore depends on arterial vascularization of a lesion relative to surrounding parenchyma.

In general, the "vascularity" of metastases is classified according to their contrast behavior in the arterial-dominant phase scan. Metastases which are hyperdense to normal liver parenchyma in this phase are called "hypervascular". Hypervascular metastases are less frequently than hypovascular metastases in the liver and typically originate from renal cell carcinomas, carcinoids, pancreatic islet cell carcinomas, sarcomas, pheochromocytomas, melanomas, thyroid carcinomas, chorion carcino-

mas, and sometime breast cancer. The best phase for detection of hypervascular metastases is the arterial phase. While they receive strong contrast enhancement via the hepatic artery, the liver parenchyma enhances only minimally in the arterial phase. Small hypervascular metastases usually present with homogeneous enhancement, whereas larger lesions appear heterogeneous or show a enhancing peripheral rim surrounding the necrosis. In the portal venous phase most hypervascular metastases show isodense/isointense attenuation, because the tumor still receive some contrast by the hepatic artery and the liver parenchyma also receive contrast by portal vein.

Most hepatic metastases are hypovascular and primary tumors that seed them are adenocarcinomas from gastrointestinal tract, lung and breast tumors. Metastases from squamous cell carcinomas (head and neck, esophagus, lung) usually show hypovascular metastases. Hypovascular metastases receive only minimal arterial and portal venous blood supply due to confluent dense cellularity, fibrosis or necrosis (SEMELKA and HELMBERGER 2001). So detection of hypovascular metastases is highest, when contrast enhancement of the normal liver parenchyma reaches its maximum in the portal venous phase and no or less arterial and venous blood supply in the metastases (Fig. 19.8). So portal venous phase shows optimal lesion to liver contrast. Some "hypovascular" metastases show a target appearance with a hyperattenuating rim and hypoat-

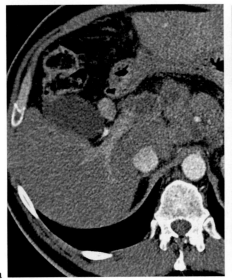
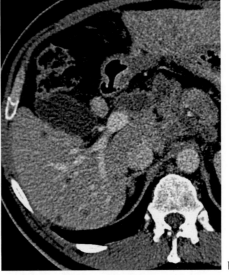

a   b

Fig. 19.8a,b. Hypovascular metastases of metastatic adenocarcinoma. **a** In the arterial phase the small lesions throughout the liver are only faintly visible. **b** In the portal-venous phase scan, diffuse metastatic spreading in the liver is well demonstrated

tenuating center in the arterial phase and the portal venous phase. In the delayed phase the outer rim may become isodense/isointense to surrounding liver parenchyma, so that the lesion appears smaller than it is in reality. This finding can lead to problems in preoperative staging or follow-up examinations after chemotherapy.

19.6
Pitfalls in Liver Imaging

Arterial phase imaging may reveal a lot of pseudolesions. Most of them result from vascular variations or changes in the normal dual blood supply of the liver (Fig. 19.9) (CHEN et al. 1999; HERTS et al. 1993; SILVERMAN et al. 1995b). Common pseudolesions are seen in the gallbladder fossa, near the falciform ligament and the porta hepatis and are either focal fatty infiltration or focal sparing in diffuse fatty infiltration of the liver. The changes in fatty infiltration of the liver near the falciform ligament are explained by the presence of systemic venous supply instead of portal blood supply (ITAI and SAIDA 2002). Presence of fat or focal fatty sparing is confirmed by comparison of in- and opposed-phase MR images.

Hepatic veins, which are not opacified due to inadequate timing of CT scan or due to delayed contrast transit in outflow obstruction, can be misinterpreted as true lesions on single images.

However, evaluation of adjacent slices in cine mode should help to differentiate between true lesions of rounded shape and non-opacified tubular venous structures. Poor hepatic parenchymal enhancement can limit the detection of hypovascular lesions, which are best seen in portal venous phase (MILLER et al. 1998). Vascular tumors can mimic the appearance of aneurysms or vascular malformations. Peripheral enhancement of hemangiomas during arterial phase could be difficult to appreciate, so nodular enhancement during additional portal-venous phase could be helpful. Lesion detection in patients with diffuse liver disease could be problematic due to inhomogeneous enhancement patterns of the whole liver. Portal hypertension can delay hepatic enhancement and underestimate parenchymal disease or mimic portal vein thrombosis. Peripheral arterioportal shunts could be sometimes seen on arterial phase and can mimic small lesions (KIM et al. 1998b). The key to the correct diagnosis is the presence of a feeding vessels seen at thin slices of arterial phase MDCT, the triangular shape of arterioportal shunt and the often only faint enhancement. However, especially early arterial phase scanning can result in different phenomena that are potential diagnostic pitfalls if not appropriately recognized. Careful analysis of unenhanced and portal-venous phase CT scans helps to avoid false diagnoses of hypervascular neoplasms. In equivocal cases contrast-enhanced MR with liver-specific agents may help to rule out malignant disease (Fig. 19.10).

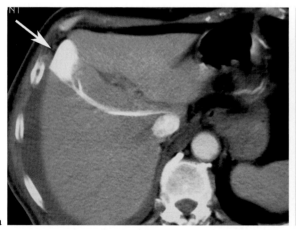

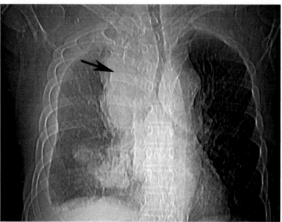

a   b

Fig. 19.9a,b. Perfusion abnormality simulating hypervascular metastasis. **a** Contrast-enhanced CT shows a very hypervascular area in IV segment close to the abdominal wall (*arrow*). There is early drainage of contrast into the liver vein. The IVC already shows much more enhancement than the aorta. **b** Topogram of CT shows a large mediastinal tumor (lymph nodes) obstructing the SVC (*arrow*), which resulted in formation of venous collaterals from the upper trunk to the IVC. One venous collateral pathway typically leads in the anterior abdominal wall through the liver parenchyma (IV segment) and into the IVC

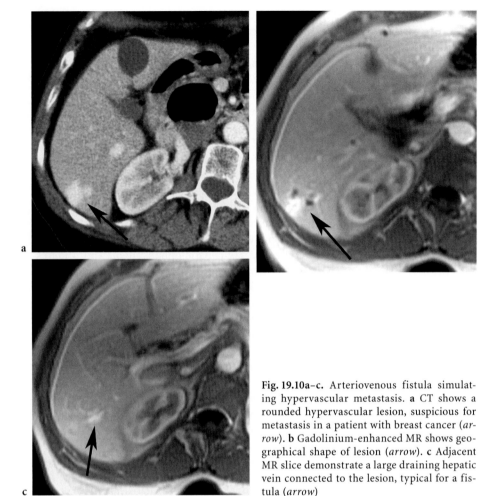

Fig. 19.10a–c. Arteriovenous fistula simulating hypervascular metastasis. **a** CT shows a rounded hypervascular lesion, suspicious for metastasis in a patient with breast cancer (*arrow*). **b** Gadolinium-enhanced MR shows geographical shape of lesion (*arrow*). **c** Adjacent MR slice demonstrate a large draining hepatic vein connected to the lesion, typical for a fistula (*arrow*)

19.7
Assessment of Small Liver Lesions

One of the most common challenges in liver imaging is the small focal lesion detected incidentally or during work-up of a patient with malignant disease. Knowledge of number, location, size and characterization of these small lesions is crucial to determine the appropriate treatment.

JONES et al. (1992) reported that in a series of more than 1400 patients referred for abdominal contrast-enhanced CT, 17% of patients had 15 mm or smaller liver lesions. In these series, 82 % of the patients had a known malignancy. Overall, 51% of lesions were classified as benign, 22% as malignant, and in 27% of patients the lesions could not be classified. In the subgroup of patients with known malignant tumors and single small hepatic lesions, only 5% of lesions were malignant. However, another 30% were deemed indeterminate.

In a study by SCHWARTZ et al. (1999), focal liver lesions 1 cm or less in diameter were found in 12.7% of 2900 cancer patients. Of these lesions 80.2% were classified as benign by follow-up, 11.6% as malignant, and 8.2% as indeterminate due to incomplete follow-up. In both studies, by dynamic incremental CT with contiguous 10-mm thick sections was used, which rendered reliable characterization of small focal lesions very difficult (JONES et al. 1992; SCHWARTZ et al. 1999). In this clinical scenario, percutaneous biopsy is often not feasible.

Since then, more advanced imaging modalities have been developed to characterize these small lesions. However, the scope of the problem has dramatically increased as the number of small focal lesions detected by helical and MDCT and MR has increased substantially. In early studies with spiral CT scanning increased the detection rate for small lesion on 74%–85% (VALLS et al. 2001; WARD et al. 1999). In these series almost all the false-negative results involved lesions smaller than 15 mm in diameter. In the study of WEG et al. (1998) the use of 2.5 mm (vs 10 mm) thick collimation in dual-slice CT scanning increased the detection rate for metastases ≤10 mm by 86%. There is no trend towards increased characterization of lesions as benign or malignant at thinner collimation (HAIDER et al. 2002). In the study of JANG et al. (2002), helical CT features of benign small lesions were smaller size, discrete margins, and markedly low attenuation, whereas a target-enhancement was specific for metastases.

Several studies have reported MR to be more sensitive and more specific than dynamic incremental CT and helical CT (RUMMENY et al. 1992; SEMELKA et al. 1992; SEMELKA et al. 1997). Ferumoxide-enhanced MR has been shown to detect more, especially small, metastatic lesions than dynamic contrast CT (Fig. 19.11) (VOGL et al. 1996a). Small lesions, which are detected at a greater frequency with this technique, likely will be particularly difficult to characterize exactly. Gadolinium-enhanced MR may help-

ful in characterization of these lesions, particularly for small hemangiomas, cysts, and biliary hamartomas (Fig. 19.12). Other studies found Mangafodipir trisodium, Gd-DTPA or Gd-EOB-DTPA superior in detection and characterization of small lesions (Fig. 19.13) (HAMM et al. 1992; PADOVANI et al. 1995; VOGL et al. 1996b).

19.7.1
Clinical Approach to Small Lesions

In a patient without known cancer and without liver cirrhosis, small lesions can be evaluated with serial follow-up imaging tests because nearly all of them will be benign (JONES et al. 1992). Small solitary liver lesions in patients with known cancer are more frequently benign than malignant, these lesions represents metastases in 5%–11.6% of the patients (JONES et al. 1992; SCHWARTZ et al. 1999).

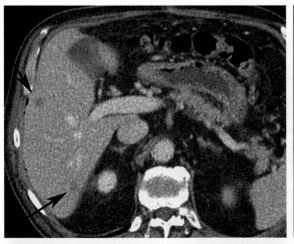

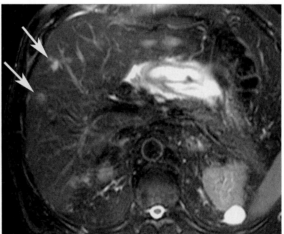

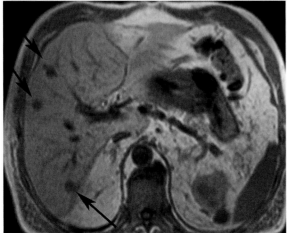

Fig. 19.11a–c. Detection of liver metastases: MDCT vs MR with liver-specific contrast agent. a Contrast-enhanced MDCT demonstrates two small metastases (*arrows*) in a patient with colorectal cancer. b T2-weighted fat saturation TSE image shows two lesions (*arrows*). There is inhomogeneity of parenchyma in the posterior part of the right lobe, but no definitive lesion is seen. c Mangafodipir-enhanced T1-weighted GRE image shows three metastases (*arrows*). The third lesion was not seen on adjacent MDCT images (not shown)

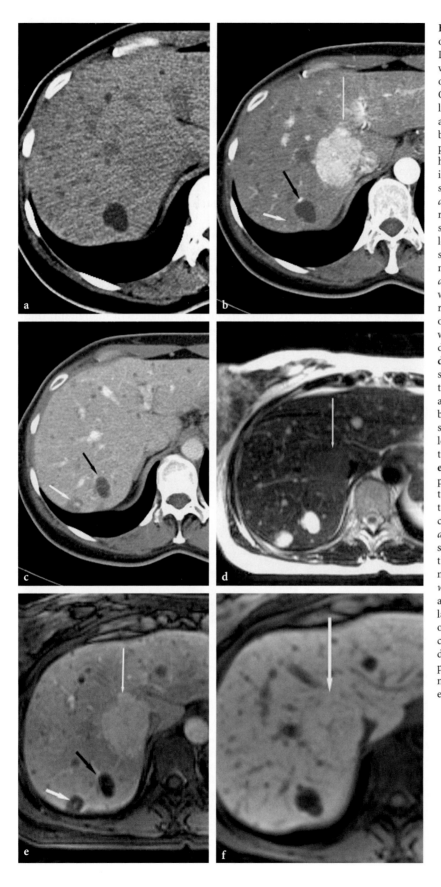

Fig. 19.12a–f. Characterization of focal lesions with Gd-EOB-DTPA-enhanced MR in a patient with breast cancer: metastases or benign lesions? **a** Unenhanced CT shows only one hypodense lesion in V segment. **b** In the arterial phase three lesions can be detected. The big lesion is hypervascular (*white arrow*), the hypodense lesion (*black arrow*) is non-enhanced and a third lesion subcapsular (*white small arrow*) shows a hyperdense rim. **c** The portal venous phase shows only the non-enhanced lesion (*black arrow*) and the small subcapsular lesion with nodular enhancement (*white arrow*). The large lesion, which was hypervascular in the arterial phase, has faded. Presence of an FNH and a hemangioma was suspected, but no definitive diagnosis could be made by CT. **d** T2-weighted TSE MR image shows the big lesion to be isointense with a central scar (*arrow*) and the two other lesions as very bright. There are multiple other small, T2-weighted very bright lesions seen, which turned out to be multiple peribiliary cysts. **e** Dynamic T1-weighted image post Gd-EOB-DTPA in the arterial phase shows the hyperintense large lesion with the typical central scar of a FNH (*white arrow*). The non-enhanced lesion is a cyst (*black arrow*) and the typical nodular enhanced mass a hemangioma (*small white arrow*). **f** T1-weighted images post Gd-EOB-DTPA in the late phase shows accumulation of contrast agent in the hepatocytes of the FNH (*arrow*). The definitive diagnosis was FNH plus hemangioma plus cyst plus multiple peribiliary cysts, but no evidence of metastasis

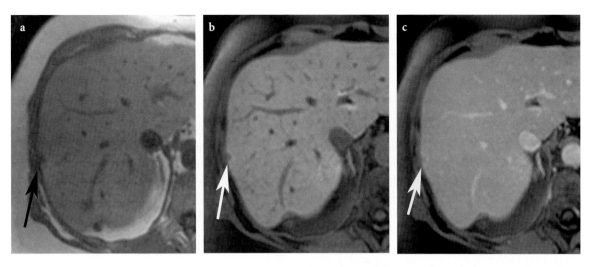

Fig. 19.13a–c. Detection of small metastases: mangafodipir-enhanced vs gadolinium-enhanced MR. **a** Unenhanced T1-weighted GRE image shows an ill-defined hypointense subcapsular lesion (*arrow*). **b** On mangafodipir-enhanced T1-weighted GRE fat saturation image the lesion is shown with better conspicuity (*arrow*). **c** The lesion is only faintly visible on the gadolinium-enhanced T1-weighted GRE fat saturation image (*arrow*)

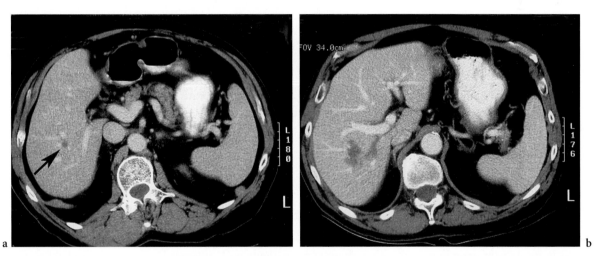

Fig. 19.14a,b. Follow-up of a small solitary lesion in a patient with known colon cancer. **a** Baseline CT study shows a small solid lesion less than 1 cm in diameter (*arrow*). The lesion could not be characterized reliably. Follow-up in 6 months was recommended, but the patient was lost to follow-up. **b** At 3 years later, follow-up CT shows considerable growth of the previously small lesion. Biopsy revealed metastasis of colon cancer

So in patients with cancer, further evaluation with MR for exact determination of the etiology of such lesions may be pivotal for defining prognosis and therapy (WARD et al. 1999). A delay in diagnosis and treatment should particularly avoided in colorectal cancer patients with small lesions, who would be candidates for liver surgery (Fig. 19.14).

19.8
Value of CT and MR

In times of limited resources, there has been considerable debate which imaging modality offers the best noninvasive examination of the liver, particularly concerning the detection and characterization of focal liver lesions. The parallel use of different diagnostic modalities is both costly and inefficient. It requires that the different imaging modalities would be placed in appropriate positions within their diagnostic pathway.

MDCT scan is well established and widely spread, and is often the first choice for a screening liver examination at many institutions. MDCT technique has improved small lesion detection by reducing respiration-related artifacts. Shortened scan time of MDCT enables exact multiphase scanning of the chest and abdomen with improved lesion characterization, but increases the radiation exposure on the other hand. Nearly isotropic voxel data acquisition enables comparable three-dimensional reconstructions, particularly for CT-angiography and demonstrating lesion location as part of surgical planning. Today 3D reconstruction modes are easy and not very time consuming to perform. At least MDCT has the big advantage for one-stop-shopping, for imaging of the liver and extrahepatic disease (both abdominal and thoracic). This ensures that MDCT will keep an important role in staging and screening.

MR imaging is at least as sensitive as CT scan in detecting focal liver lesions, and in addition some advantages over CT.

MR is more sensitive for detecting hemangiomas than CT but even more important it is able to differentiate them reliably from hepatic metastases, either by the very high signal on heavily T2-weighted images or by their characteristic enhancement pattern (Nelson et al. 1990; Yoon et al. 2003). With multiphasic scanning of MDCT typical pattern of small hemangiomas is well appreciated, however, atypically appearing hemangiomas are still a domain of MR.

Another advantage of MR vs CT is the fatty liver, which is not uncommon in patient with malignancy who have undergone chemotherapy. Focal fatty infiltrations can imitate focal lesions in CT and diffuse fatty changes severely impair the detection of focal lesions (Schertz et al. 1989). T1-weighted opposed phase imaging can readily diagnose both focal and diffuse changes (Dixon 1984) and helps differentiating focal fat from small neoplasms or metastases. Blood breakdown products have a distinctive MR appearance allowing differentiation of hematomas from more simple fluid collections or necrosis in metastases, particularly when chronic. Kinkel et al. (2002) performed a meta-analysis on the value of US, CT, MR and FDG-PET for the detection of metastases from gastrointestinal tumors. The authors found mean weighted sensitivities of 55% for US, 72% for CT, 76% for MR and 90% for FDG-PET. A limitation of this analysis is the fact that, neuroendocrine tumors, biliary malignancies and sarcomas were not included. Another point is that no CT study was performed with MDCT, so this analysis is not exactly from the actual point of view. To our knowledge there is no large study available comparing MR and MDCT in detection and characterization of focal liver lesions. Certainly, MDCT is particularly good at detecting extrahepatic tumor deposits and describing the 3D relationship of metastases to vascular and other critical structures.

19.9
Assessment of Surgical Candidates

With expanding indications for liver resection, and increasing safety of such therapies in appropriate centers, more patients are referred for evaluation and treatment of their primary and metastatic liver tumors. A total of 3%–10% of all patients with colorectal cancer will develop resectable liver metastases (August et al. 1984; Bismuth et al. 1995; Fong et al. 1999; Rose et al. 1998). The natural history of untreated patients with liver metastases shows a 5-year survival rate of 0%–3% (Wood et al. 1976). If a resection with curative intent is performed, the 5-year survival rate can be as high as 25%–40% (van Ooijen and Wiggers 1992; Bradley et al. 1999; Doci et al. 1991; Nordlinger et al. 1996; Scheele et al. 1995). The majority of liver metastases are nonresectable because of extrahepatic disease or extensive liver involvement. So extensive pre-operative assessment is indicated to exclude metastatic disease at other sites to prevent unnecessary laparotomies in patients with advanced cancer. To select those patients for a curative resection of liver metastases, a standardized pre-operative evaluation should be developed for every potential patient.

The ideal preoperative imaging modality would combine high sensitivity and specificity, with a low false-positive rate about metastases detection rate and characterization. It should provide precise anatomic information of the tumor location in relation to the major anatomic structures. In most oncologic centers, contrast-enhanced CT and/or MR are the mainstay of pre-operative staging in patients with liver tumors. However, in the retrospective study of Zacherl et al. (2002), contrast-enhanced helical CT either showed false-positive and false-negative diagnosis in 42% of surgical candidates. They concluded that intraoperative ultrasound is mandatory in surgical candidates for metastasis resection. However, state-of-the-art MDCT and MR read by radiologic specialists is likely to decrease the number of false-negative and false-positive diagnoses. MR has gained an important role in preoperative evaluation of the liver over the past decade. MANN et al. (2001) compared MR with mangafodipir with spiral CT in preoperative assessment of liver metastases for resectability, and he found MR to be more sensitive than contrast-enhanced spiral CT in the preoperative predicting of the resectability of hepatic lesions. MR detected significantly more lesions than spiral CT (sensitivity 83% vs 61%), but intraoperative ultrasound detected additional subcentimeter metastases. However, the extent of metastatic disease was under- or overestimated in only 2/20 patients by mangafodipir-enhanced MR (MANN et al. 2001). VAN ETTEN et al. (2002) found ferumoxide enhanced MR technique is safe and at least as accurate as spiral CTAP in preoperative assessment of colorectal liver metastases. Up to now no studies comparing MR with MDCT has been performed. In our experience the initial imaging should include a MDCT of the abdomen with two or three contrast phases with rapid bolus injection. In most circumstances, this imaging modality answers the clinical question, extrahepatic tumors or lymph nodes, tumor's location in relation to the major hepatic structures could be seen, and no further study is indicated.

MR imaging, enhanced with liver-specific contrast agents, is recommended if doubt regarding the intrahepatic extent or the etiology of a tumor remains.

References

Aicher KP, Laniado M, Kopp AF, et al (1993) Mn-DPDP-enhanced MR imaging of malignant liver lesions: efficacy and safety in 20 patients. J Magn Reson Imaging 3:731-737

August DA, Ottow RT, Sugarbaker PH (1984) Clinical perspective of human colorectal cancer metastasis. Cancer Metastasis Rev 3:303-324

Awai K, Takada K, Onishi H, et al (2002) Aortic and hepatic enhancement and tumor-to-liver contrast: analysis of the effect of different concentrations of contrast material at multi-detector row helical CT. Radiology 224:757-763

Bader TR, Grabenwoger F, Prokesch RW, et al (2000) Measurement of hepatic perfusion with dynamic computed tomography: assessment of normal values and comparison of two methods to compensate for motion artifacts. Invest Radiol 35:539-547

Bartolozzi C, Lencioni R, Donati F, et al (2000) Abdominal MR: liver and pancreas. Categorial Course Eur Radiol 10:121-137

Bartolozzi C, Cioni D, Donati F, et al (2001) Focal liver lesions: MR imaging-pathologic correlation. Eur Radiol 11:1374-1388

Bernardino ME, Young SW, Lee JK, et al (1992) Hepatic MR imaging with Mn-DPDP: safety, image quality, and sensitivity. Radiology 183:53-38

Bismuth H, Chiche L, Castaing D (1995) Surgical treatment of hepatocellular carcinomas in noncirrhotic liver: experience with 68 liver resections. World J Surg 19:35-41

Bradley AL, Chapman WC, Wright JK (1999) Surgical experience with hepatic colorectal metastases. Am J Surg 65:560-566

Chen WP, Chen JH, Hwang JI (1999) Spectrum of transient hepatic attenuation differences in biphasic CT. AJR Am J Roentgenol 172:419-424

Dixon WT (1984) Single proton spectroscopic imaging. Radiology 153:189-194

Doci R, Gennari L, Bignami P, et al (1991) One hundred patients with hepatic metastases from colorectal cancer treated by resection: analysis of prognostic determinants. Br J Surg 78:797-801

Engeroff B, Kopka L, Harz C, et al (2001) Impact of different iodine concentrations on abdominal enhancement in biphasic multislice helical CT. Rofo Fortschr Geb Rontgenstr Neuen Bildgeb Verfahr 173:938-941

Ernst O, Sergent G, Mizrahi D, et al (1999) Treatment of hepatocellular carcinoma by transcatheter arterial chemoembolization: comparison of planned periodic chemoembolization and chemoembolization based on tumor response. AJR Am J Roentgenol 172:59-64

Foley WD, Mallisee TA, Hohenwalter MD, et al (2000) Multiphase hepatic CT with a multirow detector CT scanner. AJR Am J Roentgenol 175:679-685

Fong Y, Sun RL, Jarnagin W, et al (1999) An analysis of 412 cases of hepatocellular carcinoma at a western center. Ann Surg 229:790-799

Frederick MG, Paulson EK, Nelson RC (1997) Helical CT for detection focal liver lesions in patients with breast carcinoma: comparison of noncontrast phase, hepatic arterial phase and portal venous phase. J Comput Assist Tomogr 21:229-235

Funke M, Kopka L, Grabbe E (2001) Biphasic contrast-enhanced multislice helical CT of the liver. In: Reiser MF, Takahashi M, Modic M, Bruening R (eds) Multislice CT. Springer-Verlag, Berlin Heidelberg New York, pp 35-38

Goldberg A, Hahn PF, Saini S, et al (1993) Value of T1 and T2 relaxation times from echoplanar imaging in the characterization of focal hepatic lesions. AJR Am J Roentgenol 160:1011-1017

Guo WJ, Yu EX, Liu LM, et al (2003) Comparison between chemoembolization combined with radiotherapy and chemoembolization alone for large hepatocellular carcinoma. World J Gastroenterol 9:1697-1701

Hahn PF, Saini S (1998) Liver-specific MR imaging contrast agents. Radiol Clin North Am 36:287-297

Haider MA, Amitai MM, Rappaport DC, et al (2002) Multidetector row helical CT in preoperative assessment of small (< or =1.5 cm) liver metastases: is thinner collimation better? Radiology 222:137-142

Hamm B, Vogl TJ, Branding G (1992) Focal liver lesions: MR imaging with Mn-DPDP – initial clinical results in 40 patients. Radiology 182:167-174

Harisinghani MG, Jhaveri KS, Weissleder R, et al (2001) MRI contrast agents for evaluating focal hepatic lesions. Clin Radiol 56:714-725

Herts BR, Einstein DM, Paushter DM (1993) Spiral CT of the abdomen: artefacts and potential pitfalls. AJR Am J Roentgenol 161:1185-1190

Ichikawa T, Kitamura T, Nakajima H, et al (2002) Hypervascular hepatocellular carcinoma: can double arterial phase imaging with multidetector CT improve tumor depiction in the cirrhotic liver? AJR Am J Roentgenol 179:751-758

Itai Y, Saida Y (2002) Pitfalls in liver imaging. Eur Radiol 12:1162-1174

Ito K, Mitchell DG, Outwater EK, et al (1997) Hepatic lesions: discrimination of nonsolid, benign lesions from solid malignant lesions with heavily T2-weighted fast spin-echo MR imaging. Radiology 204:729-737

Jang HJ, Lim HK, Lee WJ, et al (2002) Small Hypoattenuating lesions in the liver on single-phase helical CT in preoperative patients with gastric and colorectal cancer: prevalence, significance, and differentiating features. J Comput Assist Tomogr 26:718-724

Jones EC, Chezmar JL, Nelson RC, et al (1992) The frequency and significance of small (less than or equal to 15 mm) hepatic lesions detected by CT. AJR Am J Roentgenol 158:535-539

Kelekis NL, Semelka RC, Woosley JT (1996) Malignant lesions of the liver with high signal intensity on T1-weighted MR images. J Magn Reson Imaging 6:291-294

Kim T, Murakami T, Takahashi S, et al (1998a) Effects of injection rates of contrast material on arterial phase hepatic CT. AJR Am J Roentgenol 171:429-432

Kim TK, Choi BI, Han JK, et al (1998b) Nontumorous arterioportal shunt mimicking hypervascular tumor in cirrhotic liver: two-phase spiral CT findings. Radiology 208:597-603

Kinkel K, Lu Y, Both M, et al (2002) Detection of hepatic metastases from cancers of the gastrointestinal tract by using non-invasive imaging methods (US, CT, MR imaging, PET): a meta-analysis. Radiology 224:748-756

Kokubo T, Itai Y, Ohtomo K (1988) Muci-hypersecreting intrahepatic biliary neoplasms. Radiology 168:609-614

Kopka L, Funke M, Fischer U, et al (1995) Parenchymal liver enhancement with bolus-triggered helical CT: preliminary clinical results. Radiology 195:282-284

Kopka L, Rodenwaldt J, Fischer U, et al (1996) Dual-phase helical CT of the liver: effects of bolus tracking and different volumes of contrast material. Radiology 201:321-326

Kopka L, Rodenwaldt J, Hamm BK (2000) Value of hepatic perfusion imaging for indirect detection of different liver lesions: feasibility study with multi-slice helical CT. Radiology 217(P):457

Kulinna C, Helmberger T, Kessler M, et al (2001) Improvement in diagnosis of liver metastases with the multidetector CT. Radiologe 41:16-23

Llado L, Virgili J, Figueras J, et al (2000) A prognostic index of the survival of patients with unresectable hepatocellular carcinoma after transcatheter arterial chemoembolization. Cancer 88:50-57

Loyer EM, Chin H, DuBrow RA, et al (1999) Hepatocellular carcinoma and intrahepatic peripheral cholangiocarcinoma: enhancement patterns with quadruple phase helical CT. A comparative study. Radiology 212:866-875

Mahfouz AE, Hamm B, Mathieu D (1996) Imaging of metastases to the liver. Eur Radiol 6:607-614

Mann GN, Marx HF, Lai LL, et al (2001) Clinical and cost effectiveness of a new hepatocellular MRI contrast agent, mangafodipir trisodium, in the preoperative assessment of liver respectability. Ann Surg Oncol 8:573-579

Miller FH, Butler RS, Hoff FL, et al (1998) Using triphasic helical CT to detect focal hepatic lesions in patients with neoplasms. AJR Am J Roentgenol 171:643-649

Mueller GC, Hussain HK, Carlos RC, et al (2003) Effectiveness of MR imaging in characterizing small hepatic lesions: routine versus expert interpretation. AJR Am J Roentgenol 180:673-680

Nelson RC, Chezmar JL, Sugarbaker PH, et al (1990) Preoperative localization of focal liver lesions to specific liver segments: utility of CT during arterial portography. Radiology 176:89-94

Nordlinger B, Guiguet M, Vaillant JC (1996) Surgical resection of colorectal carcinoma metastases to the liver. A prognostic scoring system to improve case selection, based on 1568 patients. Cancer 77:1254-1262

Ohnesorge B, Flohr T, Schaller S, et al (1999) The technical bases and uses of multi-slice CT. Radiologe 39:923-931

Oliver JH 3rd, Baron RL, Federle MP, et al (1997) Hypervascular liver metastases: do unenhanced and hepatic arterial phase CT images affect tumor detection? Radiology 205:709-715

Oliver JH 3rd, Baron RL, Federle MP (1998) Hypervascular liver metastases: do unenhanced and hepatic arterial phase CT images affect tumor detection? Radiology 209:585-586

Padovani B, Lecesne R, Raffaelli C, et al (1995) Phase III study of MN-DPDP in MR imaging and contrast-enhanced CT. Radiology 197(P):415

Patten RM, Byun JY, Freeny PC (1993) CT of hypervascular hepatic tumors: are unenhanced scans necessary for diagnosis ? AJR Am J Roentgenol 161:979-984

Paulson EK, McDermott VG, Keogan MT, et al (1998) Carcinoid metastases to the liver: role of triple-phase helical CT. Radiology 206:143-150

Poeckler-Schoeniger C, Koepke J, Gueckel F, et al (1999) MRI with supermagnetic iron oxide: efficacy in the detection and characterization of focal hepatic lesions. Magn Reson Imaging 17:383-392

Pickren JK, Tsukada Y, Lane WW (1982) Liver metastasis. Analysis of autopsy data. In: Weiss L, Gilbert HA (eds) Liver metastasis. Hall, Boston, pp 2-18

Reimer P, Tombach B (1998) Hepatic MRI with SPIO: detection and characterization of focal liver lesions. Eur Radiol 8:1198-1204

Rose AT, Rose DM, Pinson CW, et al (1998) Hepatocellular carcinoma outcomes based on indicate treatment strategy. Am J Surg 64:1128-1134

Rummeny EJ, Wernecke K, Saini S, et al (1992) Comparison between high-field strength MR imaging and CT for screening of hepatic metastases: a receiver operating characteristic analysis. Radiology 182:879-886

Rummeny EJ, Torres CG, Kurdziel JC, et al (1997) Mn-DPDP for MR imaging of the liver. Results of an independent image evaluation of the European phase III studies. Acta Radiol 38:638-642

Scheele J, Stang R, Altendorf-Hofmann A, et al (1995) Resection of colorectal liver metastases. World J Surg 19:59-71

Schertz LD, Lee JK, Heiken JP, et al (1989) Proton spectroscopic imaging (Dixon method) of the liver: clinical utility. Radiology 173:401-405

Schima W, Saini S, Echeverri JA, et al (1997) Focal liver lesions: characterization with conventional spin-echo versus fast spin-echo T2-weighted MR imaging. Radiology 202:389-393

Schwartz LH, Gandras EJ, Colangelo SM, et al (1999) Prevalence and importance of small hepatic lesions found at CT in patients with cancer. Radiology 210:71-74

Semelka RC, Helmberger TK (2001) Contrast agents for MR imaging of the liver. Radiology 218:327-332

Semelka RC, Shoenut JP, Kroeker MA (1992) Focal liver disease: comparison of dynamic contrast-enhanced CT and T2-weighted fat-suppressed, FLASH, and dynamic gadolinium-enhanced MR imaging at 1.5T. Radiology 184:687-694

Semelka RC, Worawattanakul S, Kelekis NL (1997) Liver lesion detection, characterization and effect on patient management: comparison of single-phase spiral CT and current MR techniques. J Magn Reson Imaging 7:1040-1047

Sheafor DH, Frederick MG, Paulson EK (1999) Comparison of unenhanced, hepatic arterial-dominant and portal venous-dominant phase helical CT for the detection of liver metastases in women with breast carcinoma. AJR Am J Roentgenol 172:961-968

Sica GT, Hoon J, Pablo RR (2000) CT and MR imaging of hepatic metastases. AJR Am J Roentgenol 174:691-698

Silverman PM, Brown B, Wray H, et al (1995a) Optimal contrast enhancement of the liver using helical (spiral) CT: value of SmartPrep. AJR Am J Roentgenol 164:1169-1171

Silverman PM, Cooper CJ, Weltman DI, et al (1995b) Helical CT: practical considerations and potential pitfalls. Radiographics 15:25-36

Simon GH, Daldrup-Link HE, Rummeny EJ (2003) MR imaging of hepatic metastases. Imaging Decisions 1:19-28

Slater GJ, Saini S, Mayo-Smith WW, et al (1996) Mn-DPDP enhanced MR imaging of the liver: analysis of pulse sequence performance. Clin Radiol 51:484-486

Sugarbaker PH (1993) Metastatic inefficiency: the scientific basis for resection of liver metastases from colorectal cancer. J Surg Oncol Suppl 3:158-160

Sun HC, Tang ZY (2003) Preventive treatments for recurrence after curative resection of hepatocellular carcinoma. A literature review of randomized control trials. World J Gastroenterol 9:635-640

Tublin ME, Tessler FN, Cheng SL, et al (1999) Effect of injection rate of contrast medium on pancreatic and hepatic helical CT. Radiology 210:97-101

Valls C, Andia E, Sanchez A (2001) Hepatic metastases from colorectal cancer: preoperative detection and assessment of respectability with helical CT. Radiology 218:55-60

van Etten B, Van der Sijp JRM, Kruyt RH, et al (2002) Ferumoxide-enhanced magnetic resonance imaging techniques in preoperative assessment for colorectal liver metastases. Eur J Surg Oncol 28:645-651

van Leeuwen MS, Noordzij J, Feldberg MA, et al (1996) Focal liver lesions: characterization with triphasic spiral CT. Radiology 201:327-336

van Ooijen B, Wiggers T (1992) Hepatic resections for colorectal metastases in the Netherlands. A multi-institutional study. Cancer 70:28-34

Vogl TJ, Hammerstingl, R, Schwarz W (1996a) Supermagnetic iron oxide-enhanced versus gadolinium-enhanced MR imaging for differential diagnosis for focal liver lesions. Radiology 198:881-887

Vogl TJ, Kummel S, Hammerstingl R (1996b) Liver tumors: comparison of MR imaging with Gd-EOB-DTPA and Gd-DTPA. Radiology 200:59-67

Wang C, Ahlström H, Eriksson B, et al (1998) Uptake of mangafodipir trisodium in liver metastases from endocrine tumors. J Magn Reson Imaging 8:682-686

Ward J, Naik KS, Guthrie JA, et al (1999) Hepatic lesion detection: comparison of MR imaging after the administration of supermagnetic iron oxide with dual phase CT by using alternative free response receiver operating characteristic analysis. Radiology 210:459-466

Weg N, Scheer MR, Gabor MP (1998) Liver lesions: improved detection with dual-detector-array CT and routine 2.5 mm thin collimation. Radiology 209:417-426

Wittenberg J, Stark DD, Forman BH, et al (1988) Differentiation of hepatic metastases from hepatic hemangiomas and cysts by using MR imaging. AJR Am J Roentgenol 151:79-84

Wood CB, Gillis CR, Blumgart LH (1976) A retrospective study of the natural history of patients with liver metastases from colorectal cancer. Clin Oncol 2:285-288

Yamasaki T, Kurokawa F, Shirahashi H, et al (2002) Percutaneous radiofrequency ablation therapy for patients with hepatocellular carcinoma during occlusion of hepatic blood flow. Comparison with standard percutaneous radiofrequency ablation therapy. Cancer 95:2353-2360

Yamashita Y, Matsukawa T, Arakawa A, et al (1995) US-guided liver biopsy: predicting the effect of interventional treatment of hepatocellular carcinoma. Radiology 196:799-804

Yoon SS, Charny CK, Fong Y, et al (2003) Diagnosis, management, and outcomes of 115 patients with hepatic hemangioma. J Am Coll Surg 197:392-402

Zacherl J, Scheuba C, Imhof M, et al (2002) Current value of intraoperative sonography during surgery for hepatic neoplasms. World J Surg 26:550-554

20 Diagnostic and Staging Work-Up

THOMAS K. HELMBERGER

20.1
Introduction

In malignant diseases, diagnostics of the extent of the primary tumour and staging of the potential spread of disease is of fundamental importance. Without this information, a sufficient stage-adequate therapy is not possible. A cost- and therapeutically effective diagnostic and staging system must allow for the natural history, patterns of typical spread, and potentially therapeutic options for a specific disease. To utilize diagnostic methods, a good knowledge of their general efficacy and specific value in a particular disease is crucial. However, a significant problem in all staging examinations is the relatively high incidence of benign findings. Therefore, high diagnostic specificity is a major requirement in order to rule out many sorts of benign findings that might influence a therapeutic decision in the case of misinterpretation.

Beside the lungs and lymphatic system, the liver is the most common site of metastatic spread in malignancies. In autopsy studies, the incidence of hepatic metastases is up to 100% dependent on the primary tumour (i.e. colorectal, oesophageal, gastric carcinoma). Even if this fact represents the final status of a malignancy, about half of all patients dying from malignant disease will have apparent hepatic metastases. Nevertheless, the risk of developing hepatic metastases varies widely with respect to the primary malignancy (Table 20.1).

In the case of exclusive metastatic spread to the liver, the extent of the particular tumour manifestation mainly determines the long-term survival. This is especially true since in these cases modern surgical procedures, and increasingly minimal-invasive ablative techniques, can improve patient survival significantly (LEEN 1999). Therefore, the basic therapeutic decision and further therapeutic planning necessitates an exact identification and characterization of all hepatic lesions and exclusion of an active extrahepatic tumour manifestation.

For adequate diagnostic and therapeutic planning, a basic knowledge of the biophysiologic mechanisms of metastatic spread, efficacy of the various diagnostic methods, and reasonable staging strategies according to the primary malignancy are mandatory.

T. K. HELMBERGER, MD
Institute of Clinical Radiology, Klinikum Grosshadern, Ludwig Maximilians University, Marchioninistrasse 15, 81377 Munich, Germany

Table 20.1. Relative risk to develop hepatic metastases in various tumours

High risk	Intermediate risk	Low risk
Colonic cancer	Breast cancer	Prostatic cancer
Oesophageal cancer	Skin cancer	Cervical cancer
Gastric cancer	Ovarian cancer	Testicular cancer
Pancreatic cancer	Sarcomatous soft tissue tumour	Thyroid cancer
Pulmonary cancer	Renal cell cancer	Osseous cancer
Neuroendocrine tumour (i.e. carcinoids)		
Hepatocellular and cholangiocellular cancer		

20.2
Mechanisms of Growth and
Spread of Metastases

In some tumour entities with direct hematogenous drainage to the liver the high incidence of hepatic metastases can be explained by the "filter function" of the liver. Due to their size terminal portal venules, presinusoidal arterioles, and hepatic sinusoids represent a "filter" able to trap clusters of tumour cells. This effect probably could further be enhanced by organotropic effects related to specific tumour cell adhesion molecules (i.e. CD44). Once in place the growth of tumour cells might also be stimulated and enhanced by hepatic humoral factors (i.e. hepatic growth factor) responsible for the normal hepatic regeneration and/or angiogenic factors released by the tumour itself.

The primary tumour and its local extent, the cellular type and aggressiveness (tumour grading), the metastatic target organ, and environmental factors (i.e. well vascularized target organ, immuno-biological factors) determine the delay until potential metastases may be detected by their clinical and/or imaging manifestation if a diagnosis of primary malignancy is established. The latent period of metastatic seeding (occult metastases) where only single or clustered cells are present hampers the detection of metastases in an early stage of disease.

Malignant tumours originating from the GI tract such as colon, rectum, stomach, pancreas, and lower oesophagus typically metastasise to the liver via the portal vein and lymphatics, while other soft tissue tumours such as breast cancer, lung cancer, etc. spread via the hematogenous or even a direct transperitoneal route such as peritoneal or retroperitoneal tumours, and ovarian neoplasms generating superficial hepatic metastases.

The mechanisms of synchronous metastases are understood and are related to an early release of tumour cells with enough time for growth to gain imaging and potentially clinical relevance at the time of diagnosis. Recurrent or newly developed metastases are a common observation even years after effective treatment or resection of a primary tumour. Nevertheless, the mechanisms responsible for tumour cells becoming dormant but remaining viable to "awake" after an unpredictable period of time is not yet clarified (Leen 1999; Finlay and McArdle 1986; Leveson et al. 1985).

By definition metastases are composed of non-hepatic tissue resembling the histology of the originating tumour to various degrees. After embedding in the host tissue the developing micrometastases are nourished on diffusion from the surrounding normal hepatic tissue. At this time, this stage of metastatic spread may only be assumed by an increased ratio of hepatic arterial blood flow/portal venous blood flow (Leen 1999). The further growth of tumour cells is dependent on an increased blood supply that is promoted by angiogenic factors released by the tumour (Seto et al. 2000). In experimental animal models rerouting of the arterial inflow into the tumour via portal venules could be demonstrated. The resulting increased arterioportal pressure gradient leads to an increased arterial/portal flow ratio and might finally be responsible for the altered contrast behaviour of metastases in contrast enhanced imaging studies (Kan et al. 1993).

In general, the detection of metastases (at least at a specific size) by imaging methods is based on micro- and macrostructural changes that differentiate tumour tissue from normal hepatic tissue. These changes incorporate various pathoanatomical and physiological variances such as increased water content of tumour cells, mucinous content, and neovascularization, as well as regressive changes such as haemorrhage, necrosis, desmoplastic fibrosis, and calcification.

Planning an imaging study must take into account these tumour specific pathological properties in order to tailor a specific study protocol to best display the difference between normal and pathological tissue. The use of contrast agent is the single most important technique in all imaging modalities to intensify this difference, consequently improving detection and characterisation of focal hepatic disease.

20.3
Imaging Studies

The criteria that can be derived from imaging studies are size and composition of a lesion and its relationship to adjacent anatomical structures. The lesion's composition can be assessed regarding its fluid content (necrosis vs solid parts), degree of vascularization, and in some aspects regarding cellular components and metabolic processes (i.e. loss of Kupffer cells due to replacement by malignant cells, increased glucose utilisation of lesion cells displayed by 18-FDG-PET). Since in Chaps. 1–3 the technical specifications and properties of the different imaging modalities are discussed, and in Chaps. 18–19 the different imaging findings are extensively explained, only some specific aspects of lesion diagnostics and follow-up according to the imaging method used will be discussed briefly below.

20.3.1
Ultrasound

Modern ultrasound (US), including Doppler-, colour-coded sonography and tissue harmonic imaging, is the most commonly used modality world-wide in the diagnostic work-up of the liver and abdomen. In most guidelines (i.e. British Columbia Medical Association, Guidelines and Protocols Advisory Committee, 3/2002; German AWMF-guideline registry Nr. 032/011 Dt. Krebsgesellschaft: Kurzgefasste Interdisziplinäre Leitlinien 2002, 3. Auflage 2002) for the work-up in malignancies, ultrasound is the primarily recommended method (BENSON et al. 2000). Nevertheless, examiner dependency, as well as restricted standardisation and sensitivity are the limiting factors of this technique despite the technical directives given by various national ultrasound societies (NEUMAIER et al. 2001). Moreover, due to superimposed rips, interpolated bowel loops, and obesity, the liver in particular may elude sonographic examination.

Recent studies on the ultrasound staging of asymptomatic liver metastases in colorectal cancer patients revealed a high diagnostic specificity of 96% degraded by an insufficient low specificity of 46%, whereas the use of the hepatic perfusion index could increase the sensitivity by only 10%–15% (GLOVER et al. 2002).

Since US is surpassed by CT and MR even in the follow-up of known metastases in terms of diagnostic accuracy, US can only be regarded as suitable for approximate rather than exact staging (HAMM 1996; DELORME and VAN KAICK 1996; BENSON et al. 2000; NEUMAIER et al. 2001). Whether the clinical application of the more advanced US techniques such as contrast-enhanced US or late-phase pulse inversion harmonic imaging (PIHI) will change this situation on a broader basis has not yet been determined (HOHMANN et al. 2003; YUCEL et al. 2002).

20.3.2
Computed Tomography

At present, computed tomography (CT) is the most widely used and accepted imaging method for the diagnostic work-up of focal hepatic lesions and the abdomen. CT produces examiner independent and reproducible results and could therefore replace US for differentiated assessment of the liver.

Nevertheless, the diagnostic efficacy of CT is highly dependent on the technical realisation of the scanner (i.e. single vs multi-slice scanner) and the processing of a particular examination (i.e. unenhanced vs bi-phasic contrast-enhanced study) (KAHN 2000; FENCHEL et al. 2002; ITOH et al. 2003).

The bi-phasic contrast-enhanced scan during the arterial-dominant (15–25 s post injection) and the portal-venous (50–70 s post injection) perfusion phase after bolus-like contrast administration is widely accepted as standard for the optimised display of the complex vascularization of the liver and potential hepatic lesions. Thin-slice data acquisition by modern multi-slice scanners allows isotropic multiplanar reformations with equivalent representations as known from MR. Moreover, CT-arterioportography, also in comparison to modern MR, became less important not least due to the relatively high rate of false positive findings (VOGL et al. 2003).

20.3.3
Magnetic Resonance

Over the last 15 years magnetic resonance (MR) imaging gained increasing significance in all fields of diagnostic imaging. The unique feature of MR, depicting the proton content of tissue provides a superior contrast resolution to all other imaging modalities. With special techniques, ever more functional, physiological and physical information can be detected and differentiated together with morphological information. This is possible due to new hard- (i.e. multi-channel/multi-array technique) and software developments (i.e. navigator techniques compensating respiratory motion, parallel imaging etc.), which allow for abdominal imaging with a spatial resolution comparable to CT but with superior contrast resolution.

Based on characteristic signal behaviour a variety of lesions such as cysts or parenchymal changes like haemorrhage can already be diagnosed on unenhanced MR. Furthermore, diagnostic efficacy improves significantly with the use of MR contrast agents (HELMBERGER and SEMELKA 2001; SEMELKA and HELMBERGER 2001). MR contrast agents can be divided into non-specific, extracellular (i.e. Gd-chelates), resembling the contrast behaviour of contrast agents for CT examinations, and tissue-specific, hepatotropic contrast agents (i.e. RES-specific superparamagnetic iron oxide particles, hepatocyte specific agents) (Figs. 20.1, 20.2).

Superparamagnetic iron oxide particles (SPIO, Endorem, Guerbet, France; Resovist, Schering, Germany) are phagocytized by the Kupffer cells of the liver as is known from colloidal tracer substances in nuclear medicine studies. Since most malignant lesions contain no Kupffer cells, this specific uptake of the SPIO particles into normal and to some degree into benign focal hepatic lesions provides an greatly increased detection and characterisation rate for malignant liver lesions.

Via specific transporter mechanisms, Mn-DPDP (Teslascan, Amersham Health, UK), Gd-BOPTA (MultiHance, Bracco, Italy), and Gd-EOB-DTPA (Primovist, Schering, Germany, proposed release in 2004) are selectively taken into normal functioning hepatocytes to varying degrees, whereas an uptake into hepatocellular tumours is possible.

Although for this entire range of contrast media efficacy data from a large number of phase-trials only exist for Gd-chelates and SPIO particles, comparative results are available (HELMBERGER and SEMELKA 2001; RUMMENY and MARCHAL 1997; HELMBERGER et al. 2000; SENETERRE et al. 1996; VOGL et al. 2003; WARD et al. 2003).

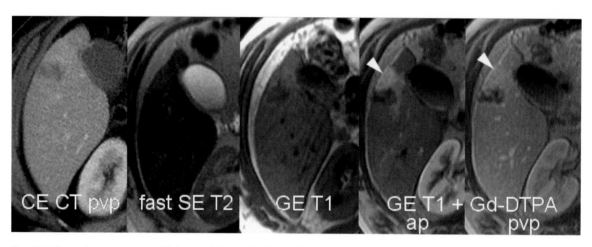

Fig. 20.1. Restaging in a patient with known history of colorectal cancer and rising tumour markers. The lesion in VI segment was already known and considered as residual, non-active metastasis after chemotherapy. While on contrast-enhanced CT and unenhanced MR only the known lesion could be appreciated, the Gd-chelate enhanced MR revealed the loco-regional recurrence (*arrowhead*)

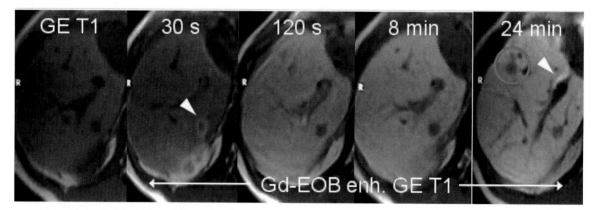

Fig. 20.2. Hepatocyte-specific contrast agents such as Gd-EOB-DTPA (Primovist, Schering, Germany) may enhance the efficacy of lesion detection. Immediately after the injection of the contrast agent perfusion phenomena known from "classic" Gd-chelates can be seen such as ring-like enhancement (*arrowhead*). Delayed imaging, during the uptake and hepatocellular storage phase, may reveal additional findings such as a further metastasis. [Note the contrast within the biliary ducts based on the biliary elimination of the contrast agent (*arrowhead*)]

20.3.4
Nuclear Medicine Studies

Morphological radiological diagnostics can be complemented by nuclear medicine (NUC) studies such as 99mTc-, 123 I-scintigraphy or F18-fluor-deoxy-glucose positron emission tomography (FDG-PET) depicting and (semi-) quantifying a variety of biochemical processes in vivo. For imaging secondary malignant tumours of the liver, mainly receptor-scintigraphy (i.e. octreotide-scintigraphy in metastases of neuroendocrine tumours) and FDG-PET are used. For the latter the dramatically increased aerobic and anaerobic glycolysis in malignant tumours builds the pathophysiological basis for the tracer up-take. In particular, the option of whole body staging makes FDG-PET increasingly popular (RESKE and KOTZERKE 2001; BALZER et al. 2003; KINKEL et al. 2002).

Nevertheless, the significantly inferior spatial and contrast resolution of NUC studies is the reason that in general these studies are not primarily clinically applied. However, the combination of a CT and a PET machine in a single scanner (CT-PET) might be sufficient to overcome these restrictions. This is because the synergistic co-registration of CT and PET data allows for a faster and more precise attenuation correction, together with a very precise anatomical correlation of CT and PET findings (ARULAMPALAM et al. 2004; FORSTER et al. 2003; OSMAN et al. 2003).

20.4
Strategies for Staging and Follow-Up

Beside the type of primary lesion and potential route of metastatic spread, local expertise, available technical equipment, workload at imaging devices, as well as advances in technology and imaging interpretation, may all influence the strategies in primary diagnostic work-up and follow-up studies.

In the case of hepatic metastases the diagnostic work-up and follow-up has to incorporate the evaluation of the site of the primary lesion and the potential metastatic sites. In the current environment of increased cost-awareness, the total extent of this evaluation has to be tailored according to the type of metastases of the respective malignancy. Therefore, for example, it makes no sense in a patient with a glioblastoma to perform hepatic or even whole body lesion staging since there is only a miniscule probability of extracerebral lesion manifestation, and if

so, the (poor) prognosis will still be determined by the primary lesion.

In this context, it is understandable that the complex situation of a wide variety of potential primary tumours, unpredictable sites of metastases, and the patient's individual situation with/without debilitation complicates the set-up of guidelines for the diagnostic work-up in lesion patients. To make diagnostics most efficient, the initial lesion stage at presentation, prior imaging studies, potential previous treatments, the timing of previous treatments, and the overall clinical situation of the individual patient needs to be incorporated.

20.4.1
Rationale for Staging and Follow-Up

Study results of the 1980s and early 1990s could not prove that imaging made a significant contribution to the survival of cancer patients with hepatic metastases. For example, KJELDSEN et al. (1997) evaluated 597 patients after surgery for colorectal cancer between 1983 and 1994 with frequent (290) and no follow-up (307). After 5 and 10 years there was the same recurrence rate of 26% without any difference regarding the total and tumour-associated survival between the two groups. WALLACE et al. (2001) reviewed 179 patients undergoing surgery for colorectal metastases between 1993 and 1999. In these 179 patients 35 CT examinations were performed, with only 45% correct staging results. However, the design of this study was so restricted that no real conclusion on the value of CT can be drawn. Probably on the basis of such data, the recent guidelines of several oncological societies are still not recommending CT, MR, and PET for staging and follow-up for hepatic metastases. These imaging modalities are considered only as "helpful in patients with a pre-existing potentially malignant abnormality", whereas it is not explained in detail how the pre-existing potentially malignant abnormality should be detected.

In contrast, recent literature paints a different picture of the value of staging and follow-up studies. There is evidence that even in high risk patients follow-up, including clinical examination, CEA, hepatic US, X-ray of the thorax, and colonoscopy, leads to chemotherapy for metastases at an earlier stage followed by improved survival (DE GOEDE et al. 1998). RENEHAN et al. (2002) reviewed five randomised studies with a total of 1342 patients who underwent an intensified follow-up (CT+CEA analysis) and demonstrated a significant reduction in total mortality, earlier detection of local recurrences and improved total survival; however, they could not clarify which follow-up component, CT or CEA, was more important. Indirect evidence that earlier detection of (potentially smaller) hepatic metastases improves survival is supported by the study of Bramhall et al. (2003) on 202 patients with colorectal cancer metastases where patients with metastases less than 5 cm in diameter had a significantly prolonged survival compared to patients with lesions greater than 5 cm. Similar data were also presented in a smaller patient group by Irie et al. (1999).

Therefore, present clinical reality appears to be changing and, according to the recent literature, clinical practice is obviously often not following guidelines. The progress in imaging is paralleled by the fact that over the last 10-15 years therapeutic options have improved significantly. Thus, a large armamentarium for the treatment of hepatic tumours has been developed, including sophisticated surgical techniques (i.e. atypical or multi-segmental resection), tailored chemotherapies, local ablative techniques such as radiofrequency ablation (RFA) and laser induced thermotherapy (LITT), transcutaneous (stereotactic) radiotherapy and percutaneous brachytherapy like after loading techniques or selective intraarterial radiotherapy (SIRT) with Yttrium-90 micro particles (Meyers et al. 2003). Even more aggressive surgical approaches as presented by Gazelle et al. (2003) and co-workers and other groups have resulted in better survival with an increased cost-effectiveness emphasising the need for a comprehensive pre-operative diagnostic work-up (Fusai and Davidson 2003a).

This wide variety of therapeutic options increasingly embedded in multi-disciplinary and modal therapeutic concepts necessitates a differentiated diagnostic work-up to customise individual therapeutic pathways (Fig. 20.3).

20.4.2
Tasks in Hepatic Diagnostics and Staging, Documentation of Findings

In general, imaging of the liver for metastases is an integral component of a whole body staging process. The findings of this staging are usually described according to the TNM classification (T, primary tumour; N, regional lymph nodes; M, distant metastasis) by the UICC, whereas the TNM classification incorporates only a rough estimate of the metastatic

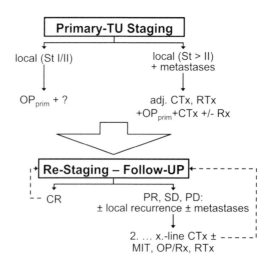

Fig. 20.3. Comprehensive stage dependent staging and follow-up regimen incorporating the extent of the primary tumour and potential metastases

presence (i.e. not present; present; undetermined) (Sobin 2003a; Sobin 2003b).

If the absence of extrahepatic tumour manifestation is established the decision on the further therapeutic management (i.e. typical or atypical segmental resection, local ablative therapy or chemotherapy) necessitates organ specific information such as:
1. Exact tumour size and number of tumours
2. Segmental allocation
3. Vascularization and relation to hepatic vasculature
4. Potential vascular invasion
5. Lymph nodes in the hepatic hilum
6. Extent beyond the hepatic capsule

Even if there is no general agreement among various surgical centres on the absolute number and size of hepatic metastases that might make a patient eligible for surgery, this information will contribute significantly to the decision as to whether the patient is a surgical or non-surgical candidate according to the centre-specific guidelines, if an alternative minimally invasive treatment such as radiofrequency, laser, local radiation beam ablation, or if chemotherapy is offered. After tumour removal/destruction, follow-up has to check for tumour recurrence and potential new metastatic spread. Therefore, follow-up studies are in principal not different from imaging in primary staging.

If the tumour extent renders a surgical or minimally invasive ablative therapy impracticable, baseline imaging is of fundamental importance to assess the time dependent efficacy of neoadjuvant/adjuvant chemo-, endocrine, or antibody therapy. In comparison to imaging after removal of a tumour, imaging addressing the potential change of a tumour or several tumour manifestations is more complex. To describe tumour response to a therapy, a standardised report system according to the WHO or RECIST criteria should be used (Tables 20.2–20.4).

20.4.3
Procedures in the Staging of Hepatic Metastases

Staging in terms of a diagnostic strategy stands for the purposeful and foresighted planning and accomplishment of a specific diagnostic task taking into account all available clinical information and the effectiveness of the available diagnostic tests. With respect to the clinical context an abnormal condition has to be identified, the diagnosis of a benign or malignant disease be established, and the decision has to be made as to whether a specific treatment is necessary and possible. If the primary malignancy is resectable, in most cases the patient's further survival is dependent on the presence of potential hepatic metastases. Therefore, it is important that potential metastases are verified as early as possible and characterised precisely (FUSAI and DAVIDSON 2003a; FUSAI and DAVIDSON 2003b; BALZER et al. 2003; GAZELLE et al. 2003).

In general, it seems easier to reveal extensive disease excluding surgical treatment than to confirm limited malignant disease still suitable for resection.

Consequently, every imaging test revealing a number, size and/or localisation of hepatic metastases that excludes a potential resection might be sufficient. Nevertheless, the imaging test must also enable an assessment of response to other treatment options during follow-up (Fig. 20.4).

Since sensitivity and specificity of percutaneous ultrasound is inferior in comparison to CT and MR, ultrasound for staging is only sufficient if extensive tumour spread or newly developed metastases are detected but exact characterisation for a surgical treatment is not needed.

CT and MR can provide a more comprehensive staging of the whole abdomen, including the liver. Nevertheless, in non-invasive staging of the liver the same dilemma exists between CT and MR in comparison to ultrasound because of the superior diagnostic efficacy of state-of-the-art contrast-enhanced MR over contrast-enhanced CT. Against this background, the critical scenario is when CT reveals no or a limited number of metastases in general suitable for resection, while the presence of one or more additional metastases would affect the decision between surgical and non-surgical treatment. In this context, the most sensitive methods of evaluation might be contrast-enhanced MR and increasingly FDG-PET. Therefore, one could think that in future (under the changing conditions of disease related management, pathways, and increased cost pressure) a combination of an orientating ultrasound study and a CT-PET study could be sufficient for comprehensive staging (Fig. 20.5).

Nevertheless, it seems astonishing that in most current guidelines of professional medical socie-

Table 20.2. Response criteria in target and non-target lesions according to the WHO and RECIST criteria (percentage in parentheses)

Response	Target lesions	Non-target lesions
Complete response (CR)	Disappearance of all target lesions	Disappearance of all non-target lesions and normalisation of tumour marker level
Partial response (PR)	At least a 50% (30%) decrease in the sum of the longest diameter (LD) of target lesions, taking as reference the baseline sum LD	Persistence of one or more non-target lesion(s) or/and tumour marker level above the normal limits
Progressive disease (PD)	At least a 25% (20%) increase in the sum of the LD of target lesions, taking as reference the smallest sum LD recorded since the treatment started or the appearance of one or more new lesions	Appearance of one or more new lesions and/or unequivocal progression of existing non-target lesions
Stable disease (SD)	Neither sufficient shrinkage to qualify for PR nor sufficient increase to qualify for PD, taking as reference the smallest sum LD since the treatment started	No change in appearance of non-target lesions and of tumour marker level

Table 20.3. Comparison of WHO and RECIST (response evaluation criteria in solid tumours) criteria for describing tumour response. [Adapted from GEHAN and TEFFT (2000)]

Characteristics/criteria	WHO	RECIST
Baseline (before any treatment, or unknown prior staging)	**1. Measurable:** bi-dimensional [product of longest diameter (LD) and greatest perpendicular diameter]	**1. Measurable:** uni-dimensional (longest diameter only, size with conventional techniques >20 mm; spiral CT >10 mm)
Measurability of lesions	**2. Non-measurable/evaluable** (i.e. lymphangitic pulmonary metastases, abdominal masses, peritoneal carcinosis)	**2. Non-measurable** (evaluable is not recommended): all other lesions, including small lesions
Objective response	**1. Measurable disease** (change in sum of products of LDs and greatest perpendicular diameters, no maximum number of lesions specified) CR: disappearance of all known disease, confirmed at ≥4 weeks PR: >50% decrease from baseline, confirmed at ≥4 weeks PD: >25% increase of one or more lesions, or appearance of new lesions NC: neither PR or PD criteria met	**1. Target lesions** (change in sum of LDs, maximum of five per organ up to ten in total CR: disappearance of all target lesions, confirmed at ≥4 weeks PR: >30% decrease from baseline, confirmed at 4 weeks PD: >20% increase over smallest sum observed, or appearance of new lesions SD: neither PR or PD criteria met
	2. Non-measurable disease CR: disappearance of all known disease, confirmed at ≥4 weeks PR: estimated decrease of ≥50%, confirmed at ≥4 weeks PD: estimated increase of ≥25% in existent lesions or appearance of new lesions NC: neither PR or PD criteria met Non-PD: persistence of one or more non-target lesions and/or tumour markers above normal limits	**2. Non-target lesions** CR: disappearance of all target lesions and normalisation of tumour markers, confirmed at ≥4 weeks PD: unequivocal progression of non-target lesions, or appearance of new lesions Non-PD: persistence of one or more non-target lesions and/or tumour markers above normal limits
Overall response	1. Best response recorded in measurable disease 2. NC in non-measurable lesions will reduce a CR in measurable lesions to an overall PR 3. NC in non-measurable lesions will not reduce a PR in measurable lesions	1. Best response recorded in measurable disease from treatment start to disease progression or recurrence 2. Non-PD in non-target lesion(s) will reduce a CR in target lesion(s) to an overall PR 3. Non-PD in non-target lesion(s) will not reduce a PR in target lesion(s)
Duration of response	1. CR From: date CR criteria first met To: date PD first noted 2. Overall response From: date of treatment start To: date PD first noted 3. In patients who only achieve a PR, only the period of overall response should be recorded	1. Overall CR From: date CR criteria first met To: date recurrent disease first noted 2. Overall response From: date CR or PR criteria first met (whichever status came first) To: date recurrent disease or PD first noted 3. SD From: date of treatment start To: date PD first noted

Note:

Measurable disease	Presence of at least one measurable lesion. In case of a solitary lesion, its neoplastic nature should be confirmed by cytology/histology
Measurable lesions	Lesions that can be accurately measured in at least one dimension with longest diameter >20 mm using conventional techniques (only in lung and bones) or >10 mm with spiral CT scan
Non-measurable lesions	All other lesions, including small lesions (longest diameter <20 mm with conventional techniques (only in lung and bones) or <10 mm with spiral CT scan), i.e. bone lesions, leptomeningeal disease, ascites, pleural/pericardial effusion, inflammatory breast disease, lymphangitis cutis/pulmonis, cystic lesions, and also abdominal masses that are not confirmed and followed by imaging techniques

Table 20.4. Assessment of "best overall response" (recorded from the start of the therapy until progression/recurrence of disease incorporating measurable imaging and clinical data)

Target lesions	Non-target lesions	New lesions		Overall response
CR	CR	No	→	CR
CR	Incomplete response/SD	No	→	PR
PR	Non-PD	No	→	PR
SD	Non-PD	No	→	SD
PD	Any	Yes or no	→	PD
Any	PD	Yes or no	→	PD
Any	Any	Yes	→	PD

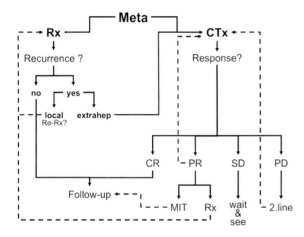

Fig. 20.4. Stage and staging-dependent therapeutic pathway in hepatic metastases

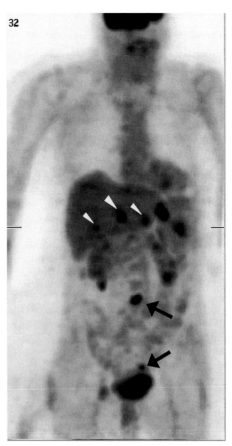

Fig. 20.5. Work-up for potential local resection of hepatic metastases (*arrowheads*) in a patient with known history of colorectal cancer. FDG-PET revealed an extraluminal recurrence plus a distant para-aortic lymph node metastasis (*arrows*), changing the prior planned therapy regimen significantly

ties, MR would be considered only an optional diagnostic adjunct in the above drafted scenario, while PET and contrast-enhanced ultrasound are not even mentioned.

20.5 Conclusion

The wide variety of differentials and the finding-related, complex therapeutic pathways still make diagnostics of focal liver lesions a challenge. An optimised, tailored, surgical, interventional, or non-surgical therapy necessitates exact staging and follow-up. In general, this is possible with current cross-sectional imaging techniques. For this purpose, ultrasound due to its ubiquitous availability, and CT due to its well accepted diagnostic reliability are mostly used. MR with and without tissue-specific contrast agents allows a further increase in diagnostic efficacy, whereas further studies have to prove to what extent PET (and more advanced CT-PET) will influence staging for hepatic metastases and, if so, how this will translate in future staging and follow-up strategies.

In general, a robust, stratified diagnostic procedure accounting for diagnostic and economic efficacy of the respective diagnostic modality will significantly contribute to the efficient therapeutic management of patients with malignant hepatic tumours.

References

Arulampalam TH, Francis DL, Visvikis D, et al (2004) FDG-PET for the pre-operative evaluation of colorectal liver metastases. Eur J Surg Oncol 30:286–291

Balzer JO, Luboldt W, Vogl TJ (2003) Importance of CT and MRI in the follow-up of patients with rectal cancer. Radiologe 43:122–127

Benson AB 3rd, Choti MA, Cohen AM, et al (2000) NCCN practice guidelines for colorectal cancer. Oncology (Huntingt) 14:203–212

Bramhall SR, Gur U, Coldham C, et al (2003) Liver resection for colorectal metastases. Ann R Coll Surg Engl 85:334–339

de Goede E, Filez L, Janssens J, et al (1998) Follow-up of colon cancer: detection of liver metastases: benefit and periodicity. Acta Gastroenterol Belg 61:8–10

Delorme S, van Kaick G (1996) Cui bono? Comments on cost-benefit analysis in ultrasound diagnosis. Radiologe 36:285–291

Fenchel S, Fleiter TR, Merkle EM (2002) Multislice helical CT of the abdomen. Eur Radiol 12 (Suppl 2):S5–10

Finlay IG, McArdle CS (1986) Occult hepatic metastases in colorectal carcinoma. Br J Surg 73:732–735

Forster GJ, Laumann C, Nickel O, et al (2003) SPET/CT image co-registration in the abdomen with a simple and cost-effective tool. Eur J Nucl Med Mol Imaging 30:32–39

Fusai G, Davidson BR (2003a) Strategies to Increase the Resectability of Liver Metastases from Colorectal Cancer. Dig Surg 20:481–496

Fusai G, Davidson BR (2003b) Management of colorectal liver metastases. Colorectal Dis 5:2–23

Gazelle GS, Hunink MG, Kuntz KM, et al (2003) Cost-effectiveness of hepatic metastasectomy in patients with metastatic colorectal carcinoma: a state-transition Monte Carlo decision analysis. Ann Surg 237:544–555

Gehan EA, Tefft MC (2000) Will there be resistance to the RECIST (response evaluation criteria in solid tumors)? J Natl Cancer Inst 92:179–181

Glover C, Douse P, Kane P, et al (2002) Accuracy of investigations for asymptomatic colorectal liver metastases. Dis Colon Rectum 45:476–484

Hamm B (1996) Cost benefit considerations in modern diagnostic sectional imaging exemplified by upper abdominal organs. Radiologe 36:292–299

Helmberger T, Gregor M, Holzknecht N, et al (2000) Effects of biphasic spiral CT, conventional and iron oxide enhanced MRI on therapy and therapy costs in patients with focal liver lesions. Rofo Fortschr Geb Rontgenstr Neuen Bildgeb Verfahr 172:251–259

Helmberger T, Semelka RC (2001) New contrast agents for imaging the liver. Magn Reson Imaging Clin N Am 9:745–766

Hohmann J, Skrok J, Puls R, et al (2003) Characterization of focal liver lesions with contrast-enhanced low MI real time ultrasound and SonoVue. Rofo Fortschr Geb Rontgenstr Neuen Bildgeb Verfahr 175:835–843

Irie T, Itai Y, Hatsuse K, et al (1999) Does resection of small liver metastases from colorectal cancer improve survival of patients? Br J Radiol 72:246–249

Itoh S, Ikeda M, Achiwa M, et al (2003) Multiphase contrast-enhanced CT of the liver with a multislice CT scanner. Eur Radiol 13:1085–1094

Kahn T (2000) Value of CT and MRI in malignant hepatobiliary tumors. Zentralbl Chir 125:610–615

Kan Z, Ivancev K, Lunderquist A, et al (1993) In vivo microscopy of hepatic tumors in animal models: a dynamic investigation of blood supply to hepatic metastases. Radiology 187:621–626

Kinkel K, Lu Y, Both M, et al (2002) Detection of hepatic metastases from cancers of the gastrointestinal tract by using noninvasive imaging methods (US, CT, MR imaging, PET): a meta-analysis. Radiology 224:748–756

Kjeldsen BJ, Kronborg O, Fenger C, et al (1997) A prospective randomized study of follow-up after radical surgery for colorectal cancer. Br J Surg 84:666–669

Leen E (1999) The detection of occult liver metastases of colorectal carcinoma. J Hepatobiliary Pancreat Surg 6:7–15

Leveson SH, Wiggins PA, Giles GR, et al (1985) Deranged liver blood flow patterns in the detection of liver metastases. Br J Surg 72:128–130

Meyers MO, Sasson AR, Sigurdson ER (2003) Locoregional strategies for colorectal hepatic metastases. Clin Colorectal Cancer 3:34–44

Neumaier CE, Cittadini G, Grasso A, et al (2001) Role of ultrasonography in the staging of gastrointestinal neoplasms. Semin Surg Oncol 20:86–90

Osman MM, Cohade C, Nakamoto Y, et al (2003) Clinically significant inaccurate localization of lesions with PET/CT: frequency in 300 patients. J Nucl Med 44:240–243

Renehan AG, Egger M, Saunders MP, et al (2002) Impact on survival of intensive follow up after curative resection for colorectal cancer: systematic review and meta-analysis of randomised trials. BMJ 324:813

Reske SN, Kotzerke J (2001) FDG-PET for clinical use. Results of the 3rd German Interdisciplinary Consensus Conference, "Onko-PET III", 21 July and 19 September 2000. Eur J Nucl Med 28:1707–1723

Rummeny EJ, Marchal G (1997) Liver imaging. Clinical applications and future perspectives. Acta Radiol 38:626–630

Semelka RC, Helmberger TK (2001) Contrast agents for MR imaging of the liver. Radiology 218:27–38

Seneterre E, Taourel P, Bouvier Y, et al (1996) Detection of hepatic metastases: ferumoxides-enhanced MR imaging versus unenhanced MR imaging and CT during arterial portography [see comments]. Radiology 200:785–792

Seto S, Onodera H, Kaido T, et al (2000) Tissue factor expression in human colorectal carcinoma: correlation with hepatic metastasis and impact on prognosis. Cancer 88:295–301

Sobin LH (2003a) TNM, sixth edition: new developments in general concepts and rules. Semin Surg Oncol 21:19–22

Sobin LH (2003b) TNM: evolution and relation to other prognostic factors. Semin Surg Oncol 21:3–7

Vogl TJ, Schwarz W, Blume S, et al (2003) Preoperative evaluation of malignant liver tumors: comparison of unenhanced and SPIO (Resovist)-enhanced MR imaging with biphasic CTAP and intraoperative US. Eur Radiol 13:262–272

Wallace JR, Christians KK, Quiroz FA, et al (2001) Ablation of liver metastasis: is preoperative imaging sufficiently accurate? J Gastrointest Surg 5:98–107

Ward J, Guthrie JA, Wilson D, et al (2003) Colorectal hepatic metastases: detection with SPIO-enhanced breath-hold MR imaging – comparison of optimised sequences. Radiology 228:709–718

Yucel C, Ozdemir H, Gurel S, et al (2002) Detection and differential diagnosis of hepatic masses using pulse inversion harmonic imaging during the liver-specific late phase of contrast enhancement with Levovist. J Clin Ultrasound 30:203–212

Image-Guided Tumor Ablation

21 Radiofrequency Ablation: Principles and Techniques

Riccardo Lencioni, Dania Cioni, Jacopo Lera, Erika Rocchi, Clotilde Della Pina, **and** Laura Crocetti

CONTENTS

21.1 Introduction

Image-guided radiofrequency (RF) ablation is a minimally invasive procedure that has emerged as the most powerful percutaneous technique for tumor destruction and is nowadays established as the primary ablative modality at most institutions (Goldberg 2002; Lencioni et al. 2003; Shibata et al. 2002). In fact, recent improvements in RF technology have permitted the creation of in vivo spherical ablation zones exceeding 5 cm in diameter with a single probe insertion, thus substantially increasing the potential of the technique in clinical application (Berber et al. 2004; Lencioni et al. 2004a). A thorough understanding of the basic principles, mechanisms of energy deposition, modulation of tissue physiologic characteristics to increase tumor destruction, and technical clues in clinical application is essential for optimal use of RF ablation.

R. Lencioni, MD; D. Cioni, MD; J. Lera, MD; E. Rocchi, MD; C. Della Pina, MD; L. Crocetti, MD
Division of Diagnostic and Interventional Radiology, Department of Oncology, Transplants and Advanced Technologies in Medicine, University of Pisa, Via Roma 67, 56126 Pisa, Italy

21.2 Radiofrequency: How it Works

21.2.1 Basic Principles

The goal of RF ablation is to induce thermal injury to the tissue through electromagnetic energy deposition. The term RF ablation applies to coagulation induced by all electromagnetic energy sources with frequencies less than 900 kHz, although most devices function in the range of 375–500 kHz. The term RF refers not to the emitted wave but rather to the alternating electric current that oscillates in this frequency range. In monopolar RF ablation, the patient is part of a closed-loop circuit that includes an RF generator, an electrode needle, and a large dispersive electrode (ground pads). An alternating electric field is created within the tissue of the patient. Because of the relatively high electrical resistance of tissue in comparison with the metal electrodes, there is marked agitation of the ions present in the target tissue that surrounds the electrode, since the tissue ions attempt to follow the changes in direction of the alternating electric current. The agitation results in frictional heat around the electrode. The discrepancy between the small surface area of the needle electrode and the large area of the ground pads causes the generated heat to be focused and concentrated around the needle electrode (Gazelle et al. 2000; Rhim et al. 2001).

The thermal damage caused by RF heating is dependent on both the tissue temperature achieved and the duration of heating. Heating of tissue at 50–55°C for 4–6 min produces irreversible cellular damage. At temperatures between 60°C and 100°C near immediate protein coagulation is induced, with irreversible damage to mitochondrial and cytosolic enzymes as well as nucleic acid-histone protein complexes (Goldberg et al. 2000a). Cells experiencing this extent of thermal damage most often, but not always, undergo coagulative necrosis over the course of several days. In fact, the zone of co-

agulation, while predominantly comprising coagulative necrosis, often lacks the classic well-defined
histologic appearance of coagulative necrosis in the
acute postablation period or even within some zones
of adequately ablated tissue for many months after
ablation. Indeed, in many cases, specialized stains
are required to confirm that cellular death has been
achieved after thermal ablation (Goldberg et al.
2000a).

For this reason and because many tumors undergo central necrosis without ablation therapy, the
term "coagulation" is preferred over the use of "necrosis" alone, because it denotes that the ablation intervention is actively leading to tumor destruction.
The more generalized term "coagulation" is preferred over the term "coagulative necrosis" because
the latter term has a well-defined meaning in the pathology literature, including the absence of visible
nuclei within the dead cells (Goldberg et al. 2003).

In a recent study, explanted livers of cirrhotic patients who had RF ablation of their hepatocellular
carcinomas were examined. A detailed histopathologic analysis showed that, unlike classic tissue
necrosis, the treated lesions all showed "thermal
fixation," with preserved tissue architecture and
microscopic cellular detail. The cellular staining
characteristics faded with time, but the treated tissue became brittle, resisted tissue breakdown, and
generated a minimal wound healing response. At
the periphery of the lesion, the fibrous septa of the
cirrhotic liver and vascular structures appeared to
demarcate or limit progression of the ablation front.
A narrow hypocellular fibrous boundary with a focal "foreign body" giant cell-type reaction developed around the edge of the ablation zone (Coad et
al. 2003).

At 110°C, tissue vaporizes and carbonizes.
These processes usually retard optimal ablation
due to a resultant decrease in energy transmission
(Goldberg et al. 1996). For adequate destruction of
tumor tissue, the entire target volume must be subjected to cytotoxic temperatures. Thus, an essential
objective of ablative therapy is achievement and
maintenance of a 50–100°C temperature throughout the entire target volume for at least 4–6 min.
However, the relatively slow thermal conduction
from the electrode surface through the tissues may
increase the duration of application to 10–30 min.
On the other hand, the tissue temperature should
not be increased over these values to avoid carbonization around the tip of the electrode due to excessive heating (Gazelle et al. 2000; Goldberg et al.
1996; Rhim et al. 2001).

21.2.2
Mechanisms of Energy Deposition

In the early experiences with RF treatment, a major
limitation of the technique was the small volume of
ablation created by conventional monopolar electrodes. These devices were capable of producing
cylindrical ablation zones not greater than 1.6 cm
in the short axis (Goldberg et al. 1995). Therefore,
multiple electrode insertions were necessary to treat
all but the smallest lesions. Subsequently, several
strategies for increasing the ablation zone achieved
with RF treatment have been used.

Heat efficacy is defined as the difference between
the amount of heat produced and the amount of heat
lost. Therefore, effective ablation can be achieved by
optimizing heat production and minimizing heat
loss within the area to be ablated. The relationship
between these factors has been characterized as the
"bio-heat equation." The "bio-heat" equation gov-
erning RF-induced heat transfer through tissue has
been previously described by Pennes (1948), with
this equation simplified to a first approximation by
Goldberg et al. (2000b) as follows:

Coagulation =
energy deposited × local tissue interactions – heat lost

Heat production is correlated with the intensity
and duration of the RF energy deposited. On the
other hand, heat conduction or diffusion is usually
explained as a factor of heat loss in regard to the
electrode tip. Heat is lost mainly through convec-
tion by means of blood circulation (Patterson et
al. 1998).

Therefore, most investigators devoted their attention to strategies that increase the energy deposited
into the tissues and several corporations have manufactured new RF ablation devices based on technologic advances that increase heating efficacy. To
accomplish this increase, the RF output of all commercially available generators has been increased to
150–200 W, which may potentially increase the intensity of the RF current deposited at the tissue.

Major progress was achieved with the introduction of modified electrode needles, including internally cooled electrodes and multitined expandable electrodes with multiple retractable prongs
on the tip (Berber et al. 2004; Lencioni et al.
1998; Lencioni et al. 2001; Lencioni et al. 2004b;
Solbiati et al. 1997). These techniques enabled a
substantial and reproducible enlargement of the ablation zone produced with a single needle insertion,

and prompted the start of clinical application of RF ablation (Fig. 21.1).

Internally cooled electrodes (Radionics, Tyco Healthcare Group, Burlington, MA) consist of dual-lumen electrodes with an exposed active tip of variable length. Internal cooling is obtained by continuous perfusion with chilled saline and is aimed at preventing overheating of tissues nearest to the electrode to minimize carbonization and gas formation around the tip. The tip contains a thermocouple for recording the temperature of the adjacent tissue. To increase the size of the ablation, the company placed three of the cooled electrodes in a parallel triangular cluster with a common hub. This device produces a significantly larger ablation than does a single cooled electrode (GOLDBERG et al. 1998a). Pulsing of RF energy (i.e. alternation of very high RF current for several seconds followed by minimal RF deposition for a defined period) has also been described as a method that allows overall increased current deposition (GOLDBERG et al. 1999).

Multitined expandable electrodes have an active surface which can be substantially expanded by prongs deployed from the tip. The number of prongs and the length of their deployment varies according to the device and to the desired volume of ablation. The commercially available devices were developed to monitor the ablation process so that high-temperature coagulation may occur without exceeding a 110°C maximum temperature threshold. One device (RITA Medical Systems, Mountain View, CA) relies on direct temperature measurement. This kind of electrode, in fact, is made by an insulated outer cannula that houses nine curved electrodes of various lengths, which deploy out from the trocar tip. Five of the electrodes are hollow and contain thermocouples in their tips that are used to measure the tissue temperature. Probe-tip temperatures, tissue impedance, and wattage are displayed on the RF generator and are graphically recorded by dedicated software. Maximum power output of the RF generator, amount of electrode array deployment from the trocar, and duration of the effective time of the ablation (time at target temperature) depend on the desired volume of ablation. In fact, the generator runs by an automated program and maintains the target temperature throughout the procedure. At the end of the procedure, the coagulation of the needle track can be done after retraction of the hooks with the aim of preventing any tumor cell dissemination (LENCIONI et al. 2001; LENCIONI et al. 2004a).

Another manufacturer (Boston Scientific, Natick, MA) produces an RF ablation device that relies on

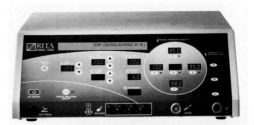

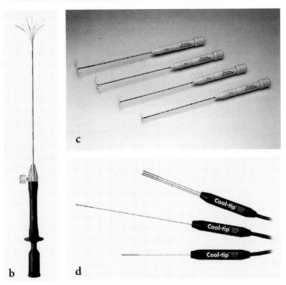

Fig. 21.1a–d. Current RF equipment: **a** RF generator Model 1500 X, with a maximum output of 200 W and **b** Model 90 StarBurst XL multitined expandable electrode with nine prongs (RITA Medical Systems, Mountain View, CA). **c** Expandable electrodes for 2.0–4.0-cm ablation Zones (Boston Scientific, Natick, MA). **d** single or cluster internally Cool-tip RF electrodes (Radionics, Tyco Healthcare Group,

electrical measurement of tissue impedance rather than on tissue temperature. The electrode is made by an insulated 14-gauge outer needle that houses ten retractable curved electrodes. The electrodes are manufactured in different lengths. In application, the tip of the needle is advanced to the target tissue and the curved electrodes are deployed to full extension. The generator is switched on and energy is administered until a rapid rise in impedance occurs. The impedance of the tissue increases as the tissue desiccates. It is assumed that an ablation is successful if the device impedes out (RHIM et al. 2001).

In addition to the previously described devices, several other designs for RF electrodes were recently developed and some of them are currently undergoing clinical investigations. These include bipolar devices with two active electrode applicators placed in proximity to achieve contiguous coagulation and perfusion electrodes that have small apertures at the tip of the prongs that allow fluids (i.e. normal or hypertonic saline) to be infused into the tissue during the ablation procedure (Fig. 21.2) (BURDIO et al. 2003; KETTENBACH et al. 2003; MIAO et al. 2001; MULIER et al. 2003).

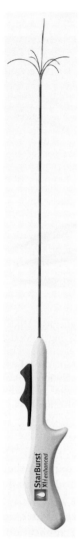

Fig. 21.2. The RITA model 100 (Starburst Xli) has five electrodes with infusion sites for hypertonic saline at the end. They alternate with four metal prongs with thermocouples at their tip to monitor the tissue temperature. Two subtypes exist to create RF lesions of up to 5 cm or 7 cm

21.3
The Bio-heat Equation: How to Increase Tumor Destruction

Despite technologic advances and electrode modifications that have effectively increased RF energy deposition and tissue heating, inadequate coagulation can represent a clinical problem in some circumstances. Specifically, there are multiple and often tissue specific limitations which may cause heterogeneity of heat deposition throughout a given lesion to be treated. This has led some investigators to study modifications of the underlying tumor characteristics in an attempt to improve RF thermal ablation. These modifications can be divided, on the basis of the bio-heat equation, as (a) strategies that permit an increase in the overall deposition of energy through an alteration in tissue electrical conductivity, (b) strategies that improve heat retention within the tissue, and (c) strategies that decrease the tolerance of tumor tissue to heat (GOLDBERG et al. 2000b).

For a given RF current, power deposition is strongly dependent on local electrical conductivity. Intratumoral injection of saline solution prior to or during the application of RF current alters tissue conductivity and thereby allows greater deposition of RF current and increased tissue heating and coagulation (GOLDBERG et al. 2001a; LIVRAGHI et al. 1997). Experimental findings demonstrated that ablative temperatures can be generated farther from an RF electrode by increasing tissue electrical conductivity with NaCl solution injection. However, because both volume and concentration of saline solution influence tissue heating and the coagulation diameter in a nonlinear fashion, optimal parameters for injection of saline solution must be determined for each type of RF apparatus used and for the different types of tumors and tissues to be treated. In an experimental study performed in a controlled system of agar phantoms (LOBO et al. 2004), excessive increase of tissue electrical conductivity obtained with very high saline concentrations decreased the extent of heating. Increased electrical conductivity, in fact, has competing effects on RF ablation: it enables increased energy deposition and greater heating, but it also increases the energy required to heat a given volume of tissue. If this amount of energy cannot be delivered, that is, it is beyond the maximum generator output, then less actual heating, and thus less coagulation, is achieved (LOBO et al. 2004). A major concern for the clinical application of percutaneous injection strategies is the possibility of determining a nonuniform alteration of tissue electrical conductivity because of the difficulty of achieving uniform fluid diffusion and distribution. Irregularly shaped areas of coagulation have been observed with RF performed during simultaneous saline injection (LIVRAGHI et al. 1997). Also, saline-enhanced ablation may potentially lead to distortions of the ablation zone shape because of the spread of fluid outside the target, along paths of least resistance (AHMED et al. 2002; BOEHM et al. 2002). GOLDBERG et al. (2001a) have observed this phenomenon in tissue samples in which large volumes of saline (25 ml) were injected. These results suggested that infusion of very small volumes of fluid could increase the ablation volume without risks of undesired leakage.

Perfusion-mediated tissue cooling reduces the extent of coagulation produced by thermal ablation (GOLDBERG et al. 1998b). Modeling of the bio-heat equation shows that for a given tissue and power deposition, the effects of tissue blood flow predominate. RF-induced coagulation is also more limited and variable in vivo than ex vivo. Coagulation in vivo is often shaped by vasculature in the vicinity of the ablation. Experiments in which hepatic perfusion is altered by mechanical or pharmacologic means during RF ablation of normal liver tissue and tumors show that blood flow is largely responsible for this reduction in observed coagulation (GOLDBERG et al. 1998c; ROSSI et al. 2000). Several strategies for reducing blood flow during ablation therapy have been proposed. Total portal inflow occlusion (Pringle maneuver) has been used at open laparotomy and at laparoscopy. Angiographic balloon occlusion of the hepatic artery can be used but proved useful for hypervascularized tumors only (ROSSI et al. 2000). de BAERE et al. (2002) published promising results showing that temporary hepatic vein or portal branch occlusion during RF ablation can facilitate the treatment of large tumors (>3.5 cm in maximum diameter) or tumors in contact with the walls of large vessels. However, RF ablation performed during vascular occlusion can increase the risks associated with the treatment. In one study, portal vein thrombosis was significantly more frequent after RF ablation performed during a Pringle maneuver in patients with liver cirrhosis (DE BAERE et al. 2003). Pharmacologic modulation of blood flow and antiangiogenesis therapy are theoretically possible but should currently be considered experimental (GOLDBERG et al. 1998c).

As far as decreasing tissue resistance to heat, based upon the well-documented relationship between the effects of some chemotherapeutic agents and hyperthermia, recent studies began to explore the potentiation of effects that can be achieved with a combination of chemotherapy and RF ablation (GOLDBERG et al. 2001b; GOLDBERG et al. 2002). These advances have already raised substantial clinical interest because preliminary results from a randomized study using combined RF/liposomal doxorubicin therapy in patients with primary and secondary liver tumors demonstrated significant increases in tumor necrosis compared with RF ablation alone (GOLDBERG et al. 2002). AHMED et al. (2003) provided insight into the factors that can potentially improve the outcome of this combination therapy. Validation in tumor models of larger size and different histological types will be a necessary next step to confirm the utility of this combination therapy before its adoption in a wider clinical setting. Further research exploring all of the factors that influence intratumoral liposome delivery, including liposome size, charge, circulation time, and composition, is ongoing. Other combination therapies, such as combined treatment of RF ablation and acid acetic injection, are currently under investigation (LEE et al. 2004).

21.4
Technical Clues for Clinical Application

21.4.1
Imaging

Imaging is used in five separate and distinct ways in RF ablation: planning, targeting, monitoring, controlling, and assessing treatment response (GOLDBERG et al. 2003). Imaging techniques, including ultrasound (US), CT, MR imaging, and more recently positron emission tomography (PET), are used to help determine whether patients are suitable candidates for RF ablation. Pre-treatment imaging planning must define tumor size and shape, number, and location within the liver relative to blood and biliary vessels, as well as critical structures (i.e. gallbladder, gastrointestinal tract) that might be at risk for injury during the ablation (GOLDBERG et al. 2003). Targeting refers to the placement of the RF electrode into the tumor, which can be achieved by using US, CT, or MR imaging. The guidance system is chosen largely on the basis of operator preference and local availability of dedicated equipment such as CT fluoroscopy or open MR systems. Monitoring is the term used to describe the process with which ablation effects are viewed during the procedure. Important aspects to be monitored include how well the tumor is being covered and whether any adjacent normal structures are being affected at the same time (GOLDBERG et al. 2003). While the transient hyperechoic zone that is seen on US within and surrounding a tumor during and immediately after RF ablation can be used as a rough guide to the extent of tumor destruction, MR is currently the only imaging modality with validated techniques for real-time temperature monitoring (QUESSON et al. 2000). The term "controlling" is used to describe the intraprocedural tools and techniques that are used to control the treatment. To control an image-guided ablation procedure, the operator can utilize the image-based information obtained during monitoring or automated systems that terminates the ablation at a critical point in the procedure (GOLDBERG et al. 2003). Finally, imaging is used to assess the outcome of the procedure. Contrast-enhanced US performed after the end of the procedure may allow an initial evaluation of treatment effects. Contrast-enhanced CT and MR imaging are recognized as the standard modalities to assess treatment outcome, although promising initial results have been reported by using PET after RF ablation of liver metastases (DONCKIER et al. 2003). CT and MR images obtained after treatment show successful ablation as a non-enhancing area surrounded by an enhancing rim. The enhancing rim appears a relatively concentric, symmetric, and uniform process in an area with smooth inner margins. This is a transient finding that represents a benign physiologic response to thermal injury (initially, reactive hyperemia; subsequently, fibrosis and giant cell reaction) (GOLDBERG et al. 2000a). Benign periablational enhancement needs to be differentiated from irregular peripheral enhancement due to residual tumor that occurs at the treatment margin. In contrast to benign periablational enhancement, residual unablated tumor often grows in scattered, nodular, or eccentric patterns (GOLDBERG et al. 2003). Later follow-up imaging studies should be aimed at detecting the recurrence of the treated lesion (i.e. local tumor progression), the development of new hepatic lesions, or the emergence of extrahepatic metastases.

21.4.2
Anesthesiology Care

Patient candidates to RF ablation can have a medium-to-high anesthesiology risk. Most of them, in fact, have been rejected for surgery for associated diseases involving the cardiovascular system. There is no consensus on the best anesthesiology care for RF ablation. Local anesthesia does not produce adequate pain relief. Some centers use general anesthesia and endotracheal intubation. Others, including our own, prefer to perform liver RF under conscious sedation. The association of an hypnotic drug with an ultrashort half-life analgesic drug allows a mild sedation of the patient, who can cooperate with the operator and bear the pain induced by treatment. One possible protocol consists of administering a bolus

of ketorolac (0.5-0.8 mg/kg) followed by infusion of propofol (1-2 mg/kg/h) and remifentanil (0.1 µg/kg/min). However, drug posology has to be modulated in relation to the individual patient compliance and to the different phases of the procedure. The infusion of the hypnotic drug can be varied between 0.5 and 2 mg/kg/h to achieve a patient sedation that preserves the ability to do easy actions. The infusion of remifentanil can be varied between 0.05 and 0.15 µg/kg/min to obtain an optimal analgesia. Attention has to given to avoiding bolus administration of remifentanil, as this may cause respiratory depression. The procedure is performed under standard cardiac, pressure, and oxygen monitoring. A careful post-treatment protocol is to be recommended following RF ablation. The patient is kept under close medical observation and re-scanned with US 1–2 h after treatment to detect any bleeding. An overnight hospital stay is scheduled. In most of the cases, patients may be discharged the day after the procedure.

21.4.3
Ablation Protocols

An important factor that affects the success of RF ablation is the ability to ablate all viable tumor tissue and an adequate tumor-free margin. The most important difference between surgical resection and RF ablation of hepatic tumors is the surgeon's insistence on a 1-cm-wide tumor-free zone along the resection margin. To achieve rates of local tumor recurrence with RF ablation that are comparable to those obtained with hepatic resection, physicians should produce a 360°, 1-cm-thick tumor-free margin around each tumor (CADY et al. 1998). This cuff is necessary to ensure that all microscopic invasions around the periphery of a tumor have been eradicated. Thus, the target diameter of an ablation must be ideally 2 cm larger than the diameter of the tumor that undergoes treatment (Fig. 21.3) (DODD et al. 2000; PATTERSON et al. 1998). Eradication of a tumor can therefore be achieved with a single ablation if the diameter of the tumor is 2 cm less than the diameter of tissue ablated. Currently, the maximum diameter of the in vivo ablation sphere produced by RF is 5.5–5.6 cm (BERBER et al. 2004). Therefore the tumor to be treated should not exceed 3.5 cm in longest axis to obtain a safety margin of 1 cm all around the lesion.

Despite technological advances and all the efforts made to obtain larger zones of ablation, moderate to high rates of local tumor recurrence have been

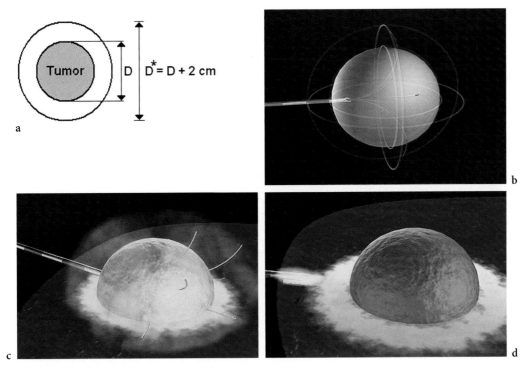

Fig. 21.3a–d. Schematic model of an RF ablation protocol. **a,b** A 360°, 1-cm-thick tumor-free margin around each tumor must be achieved for successful ablation. Thus, the target diameter (D*) of an ablation must be ideally 2 cm larger than the diameter (D) of the tumor that undergoes treatment. **c,d** The multitined electrode needle is placed in the tumor and deployed gradually to encompass the tumor itself and 1 cm of tissue all around it

reported, especially in larger tumors (LIVRAGHI et al. 2000; SOLBIATI et al. 1997). A possible reason for failures in the treatment of large tumors is the inability to determine the optimal number of ablations and the exact location of electrode placement needed to completely destroy tumors larger than the size of a single ablation zone. Thus, appropriate protocols to determine the correct number of RF ablations have been devised (CHEN et al. 2004; DODD et al. 2000). In one model, developed for treatment of tumors larger than 3.5 cm in diameter, the regular prism and the regular polyhedron were used to generate mathematical models for determining the correct preoperative protocol. Number of ablations ranged from 4 to 12 for spherical tumors with diameters respectively of 4.0–4.3 cm and 5.7–6.5 cm. In some cases, however, fewer electrodes were placed than were calculated mathematically because of the particular characteristics of the tumors (CHEN et al. 2004). In this study, local recurrence rate did not exceed 24% in a series of 121 tumors with a mean diameter of 4.7±0.9 cm (range 3.6–7.0 cm) (CHEN et al. 2004).

In addition to size, tumor location is one of the important factors that influence the likely outcome of therapy. Treatment of lesions adjacent to the gallbladder or to the hepatic hilum is at risk of thermal injury of the biliary tract. Nevertheless, in experienced hands, RF ablation of tumors adjacent to the gallbladder was shown to be feasible although associated in most cases with self-limited iatrogenic cholecystitis (CHOPRA et al. 2003). In contrast, treatment of lesions located in the vicinity of hepatic vessels is possible, since flowing blood usually "refrigerates" the vascular wall, protecting it from thermal injury: in these cases, however, the risk of incomplete ablation of the neoplastic tissue adjacent to the vessel may increase because of the heat loss caused by the vessel itself. Lesions located along the surface of the liver can be considered for RF ablation, although their treatment requires experienced hands and may be associated with a higher risk of complications. Percutaneous treatment of superficial lesions that are adjacent to any part of the gastrointestinal tract must be avoided because of the risk of thermal injury of the gastric or bowel wall (BUSCARINI and

Buscarini 2004; Livraghi et al. 2003). The colon appears to be at greater risk than the stomach
or small bowel for thermally mediated perforation
(Rhim et al. 2004). Gastric complications are rare,
likely owing to the relatively greater wall thickness
of the stomach or the rarity of surgical adhesions
along the gastrohepatic ligament. The mobility of the
small bowel may also provide the bowel with greater
protection compared with the relatively fixed colon.
The potential risk of thermal damage to adjacent
structures should be weighed against benefits on a
case-by-case basis. A laparoscopy approach can also
be considered in such instances, as the bowel may be
lifted away from the tumor (Rhim et al. 2004).

References

Ahmed M, Lobo SM, Weinstein J, et al (2002) Improved
coagulation with saline solution pretreatment during
radiofrequency tumor ablation in a canine model. J Vasc
Interv Radiol 13:717–724

Ahmed M, Monsky WE, Girnum G, et al (2003) Radiofrequency thermal ablation sharply increases intratumoral
liposomal doxorubicin accumulation and tumor coagulation. Cancer Res 63:6327–6333

Berber E, Herceg NL, Casto KJ, et al (2004) Laparoscopic
radiofrequency ablation of hepatic tumors: prospective
clinical evaluation of ablation size comparing two treatment algorithms. Surg Endosc 18:390–396

Boehm T, Malich A, Goldberg SN, et al (2002) Radio-frequency tumor ablation: internally cooled electrode
versus saline-enhanced technique in an aggressive
rabbit tumor model. Radiology 222:805–813

Burdio F, Guemes A, Burdio JM, et al (2003) Bipolar saline-
enhanced electrode for radiofrequency ablation: results
of experimental study of in vivo porcine liver. Radiology
229:447–456

Buscarini E, Buscarini L (2004) Radiofrequency thermal
ablation with expandable needle of focal liver malignancies: complication report. Eur Radiol 14:31–37

Cady B, Jenkins RL, Steele GD Jr, et al (1998) Surgical margin
in hepatic resection for colorectal metastasis: a critical
and improvable determinant of outcome. Ann Surg
227:566–571

Chen MH, Yang W, Yan K, et al (2004) Large liver tumors:
protocol for radiofrequency ablation and its clinical
application in 110 patients. Mathematical model, overlapping mode, and electrode placement process. Radiology 232:260–271

Chopra S, Dodd GD 3rd, Chanin MP, et al (2003) Radiofrequency ablation of hepatic tumors adjacent to the gallbladder: feasibility and safety. AJR Am J Roentgenol
180:697–701

Coad JE, Kosari K, Humar A, et al (2003) Radiofrequency
ablation causes "thermal fixation" of hepatocellular carcinoma: a post-liver transplant histopathologic study.
Clin Transplant 17:377–384

de Baere T, Bessoud B, Dromain C, et al (2002) Percutaneous radiofrequency ablation of hepatic tumors during
temporary venous occlusion. AJR Am J Roentgenol
178:53–59

de Baere T, Risse O, Kuoch V, et al (2003) Adverse events
during radiofrequency treatment of 582 hepatic tumors.
AJR Am J Roentgenol 181:695–700

Dodd GD 3rd, Soulen M, Kane R, et al (2000) Minimally
invasive treatment of malignant hepatic tumors: at
the threshold of major breakthrough. Radiographics
20:9–27

Donckier V, Van Laethem JL, Goldman S, et al (2003) [F-
18]fluorodeoxyglucose positron emission tomography
as a tool for early recognition of incomplete tumor
destruction after radiofrequency ablation for liver
metastases. J Surg Oncol 84:215–223

Gazelle GS, Goldberg SN, Solbiati L, et al (2000) Tumor ablation with radio-frequency energy. Radiology 217:633–
646

Goldberg SN (2002) Comparison of techniques for image-
guided ablation of focal liver tumors. Radiology
223:304–307

Goldberg SN, Gazelle GS, Dawson SL, et al (1995) Tissue
ablation with radiofrequency: effect of probe size, ablation duration, and temperature on lesion volume. Acad
Radiol 2:399–404

Goldberg SN, Gazelle GS, Halpern EF, et al (1996) Radiofrequency tissue ablation: importance of local temperature
along the electrode tip exposure in determining lesion
shape and size. Acad Radiol 3:212–218

Goldberg SN, Solbiati L, Hahn PF, et al (1998a) Large volume
tissue ablation with radiofrequency by using a clustered, internally cooled electrode technique: laboratory
and clinical experience in liver metastases. Radiology
209:371–379

Goldberg SN, Hahn PF, Tanabe KK, et al (1998b) Percutaneous radiofrequency tissue ablation: does perfusion-
mediated tissue cooling limit coagulation necrosis? J
Vasc Interv Radiol 9:101–115

Goldberg SN, Hahn PF, Halpern E, et al (1998c) Radio-frequency tissue ablation: effect of pharmacologic modulation of blood flow on coagulation diameter. Radiology
209:761–767

Goldberg SN, Stein MC, Gazelle GS, et al (1999) Percutaneous
radiofrequency tissue ablation: optimization of pulsed-
technique to increase coagulation necrosis. J Vasc Interv
Radiol 10:907–916

Goldberg SN, Gazelle GS, Compton CC, et al (2000a) Treatment of intrahepatic malignancy with radiofrequency
ablation: radiologic-pathologic correlation. Cancer
88:2452–2463

Goldberg SN, Gazelle GS, Mueller PR (2000b) Thermal ablation therapy for focal malignancy: a unified approach to
underlying principles, techniques, and diagnostic imaging guidance. AJR Am J Roentgenol 174:323–331

Goldberg SN, Ahmed M, Gazelle GS, et al (2001a) Radio-frequency thermal ablation with NaCl solution injection:
effect of electrical conductivity on tissue heating and
coagulation-phantom and porcine liver study. Radiology 219:157–165

Goldberg SN, Saldinger PF, Gazelle GS, et al (2001b) Percutaneous tumor ablation: increased necrosis with combined radio-frequency ablation and intratumoral doxo-

rubicin injection in a rat breast tumor model. Radiology 220:420–427

Goldberg SN, Kamel IR, Kruskal JB, et al (2002) Radiofrequency ablation of hepatic tumors: increased tumor destruction with adjuvant liposomal doxorubicin therapy. AJR Am J Roentgenol 179:93–101

Goldberg SN, Charboneau JW, Dodd GD 3rd, et al; International Working Group on Image-Guided Tumor Ablation (2003) Image-guided tumor ablation: proposal for standardization of terms and reporting criteria. Radiology 228:335–345

Kettenbach J, Kostler W, Rucklinger E, et al (2003) Percutaneous saline-enhanced radiofrequency ablation of unresectable hepatic tumors: initial experience in 26 patients. AJR Am J Roentgenol 180:1537–1545

Lee JM, Lee YH, Kim YK, et al (2004) Combined treatment of radiofrequency ablation and acetic acid injection: an in vivo feasibility study in rabbit liver. Eur Radiol 14:1303–1310

Lencioni R, Goletti O, Armillotta N, et al (1998) Radiofrequency thermal ablation of liver metastases with a cooled-tip electrode needle: results of a pilot clinical trial. Eur Radiol 8:1205–1211

Lencioni R, Cioni D, Bartolozzi C (2001) Percutaneous radiofrequency thermal ablation of liver malignancies: techniques, indications, imaging findings, and clinical results. Abdom Imaging 26:345–360

Lencioni R, Allgaier HP, Cioni D, et al (2003) Small hepatocellular carcinoma in cirrhosis: randomized comparison of radiofrequency thermal ablation versus percutaneous ethanol injection. Radiology 228:235–240

Lencioni R, Cioni D, Crocetti L, et al (2004a) Percutaneous ablation of hepatocellular carcinoma: state-of-the-art. Liver Transpl 10:S91–97

Lencioni R, Crocetti L, Cioni D, et al (2004b) Percutaneous radiofrequency ablation of hepatic colorectal metastases: technique, indications, results, and new promises. Invest Radiol (in press)

Livraghi T, Goldberg SN, Lazzaroni S, et al (1997) Saline-enhanced radio-frequency tissue ablation in the treatment of liver metastases. Radiology 202:205–210

Livraghi T, Goldberg SN, Lazzaroni S, et al (2000) Hepato-cellular carcinoma: radiofrequency ablation of medium and large lesions. Radiology 241:761–768

Livraghi T, Solbiati L, Meloni MF, et al (2003) Treatment of focal liver tumors with percutaneous radio-frequency ablation: complications encountered in a multicenter study. Radiology 226:441–451

Lobo SM, Afzal KS, Ahmed M, et al (2004) Radiofrequency ablation: modeling the enhanced temperature response to adjuvant NaCl pretreatment. Radiology 230:175–182

Miao Y, Ni Y, Yu J, et al (2001) An ex vivo study on radiofrequency tissue ablation: increased lesion size by using an "expandable-wet" electrode. Eur Radiol 11:1841–1847

Mulier S, Ni Y, Miao Y, et al (2003) Size and geometry of hepatic radiofrequency lesions. Eur J Surg Oncol 29:867–878

Patterson EJ, Scudamore CH, Owen DA, et al (1998) Radiofrequency ablation of porcine liver in vivo: effects of blood flow and treatment time on lesion size. Ann Surg 227:559–565

Pennes HH (1948) Analysis of tissue and arterial blood temperatures in the resting human forearm. J Appl Physiol 1:93–122

Quesson B, de Zwart JA, Moonen CTW (2000) Magnetic resonance temperature imaging for guidance of thermotherapy. J Magn Reson Imaging 12:525–533

Rhim H, Goldberg SN, Dodd GD 3rd, et al (2001) Essential techniques for successful radio-frequency thermal ablation of malignant hepatic tumors. Radiographics 21:S17–S35

Rhim H, Dodd GD3rd, Chintapalli KN, et al (2004) Radiofrequency thermal ablation of abdominal tumors: lessons learned from complications. Radiographics 24:41–52

Rossi S, Garbagnati F, Lencioni R, et al (2000) Percutaneous radio-frequency thermal ablation of nonresectable hepatocellular carcinoma after occlusion of tumor blood supply. Radiology 217:119–126

Shibata T, Iimuro Y, Yamamoto Y, et al (2002) Small hepatocellular carcinoma: comparison of radio-frequency ablation and percutaneous microwave coagulation therapy. Radiology 223:331–337

Solbiati L, Goldberg SN, Ierace T, et al (1997) Hepatic metastases: percutaneous radio-frequency ablation with cooled-tip electrodes. Radiology 205:367–373

22 Imaging Guidance, Monitoring, and Follow-Up

Alice R. Gillams

CONTENTS

22.1
Introduction

Radio-frequency ablation (RFA) is now widely practised with thousands of treatments being performed in hundreds of centres annually. Ablation efficacy is improved by accurate on line monitoring. The production of necrosis is dependant on multiple different factors, some technical, some physiological. Therefore necrosis is not predictable and monitoring is very important. This chapter will apprise you of the different CT and MR techniques currently used to guide and monitor ablation, the appearances of successful and unsuccessful ablation on follow-up and describe some new developments which have not yet reached clinical practice.

A.R. Gillams, MD
Department of Medical Imaging, The Middlesex Hospital, Mortimer Street, London, W1T 3AA, UK

22.2
Image Guidance

22.2.1
Lesion Visualisation

Any guidance technique requires the accurate depiction of the lesion to be targeted and of the device to be deployed. Wherever possible ultrasound (US) guidance is preferred as the quickest, easiest, real-time, interactive technique. However, not all patients are good US subjects particularly the obese and even in patients who are good subjects not all tumours are US visible. Approximately 10%–15% of colorectal metastases are occult on trans-abdominal US. In part this is anatomical, i.e. the dome of the liver is often obscured by overlying lung, a problem that is exacerbated in the sedated patient when the liver moves up into the chest. Ribs may obscure superficial lesions. Hepato-steatosis can make US assessment difficult yet: it is common to be referred patients who have already received chemotherapy, a proportion of whom will have developed a fatty liver. Computed tomography (CT) and magnetic resonance (MR) visualisation of colorectal metastases have already been dealt with in detail elsewhere in this volume. Both are superior to US.

22.2.2
Device Compatibility: CT

Needle compatibility and visualisation are both easy on CT. Volumetric acquisitions and multi-planar reformats aid appreciation of the needle position relative to the whole tumour volume in 3D (Antoch et al. 2002). This is particularly valuable for steep oblique, long trajectory needle placement (Fig. 22.1). CT will also show each of the multiple tines/prongs of the expandable electrodes, which can be difficult on US, i.e. there have been reports of a tine being advanced inadvertently into small bowel and this misplacement was not appreciated

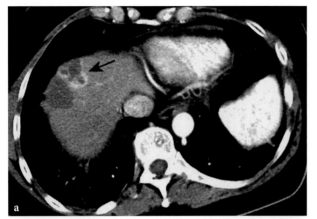

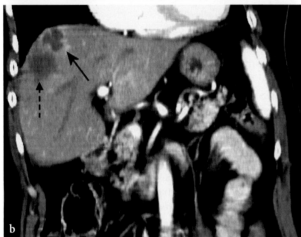

Fig. 22.1a–i. Female patient with three colorectal metastases. Two tumours had been treated at a previous session 1 month earlier. **a** Axial contrast enhanced CT showing the active colorectal metastasis with rim enhancement (*black arrow*) lying anteromedial to an ablated metastasis. **b** Coronal reformat of the same tumour (*black arrow*). The *dashed arrow* indicates one of the previously ablated metastases. **c** Sagittal reformat shows the metastasis (*black arrow*) anteriorly with the two old ablation zones posteriorly. **d** Sagittal reformat of the electrode positioned posterior to the untreated tumour. **e** Sagittal reformat shows the electrode in the region of the untreated tumour. **f** Coronal reformat of the same. **g** Coronal reformat from CT scans performed during the treatment, after the ablation is thought to be complete but whilst the patient is still under general anaesthesia so that further ablation can be performed if necessary. This scan shows a large area of necrosis with no residual tumour. Note gas bubbles in the ablated zone. A total of 5% dextrose has been instilled around the liver to protect lung and diaphragm (*arrow*). **h** Sagittal reformat of (**g**). The electrode can be seen pulled back out of the liver to avoid artefact across the ablation zone. **i** Sagittal reformat from CT scans obtained 1 day post ablation showing complete ablation

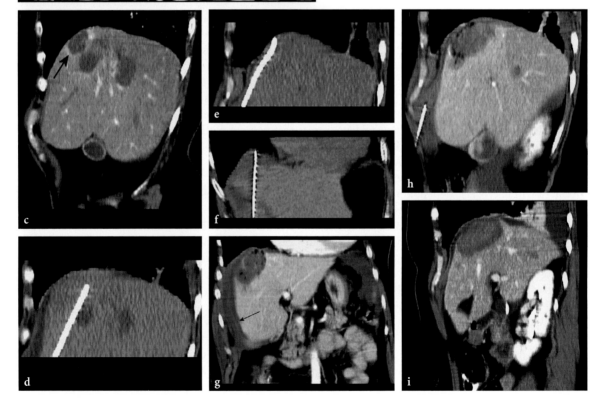

on US. CT fluoroscopy facilitates needle insertion and positioning. Technological refinements include the introduction of a flexible shaft electrode (RITA Medical Systems) to overcome the problem of scanning long electrodes within a narrow gantry and the introduction of large (<83 cm) gantry interventional CT scanners (Siemens, Erlangen, Germany).

22.2.3
Device Compatibility: MR

Laser fibres and applicators are MR compatible whereas in the early days of RF ablation, the electrodes were not MR compatible and were readily deflected within even low field systems. The first MR compatible RF device was a straight, saline perfusion electrode produced by Berchtold, (Tuttlingen, Germany); latterly other RF manufacturers (Valleylab, Boulder, Colorado, USA and RITA Medical Systems, California, USA) have produced MR compatible electrodes (Fig. 22.2) (HUPPERT et al. 2000; KELEKIS et al. 2003; KETTENBACH et al. 2003). These electrodes are less sharp and more flexible than their CT equivalent.

Electronic noise produced by generators interferes with the MR image acquisition and can significantly degrade image quality. Simultaneous RF ablation and image acquisition is not possible. Different methods of noise reduction have been explored but the easiest technique has been a simple switching circuit that permits alternating MR acquisition and ablation (OSHIRO et al. 2002; ZHANG et al. 1998).

The open configuration of interventional MR scanners, required to allow access to the patient, are only feasible at low field strengths i.e. 0.2 or 0.5 T (Fig. 22.3). Plans to develop higher field strength (1.0 T) open MR systems have not yet been realised. As with all MR systems there is a trade-off between time, contrast and spatial resolution. Achieving all three, as required in intervention, has been difficult at low field strengths. For needle/electrode visualisation the optimal situation is a small but accurate magnetic susceptibility artefact. The artefact will depend on the material used, the relationship of the needle to the main magnetic field, the relationship of the needle to the phase-encoding direction and the MR sequence. The operator can manipulate the various parameters to get more or less artefact, i.e. more artefacts may be better for needle visualisation during insertion but fewer artefacts is preferred during temperature monitoring. Needle artefact is reduced

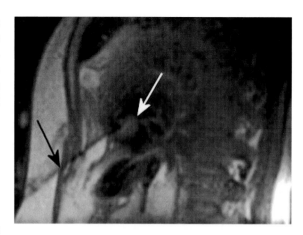

Fig. 22.2. Sagittal localising scan showing a single 17-G MR compatible Cool Tip RF electrode (Valleylab, Boulder, Colorado, USA) inserted into the left lobe of the liver. The electrode is seen as a thin low signal intensity line (*black arrow*). The tip lies in the proximal part of the metastasis (*white arrow*)

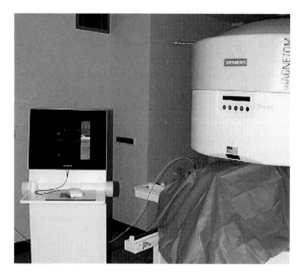

Fig. 22.3. Clinical set up in the interventional MR suite – open 0.2-T MR (Siemens, Erlangen, Germany)

when the needle is parallel to the main magnetic field, i.e. a needle inserted vertically for treatment of a left lobe liver lesion will be harder to see in the C shaped open system where the main magnetic field is vertical. An oblique needle insertion may be better in this situation. Apparent needle width will be thinner and the tip more accurately localised if the needle is inserted parallel to the phase encoding direction, i.e. perpendicular to the read out direction (HWANG et al. 1999). For needle visualisation T2-weighted fast spin echo (FSE) sequences are preferable to steady state precession sequences (FISP or PSIF) (ASCHOFF et al. 2001). Alternatively T1-weighted gradient echo sequences are often adequate for needle insertion.

Some MR systems provide real-time interactive multi-planar imaging during needle insertion and 3D navigator tools have been developed to facilitate this. Images refresh every 5–7 s permitting a stuttering needle advance. Liver specific contrast agents are useful to improve the poor inherent tissue contrast of low field systems. A T1 shortening agent that will increase normal liver signal is preferable. The loss of signal in normal liver parenchyma produced by super paramagnetic iron oxide particle contrast agents may make needle depiction harder.

22.3
Imaging Monitoring

The final volume of necrosis is the result of a delicate interplay of multiple independent variables i.e. electrode shape at deployment, current density, current pathways, applied power, tumour type and location, tissue perfusion which in turn varies with cardiac output and more. The main cause for "failure" is incomplete or inadequate ablation. Treatment without monitoring is likely to result in incomplete ablation in all but the smallest lesions i.e. <1 cm. Much effort has gone into improving monitoring. Ideally ablation monitoring would provide immediate feedback in 3D of the volume of tissue successfully treated. Monitoring can be divided into two types those that monitor temperature and extrapolate the volume of successful ablation and those that look at changes in tissue T1, T2 or contrast enhancement on either CT or MR.

22.4
Temperature Measurement

The induction of necrosis is both time and temperature dependent i.e. cell death requires a longer period of modestly elevated temperature but occurs within 1 min at temperatures over 80°C. Spot temperature measurements can be gathered from thermo-sensors at the tip of the electrodes either during treatment, at the end of treatment or after a cool-down period. Recent innovations include the incorporation of a thermo-sensor that is deployed perpendicular to the electrode shaft and can be repetitively deployed in different areas as required. US have been used to measure temperature but most clinical research has centred on MR monitoring

(VARGHESE et al. 2002). There are several different methods available including diffusion imaging, proton frequency shift (also termed proton resonance frequency), changes in T1 and spectroscopy. Diffusion requires a stationary area of interest and therefore has no utility in liver ablation.

22.5
Proton Frequency Shift

It has been experimentally determined that temperature causes the proton frequency to shift by 0.01 ppm/°C in water. Based on this, temperature maps can be created by observing the phase difference produced by the temperature induced frequency shift in gradient-echo sequences. Proton frequency shift (PFS) shows good temperature sensitivity, and importantly both linearity and near independence of tissue type. PFS is both field strength and TE dependent, therefore it is said to be the preferred technique at higher field strengths i.e. ≥1 T. Working at 0.5 T the temperature uncertainty has been estimated to be ±2.7°C ex vivo and ±4.3°C in animal experiments (BOTNAR et al. 2001). Echo shifted gradient echo sequences have successfully been implemented ex-vivo at 0.2 T (CHUNG et al. 1999).

22.6
T1 Thermometry

Changes in T1 in response to temperature are more complex. Exchange processes between mobile bulk water and relatively immobilised water in membranes is thought to play an important role. T1 changes are linear within a small temperature range (45 –65°C) but both T1 and the temperature-induced changes vary between tissues. Increasing temperature causes a progressive loss of signal on T1-weighted images. This loss of signal reflects both a permanent and a transient change in tissue. During ablation vaporisation of tissue water results in gas bubbles, readily depicted on US and CT (Fig. 22.1). Gas will alter T1 signal, as will small amounts of haemorrhage, dehydration, charring and protein denaturation, all of which occur during ablation.

Changes in T1 are easier to visualise and are more readily implemented at low field strength compared to PFS. Other groups have used changes in T1-weighted at high field (1.5 T) (VOGL et al. 1995). Two

2D flash sequences were used with image subtraction from baseline and updates at 30-s intervals. The information provided was used to direct the length of treatment and was then supplemented by contrast enhanced imaging at the end of the ablation. Precision in vivo is of the order of 3°C in 13 s for a voxel 1.5×1.5×7 mm at 1.5 T (GERMAIN et al. 2001). As high field systems have limited patient access, needle placement was performed in CT prior to transfer to the MR unit. Comparisons of the volume of low signal intensity on T1 with histopathology show that the maximum distribution of reduced signal on T1 during treatment tends to overestimate the area of necrosis but that the distribution of T1 signal after cool down is more accurate (BREMER et al. 2002). Nevertheless loss of signal on T1 during treatment can be used as an approximate guide to ablation.

Both proton-frequency shift (PFS) MR and T1-weighted changes require a subtraction technique that in turn requires accurate image registration without tissue deformation. This is hard to achieve in the liver ablation patient. One attempt at co-registration showed a 13% increase in error between the top and bottom of the liver due to liver motion, rotation and deformation in different phases of respiration (WILSON et al. 1998). An attempt to estimate the impact of respiration showed that PFS had an accuracy of ±3.5°C in ex vivo models with simulated respiration (HEISTERKAMP et al. 1999). There have been few comparisons of T1 temperature sensitivity and PFS but one comparison in porcine paravertebral muscle and liver at 0.5 T showed PFS to be superior. PFS depicted 9/12 liver lesions as compared to T1, which only showed 3/12 (STEINER et al. 1998).

22.7
Parenchymal Changes at MR

Ablated tumour is seen as low signal on T2, residual tumour is high signal and vice versa on T1 (Fig. 22.4a, b). There have been a number of papers that have compared different MR sequences with histopathology in animal experiments, mostly in normal tissue. Within the actual ablated region two zones can be identified, a dominant, central zone and a thin, peripheral penumbra. On T2-weighted sequences the central zone is of low signal and the penumbra of high signal, the reverse is true on T1 weighted images. Pathological correlation shows that the area of ablation encompasses the central zone and some but not the entire peripheral zone. Therefore measurement of the central zone will underestimate and measurement of the whole zone will overestimate. The degree of error is small, i.e. the mean overestimate was 1.17 mm and the mean underestimate was 0.85 mm in one paper and in another the overestimate was not more than 2 mm with a correlation co-efficient of 0.9 (BREEN et al. 2003). The development of low signal intensity within the ablated zone on STIR imaging can be monitored during ablation (Fig. 22.4c-f).

We have compared STIR and T1-weighted images obtained at low field 18 h post-ablation with contrast enhanced CT in 14 tumours in 11 patients (GILLAMS et al. 2001). The rationale is that contrast enhanced CT has been verified with pathological specimens and shown to have 1–2 mm accuracy. In addition the opportunity to obtain histological data in a patient population is not common. Our results were similar, namely that the actual cell death zone lay beyond the central MR zone but was slightly less than the diameter of both zones (Fig. 22.5). The differences between CT and MR were small (Table 22.1). For all work at low field there is a constant pressure to chose between spatial, temporal and contrast resolution. One solution to this problem is to prolong the image acquisition times up to 2 min. This requires a period of hyperventilation followed by suspension of respiration in the anaesthetised, paralysed and ventilated patient.

Table 22.1 Mean differences between low-field (0.2 T) open MR sequences and contrast enhanced CT

	STIR (whole lesion)	STIR (central low signal only)	T1 (whole lesion)	T1 (central high signal only)
Maximum diameter (cm)	-0.3 (p=0.13)	1.0 (p=0.00)	–0.1	0.76 (p=0.052)
Cross-sectional area (cm2)	-2.6 (p=0.15)	10 (p=0.001)	–0.9	9.4 (p=0.031)

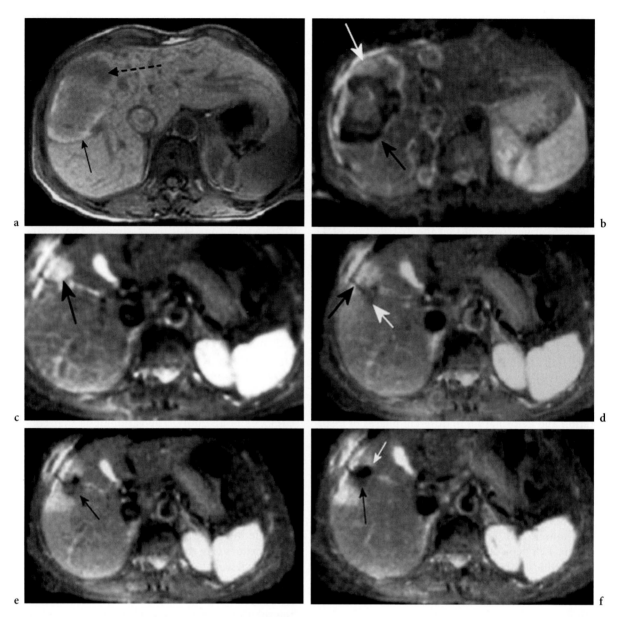

Fig. 22.4. a Axial T1-weighted image showing the ablation zone has high signal intensity posteriorly (*arrow*) and active residual tumour as low signal intensity anteriorly (*dashed arrow*). **b** Same level axial STIR image shows the ablation zone as low signal intensity (*black arrow*) and the residual tumour as high signal (*white arrow*). Sequential axial STIR images at 0.2 T performed during treatment in another patient. **c** High signal intensity colorectal metastasis in V segment (*black arrow*). The high signal intensity over the surface of the liver and in the chest wall is local anaesthetic. **d** The low intensity line (*black arrow*) represents the MR needle carrying the bare tip laser fibre. There is mild loss of signal around the needle tip (*white arrow*) consistent with heating. **e-f** Progressive loss of signal develops centrally during treatment (*black arrows*). There is also increased signal around the heated zone presumably oedema. The signal void lying anteriorly (*white arrow*) within the ablation zone may be gas

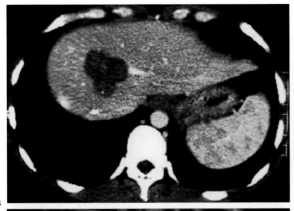

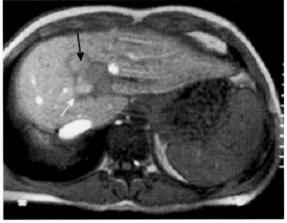

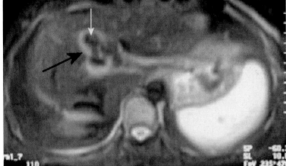

Fig. 22.5a–c. Correlation between contrast enhanced CT and low field MR imaging 24 h post ablation. **a** Contrast enhanced CT during the portal venous phase shows three overlapping spheres of necrosis. **b** Axial T1-weighted image shows two zones of signal intensity: a central high signal area (*black arrow*) and a thin rim of low signal (*white arrow*). **c** Axial STIR image at the same level showing a smaller central zone of low signal (*white arrow*) and a rim of high signal intensity (*black arrow*). Measurement analysis shows that at 24 h the T1-weighted image correlates best with the CT scan

22.8
Parenchymal Changes at CT

Areas of necrosis are seen as absent contrast enhancement. This has been verified post ablation by comparing imaging with pathological specimens obtained at resection (GOLDBERG et al. 2000; SCUDAMORE et al. 1999). During ablation interpretation of the CT image is complicated by focal gas, mild hyperattenuation in the ablation zone from small amounts of haemorrhage and hyperperfusion injury superimposed on focal ablated tumours, ablation tracts and potentially residual tumour (Figs. 22.1, 22.6) (LIMANOND et al. 2003). Nevertheless contrast enhanced CT scans performed during the ablation, whilst the patient is still under anaesthesia, provide useful information as to the completeness of treatment. Multi-planar reformats are invaluable in assessing the whole tumour volume in 3D (Fig. 22.1). If residual tumour is seen or an inadequate margin identified then it is possible to perform further ablation during the same treatment session. This improves complete ablation rates, reduces the number of hospital visits and overall is more economic.

Ideally the tumour and the ablation zone would be co-registered so that complete ablation and the relationship of the margin of the ablation zone to the tu-

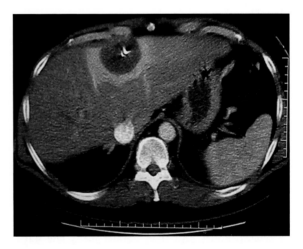

Fig. 22.6. Contrast enhanced CT scans performed during ablation. A triple electrode lies within the area of ablation surrounded by an area of hyper-perfusion

mour could be appreciated in 3D. In CT the number of scans performed during a treatment is limited by total contrast dosage and by reduced tissue contrast on later scans due to the persistence of i.v. contrast in normal parenchyma from earlier injections. As gadolinium behaves like iodine, the same technique can be applied at high field MR (VOGL et al. 1995). It has not been possible to achieve the necessary temporal and spatial resolution to perform dynamic gadolinium enhanced imaging at low field.

22.9
Parenchymal Changes at US

A transient hyperechoic zone is seen at US within and surrounding a tumor during and immediately after ablation. However, this finding can be used only as a rough guide to the extent of tumor destruction. Contrast-enhanced US performed after the end of the procedure may allow an initial evaluation of treatment effect. Residual viable tumor can be easily identified in hypervascular lesions, such as hepatocellular carcinoma (HCC), as it stands out in the arterial phase against the unenhanced ablated area. However, interpretation of contrast-enhanced US findings is more difficult in hypovascular lesions.

22.10
New Developments

Gadolinium encapsulated liposomes are under development (FOSSHEIM et al. 2000). The idea is to develop liposomes that undergo gel to liquid phase transition at a particular temperature i.e. they would behave as an on-off messenger, switched on when a particular temperature has been reached. Different liposomes would be sensitive to different temperatures so a specific liposome would be specific to an application either ablation or hyperthermia. Other contrast agents in development are necrosis avid agents (NI et al. 2002). These are injected i.v. and taken up within areas of necrosis over a period of several hours and then persist for a few days. Correlation with histopathology shows that these agents can provide same day assessment but not same-session of treatment efficacy.

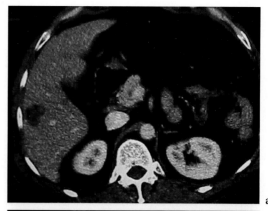

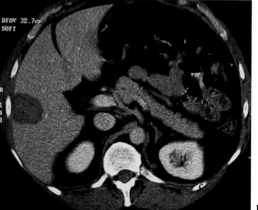

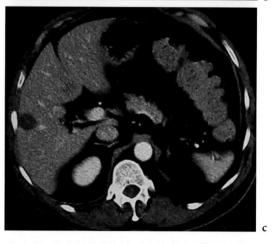

Fig. 22.7a–c. Successful ablation. **a** CT scans of a solitary metastasis immediately prior to treatment. **b** CT scans 1 day post treatment showing complete ablation with a margin of normal liver. **c** CT scans 2 years later showing that the ablation is slowly reducing in size with no evidence of active tumour

22.11
Post-ablation Appearances and Follow-Up at Contrast Enhanced CT

Immediately after ablation it is common to see a hyper-attenuating area around the ablation (Fig. 22.6). This is caused by a several factors including an increase in hepatic arterial perfusion as a response to ischaemic injury. This increase has been quantified using CT in a group of 32 patients who underwent laser ablation (GILLAMS and LEES 1999). There was a mean 3.3-fold increase immediately adjacent to the ablated area. Other components of the hypervascular rim, which presumably develop after a delay, include an inflammatory response and granulation tissue (GOLDBERG et al. 2000). TSUDA et al. (2001) studied the temporal changes on CT in 22 HCC in 20 patients post-RFA. The hypervascular rim was seen in 89% of 20 treated tumours at 1 month, 56% between 1 and 3 months and 22% between 3 and 6 months. Some authors have found it difficult to differentiate this zone of hyperperfusion from re-

sidual hypervascular tumour. In general a thin rim is usually reactive but a nodular or an irregular thick rim indicates active tumour (NGHIEM et al. 2002). The necrotic zone shows absent enhancement which if necessary can be confirmed by measuring attenuation values (BERBER et al. 2000).

Over time the completely ablated zone will become better defined, more homogeneous and start to reduce in size (Fig. 22.7). The rate of liver regeneration varies with the age of the patient and the underlying pathology. More rapid regeneration is seen in cirrhosis than in patients with normal background parenchyma. Eventually some lesions will shrink to a linear scar or disappear completely.

22.12
Recognising Recurrence

Despite the appearance of complete ablation on scans performed immediately after treatment, it is

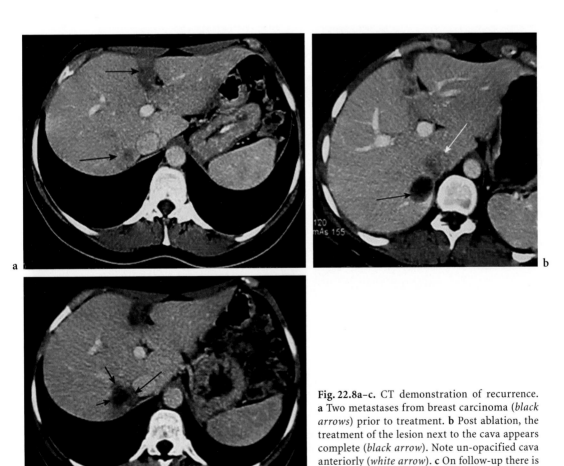

Fig. 22.8a–c. CT demonstration of recurrence. **a** Two metastases from breast carcinoma (*black arrows*) prior to treatment. **b** Post ablation, the treatment of the lesion next to the cava appears complete (*black arrow*). Note un-opacified cava anteriorly (*white arrow*). **c** On follow-up there is nodular recurrence at the periphery of the ablation (*black arrows*)

possible for some microscopic cells to persist and eventually some of these will enlarge and present as recurrence (Figs. 22.8, 22.9). Recurrence is most common adjacent to vessels, >3 mm in diameter. This is because flowing blood can cool the surrounding tissue and protect tumour cells and because vessels can act as a conduit carrying the radio-frequency current away from the treatment zone. Tissue perfusion mediated cooling, not to be confused with cooling from nearby blood vessels, can also protect tumour. Tissue perfusion mediated cooling occurs at the interface between normal liver and tumour and can result in the ablation zone mapping the original tumour size and shape. As there are often small amounts of tumour in the normal appearing liver adjacent to metastases these are protected and can present as edge recurrence. The most common appearance of recurrence is a small nodule of hypo- or hyper-vascular tumour at the periphery of the ablated zone. Recurrence has been divided into three types: a circumferential halo, i.e. active tumour on all edges of the ablation zone, nodular recurrence, i.e. nodules at the periphery or recurrence associated with an overall increase in the ablation zone (CHOPRA et al. 2001). Only a proportion of patients develop the latter type of recurrence. Very occasionally it is possible to see tumour recurrence as filling in of the ablation zone without an increase in lesion size, a halo or a nodule.

Standard oncologic assessment of treatment (RECIST criteria) uses lesion size. This cannot be applied to ablation as ideally there is an initial increase in lesion size on imaging and then a slow reduction in size as healing occurs. DROMAIN et al. (2002) measured the decrease in size in successfully treated tumours over time. The mean decrease was 15% (range 10%–30%) at 6 months and 35% (15%–90%) at 12 months. As healing results in shrinkage of most of the lesion but small areas of recurrence will produce focal areas of enlargement it is possible to have recurrence without an overall increase in tumour size. VILANA et al. (2003) have suggested

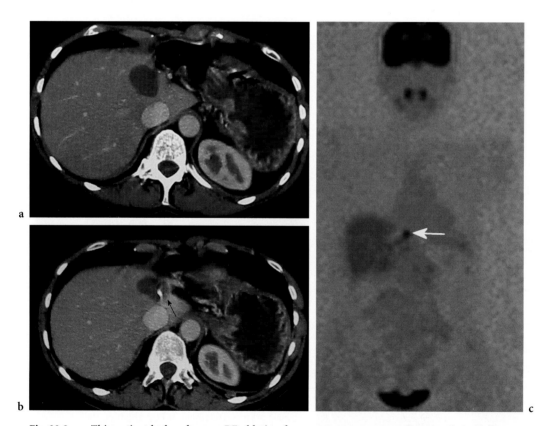

Fig. 22.9a–c. This patient had undergone RF ablation for recurrence on a resection margin. **a** Follow-up scans show absent enhancement inferiorly. **b** More cranial slices show subtle increased attenuation (*black arrow*) in the medial portion of the ablation, to the left of the surgical sutures, immediately inferior to the heart. **c** PET confirms increased activity in this area (*white arrow*). The photopaenic area correlates with the ablation zone. This recurrence was confirmed histologically

that measurement of viable tumour is used instead as the whole ablation zone. The detection of early recurrence is best achieved by careful comparison of CT scans performed immediately or soon after ablation and on follow-up. Even then interpretation can be difficult and correlation with tumour markers or the use of PET (Fig. 22.9) or even biopsy may be necessary in equivocal cases (ANDERSON et al. 2003; FOSSHEIM et al. 2000). An alternative approach is to repeat imaging at a reduced follow-up interval.

22.13
Timing of Recurrence

Most centres perform contrast-enhanced studies at 3-month intervals in patients with colorectal metastases. The follow-up interval should be tailored to the underlying primary tumour and the biological behaviour, i.e. most of our patients with breast metastases have follow-up scans at 4- 6-month intervals and most patients with more indolent neuro-endocrine metastases have scans at 6- to 12-month intervals.

Different papers have reported different time-scales for the detection of recurrence. Mean time to recurrence in one series of patients with hepato-cellular carcinoma treated with a range of ablation techniques was 4 months (CATALANO et al. 2001). In our experience using thermal ablation techniques the median time to recurrence is 8 months but in some slow growing tumours or patients who respond to chemotherapy recurrence may be delayed until as late as 20 months. Other authors have also seen examples of late recurrence up to 14 months post treatment (CHOPRA et al. 2001).

22.14
CT vs MR for Detection of Recurrence

DROMAIN et al. (2002) compared the performance of CT and MR in the detection of recurrence in a group of 31 patients. CT and MR were performed at 2, 4 and 6 months post ablation. MR detected local recurrence in 8/9 patients at 2 months as compared with CT that was positive in 4 of 9. This difference did not reach significance. They found the optimal sequence for the detection of recurrence was the T2-weighted sequence where active tumour is seen as high signal intensity. All areas of recurrence could be seen at 4 months on both techniques. Therefore

although MR is probably slightly better than CT the difference is marginal and time limited. For most patients good quality, fine collimation, uni- or biphasic multi-detector CT with assessment of interval change will be adequate. If MR is used then either dynamic gadolinium enhanced images at high field or T2-weighted sequences are effective in showing recurrence. Liver specific contrast agent MR is preferred in patients with altered perfusion (i.e. post chemotherapy) or hepato-steatosis particularly if this is patchy.

22.15
Conclusion

Although the development of interventional MR has been challenging, many of the problems, i.e. material compatibility issues, have now been overcome. More predictable ablation would reduce the need for monitoring but this is unlikely to be realised in the foreseeable future. Therefore monitoring will remain an important part of ablation treatment. 3D image registration must become a routine for both CT and MR. Some of the more innovative developments described in this article should reach the clinical arena in the next few years.

References

Anderson GS, Brinkmann F, Soulen MC, et al (2003) FDG positron emission tomography in the surveillance of hepatic tumors treated with radiofrequency ablation. Clin Nucl Med 28:192–197

Antoch G, Kuehl H, Vogt FM, et al (2002) Value of CT volume imaging for optimal placement of radiofrequency ablation probes in liver lesions. J Vasc Interv Radiol 13:1155–1161

Aschoff AJ, Wendt M, Merkle EM, et al (2001) Comparison of susceptibility artefacts of different radiofrequency electrodes at 0.2 T. Influence of electrode positioning, pulse sequence and image reconstruction methods. Rofo Fortschr Geb Rontgenstr Neuen Bildgeb Verfahr 173:257–262

Berber E, Foroutani A, Garland AM, et al (2000) Use of CT Hounsfield unit density to identify ablated tumour after laparoscopic radiofrequency ablation of hepatic tumors. Surg Endosc 14:799–804

Botnar R, Steiner P, Dubno B, et al (2001) Temperature quantification using the proton frequency shift technique: in vitro and in vivo validation in an open 0.5 tesla interventional MR scanner during RF ablation. J Magn Reson Imaging 13:437–444

Breen MS, Lancaster TL, Lazebnik RS, et al (2003) Three-dimensional method for comparing in vivo interventional MR images of thermally ablated tissue with tissue response. J Magn Reson Imaging 18:90–102

Bremer C, Kreft G, Filler T, et al (2002) Accuracy of non-enhanced MRI to monitor histological lesion size during laser-induced interstitial thermotherapy. Eur Radiol 12:237–244

Catalano O, Lobianco R, Esposito M, et al (2001) Hepatocellular carcinoma recurrence after percutaneous ablation therapy: helical CT patterns. Abdom Imaging 26:375–383

Chopra S, Dodd GD 3rd, Chintapalli KN, et al (2001) Tumour recurrence after radiofrequency thermal ablation of hepatic tumours: spectrum of findings on dual-phase contrast-enhanced CT. AJR Am J Roentgenol 177:381–387

Chung YC, Duerk JL, Shankaranarayanan A, et al (1999) Temperature measurement using echo-shifted FLASH at low field for interventional MRI. J Magn Reson Imaging 10:108

Dromain C, de Baere T, Elias D, et al (2002) Hepatic tumors treated with percutaneous radio-frequency ablation: CT and MR imaging follow-up. Radiology 223:255–262

Fossheim S, Il'yasov K, Hennig J, (2000) Thermosensitive paramagnetic liposomes for temperature control during MR imaging-guided hyperthermia: in vitro feasibility studies. Acad Radiol 12:1107–1115

Germain D, Chevallier P, Laurent A, et al (2001) MR monitoring of tumour thermal therapy. MAGMA 13:47–59

Gillams A, Lees WR (1999) Thermal ablation induced changes in hepatic arterial perfusion. Radiology 213P

Gillams A, Lees W, Sellars P (2001) Correlation of ablation size as depicted on contrast enhanced CT and on low field, open MR. Cardiovasc Intervent Radiol 24 [Suppl 1]:S124

Goldberg SN, Gazelle GS, Compton CC, et al (2000) Treatment of intrahepatic malignancy with radiofrequency ablation: radiologic-pathologic correlation. Cancer 88:2452–2463

Heisterkamp J, Matheijssen N, van Hillegersberg R, et al (1999) Accuracy of MR phase mapping for temperature monitoring during interstitial laser coagulation (ILC) in the liver at rest and simulated respiration. Magn Reson Imaging 41:919–925

Huppert PE, Trubenbach J, Schick F, et al (2000) MRI-guided percutaneous radiofrequency ablation of hepatic neoplasms; first technical and clinical experiences. Rofo Fortschr Geb Rontgenstr Neuen Bildgeb Verfahr 172:692–700

Hwang KP, Lim J, Wendt M, et al (1999) Improved device definition in interventional magnetic resonance imaging using a rotated stripes keyhole acquisition. Magn Reson Med 42:554-560

Kelekis AD, Terraz S, Roggan A, et al (2003) Percutaneous treatment of liver tumors with an adapted probe for cooled-tip, impedance-controlled radio-frequency ablation under open-magnet MR guidance: initial results. Eur Radiol 13:1100–1105

Kettenbach J, Kostler W, Rucklinger E, et al (2003) Percutaneous saline-enhanced radiofrequency ablation of unresectable hepatic tumors: initial experience in 26 patients. AJR Am J Roentgenol 180:1537–1545

Limanond P, Zimmerman P, Raman SS, et al (2003) Interpretation of CT and MRI after radiofrequency ablation of hepatic malignancies. AJR Am J Roentgenol 181:1635–1640

Nghiem HV, Francis IR, Fontana R, et al (2002) Computed tomography appearances of hypervascular hepatic tumors after percutaneous radiofrequency ablation therapy. Curr Probl Diagn Radiol 31:105–111

Ni Y, Cressen E, Adriaens P (2002) Necrosis avid contrast agents: introducing nonporphyrin species. Acad Radiol 9 (Suppl 1):S98–S101

Oshiro T, Sinha U, Lu D, et al (2002) Reduction of electronic noise from radiofrequency generator during radiofrequency ablation in interventional MRI. J Comput Assist Tomogr 26:308–316

Scudamore CH, Lee SI, Patterson EJ, et al (1999) Radiofrequency ablation followed by resection of malignant liver tumors. Am J Surg 177:411–417

Steiner P, Botnar R, Dubno B, et al (1998) Radio-frequency-induced thermoablation: monitoring with T1-weighted and proton-frequency-shift MR imaging in an interventional 0.5 T environment. Radiology 206:803–810

Tsuda M, Majima K, Yamada T, et al (2001) Hepatocellular carcinoma after radiofrequency ablation therapy: dynamic CT evaluation of treatment. Clin Imaging 25:409–415

Varghese T, Zagzebski JA, Chen Q, et al (2002) Ultrasound monitoring of temperature change during radiofrequency ablation: preliminary in-vivo results. Ultrasound Med Biol 28:321–329

Vilana R, Llovet JM, Bianchi L, et al (2003) Contrast-enhanced power Doppler sonography and helical computed tomography for assessment of vascularity of small hepatocellular carcinomas before and after percutaneous ablation. J Clin Ultrasound 31:119–128

Vogl T, Muller PK, Hammerstingl R (1995) Malignant liver tumors treated with MR imaging-guided laser-induced thermotherapy. Radiology 196:257–265

Wilson DL, Carrillo A, Zheng L, et al (1998) Evaluation of 3D image registration as applied to MR-guided thermal treatment of liver cancer. J Magn Reson Imaging 8:77–84

Zhang Q, Chung YC, Lewin JS, et al (1998) A method for simultaneous RF ablation and MRI. J Magn Reson Imaging 8:110–114

23 Percutaneous Ablation of Hepatocellular Carcinoma

Riccardo Lencioni, Laura Crocetti, Dania Cioni, Elisa Batini, Clotilde Della Pina, and Carlo Bartolozzi

23.1
Introduction

Hepatocellular carcinoma (HCC) is the fifth most common cancer, and its incidence is increasing worldwide because of the dissemination of hepatitis B and C virus infection (Llovet et al. 2003). Patients with cirrhosis are at the highest risk of developing HCC. Currently, HCC is the leading cause of death among cirrhotic patients. Screening can lead to diagnosis at an early stage, when the tumor may be curable by resection, liver transplantation, or percutaneous ablation (Bruix and Llovet 2002; Bruix et al. 2001).

Resection is currently indicated among patients with single asymptomatic HCC and extremely well-preserved liver function, who have neither clinically significant portal hypertension nor abnormal bilirubin (Bruix and Llovet 2002; Llovet et al. 2003). However, less than 5% of cirrhotic patients with HCC fit these criteria (Llovet et al. 1999). Liver transplantation benefits patients who have decompensated cirrhosis and one tumor smaller than 5 cm or up to three nodules smaller than 3 cm, but donor shortage greatly limits its applicability (Bruix and

R. Lencioni, MD; L. Crocetti, MD; D. Cioni, MD;
D. Cioni, MD; E. Batini, MD; C. Della Pina, MD;
C. Bartolozzi, MD
Division of Diagnostic and Interventional Radiology, Department of Oncology, Transplants and Advanced Technologies in Medicine, University of Pisa, Via Roma 67, 56100 Pisa, Italy

Llovet 2002; Llovet et al. 2003). This difficulty might be overcome by living donation; this, however, is still at an early stage of clinical application.

As a result, image-guided techniques for percutaneous tumor ablation play a major role in the therapeutic management of HCC. While percutaneous ethanol injection (PEI) is a well-established technique for percutaneous treatment, several newer methods of tumor destruction have been developed and clinically tested over the past few years (Lencioni et al. 2004a). Among these methods, radiofrequency (RF) ablation constitutes the most extensively studied alternative to PEI (Galandi and Antes 2004).

23.2
General Eligibility Criteria

A careful clinical, laboratory, and imaging assessment has to be performed on each individual patient by a multidisciplinary team to evaluate eligibility for percutaneous ablation (Lencioni et al. 2001). Patients classified as stage 0 (very early stage) or stage A (early stage) according to the Barcelona-Clinic Liver Cancer staging classification for treatment schedule may qualify for percutaneous ablation if surgical resection and liver transplantation are not suitable options (Llovet et al. 2003). Patients are required to have either a single tumor smaller than 5 cm or as many as three nodules smaller than 3 cm each in the absence of vascular involvement and extrahepatic spread, a performance status test of 0, and liver cirrhosis in Child-Pugh class A or B.

Imaging techniques, including ultrasound plus spiral computed tomography (CT) or dynamic magnetic resonance (MR) imaging, are used to help determine whether patients are suitable candidates for percutaneous treatment. Pre-treatment imaging planning must carefully define size, shape, and location of each lesion. Percutaneous ablation is best indicated for expanding, nodular-type tumors smaller than 3–5 cm. Lesions located along the surface of the liver can be considered for percutaneous ablation, although their treatment requires adequate expertise and may be associated with a higher risk of complications. Thermal ablation of superficial lesions that are adjacent to any part of the gastrointestinal tract must be avoided because of the risk of thermal injury of the gastric or bowel wall (RHIM et al. 2004). The colon appears to be at greater risk than the stomach or small bowel for thermally mediated perforation. Gastric complications are rare, likely owing to the relatively greater wall thickness of the stomach or the rarity of surgical adhesions along the gastrohepatic ligament. The mobility of the small bowel may also provide the bowel with greater protection compared with the relatively fixed colon. Treatment of lesions adjacent to the gallbladder or to the hepatic hilum is at risk of thermal injury of the biliary tract. In experienced hands, RF ablation of tumors located in the vicinity of the gallbladder was shown to be feasible, although associated in most cases with self-limited iatrogenic cholecystitis (CHOPRA et al. 2003). In contrast, thermal ablation of lesions adjacent to hepatic vessels is possible, since flowing blood usually protects the vascular wall from thermal injury: in these cases, however, the risk of incomplete treatment of the neoplastic tissue close to the vessel may increase because of the heat loss. The potential risk of thermal damage to critical structures should be weighed against benefits on a case-by-case basis.

A careful assessment of the coagulation status is mandatory before percutaneous ablation. A prothrombin time ratio (normal time/patient's time) greater than 50% as well as a platelet count higher than 50,000/µl are required to keep the risk of bleeding at an acceptably low level.

23.3
Percutaneous Ethanol Injection

PEI is a well-established technique for tumor ablation (BARTOLOZZI and LENCIONI 1996). It induces tumor necrosis as a result of cellular dehydration, protein denaturation, and chemical occlusion of tumor vessels. It is best administered by using ultrasound guidance because ultrasound allows for continuous real-time monitoring of the injection. This is crucial to realize the pattern of tumor perfusion and to avoid excessive ethanol leakage outside the lesion. Fine noncutting needles, with either a single end hole or multiple side holes, are commonly used for PEI. PEI is usually performed under local anesthesia and does not require routine patient hospitalization. The treatment schedule includes four to six sessions performed once or twice weekly. The number of treatment sessions, as well as the amount of injected ethanol per session, may vary greatly according to the size of the lesion, the pattern of tumor perfusion, and the compliance of the patient.

Several studies have shown that PEI is an effective treatment for small, nodular-type HCC. HCC nodules have a soft consistency and are surrounded by a firm cirrhotic liver. Consequently, injected ethanol diffuses within them easily and selectively, leading to complete tumor necrosis in about 70% of the cases (SHIINA et al. 1991). Although there have not been any prospective randomized trials comparing PEI and best supportive care or PEI and surgical resection, several series have provided indirect evidence that PEI improves the natural history of HCC: the long-term outcome of patients with early-stage tumors who were treated with PEI was shown to be similar to that of patients who had undergone resection, with 5-year survival rates ranging from 32% to 52% (Table 23.1) (CASTELLS et al. 1993; LENCIONI et al. 1995; LENCIONI et al. 1997; LIVRAGHI et al. 1995; SHIINA et al. 1993). In a recent prospective comparative study, the 1-, 3-, and 5-year survival rates were almost identical between two cohorts of patients who received surgical resection (97%, 84%, and 61%, respectively) or PEI (100%, 82%, and 59%, respectively) (YAMAMOTO et al. 2001).

Despite PEI being a low-risk procedure, severe complications have been reported. In a multicenter survey including 1,066 patients (8,118 PEI sessions), one death (0.1%) and 34 complications (3.2%), including seven cases of tumor seeding (0.7%), were reported (DI STASI et al. 1997). The major limitation of PEI, besides the uncertainty of tumor ablation and the long treatment times, is the high local recurrence rate, which may reach 33% in lesions smaller than 3 cm and 43% in lesions exceeding 3 cm (KHAN et al. 2000; KODA et al. 2000). The injected ethanol does not always achieve complete tumor necrosis because of its inhomogeneous distribution within the lesion, especially in the presence of intratumoral septa, and the limited effect on extracapsular cancerous spread. Also, PEI is unable to create a safety margin of ablation in the liver parenchyma surrounding the nodule, and therefore may not destroy tiny satellite nodules that, even in small tumors, may be located in close proximity to the main lesion (OKUSAKA et al. 2002).

Table 23.1 Survival outcomes of patients with early-stage hepatocellular carcinoma receiving percutaneous ablation

Treatment	No. Patients	Survival Rates (%)		
		1-yr	3-yr	5-yr
Percutaneous ethanol injection				
CASTELLS et al. (1993)	30	83	55	N/A
SHIINA et al. (1993)	98	85	62	52
LENCIONI et al. (1995)	105	96	68	32
LIVRAGHI et al. (1995)				
Child class A, single HCC	293	98	79	47
Child class B, single HCC	149	93	63	29
Radiofrequency ablation				
LENCIONI et al. (2004b)				
Child class A	144	100	76	51
Child class A, single HCC	116	100	89	61
Child class B	43	89	46	31
Microwave coagulation				
SHIINA et al. (2002)	122	90	68	N/A

N/A=not available. HCC=hepatocellular carcinoma.

23.4
Radiofrequency Ablation

Early clinical experiences with RF ablation were conducted in the framework of feasibility studies (CURLEY et al. 1999; ROSSI et al. 1998). These investigations had merit in showing the efficacy and the safety of the procedure. However, the data were heterogeneous and unsystematically presented (GALANDI and ANTES 2004). Moreover, RF treatment was not compared to any established treatment for HCC. The European Association for the Study of the Liver has recommended comparing newer methods of tumor destruction, such as RF ablation, with the well-established and accepted PEI method through randomized trials (BRUIX et al. 2001). In fact, methodological research has given convincing evidence that less rigorous study designs are likely to produce biased results and to exaggerate the estimated effect of a new therapy (GALANDI and ANTES 2004).

One randomized study compared RF ablation versus PEI for the treatment of early-stage HCC (LENCIONI et al. 2003). In this trial, 104 patients with 144 HCC lesions were randomly assigned to receive RF ablation or PEI. No statistically significant differences between RF ablation and PEI groups were observed with respect to baseline characteristics, except for patients' age and albumin concentration. At the time of the analysis, the mean follow-up was 22 months. The overall survival rates at 1 and

2 years were 100% and 98%, respectively, in the RF group, and 96% and 88%, respectively, in the PEI group. Despite the tendency to favor RF ablation, the observed difference did not reach statistical significance (hazard ratio, 0.20; 95% confidence interval, 0.02–1.69; $p=0.138$). However, 1- and 2-year recurrence-free survival rates were clearly higher in RF-treated patients than in PEI-treated patients (86% and 64%, respectively, in the RF ablation group versus 77% and 43%, respectively, in the PEI group; hazard ratio, 0.48; 95% confidence interval, 0.27–0.85; $p=0.012$) (Fig. 23.1). RF treatment was confirmed as an independent prognostic factor for local recurrence-free survival by multivariate analysis.

This trial suggested that RF ablation can achieve higher recurrence-free survival rates than PEI, thereby confirming findings in two previous comparative studies, in which higher complete tumor response rates were observed in tumors treated with RF ablation with respect to those submitted to PEI (IKEDA et al. 2001; LIVRAGHI et al. 1999). However, likely because of the short follow-up period and the limited sample size, no difference with respect to overall survival was found. Recently, a prospective intention-to-treat clinical trial reported the long-term survival outcomes of RF ablation-treated patients (LENCIONI et al. 2004b). In this study, 206 patients with early-stage HCC who were not candidates for resection or transplantation were enrolled. RF ablation was considered as the first-line nonsurgical treatment and was actually performed in 187

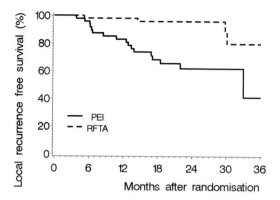

Fig. 23.1. Probability of local recurrence-free survival of HCC patients treated by PEI (*n*=50) or RF thermal ablation (*n*=52). The difference between the groups was statistically significant (*p*=0.0016). The number of patients in follow-up at 6, 12, 18, 24, and 30 months was 46, 37, 24, 16, and 5, respectively, for the PEI group; and 49, 46, 33, 24, and 10, respectively, for the RF group

(91%) of 206 patients. Nineteen (9%) of 206 patients had to be excluded from RF treatment because of the unfavorable location of the tumor. Non-compliant patients were treated with either PEI or segmental transcatheter arterial chemoembolization. The overall survival rates in the intention-to-treat analysis including all the 206 patients enrolled in the study (67% at 3 years and 41% at 5 years) were not significantly different from those achieved in the 187 compliant patients who received RF ablation (71% at 3 years and 48% at 5 years; *p*=0.5094) (Fig. 23.2). In patients who underwent RF ablation, survival depended on the severity of the underlying cirrhosis and the tumor multiplicity. Patients in Child class A had 3- and 5-year survival rates of 76%, and 51%, respectively. These figures were significantly higher than those obtained in Child class B patients (46% at 3 years and 31% at 5 years; *p*=0.0006) (Table 23.1) (Fig. 23.3). Patients with a solitary HCC had 3- and 5-year survival rates of 75% and 50%, respectively, while those with multiple tumors had 3- and 5-year survival rates of 51% and 34%, respectively. Such a difference was also statistically significant (*p*=0.0133). Of interest, a subgroup of 116 patients in Child class A who had a solitary HCC showed 3- and 5-year survival rates of 89% and 61%, respectively (Table 23.1).

In this series, recurrence of the tumor treated by RF ablation occurred in 10 of 187 patients. Despite the absence of viable neoplastic tissue on post-treatment spiral CT images, residual microscopic nests of tumor or small undetected satellite nodules led to a

local tumor progression. The actuarial 5-year local tumor progression rate was 10% (Fig. 23.4). However, new HCC tumors developed in 93 patients during the follow-up. The rate of recurrence with new tumors reached 81% at 5 years (Fig. 23.4). Such a high rate of new tumors is the expression of the inherent multicentric nature of HCC in cirrhosis and does not seem to represent a drawback of RF ablation, being found in cirrhotic HCC patients treated with either percutaneous therapies or surgical resection.

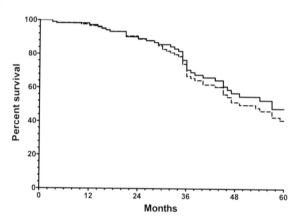

Fig. 23.2. Survival outcomes of patients with liver cirrhosis and early-stage HCC in whom RF ablation was used as the sole first-line anticancer treatment. The difference between the survival curve obtained in intention-to-treat analysis (*dotted line*) and the survival curve of compliant patients (*continuous line*) is not statistically significant (*p*=0.5094). (Courtesy of LENCIONI et al. 2004b)

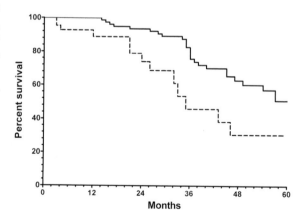

Fig. 23.3. Survival of early-stage HCC patients treated with RF ablation according to the severity of the underlying cirrhosis. Patients in Child class A (*n*=144) (*continuous line*) showed significantly better survival (*p*=0.0006) than those in Child class B (*n*=43) (*dotted line*). (Courtesy of LENCIONI et al. 2004b)

The data on long-term outcome of RF ablation must be compared with those obtained in patients with early-stage tumors who received other potentially curative treatments. Liver transplantation was shown to be the only treatment option that consistently provided 5-year survival rates in the range of 71–75% (BISMUTH et al. 1999; JONAS et al. 2001; LLOVET et al. 1999; MAZZAFERRO et al. 1996). Surgical resection of early-stage HCC resulted in 5-year survival rates in the range of 41–51% (FONG et al. 1999; JONAS et al. 2001; LLOVET et al. 1999; WAYNE et al. 2002). Resection achieved substantially higher survival rates only when patients with a solitary tumor and extremely well preserved liver function, who had neither clinically significant portal hypertension nor abnormal bilirubin, were selected (LLOVET et al. 1999). In large series, PEI achieved 5-year survival rates ranging from 32% to 52%. In a multicenter study, survival of 293 patients with Child class A cirrhosis and a solitary tumor smaller than 5 cm who received PEI was 47% at 5 years (LIVRAGHI et al. 1995). Comparison of results obtained with RF ablation with those achieved in the past by using PEI, however, may be biased by the ability to better select patients with early-stage tumors owing to the improvement in imaging techniques.

In most of the reported series, RF ablation was associated with acceptable morbidity. In a multicenter survey in which 2,320 patients with 3,554 lesions were included, six deaths (mortality rate, 0.3%) were noted, including two caused by multiorgan failure following intestinal perforation; one case each of septic shock following *Staphylococcus aureus*-caused peritonitis, massive hemorrhage following tumor rupture, liver failure following stenosis of right bile duct; and one case of sudden death of unknown cause 3 days after the procedure. Fifty (2.2%) patients had additional major complications. Tumor seeding, in particular, occurred in only 12 (0.5%) of 2,320 patients (LIVRAGHI et al. 2003). However, lesions with subcapsular location or an invasive tumoral pattern, as shown by a poor differentiation degree, may be at risk for such a complication (LLOVET et al. 2001).

Recently, following advances in RF technology, RF ablation has also been used to treat patients with intermediate stage tumors. However, results obtained by RF ablation alone were not entirely satisfactory. LIVRAGHI et al. (2000) treated 114 patients with 126 HCC lesions greater than 3 cm in diameter. Complete necrosis (on imaging) was attained in only 60 lesions (47.6%), nearly complete (90–99%) necrosis in 40 lesions (31.7%), and partial (50–89%) necrosis in

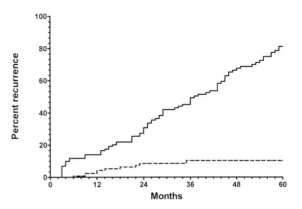

Fig. 23.4. Tumor recurrence in patients with early-stage HCC who received RF ablation. Rates of recurrence within the treated tumor (*dotted line*) were 4% at 1 year, 10% at 3 years, and 10% at 5 years. Rates of recurrence with new tumors (*continuous line*) were 14% at 1 year, 49% at 3 years, and 81% at 5 years. (Courtesy of LENCIONI et al. 2004b)

the remaining 26 lesions (20.6%). Therefore, there is currently a focus on a multimodality strategy in attempts to ensure a more effective percutaneous ablation of large HCC tumors.

Of interest, recent studies have proved the influence of perfusion-mediated tissue cooling on the area of thermal necrosis achievable with RF treatment. GOLDBERG et al. (1998) applied RF in vivo to normal porcine liver without and with balloon occlusion of the portal vein, celiac artery, or hepatic artery, and to ex vivo calf liver: RF application during vascular occlusion produced larger areas of coagulation necrosis than RF with unaltered blood flow. LEES et al. (2000) showed that hypotensive anesthesia improved the effectiveness of liver RF ablation in a human study. Assuming that the volume of thermal necrosis produced by RF treatment is strongly dependent on blood flow, and considering that in HCC blood flow is mainly sustained by the hepatic artery, we performed a multicenter clinical trial aimed at investigating whether interruption of the tumor arterial blood supply by means of occlusion of either the hepatic artery with a balloon catheter or the feeding arteries with gelatin sponge particles could increase the extent of RF-induced coagulation necrosis (ROSSI et al. 2000). A series of 62 consecutive patients with a single, large HCC ranging from 3.5 to 8.5 cm in diameter (mean 4.7 cm) accompanying cirrhosis underwent RF ablation after occlusion of the tumor arterial supply. The RF energy was delivered by using an expandable electrode needle at the time of balloon catheter occlusion of the hepatic artery (n=40), at the time of occlusion of the

HCC feeding arteries with gelatin sponge particles (*n*=13), or 2–5 days thereafter (*n*=9). Two patients underwent liver resection after the thermal ablation; the remaining 60 patients were followed up for a mean of 12.1 months (range 3–26 months). During the follow-up, 49 (82%) of the 60 treated HCC nodules showed a stable complete response, while the remaining 11 (18%) nodules showed local progression. Histopathologic analysis of one autopsy and of the two surgical specimens revealed more than 90% necrosis in one specimen and 100% necrosis in two. No fatal or major complications related to the treatment occurred, despite the more aggressive RF treatment protocol.

Results of this study provide evidence that areas of coagulative necrosis that are much larger than those previously reported can be created if RF thermal ablation is performed in HCC nodules after occlusion of their arterial supply. The results achieved with this technique were confirmed by two recent studies. YAMASAKI et al. (2002) compared the coagulation diameters obtained with balloon-occluded RF and standard RF in 31 patients with 42 HCC lesions measuring less than 4 cm in the greatest dimension. There were no significant differences in the ablation conditions such as the frequency of a fully expanded electrode, the number of needle insertions, application cycles, or treatment times between the two groups. However, the greatest dimension of the area coagulated by balloon-occluded RFA was significantly larger than that coagulated by standard RFA. YAMAKADO et al. (2002) evaluated the local therapeutic efficacy of RF ablation after transarterial chemoembolization in 64 patients with 108 lesions. Sixty-five lesions were small (3 cm or less), 32 were intermediate in size (3.1–5 cm), and 11 were large (5.1–12 cm). Complete necrosis was achieved in all lesions, and there were no local recurrences in small and intermediate-sized lesions during a mean follow-up of 12.5 months.

Despite these encouraging preliminary results, there are no reports showing that RF ablation, performed alone or in combination with intra-arterial procedures, results in improved survival in patients with intermediate stage HCC. A randomized trial comparing an optimized RF technology with chemoembolization would be needed to establish the potential role of the technique in this patient population.

23.5
Other Methods of Percutaneous Ablation

Other methods of percutaneous ablation have been clinically tested over the past few years. One group compared percutaneous acetic acid injection and PEI (OHNISHI et al. 1998). Sixty patients with one to four HCC lesions smaller than 3 cm were entered into a randomized trial. All original tumors were treated successfully by either therapy. However, 8% of 38 tumors treated with percutaneous acetic acid injection and 37% of 35 tumors treated with PEI developed a local recurrence ($p<0.001$) during the follow-up. The 1- and 2-year survival rates were 100% and 92% in the percutaneous acetic acid injection group and 83% and 63% in the PEI group ($p=0.0017$). A multivariate analysis of prognostic factors revealed that treatment was an independent predictor of survival. The authors concluded that percutaneous acetic acid injection was superior to PEI in the treatment of small HCC. However, the results of acetic acid injection were not established in large series of patients.

Other investigators investigated the usefulness of percutaneous microwave coagulation therapy (MCT). A 3-year survival of 68% was reported in a retrospective analysis of 122 patients with early-stage HCC who received MCT (SHIINA et al. 2002). Another study compared MCT and PEI in a retrospective analysis of 90 patients with small HCC (SEKI et al. 1999). The overall 5-year survival rates for patients with well-differentiated HCC treated with MCT and PEI were not significantly different. However, among the patients with moderately or poorly differentiated HCC, overall survival with MCT was significantly better than with PEI ($p=0.03$). The authors concluded that MCT may be superior to PEI for the local control of moderately or poorly differentiated small HCC. Other authors compared the effectiveness of MCT with that of RF ablation in a randomized trial (SHIBATA et al. 2002). The data were analyzed with respect to lesions and not to patients. Although no statistically significant differences were observed with respect to the efficacy of the two procedures, a tendency to favor RF ablation was recognized with respect to local recurrences and complication rates (GALANDI and ANTES 2004).

23.6
Conclusion

From the early studies with PEI to the latest reports on RF ablation, percutaneous techniques have been refined and their clinical efficacy better defined. While PEI is a valuable and accepted treatment for nonsurgical patients with early-stage HCC, RF ablation seems to achieve more effective local control of disease. Appropriate experience and optimized techniques are needed in RF ablation to keep complications at an acceptably low rate. Further randomized trials will be needed to fully establish the clinical role of RF ablation with respect to other percutaneous treatments and to devise an unbiased therapeutic strategy.

References

Bartolozzi C, Lencioni R (1996) Ethanol injection for the treatment of hepatic tumours. Eur Radiol 6:682–696

Bismuth H, Majno PE, Adam R (1999) Liver transplantation for hepatocellular carcinoma. Semin Liver Dis 19:311–322

Bruix J, Llovet JM (2002) Prognostic prediction and treatment strategy in hepatocellular carcinoma. Hepatology 35:519–524

Bruix J, Sherman M, Llovet JM (2001) EASL Panel of Experts on HCC. Clinical management of hepatocellular carcinoma. Conclusions of the Barcelona-2000 EASL Conference. European Association for the Study of the Liver. J Hepatol 35:421–430

Castells A, Bruix J, Bru C, et al (1993) Treatment of small hepatocellular carcinoma in cirrhotic patients: a cohort study comparing surgical resection and percutaneous ethanol injection. Hepatology 18:1121–1126

Chopra S, Dodd GD 3rd, Chanin MP, et al (2003) Radiofrequency ablation of hepatic tumors adjacent to the gallbladder: feasibility and safety. AJR Am J Roentgenol 180:697–701

Curley SA, Izzo F, Delrio P, et al (1999) Radiofrequency ablation of unresectable primary and metastatic malignancies: results in 123 patients. Ann Surg 230:1–8

Di Stasi M, Buscarini L, Livraghi T, et al (1997) Percutaneous ethanol injection in the treatment of hepatocellular carcinoma. A multicenter survey of evaluation practices and complication rates. Scand J Gastroenterol 32:1168–1173

Fong Y, Sun RL, Jarnagin W, et al (1999) An analysis of 412 cases of hepatocellular carcinoma at a Western center. Ann Surg 229:790–800

Galandi D, Antes G (2004) Radiofrequency thermal ablation versus other interventions for hepatocellular carcinoma (Cochrane Review). In: The Cochrane Library, Issue 2. John Wiley & Sons, Chichester, UK

Goldberg SN, Hahn PF, Tanabe KK, et al (1998) Percutaneous radiofrequency tissue ablation: does perfusion-mediated tissue cooling limit coagulation necrosis? J Vasc Interv Radiol 9:101–115

Ikeda M, Okada S, Ueno H, et al (2001) Radiofrequency ablation and percutaneous ethanol injection in patients with small hepatocellular carcinoma: a comparative study. Jpn J Clin Oncol 31:322–326

Jonas S, Bechstein WO, Steinmuller T, et al (2001) Vascular invasion and histopathologic grading determine outcome after liver transplantation for hepatocellular carcinoma in cirrhosis. Hepatology 33:1080–1086

Khan KN, Yatsuhashi H, Yamasaki K, et al (2000) Prospective analysis of risk factors for early intrahepatic recurrence of hepatocellular carcinoma following ethanol injection. J Hepatol 32:269–278

Koda M, Murawaki Y, Mitsuda A, et al (2000) Predictive factors for intrahepatic recurrence after percutaneous ethanol injection therapy for small hepatocellular carcinoma. Cancer 88:529–537

Lees WR, Schumillian C, Gillams AR (2000) Hypotensive anesthesia improves the effectiveness of radiofrequency ablation in the liver. Radiology 217(P):228

Lencioni R, Bartolozzi C, Caramella D, et al (1995) Treatment of small hepatocellular carcinoma with percutaneous ethanol injection. Analysis of prognostic factors in 105 Western patients. Cancer 76:1737–1746

Lencioni R, Pinto F, Armillotta N, et al (1997) Long-term results of percutaneous ethanol injection therapy for hepatocellular carcinoma in cirrhosis: a European experience. Eur Radiol 7:514–519

Lencioni R, Cioni D, Bartolozzi C (2001) Percutaneous radiofrequency thermal ablation of liver malignancies: techniques, indications, imaging findings, and clinical results. Abdom Imaging 26:345–360

Lencioni R, Allgaier HP, Cioni D, et al (2003) Small hepatocellular carcinoma in cirrhosis: randomized comparison of radiofrequency thermal ablation versus percutaneous ethanol injection. Radiology 228:235–240

Lencioni R, Cioni D, Crocetti L, et al (2004a) Percutaneous ablation of hepatocellular carcinoma: state-of-the-art. Liver Transpl 10:S91–S97

Lencioni R, Cioni D, Crocetti L, et al (2004b) Early-stage hepatocellular carcinoma in cirrhosis: long-term results of percutaneous image-guided radiofrequency ablation. Radiology 2004 (in press)

Livraghi T, Giorgio A, Marin G, et al (1995) Hepatocellular carcinoma and cirrhosis in 746 patients: long-term results of percutaneous ethanol injection. Radiology 197:101–108

Livraghi T, Goldberg SN, Lazzaroni S, et al (1999) Small hepatocellular carcinoma: treatment with radio-frequency ablation versus ethanol injection. Radiology 210:655–661

Livraghi T, Goldberg SN, Lazzaroni S, et al (2000) Hepatocellular carcinoma: radio-frequency ablation of medium and large lesions. Radiology 214:761–768

Livraghi T, Solbiati L, Meloni MF, et al (2003) Treatment of focal liver tumors with percutaneous radio-frequency ablation: complications encountered in a multicenter study. Radiology 226:441–451

Llovet JM, Fuster J, Bruix J (1999) Intention-to-treat analysis of surgical treatment for early hepatocellular carcinoma: resection versus transplantation. Hepatology 30:1434–1440

Llovet JM, Vilana R, Bru C, et al (2001) Barcelona Clinic Liver Cancer (BCLC) Group. Increased risk of tumor seeding after percutaneous radiofrequency ablation for single hepatocellular carcinoma. Hepatology 33:1124–1129

Llovet JM, Burroughs A, Bruix J (2003) Hepatocellular carcinoma. Lancet 362:1907–1917

Mazzaferro V, Regalia E, Doci R, et al (1996) Liver transplantation in the treatment of small hepatocellular carcinomas in patients with cirrhosis. N Engl J Med 334:693–699

Ohnishi K, Yoshioka H, Ito S, et al (1998) Prospective randomized controlled trial comparing percutaneous acetic acid injection and percutaneous ethanol injection for small hepatocellular carcinoma. Hepatology 27:67–72

Okusaka T, Okada S, Ueno H, et al (2002) Satellite lesions in patients with small hepatocellular carcinoma with reference to clinicopathologic features. Cancer 95:1931–1937

Rhim H, Dodd GD 3rd, Chintapalli KN, et al (2004) Radiofrequency thermal ablation of abdominal tumors: lessons learned from complications. Radiographics 24:41–52

Rossi S, Garbagnati F, Lencioni R, et al (2000) Percutaneous radio-frequency thermal ablation of nonresectable hepatocellular carcinoma after occlusion of tumor blood supply. Radiology 217:119–126

Seki T, Wakabayashi M, Nakagawa T, et al (1999) Percutaneous microwave coagulation therapy for patients with small hepatocellular carcinoma: comparison with percutaneous ethanol injection therapy. Cancer 85:1694–1702

Shibata T, Iimuro Y, Yamamoto Y, et al (2002) Small hepatocellular carcinoma: comparison of radio-frequency ablation and percutaneous microwave coagulation therapy. Radiology 223:331–337

Shiina S, Tagawa K, Unuma T, et al (1991) Percutaneous ethanol injection therapy for hepatocellular carcinoma: a histopathologic study. Cancer 68:1524–1530

Shiina S, Tagawa K, Niwa Y, et al (1993) Percutaneous ethanol injection therapy for hepatocellular carcinoma: results in 146 patients. AJR Am J Roentgenol 160:1023–1028

Shiina S, Teratani T, Obi S, et al (2002) Nonsurgical treatment of hepatocellular carcinoma: from percutaneous ethanol injection therapy and percutaneous microwave coagulation therapy to radiofrequency ablation. Oncology 62(Suppl 1):64–68

Wayne JD, Lauwers GY, Ikai I, et al (2002) Preoperative predictors of survival after resection of small hepatocellular carcinomas. Ann Surg 235:722–731

Yamakado K, Nakatsuka A, Ohmori S, et al (2002) Radiofrequency ablation combined with chemoembolization in hepatocellular carcinoma: treatment response based on tumor size and morphology. J Vasc Interv Radiol 13:1225–1232

Yamamoto J, Okada S, Shimada K, et al (2001) Treatment strategy for small hepatocellular carcinoma: comparison of long-term results after percutaneous ethanol injection therapy and surgical resection. Hepatology 34:707–713

Yamasaki T, Kurokawa F, Shirahashi H, et al (2002) Percutaneous radiofrequency ablation therapy for patients with hepatocellular carcinoma during occlusion of hepatic blood flow. Comparison with standard percutaneous radiofrequency ablation therapy. Cancer 95:2353–2360

24 Percutaneous Ablation of Hepatic Metastases

J. Antony Goode, Tarun Sabharwal, and Andreas Adam

CONTENTS

J. A. GOODE, MD; T. SABHARWAL, MD;
A. ADAM, MB, BS, FRCP, FRCR, FRCS
Department of Interventional Radiology, St Thomas'
Hospital, Lambeth Palace Road, London SE1 7EH, UK

24.1
Introduction

The liver is the most common site of metastatic disease. Hepatic metastases most commonly occur from colorectal cancer and, less frequently, from neuroendocrine tumours, gastrointestinal sarcoma, ocular melanoma, and others. Complete evaluation of the extent of metastatic disease, both within and outside the liver, is important before considering treatment options.

Approximately 25% of patients with liver metastases from colorectal cancer have no other site of metastasis and can be treated with regional therapies directed towards their liver tumours. Hepatic resection results in survival rates ranging from 55%–80% at 1 year and 25%–50% at 5 years (NAGORNEY et al. 1989). However, because of advanced disease, unfavourable location of the metastases, or poor physical condition, fewer than 20% of patients are eligible for hepatic resection (FOSTER 1978; ADSON et al. 1984; COBOURN et al. 1987; FONG et al. 1995; NORDLINGER et al. 1987; STEELE et al. 1991). In general, only patients with fewer than four or five metastases, limited to one lobe and with no evidence of extrahepatic disease, are eligible for surgery. Without resection, patients with hepatic metastases from colorectal carcinoma have a median survival of less than 1 year (BADEN and ANDERSEN 1975; BENGTSSON et al. 1981; WOOD et al. 1976). Recently developed minimally invasive techniques for local ablation of hepatic metastases may provide reasonable alternatives for patients who are not candidates for surgery. Such techniques include cryotherapy, thermal ablation, microwave therapy and intra-arterial chemoembolization.

24.2
Cryotherapy

Cryotherapy is the oldest of the local thermal ablation techniques. The application of cryotherapy was first suggested by COPPER (1963). Since then, there have been multiple clinical reports detailing its use for the treatment of primary and secondary hepatic tumours (McPHEE and KANE 1997; HADDAD et al. 1998). Subfreezing temperatures are delivered through penetrating cryoprobes in which a cryogen is circulated. Thermally conducted material allows cooling of the probe tip while the shaft and delivery hoses are insulated. Irreversible destruction of tissue occurs at temperatures below −20°C to −30°C. Direct freezing, denaturation of cellular proteins, cell membrane rupture, cell dehydration, and ischaemic hypoxia cause cell death. Cryolesions as large as 6–8 cm in diameter can be created safely.

The cost of a cryoablation unit ranges from £80,000 to £110,000. The cryoprobes are typically 2–10 mm in diameter and cost approximately £800 for single use. Because of the size of the probes, cryotherapy is often used at open or laparoscopic surgery, although smaller probes are now becoming available which may enable percutaneous cryotherapy to be carried out routinely in the future.

Generally, treatment is limited to those with four or fewer metastases, although patients with slow-growing neuroendocrine tumours may have a slightly higher number of lesions and still be candidates for cryoablation. Contraindications include the presence of extrahepatic metastatic disease and inability to undergo general anaesthesia and laparotomy.

At present, cryoablation is primarily an open surgical technique, with fewer than 10% of patients treated laparoscopically. Ultrasound (US) is the most frequently used method of guiding the procedure. Depending on tumour size, one or two probes are placed centrally within the lesion with the tips of the probes touching the deep edge of the tumour. The cryogenic material (–196°C) is circulated through the probes. The ice wall is visualised as an echogenic, expanding, hemispherical rim. Freezing is continued until the cryolesion extends through the tumour and into the adjacent normal tissue, with a goal of achieving a 5–10 mm ablation margin. This first freeze takes 5–15 min and is followed by a spontaneous thaw and a second freeze to reach and slightly exceed the original cryoablation margin. After the second freeze the cryoprobe is heated and removed and the track is packed for hemostasis.

Patients are followed up with computed tomography (CT) performed immediately before discharge, at 6 and 12 months after ablation, and yearly thereafter. The thermal injury caused by cryoablation appears on CT images as an avascular, low-attenuation lesion that slowly decreases in size over time. FDG-PET performed three weeks following ablation is not only able to assess the efficacy of treatment, but it may also have a future role in follow-up of patients treated with cryosurgery as it can detect recurrent disease earlier than CT (LANGENHOFF et al. 2002).

24.2.1
Patient Outcome

The reported survival rates are 90% at 1 year, 40% at 3 years and 20% at 5 years, with a mean overall survival of 38 months (DODD et al. 2000).

Major complications occur in fewer than 20% of patients, the most common being intraperitoneal haemorrhage. No tumour seeding has been reported. Tumour recurrence at the cryotherapy site has been observed in 13% of patients (McPHEE and

KANE 1997). Minor complications, such as fever, leukocytosis and transient elevation of liver function tests are seen in the majority of patients. However, when compared with radiofrequency (RF) ablation therapy, although similar rates of treatment success and complications have been obtained, local recurrence occurred more frequently with cryoablation (ADAM et al. 2002).

24.3
Percutaneous Injection of Ethanol

Percutaneous ethanol injection (PEI) is effective in the treatment of hepatocellular carcinoma (HCC), and long-term survival rates of PEI-treated patients with HCC are similar to those of patients treated surgically (LIVRAGHI et al. 1995).

PEI is more effective in the treatment of HCC than in that of liver metastases. This is because most hepatocellular carcinomas occur in the setting of cirrhosis. In this situation the tumour is "soft", whereas the surrounding liver parenchyma is "hard". This promotes the distribution of ethanol or heat within the tumour, particularly when the HCC is encapsulated. Patients with liver metastases typically have normal (soft) underlying hepatic parenchyma, whereas the metastasis is "hard", a situation which promotes the egress of ethanol from the lesion into the normal liver. Metastases also tend to be more infiltrative than HCC.

24.4
Radiofrequency Ablation

Radiofrequency (RF) ablation uses radiofrequency energy to produce local heat in tissues. Needle-like electrodes are placed percutaneously directly into the tumour, with the use of ultrasound, computed tomography or magnetic resonance imaging guidance. The RF electrode typically is comprised of a metal shaft, which is insulated except for an exposed conductive tip that is in direct electrical contact with the targeted tissue volume. The RF generator supplies RF power to the tissue through the electrode. It is connected both to the shaft(s) of the RF electrode and to the reference electrode, usually a large conductive pad in contact with the patient's skin in an area of relatively good electrical thermal conductivity (such as the thigh). The RF generator produces RF voltage between the active electrode and the reference electrode, thereby establishing an electric field within the patient's body between the two electrodes. At the low RF frequencies used for this procedure (less than 1 MHz), the electric field pattern is governed essentially by electrostatic equations and oscillates with the alternating RF current, which causes movement of ions in the tissue in proportion to the field intensity. The mechanism of tissue heating for RF ablation is frictional, or resistive, energy loss caused by the motion of the ionic current (ORGAN 1976; COSMAN et al. 1984). All RF generators are operated at 460 kHz at a power setting of 50–200 W. The cost of the generators ranges from £8,000–£25,000. The needle electrodes cost £300–£1000 and are not reusable. There are now several different types of RF ablation systems available.

Many of these machines differ in generator power, needle size and configuration. There are also differences in the methods for monitoring of energy deposition and for maximising the volume of tumour coagulated.

Two systems (RITA Medical Systems, Inc. Mountain View, CA, and RadioTherapeutics Corp. Mountain View, CA) use coaxially deployed inner tines, which expand into the tumour after the outer needle is in place. The degree of deployment of the inner tines can be adjusted according to tumour size. The RITA system uses continuous monitoring of temperature to guide ablation, whereas the RadioTherapeutics machine uses monitoring of impedance. A third system (Radionics, Inc. Burlington, MA) has probes with either single needle or triple parallel needles; this system utilises perfusion of cold saline within the needle probe(s) to cool the electrode tip (Fig. 24.1). This minimises charring

around the needle tip thus preventing a rise in impedance and enabling the creation of a larger area of coagulation. The Berchtold system (Berchtold Medizinelektronik, Tuttlingen, Germany) is different from the above three in that (a) it can be used as a monopolar or a bipolar system and (b) it uses continuous infusion of saline from the needle tip into the tumour.

24.4.1
Patient Selection and Technique

Most investigators are limiting treatment with RF ablation to patients with four or fewer, 5-cm or smaller, primary or secondary malignant hepatic tumours, with no evidence of extrahepatic disease. However, patients with a small number of pulmonary metastases are sometimes treated, as such metastases do not usually have a significant impact on survival. RF ablation is also being used in combination with hepatic resection in the treatment of patients who would not be candidates for resection alone (PAWLIK et al. 2003). In some centres there is a waiting period for patients prior to transplantation; RF ablation is being applied to control tumour growth during this time. In addition, RF ablation is sometimes used as a test of time prior to hepatic resection in patients who are fit for surgery and in whom cross-sectional imaging reveals between one to five metastases. As new lesions can develop fairly quickly, some centres are now delaying surgery to see if this occurs. In such cases the old lesions are treated with RF ablation during the period of waiting (LIVRAGHI et al. 2003a).

In some patients with a large volume of tumour in the liver, not suitable for potentially curative surgery or treatment with radiofrequency, RF ablation is increasingly being requested by the oncologists to reduce tumour bulk in the hope that this will increase the effectiveness of chemotherapy. The effectiveness of RF for this purpose requires further investigation.

RF ablation is a good method of palliation in patients who have severe pain caused by distension of the liver capsule by large tumours. In such cases, coagulation of the tumour often provides rapid relief of pain (Fig. 24.2).

Ideal tumours for RF ablation are smaller than 3 cm in diameter, completely surrounded by hepatic parenchyma, 1 cm or more deep to the liver capsule, and 2 cm or more away from large hepatic or portal veins. Subcapsular liver tumours can be ablated, but

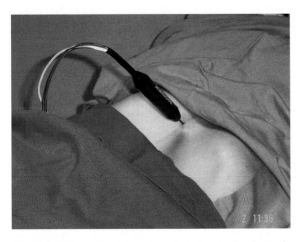

Fig. 24.1. This patient has a cooled tip single electrode (Radionics) sited in a left lobe metastasis, under CT guidance

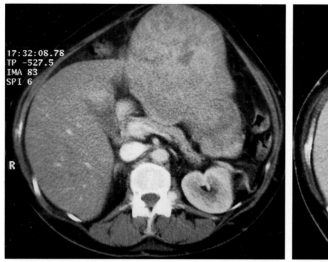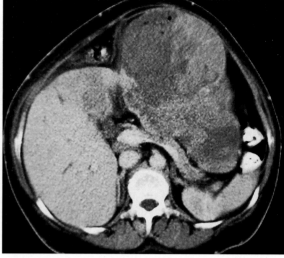

a   b

Fig. 24.2. a CT image of a large colorectal metastasis in the left lobe of the liver, which was causing local discomfort. **b** CT performed 2 weeks following RF ablation of the left lobe tumour shows reduction in size of the mass, with evidence of necrosis

their treatment is usually associated with greater procedural and post-procedural pain. Tumours adjacent to large blood vessels are more difficult to ablate completely because the blood flow in the vessels causes cooling of the adjacent tumour, and it has been shown that vessels as small as 3 mm adjacent to a tumour can result in incomplete tumour coagulation. (Lu et al. 2003). Temporary occlusion of the hepatic arterial supply to the tumour, of the portal vein and of the hepatic veins have all been used with good effect to decrease this cooling effect and allow tumours adjacent to large blood vessels to be ablated (Figs. 24.3, 24.4) (DE BAERE et al. 2002; ROSSI et al. 2000; YAMASAKI et al. 2002). Ablation of tumours adjacent to the large portal triads causes increased pain and poses the risk of damage to the associated bile duct. It is generally recognised that treating lesions close to the gallbladder, stomach, diaphragm or colon can be associated with increased risk of diaphragmatic injury, bowel perforation and peritonitis. Contraindications to treatment include sepsis, severe debilitation, and uncorrectable coagulopathies. The presence of an enterobiliary fistula or prior sphincterotomy increases the risk of biliary sepsis after the procedure, as does the presence of intrahepatic biliary dilatation.

Percutaneous RF ablation is usually carried out with the use of conscious sedation alone and can be performed on an outpatient basis. However, many operators prefer to keep the patients in hospital overnight, partly in order to treat any discomfort and partly because of the small risk of haemorrhage accompanying the procedure.

For patients who cannot tolerate sedation or in whom multiple tumour lesions are to be treated during a single session general anaesthesia is advocated. Before the procedure, adequate hydration is ensured; this is believed to reduce the incidence of the post-embolization syndrome. Antibiotics are not routinely given but in some patients at high risk of infection they should be administered prophylactically. These high-risk groups include patients with diabetes, immunosuppression, biliary-enteric anastomoses, ascites and biliary duct dilatation (DE BAERE et al. 2003; LIVRAGHI et al. 2003b).

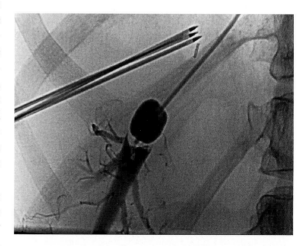

Fig. 24.3. Fluoroscopic image of an occlusion balloon inflated in hepatic vein adjacent to a metastasis to reduce cooling from blood flow during RF ablation with a triple, cooled electrode (Radionics)

Fig. 24.4. a CT image of a colorectal metastasis adjacent to the middle hepatic vein. **b** Under CT guidance, a needle is inserted into the metastasis to enable a coil to be sited within the tumour. **c** The coil is now demonstrated within the tumour. **d** Under fluoroscopic guidance a triple, cooled electrode (Radionics) is introduced into the tumour, using the coil as the target. An occlusion balloon is inflated in the adjacent hepatic artery to reduce cooling from blood flow. **e** A subsequent CT shows an area of coagulation produced by the RF ablation

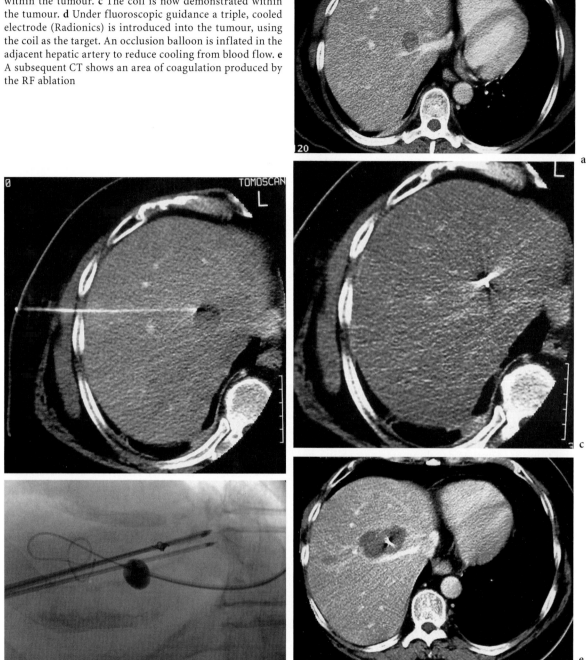

Detailed study of the imaging investigations and careful planning of the procedure are needed. Blood samples should be taken to test the renal function and coagulation status.

When using RF ablation, the operator aims to destroy the tumour and a 5–10 mm circumferential cuff of adjacent normal hepatic parenchyma. Each ablation requires exact placement of the electrode tip in relation to the tumour. A single ablation treatment raises local tissue temperatures to 60–100°C and produces an approximate 2–5 cm spherical or oval area of coagulation.

Monitoring of thermal ablation is usually carried out by measuring parameters such as temperature and impedance. The use of imaging for this purpose has not shown to be very reliable. On ultrasound lesions become more echogenic because of microbubbles produced during the ablation. However, the size of the echogenic lesion does not correspond closely with the area of coagulation. On CT, air may be produced due to vaporisation of tissue. However, the process of coagulation takes some hours to become complete and immediate CT is not a reliable guide. In theory, MR thermometry provides an accurate method of monitoring thermal ablation. However, few operators rely on this method to guide treatment.

Tumours smaller than 2 cm in diameter can be treated with one or two ablations. Larger tumours usually require several overlapping ablations for complete coagulation. However, depending on the patient's tolerance these may be administered in more than a single session of treatment. Each ablation usually lasts 12–15 min. Usually, two or three ablations are carried out during the same session when local anaesthesia is used.

The size of the coagulated area produced in a single ablation session can be increased by the use of multiple electrodes or of a "cluster" probe (Xu et al. 2004). This may have up to nine separate electrode tips, which are deployed within the lesion. One system uses a cooled tip electrode, where cold saline is used to prevent overheating of the electrode tip, and thus prevent local charring which would otherwise limit the energy deposition into the tumour. Another development is of saline-enhancement during RF ablation (Kettenbach et al. 2003; Livraghi et al. 1997). In this technique, saline is continuously perfused through a specially designed electrode into the tumour tissue during the radiofrequency ablation. The rationale is that saline in the lesion increases conductivity of current away from the needle tip, enabling a larger volume of tissue coagulation. Neoadjuvant chemotherapy in combination with radiofrequency ablation may also result in larger areas of coagulation; intravenous liposomal doxorubicin has been shown to result in increased coagulation diameter in an animal model (Goldberg et al. 2002). Chemoembolization in conjunction with radiofrequency ablation has also been used to achieve increased tumour necrosis (Kitamoto et al. 2003). Chemoembolization, proposed by Kato et al. (1981), is a technique that combines intra-arterial infusion of chemotherapeutic agents with arterial embolization of the vascular supply to the neoplasm. The vascular occlusion prolongs the transit time through the tumour

vascular bed, theoretically increasing the contact time between the infusate and the neoplastic cells to increase tumour cell kill and programmed cell death.

In most patients, thermal ablation of hepatic metastases is guided by US or CT (Pedro et al. 2002; Sica et al. 2002; Skjoldbye et al. 2002). However, some tumours are very poorly visible on either US or unenhanced CT. Furthermore, they may appear only transiently on CT images following enhancement with intravenous contrast medium, only to disappear on images obtained a few minutes later. Such lesions are difficult to treat with thermal ablation as accurate positioning of radiofrequency electrodes cannot always be accomplished during the short period during which they are visible on CT following i.v. contrast medium enhancement. It is much easier to perform the procedure under CT guidance when the tumour is visible on unenhanced images, as this allows sufficient time for accurate placement of the RF electrode. However, even when the tumour is easily visible, thermal ablation under CT guidance can be very difficult when a steeply oblique approach has to be used, for example when treating lesions located immediately below the dome of the diaphragm. For such tumours, ultrasound guidance is preferable, provided that the tumour is reasonably well seen on ultrasound images. Poor visualisation on ultrasound or CT images is a formidable obstacle to percutaneous thermal ablation. Ultrasound contrast media are very helpful in visualising hepatic tumours but some masses, especially relatively avascular ones such as colorectal metastases, are not always seen clearly. Livraghi (2001) recommend transcatheter segmental chemoembolization for hepatocellular carcinomas not recognisable on US examination. However, this approach would be unhelpful in colorectal metastases, in which chemoembolization has not been shown to be of benefit. MR-compatible RF electrodes have been developed (Kettenbach et al. 2003). However, magnetic resonance (MR) is cumbersome and time-consuming as a method of guidance in thermal ablation procedures. We have developed a technique that facilitates RF ablation of tumours poorly visualised on ultrasound or unenhanced CT (Adam et al. 2004). This involves inserting a small metallic coil into the tumour during the short period of visualisation on enhanced CT images. This can be accomplished by placing a needle in the vicinity of the tumour using anatomical landmarks prior to intravenous injection of contrast medium. The position of the needle is then adjusted appropriately during contrast enhancement and a microcoil is advanced into the centre of the tumour via the needle. This enables the radiofrequency electrode to be guide into position using fluoroscopic guidance, usually in combination with ultrasound guidance. This technique allows accurate placement of RF electrodes irrespective of the degree of visibility of tumours on ultrasound or unenhanced CT images. Provided the mass is visible, if only transiently, on enhanced CT, it can be accessed under fluoroscopic guidance following placement of the metallic coil (Fig. 24.4).

If a tumour is visible on MR but cannot be visualised on ultrasound or CT images it may be possible to use MR to place an MR-compatible metallic coil, which can be used subsequently to guide the procedure under fluoroscopic guidance as described above.

24.4.2
Complications

Complications are unusual. The main ones are intraperitoneal haemorrhage, liver abscess, intestinal perforation and seeding along the tumour tract. Two recent series reported rates of major complications of 2.2% and 5.7%, with mortality of 0.3% and 1.4% (DE BAERE et al. 2003; LIVRAGHI et al. 2003b). These compare favourably to perioperative mortality of 4.4%–10% following hepatic resection for colorectal liver metastases.

Complications are more likely (a) where the tumour is superficial (within 1 cm of the liver capsule) or close to hilar structures, (b) with prolonged ablation time and (c) when several lesions are treated during the same session. Perforation of a viscus is more likely in patients with advanced cirrhosis and/or poor performance status, when the tumour is adjacent to the gastrointestinal tract and when there has been previous right upper quadrant surgery or chronic cholecystitis, due to the increased development of adhesions in this latter group.

A number of techniques have been used to minimise the risk of injury to adjacent structures. These include infusion of intrathoracic or subphrenic saline which has been described to limit diaphragmatic injury for tumours high in the hepatic dome (KAPOOR and HUNTER 2003; SHIBATA et al. 2002a). Tumours adjacent to the gastrointestinal tract have been treated with RF ablation after percutaneous interposition of a balloon between the mass and the gastrointestinal tract, in order to prevent perforation (YAMAKADO et al. 2003). Percutaneous drainage of ascites and percutaneous drainage of a dilated biliary tree minimise the risk of haemorrhage and infection. Evidence from one case series suggests that RF ablation of tumours adjacent to the gallbladder can be performed safely and effectively; iatrogenic cholecystitis occurs frequently but it resolves spontaneously (CHOPRA et al. 2003). As described above, antibiotics should be given to patients at increased risk of infection. "Hot" withdrawal of the needle may reduce tumour seeding and haemorrhage. When a percutaneous approach is contraindicated, it may be possible to carry out RF during laparoscopic or open surgery.

There is often some pain after the procedure, but this usually settles within 24 h. Approximately 10%–20% of patients have a 1–3°C rise in temperature, as a response to tumour necrosis; this mild pyrexia usually begins the day after the procedure and can last up to 1 week. However, prolonged, marked pyrexia should always raise the suspicion of infection and merits further investigation.

24.4.3
Assessment of Treatment Effectiveness

CT and ultrasound cannot demonstrate the result of the procedure at the time of treatment. Contrast-enhanced ultrasound has been shown in animal models to be useful in guiding and monitoring ablation, and has been used in patients with hepatocellular carcinoma where it appears effective in guiding and monitoring therapy (LIU et al. 2001; MELONI et al. 2001; VILANA et al. 2003). However, CT is more sensitive than contrast-enhanced ultrasound in assessing the response to ablative therapy (MELONI et al. 2001; VILANA et al. 2003). MR has the potential of measuring temperature and providing "online" monitoring, but this capability is limited by several other practical considerations, including the difficulty of using RF in an MR machine.

In practice, patients are followed up with contrast-enhanced CT or MR carried out the day after the procedure or later. Remaining viable tumour appears as an enhancing area, which can be targeted at a subsequent session of treatment.

As with cryoablation, FDP-PET may be used to assess the efficacy of treatment and in the follow-up of patients who have been treated with RF ablation (LANGENHOFF et al. 2002).

24.4.4
Patient Outcome

In the United Kingdom, the National Institute for Clinical Excellence (2003) has recently appraised the use of radiofrequency ablation in the treatment of hepatic tumours; it has made recommendations for RF ablation in hepatocellular carcinoma and is currently working on guidelines for RF ablation in the treatment of colorectal hepatic metastases. The results of several clinical series, which have used different methods of radiofrequency ablation appear promising, with a 52%–67% complete ablation rate at 1 year and survival rates of 96%, 64% and 40% at 1, 3 and 5 years, respectively (LIVRAGHI et al. 1997; ROSSI et al. 1996, 1998; SOLBIATI et al. 1997a, 1997b, 2001). More recently, OSHOWO et al. (2003) have compared RF ablation and resection for the treatment of solitary colorectal hepatic metastases in an uncontrolled study. They found comparable median survival and 3-year survival for resection (41 months and 55.4%) and RF ablation (37 months and 52.6%). Approximately 39% of lesions develop local recurrence following treatment (SOLBIATI et al. 2001). The frequency and time to local recurrence are related to the size of the lesion. In a recent series of 117 patients survival was not found to be influenced by the number of metastases at the time of initial therapy (SOLBIATI et al. 2001). This differs from the results of some surgical series, which reported that tumour recurrence and/or survival were negatively influence by the number of metastases resected (CADY et al. 1970; EKBERG et al. 1987; GAYOWSKI et al. 1994). However, authors of larger and/or more recent reports have failed to confirm this correlation and have suggested that – in the range of the analyses (generally one to eight metastases removed) – survival following surgical resection is not correlated with the number of metastases removed (ADSON et al. 1984; BUTLER et al. 1986; FONG et al. 1997; FORTNER et al. 1984; HUGHES et al. 1986; IWATSUKI et al. 1986; NORDLINGER et al. 1987; PETRELLI et al. 1991; ROSEN et al. 1992; SCHEELE et al. 1991). These findings suggest that the decision to treat should be guided more by the likelihood of achieving tumour control than the number of lesions present.

RF ablation also appears to be a safe and effective technique for the treatment of patients with systemic symptoms from neuroendocrine metastases, although an effect on survival has not been established in this clinical setting (HENN et al. 2003).

24.5
Laser Ablation

Laser light can be converted into heat thus leading to tissue coagulation. The use of laser for thermal ablation was described by BOWN (1983). Subsequently, experimental studies showed that a reproducible thermal injury can be produced with neodymium yttrium aluminium garnet (Nd:YAG) laser (MATTHEWSON et al. 1987). The use of laser to treat patients with hepatic metastases was described by STEGER et al. (1989).

From a single, bare 400 µm laser fibre, light at optical or near-infrared wavelengths scatters within tissue and is converted into heat. Light energy of 2.0–2.5 W produces a focal volume of coagulation 2 cm in diameter. Two methods have been developed for producing larger volumes of necrosis: the first uses multiple bare fibres arrayed at 2-cm spacing throughout a target lesion (STEGER et al. 1989). The second uses cooled-tip fibres that can deposit up to 30 W over a surface area, thus diminishing local overheating (NOLSOE et al. 1993). Portable solid-state lasers are now available with outputs up to 30 W.

24.5.1
Patient Selection and Technique

The indications and contraindications for laser ablation, and the main complications and methods of follow-up are the same as for radiofrequency ablation and microwave coagulation. The procedures are usually guided with CT or ultrasound although MR is sometimes used as well. By inserting up to eight fibres simultaneously it is possible to achieve confluent necrosis of 6–7 cm in diameter. The ultimate burn size is governed by the tumour vascularity and by the vasodilatory response of surrounding normal liver parenchyma.

24.5.2
Patient Outcome

The survival data for patients undergoing laser ablation of hepatic metastases is similar to that following radiofrequency ablation. GILLAMS and LEES (2000) have reported a median survival rate of 27 months and a 5-year survival rate of 26%, and more recently VOGL et al. (2002) have published a study of 603 patients with colorectal metastases, with median survival of 3.5 years and 5-year survival of 37%. In a further large series of 2132 laser ablations performed in 899 patients the rate of major complications was 1.8% and mortality was 0.1% (Vogl et al. 2004). Survival of patients with colorectal metastases is governed by technical success in ablating the tumour and a 5- to 10-mm margin of normal liver around the tumour and by the biologic behaviour of the neoplasms.

24.6
Microwave Coagulation

In microwave coagulation therapy, molecular dipoles are vibrated and rotated, resulting in thermal coagulation of the target tissue. The basic mechanism of heat generation in living tissue consists of rotation of water molecules. The rotation follows the alternating electric field component of the ultra-high-speed (2450 MHz) microwaves (Murakami et al. 1995). Microwaves emitted from the distal segment of the percutaneous probe cause thermal coagulation of the adjacent tissues. The equipment for microwave ablation consists of a microwave generator and reusable needle electrodes. The electrodes are 25 cm long, 18-gauge monopolar units that are placed through 14-gauge access needles. Each needle electrode costs approximately £300 and the generator costs approximately £30,000.

24.6.1
Patient Selection and Technique

The technique, patient selection and main complications are similar to those for radiofrequency and laser ablation. The procedure is usually guided with ultrasound or CT. Microwave treatment produces coagulation within 60 s at a power setting of 60 W. However, the area of coagulation is smaller than that achieved after laser or radiofrequency and it is necessary to repeat the treatments several times a week in order to achieve a sufficiently large area of tumour necrosis. As with RF ablation, occlusion of segmental hepatic blood flow has been used with microwave ablation in the treatment of hepatocellular carcinoma to increase the size of the ablative lesion (Ishida et al. 2002). The use of multiple antennae is another technique, which has been described to achieve an increased volume of tumour necrosis (Wright et al. 2003; Xu et al. 2004).

24.6.2
Patient Outcome

Dong et al. (2003) report a 5-year survival of 56.7% in 234 patients with hepatocellular carcinoma treated with microwave ablation therapy. Shibata et al. (2002b) compared RF and microwave ablation in the treatment of small hepatocellular carcinomas and found no difference in therapeutic effect or complication rates between the two techniques, although RF ablation was completed with fewer sessions. There is less evidence for the therapeutic effect of microwave ablation in patients with colorectal liver metastases. In one series of 74 patients with colorectal liver metastases a 5-year survival rate of 29% was achieved, with no major complications observed (Liang et al. 2003). At present, there is, however no substantial series of patients with hepatic metastases treated with microwave coagulation.

24.7
Conclusion

When attempting to evaluate the benefits of interventional radiological treatments for hepatic metastases, the questions that must be asked are:

1. Can they reliably ablate liver metastases?
2. Can they improve survival?
3. Are they safe?

Interpreting the results of methods of ablation is more difficult than assessing the outcome of hepatic resection (Primrose 2002).

Cryotherapy and radiofrequency treatment can ablate metastases in 50%–90% of cases and are relatively safe compared to hepatic resection. With respect to overall survival, there has been no randomised comparison to show that either cryotherapy or radiofrequency treatment alter long-term survival compared with chemotherapy alone. However, this may be related to the fact that most patients being referred for ablation are considered unsuitable for hepatic resection. The ideal patient for ablative therapy would be one who, several years after a curative colonic resection for an early-stage well-differentiated cancer develops a small metastasis in the middle of a lobe of the liver (Primrose 2002). Such a patient is, however, also ideally suited to surgical treatment and for such a patient the long-term results of surgery are good. Interventional therapy tends to be used in patients who are otherwise considered to be beyond the scope of conventional surgical treatment. It is possible that ablative therapy would achieve similar results to surgery if only similar patients were referred for this method of treatment.

At present, partial hepatic resection remains the method against which all interventional radiological methods of treatment have to be compared. It is important that prospective randomised trials comparing surgery with cryotherapy and radiofrequency treatment are carried out in order to determine the precise role of these modalities in patients with hepatic metastases.

References

Adam R, Hagopian EJ, Linhares M, et al (2002) A comparison of percutaneous cryosurgery and percutaneous radiofrequency for unresectable hepatic malignancies. Arch Surg 137:1332–1340

Adam A, Hatzidakis A, Hamady M, et al. (2004) Percutaneous coil placement prior to liver radiofrequency ablation of poorly visible lesions. Eur Radiol (in press)

Adson MA, van Heerden JA, Adson MH, et al (1984) Resection of hepatic metastases from colorectal cancer. Arch Surg 119:647–651

Baden H, Andersen B (1975) Survival of patients with untreated liver metastases from colorectal cancer. Scand J Gastroenterol 10:221–223

Bengtsson G, Carlsson G, Hafstrom L, et al (1981) Natural history of patients with untreated liver metastases from colorectal cancer. Am J Surg 141:586–589

Bown SG (1983) Phototherapy in tumors. World J Surg 7:700–709

Butler J, Attiyek FF, Daly JM (1986) Hepatic resection for metastases of the colon and rectum. Surg Gynecol Obstet 162:109–113

Cady B, Monson DO, Swinton NW (1970) Survival of patients after colonic resection for carcinoma with simultaneous liver metastases. Surg Gynecol Obstet 131:697–700

Chopra S, Dodd GD, Chanin MP, et al (2003) Radiofrequency ablation of hepatic tumors adjacent to the gallbladder: feasibility and safety. AJR Am J Roentgenol 183:697–701

Cobourn CS, Makowka L, Langer B, et al (1987) Examination of patient selection and outcome for hepatic resection for metastatic disease. Surg Gynecol Obstet 165:239–246

Copper IS (1963) Cryogenic surgery: a new method of destruction or extirpation of benign or malignant tissues. N Engl J Med 268:743–749

Cosman ER, Naswhold BS, Ovelman-Levitt J (1984) Theoretical aspects of radiofrequency lesions in the dorsal root entry zone. Neurosurgery 15:945–950

de Baere T, Bessoud B, Dromain C, et al (2002) Percutaneous radiofrequency ablation of hepatic tumors during temporary venous occlusion. AJR Am J Roentgenol 178:53–59

de Baere T, Risse O, Kuoch V, et al (2003) Adverse events during radiofrequency treatment of 582 hepatic tumors. AJR Am J Roentgenol 181:695–700

Dodd GD, Soulen MC, Kane RA, et al (2000) Minimally invasive treatment of malignant hepatic tumors: at the threshold of a major breakthrough. Radiographics 20:9–27

Dong B, Liang P, Yu X, et al (2003) Percutaneous sonographically guided microwave coagulation therapy for hepatocellular carcinoma: results in 234 patients. AJR Am J Roentgenol 180:1547–1555

Ekberg H, Tranberg KG, Andersson R, et al (1987) Pattern of recurrence in liver resection for colorectal secondaries. World J Surg 11:541–547

Fong Y, Blumgart LH, Cohen AM (1995) Surgical treatment of colorectal metastases to the liver. CA Cancer J Clin 45:50–62

Fong Y, Cohen AM, Fortner JG, et al (1997) Liver resection for colorectal metastases. J Clin Oncol 15:938–946

Fortner JG, Silva JS, Cox EB, et al (1984) Multivariate analysis of a personal series of 247 consecutive patients with liver metastases from colorectal cancer. Ann Surg 199:317–324

Foster JH (1978) Survival after liver resection for secondary tumors. Am J Surg 135:390–394

Gayowski TJ, Iwatsuki S, Madariaga JR, et al (1994) Experience in hepatic resection for metastatic colorectal cancer: analysis of clinical and pathologic risk factors. Surgery 116:703–711

Gillams AR, Less WR (2000) Survival after percutaneous, image-guided, thermal ablation of hepatic metastases from colorectal cancer. Dis Colon Rectum 43:656–661

Goldberg SN, Girnan GD, Lukyanov AN, et al (2002) Percutaneous tumor ablation: increased necrosis with combined radio-frequency ablation and intravenous liposomal doxorubicin in a rat breast tumor model. Radiology 222:797–804

Haddad FF, Chapman WC, Wright JK, et al (1998) Clinical experience with cryosurgery for advanced hepatobiliary tumors. J Surg Res 75:104–108

Henn AR, Levine EA, McNulty W, et al (2003) Percutaneous radiofrequency ablation of hepatic metastases for symptomatic relief of neuroendocrine syndromes. AJR Am J Roentgenol 181:1005–1010

Hughes KS, Simon R, Songhorabodi S, et al (1986) Resection of the liver for colorectal carcinoma metastases: a multi-institutional study of patterns of recurrence. Surgery 100:278–284

Ishida T, Murakami T, Shibata T, et al (2002) Percutaneous microwave tumor coagulation for hepatocellular carcinomas with interruption of segmental hepatic blood flow. J Vasc Interv Radiol 13:185–191

Iwatsuki S, Esquivel CO, Gordon RD, et al (1986) Liver resection for metastatic colorectal cancer. Surgery 100:804–810

Kapoor BS, Hunter DW (2003) Injection of subphrenic saline during radiofrequency ablation to minimize diaphragmatic injury. Cardiovasc Interv Radiol 26:302–304

Kato T, Nemoto R, Mori H, et al (1981) Arterial chemoembolization with microencapsulated anticancer drug. An approach to selective cancer chemotherapy with sustained effects. JAMA 245:1123–1127

Kettenbach J, Kostler W, Rucklinger E, et al (2003) Percutaneous saline-enhanced radiofrequency ablation of unresectable hepatic tumors: initial experience in 26 patients. AJR Am J Roentgenol 180:1537–1545

Kitamoto M, Imagawa M, Yamada H, et al (2003) Radiofrequency ablation in the treatment of small hepatocellular carcinomas: comparison of the radiofrequency effect with and without chemoembolization. AJR Am J Roentgenol 181:997–1003

Langenhoff BS, Oyen WJ, Jager GJ, et al (2002) Efficacy of fluorine-18-deoxyglucose positron emission tomography in detecting tumor recurrence after local ablative therapy for liver metastases: a prospective study. J Clin Oncol 20:4453–4458

Liang P, Dong B, Yu X, et al (2003) Prognostic factors for percutaneous microwave coagulation therapy of hepatic metastases. AJR Am J Roentgenol 181:1319–1325

Liu JB, Goldberg BB, Merton DA, et al (2001) The role of contrast-enhanced sonography for radiofrequency ablation of liver tumors. J Ultrasound Med 20:517–523

Livraghi T (2001) Guidelines for treatment of liver cancer. Eur J Ultrasound 13:167–176

Livraghi T, Giorgio A, Marin G, et al (1995) Hepatocellular carcinoma and cirrhosis in 746 patients: long-term results of percutaneous ethanol injection. Radiology 197:101–108

Livraghi T, Goldberg SN, Monti F, et al (1997) Saline-enhanced radiofrequency tissue ablation in the treatment of liver metastases. Radiology 202:205–210

Livraghi T, Solbiati L, Meloni F, et al (2003a) Percutaneous radiofrequency ablation of liver metastases in potential candidates for resection : the "test-of-time approach". Cancer 97:3027–3035

Livraghi T, Solbiati L, Meloni MF, et al (2003b) Treatment of focal liver tumors with percutaneous radio-frequency ablation: complications encountered in a multicenter study. Radiology 226:441–451

Lu DS, Raman SS, Limanond P, et al (2003) Influence of large peritumoral vessels on outcome of radiofrequency ablation of liver tumors. J Vasc Interv Radiol 14:1267–1274

Matthewson K, Coleridge-Smith P, O'Sullivan JP, et al (1987) Biological effects of intrahepatic neodymium: yttrium-aluminum-garnet laser photocoagulation in rats. Gastroenterology 93:550–557

McPhee MD, Kane RA (1997) Cryosurgery for hepatic tumor ablation. Semin Interv Radiol 14:285–293

Meloni MF, Goldberg SN, Livraghi T, et al (2001) Hepatocellular carcinoma treated with radiofrequency ablation: comparison of pulse inversion contrast-enhanced harmonic sonography, contrast-enhanced power Doppler sonography, and helical CT. AJR Am J Roentgenol 177:375–380

Murakami R, Yoshimatsu S, Yamashita Y, et al (1995) Treatment of hepatocellular carcinoma: value of percutaneous microwave coagulation. AJR Am J Roentgenol 164:1159–1164

Nagorney DM, van Heerden JA, Ilstrup DM, et al (1989) Primary hepatic malignancy: surgical management and determinants of survival. Surgery 106:740–749

National Institute for Clinical Excellence (2003) Radiofrequency ablation of hepatocellular carcinoma. July 2003

Nolsoe CP, Torp-Pedersen S, Burcharth F, et al (1993) Interstitial hyperthermia of colorectal liver metastases with a US-guided Nd-YAG laser with a diffuser tip: a pilot clinical study. Radiology 187:333–337

Nordlinger B, Quilichini MA, Parc R, et al (1987) Hepatic resection for colorectal liver metastases. Influence on survival of preoperative factors and surgery for recurrences in 80 patients. Ann Surg 205:256–263

Organ LW (1976) Electrophysiologic principles of radiofrequency lesion making. Appl Neurophysiol 39:69–76

Oshowo A, Gillams A, Harrison E, et al (2003) Comparison of resection and radiofrequency ablation for treatment of solitary colorectal liver metastases. Br J Surg 90:1240–1243

Pawlik TM, Izzo F, Cohen DS, et al (2003) Combined resection and radiofrequency ablation for advanced hepatic malignancies: results in 172 patients. Ann Surg Oncol 10:1059–1069

Pedro MS, Semelka RC, Braga L (2002) MR imaging of hepatic metastases. Magn Reson Imaging Clin N Am 10:15–29

Petrelli N, Gupta B, Piedmonte M, et al (1991) Morbidity and survival of liver resection for colorectal adenocarcinoma. Dis Colon Rectum 34:988–904

Primrose JN (2002) Treatment of colorectal metastases: surgery, cryotherapy, or radio-frequency ablation. Gut 50:1–5

Rosen CB, Nagorney DM, Taswell HF, et al (1992) Perioperative blood transfusion and determinants of survival after liver resection for metastatic colorectal carcinoma. Ann Surg 216:493–505

Rossi S, Di Stasi M, Buscarini E, et al (1996) Percutaneous RF interstitial thermal ablation in the treatment of hepatic cancer. AJR Am J Roentgenol 167:759–768

Rossi S, Buscarini E, Garbagnati F, et al (1998) Percutaneous treatment of small hepatic tumors by an expandable RF needle electrode. AJR Am J Roentgenol 170:1015–1022

Rossi S, Garbagnati F, Lencioni R, et al (2000) Percutaneous radio-frequency thermal ablation of nonresectable hepatocellular carcinoma after occlusion of tumor blood supply. Radiology 217:119–126

Scheele J, Stangl R, Altendorf-Hofmann A, et al (1991) Indicators of prognosis after hepatic resection for colorectal secondaries. Surgery 110:13–29

Shibata T, Iimuro Y, Ikai I, et al (2002a) Percutaneous radiofrequency ablation therapy after intrathoracic saline solution infusion for liver tumor in the hepatic dome. J Vasc Interv Radiol 13:313–315

Shibata T, Iimuro Y, Yamamoto Y, et al (2002b) Small hepatocellular carcinoma: comparison of radio-frequency ablation and percutaneous microwave coagulation therapy. Radiology 223:331–337

Sica GT, Ji H, Ros PR (2002) Computed tomography and magnetic resonance imaging of hepatic metastases. Clin Liver Dis 6:165–179

Skjoldbye B, Pedersen MH, Struckmann J, et al (2002) Improved detection and biopsy of solid liver lesions using pulse-inversion ultrasound scanning and contrast agent infusion. Ultrasound Med Biol 28:439–444

Solbiati L, Goldberg SN, Ierace T, et al (1997a) Hepatic metastases: percutaneous radio-frequency ablation with cooled-tip electrodes. Radiology 205:367–373

Solbiati L, Ierace T, Goldberg SN, et al (1997b) Percutaneous US-guided radio-frequency tissue ablation of liver metastases: treatment and follow-up in 16 patients. Radiology 202:195–203

Solbiati L, Livraghi T, Goldberg SN, et al (2001) Percutaneous radio-frequency ablation of hepatic metastases from colorectal cancer: long-term results in 117 patients. Radiology 221:159–166

Steele G Jr, Bleday R, Mayer RJ, et al (1991) A prospective evaluation of hepatic resection for colorectal carcinoma metastases to the liver: gastrointestinal tumor study group protocol 6584. J Clin Oncol 9:1105–1112

Steger AC, Lees WR, Walmsley K, et al (1989) Interstitial laser hyperthermia: a new approach to local destruction of tumors. BMJ 299:362–365

Vilana R, Llovet JM, Bianchi L, et al (2003) Contrast-enhanced power Doppler sonography for assessment of vascularity of small hepatocellular carcinomas before and after percutaneous ablation. J Clin Ultrasound 31:119–128

Vogl TJ, Straub R, Eichler K, et al (2002) Malignant liver tumors treated with MR imaging-guided laser-induced thermotherapy: experience with complications in 899 patients (2,520 lesions). Radiology 225:367–377

Vogl TJ, Straub R, Eichler K, et al (2004) Colorectal carcinoma metastases in liver: laser-induced interstitial thermotherapy-local tumor control rate and survival data. Radiology 230:450–458

Wood CB, Gillis CR, Blumgart LH (1976) A retrospective study of the natural history of patients with liver metastases from colorectal cancer. Clin Oncol 2:285–288

Wright AS, Lee FT, Mahvi DM (2003) Hepatic microwave ablation with multiple antennae results in synergistically larger zones of coagulation necrosis. Ann Surg Oncol 10:275–283

Xu HX, Xie XY, Lu MD, et al (2004) Ultrasound-guided percutaneous thermal ablation of hepatocellular carcinoma using microwave and radiofrequency ablation. Clin Radiol 59:53–61

Yamakado K, Nakatsuka A, Akeboshi M, et al (2003) Percutaneous radiofrequency ablation of liver neoplasms adjacent to the gastrointestinal tract after balloon catheter interposition. J Vasc Interv Radiol 14:1183–1186

Yamasaki T, Kurokawa F, Shirahashi H, et al (2002) Percutaneous radiofrequency ablation therapy for patients with hepatocellular carcinoma during occlusion of hepatic blood flow. Comparison with standard percutaneous radiofrequency ablation therapy. Cancer 95:2353–2360

25 Laser-Induced Thermotherapy

Thomas J. Vogl, Kathrin Eichler, Thomas Lehnert, Ralf Straub, and Martin Mack

25.1
Introduction

The liver plays a central role in the human metabolism and thus represents one of the organ systems most often affected, especially by tumor diseases. In the following the basics and data will be presented for treatment aspects of both secondary and primary liver tumors.

Two thirds of patients with colorectal carcinoma (CRC) have liver metastases by the time of death (Vogl et al. 2004). For CRC hepatic metastases, survival is determined by the number and extent of metastases. In untreated patients with liver metastases of CRC the median survival time is from 4.5 to 15 months (Vogl et al. 2004). Only 5%–10% of all patients with liver metastases of CRC are suitable for resection (Nordlinger et al. 1996; Petrelli et al. 1985; Hughes et al. 1988). After resection, the 5-year survival time improves from 16% to 40%. Only 20%–30% of patients undergoing liver resection will remain free from tumor recurrence (Vogl et al. 2004).

T. J. Vogl, MD; K. Eichler, MD; T. Lehnert, MD;
R. Straub, MD; M. Mack, MD
Department of Diagnostic and Interventional Radiology, University Hospital Frankfurt, Theodor-Stern-Kai 7, 60590 Frankfurt/Main, Germany

Up to now the liver resection of solitary lesions has been the only potential curative treatment (Scheele et al. 1996). However, the high rate of intrahepatic relapses and a possible potentiating of the intrahepatic growth in metastases as part of the tumor stimulation process by released tumor cells is considered problematic. In modern oncology systemic treatment, options like chemotherapy and immunotherapy are increasingly supplemented by regional treatment options such as surgery and radiotherapy, and interventional oncological options such as thermal ablation and locoregional chemotherapy (Lorenz et al. 2000; Rossi et al. 1996).

Hepatocellular carcinoma (HCC) is one of the most common malignant neoplasms. In the case of hepatocellular carcinoma (HCC), when the tumor is at an appropriate stage, liver resection or hemihepatic resection or liver transplantation is the essential curative treatment (Bismuth et al. 1993; Fong et al. 1997; Maksan et al. 2000). In patients with a single small HCC and well-preserved liver function surgical resection provides 5-year survival ranging from 47.1%–60.5% (Bismuth et al. 1993; Fong et al. 1997; Maksan et al. 2000). However, most HCCs are unresectable because of underlying poor liver function or tumor multifocality. For small, unresectable HCC nodules the transplantation is effective with 83% remaining free of recurrence at 4 years with a 6% peri-operative mortality. If there are contraindications, transarterial chemoembolization is used as a palliative therapeutic strategy (Lorenz et al. 1996). Interstitial procedures such as MR-guided laser-induced thermotherapy or radiofrequency ablation show a high rate of controlling the site of the tumor.

Within the last decade thermal ablations have been developed and clinically improved. Different technologies have been evaluated like magnetic resonance-guided laser-induced thermotherapy (MR-guided LITT), radiofrequency ablation (RF), microwave and cryotherapy. For this reason, there has been great interest in further developments of interstitial procedures such as laser coagulation or radiofrequency ablation over the last few years.

Laser-induced interstitial thermotherapy (LITT) is a minimally invasive locoregional form of treatment, the coagulative effects of which lead to tumor destruction in solid organs (WEISS 1994; YOON and TANABE 1999; VOGL et al. 2000a, 2000b, 2000c, 2002, 2003, 2004; WANG et al. 2000; WEISS et al. 1986). Due to the comparatively high penetrative depth of the photons and the possibility of problem-free radiation transmission by fiber-optic waveguides, nearly infra-red lasers (NIR) are used for LITT.

LITT provides a photothermal tumor destruction technique, permitting solid tumor configurations inside parenchymatous organs to be destroyed. The expansion of the tissue-destroying effect is dependent on the choice of radiation capacity and radiation time. This means that the parameters must be pre-selected in such a way that all tumor cells, if possible, are exposed to the coagulative effect. Besides, there must also be a safety margin of at least 5–10 mm in width.

In order to do justice to the coagulation of a 3D tumor geometry, it must be possible to heat an approximately spherical volume of tissue at the same time. For this reason application systems of defined space radiation characteristics have been developed, the distal ends of which are prepared in such a way that the result is an even circumference of radiation.

In the following we will present the experimental and clinical data for the MR-guided laser-induced thermotherapy of malignant liver tumors, focusing on liver metastases and HCC.

Table 25.1. Documentation of the application data for the total patient material including all patients with malignant liver lesions. The number of applicators represents the number of applicators per patient. The number of applications indicates how many LITT treatments were performed per patient (an LITT treatment with one laser applicator at one certain location is one laser application). If the laser fiber is pulled back in order to enlarge the volume of coagulative necrosis a second laser application will be performed. One LITT session is the LITT treatment performed on one day with between one and seven laser applicators simultaneously. One LITT round includes all LITT sessions which are necessary to get all visible metastases treated. If new metastases are detected by MR during follow-up control studies 3 months after initial LITT treatment or later, these lesion will be treated again by LITT. This was counted as a second LITT session

Parameter	Mean	Median	Minimum	Maximum
Age	59.5	60.0	28.4	88.7
Applicators	6.8	5	1	34
Applications	11.4	9	1	56
Metastases	2.8	2	1	21
LITT session	2.4	2	1	13
LITT round	1.5	1	1	9
Applicator per metastasis	2.5	2	1	9
Session per metastasis	1.05	1	1	3
Energy per metastasis	104 KJ	82.9 KJ	5.9 KJ	502.4 KJ

25.2
Technique of Laser-Induced Thermometry (LITT)

Between June 1993 and May 2003 LITT was performed in 1421 patients (741 male, 680 female, mean age 59.5 years, range 24 to 89 years) with a total of 3122 liver metastases and 83 HCC. We included patients with different primary tumors like colorectal liver metastases, liver metastases from breast cancer, hepatocellular carcinomas, liver metastases from pancreatic cancer and a variety of other tumors.

A laser application was defined as a laser treatment at one certain position. If the laser applicator was pulled back and another laser treatment was performed to enlarge the coagulative necrosis a second laser application was performed (Table 25.1) (RAMSEY and WU 1995).

We also included patients with recurrent liver metastases after partial liver resection, patients with metastases in both liver lobes, patients with locally non-resectable lesions, and patients who had general contraindications for surgery or who refused surgical resection. The distribution for the different indications varied for different primary tumors (Fig. 25.1).

25.2.1
Laser Equipment and Application Set

Laser coagulation is accomplished using a Neodymium-YAG laser light with a wavelength of 1064 nm (MediLas 5060, MediLas 5100, Dornier Germering, Germany), delivered through optic fibers terminated by a specially developed diffusor. In the beginning a diffusor tip with a glass dome of 0.9 mm in diameter, which was mounted at the end of a silica fiber (diameter 400 μm) was used. Since the year 2000 a flexible diffuser tip has been used with a diameter of 1.0 mm, which makes the laser applications much easier due to the fact that

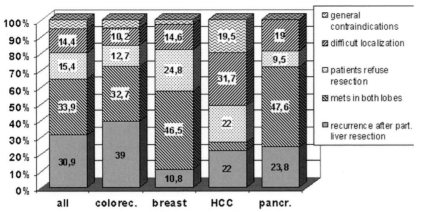

Fig. 25.1. Documentation of the distribution of the indications for LITT treatment for all patients (*all*), patients with colorectal liver metastases (*colorec.*), liver metastases from breast cancer (*breast*), hepatocellular carcinoma (*HCC*), and patients with liver metastases from pancreatic cancer (*pancr.*)

the risk of damage to the diffuser tip has dropped to almost zero. The active length of the diffusor tip ranges between 20 and 40 mm in length. The laser power is adjusted to 12 Watts per cm active length of the laser applicator.

The laser application kit (SOMATEX company, Berlin, Germany) consists of a cannulation needle, a sheath system, and a protective catheter which prevents direct contact of the laser applicator with the treated tissues and allows cooling of the tip of the laser applicator. The closed end of the protective catheter enables complete removal of the applicator even in the unlikely event of damage to the fiber during treatment. This simplifies the procedure and makes it safer for the patient.

The laser itself is installed outside of the MR examination room, and the light is transmitted through an optical fiber. All patients are examined using an MR imaging protocol including gradient recalled echo (GRE) T1-weighted plain and contrast-enhanced GD-DTPA 0.1 mmol/kg body weight (b.w). T2- and T1-weighted images are obtained for localizing the target lesion and planning the interventional procedure. The scanners are a conventional 1.5-T system (Siemens, Erlangen, Germany) and a 0.5-T system (Escint).

25.2.2
Imaging During Therapy

After informing the patients about potential complications, benefits, and disadvantages of LITT, consent is obtained. The metastases are localized on ultrasound or computed tomographic scans and the injection site is infiltrated with 20 ml of 1% lidocaine (SATO et al. 2000). Under CT guidance the laser application system is inserted using the Seldinger

technique. After the patient is positioned on the MR table, the laser catheter is inserted into the protective catheter. MR sequences are performed in three perpendicular orientations before and during LITT (Fig. 25.2).

MR sequences are performed every 30 s to assess the progress in heating the lesion and the surrounding tissue. Heating is revealed as signal loss in the T1-weighted GRE images as a result of the heat-induced increase of the T1 relaxation time. Depending on the geometry and intensity of the signal loss and the speed of heat distribution the position of the laser fibers, the laser power and the cooling rate are readjusted. Treatment is stopped after total coagulation of the lesion, and a safety margin from 5 to 15 mm surrounding the lesion can be visualized in MR images.

After switching off the laser, T1-weighted contrast-enhanced GRE-2D images are obtained for verifying the induced necrosis. After the procedure the puncture channel is sealed with fibrin glue. Follow-up examinations using plain and contrast-enhanced sequences are performed after 24–48 h, and every 3 months following the LITT procedure. Quantitative and qualitative parameters, including size, morphology, signal behavior, and contrast enhancement are evaluated for deciding whether treatment can be considered successful, or whether subsequent treatment sessions are required.

Laser-induced effects are evaluated by comparing images of lesions and surrounding liver parenchyma obtained before and after laser treatment with each other, and with those obtained at follow up examinations. Tumor volume and volume of coagulative necrosis are calculated using 3D MR images and measurements of the maximum diameter in three planes.

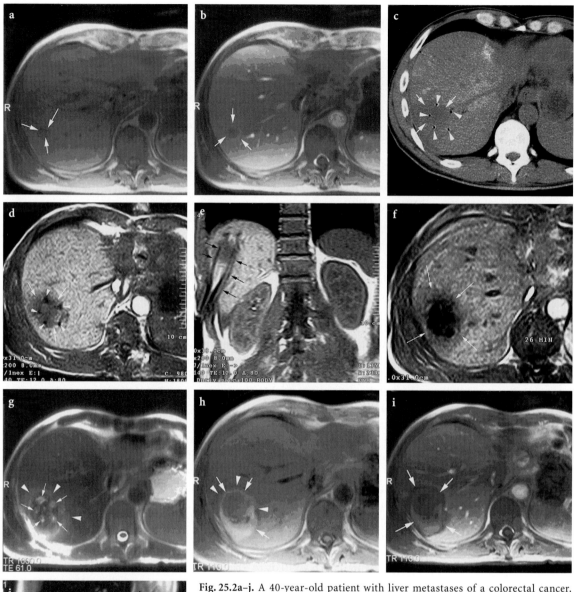

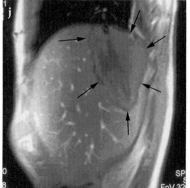

Fig. 25.2a–j. A 40-year-old patient with liver metastases of a colorectal cancer. **a** Transverse non-contrast T1-weighted GE image (TR/TE = 110/5) obtained 3 weeks before laser treatment shows a liver metastasis (*arrows*) in segments VII/VIII with a maximum diameter of 2.5 cm. **b** Transverse contrast-enhanced T1-weighted GE image (TR/TE = 110/5) 3 weeks before LITT treatment shows contrast enhancement in the periphery of the metastasis (*arrows*). **c** CT image obtained at the day of treatment shows an obvious progression of the lesion (*arrows*) in segments VII/VIII with a maximum diameter of 4.5 cm compared to pre-treatment images (Figs. 25.8a, 25.8b). Note the placement of five laser fibers (*arrowheads*) in the peripheral zone of the metastases. **d** Transverse non-contrast image immediately before starting the LITT treatment shows the metastases (*arrows*) and the positioned laser fibers (*arrowheads*). **e** Coronal non-contrast T1-weighted GE image shows the access to the metastases from caudal to cranial. For better visualization of the application systems a magnetite marker (*arrows*) was placed in the protective catheter. The course of two application systems is shown on this image. **f** Transverse non-contrast T1-weighted image obtained 26 min after starting the laser treatment demonstrates an obvious signal decrease of the lesion and the surrounding tissue (*arrows*) due to the increase of tissue temperature (compare Fig. 25.8d). The temperature in the center of the lesion is around 110°C, in the peripheral zone the temperature is around 60–70°C. **g** Transverse ▷▷

25.3
Clinical Data

All treatments can be performed under local anesthesia and are well tolerated by the patients. All patients treated between June 1993 and September 1998 (*n*=278) were hospitalized for 24–48 h after the intervention. All patients treated between October 1998 and now (*n*=613) have been treated strictly on an outpatient basis.

Evaluation of the MR thermometry data during MR-guided laser-induced thermotherapy demonstrates that metastatic tissue is very sensitive to heat, showing earlier and more widespread temperature distribution of the delivered thermal energy than does surrounding liver parenchyma. The area of obviously decreased signal intensity during LITT treatment is identical with the area classified as coagulative necrosis on MR images 24 h after laser treatment. In the minority of cases the size of the coagulative necrosis obtained 24 h after LITT treatment is larger compared to MR thermometry images. The difference is 17% in maximum.

The mean number of treated metastases per patient is three (Fig. 25.3). The evaluation of the application details is presented in Table 25.1. The localization of the metastases with respect to the different liver segments shows a quite homogenous distribution of the metastases in the different liver segments taking into account the different volumes of the liver segments (Fig. 25.4).

The mean number of inserted laser applicators for the treatment of one metastasis with a reliable safety margin with respect to the size of the metastases is shown in Fig. 25.5.

non-contrast T2-weighted image obtained 24 h after laser treatment shows the induced coagulation area (*arrows*) with some inflammatory changes and edema in the surrounding area (*arrow heads*). **h** Transverse noncontrast T1-weighted GE image 24 hours after LITT demonstrates the typical pattern of a coagulation area after LITT with hyperintense pattern (*arrows*) in the peripheral zone probably due to some slight hemorrhagic diffusion into the lesion. Corresponding to the hyperintense signal on the T2-weighted image (see Fig. 25.8g) the lesion is surrounded by a hypointense rim (*arrow head*) due to edema and inflammatory changes. **i** Transverse contrast-enhanced T1-weighted image 24 hours after laser treatment shows the induced coagulation area (*arrows*). **j** Sagittal contrast-enhanced T1-weighted GRE obtained 24 hours after LITT demonstrates the extension of the necrosis (*arrows*), which exceeds the initial tumor size by a factor of 4

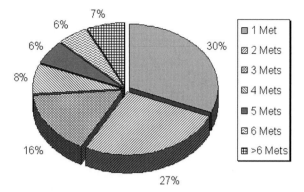

Fig. 25.3. The graph shows the total number of treated metastases per patient, including recurrent metastases during follow-up examinations

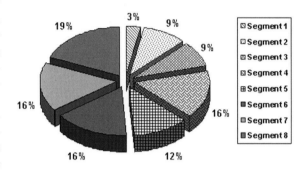

Fig. 25.4. The graph shows the distribution of the treated metastases with respect to the different liver segments

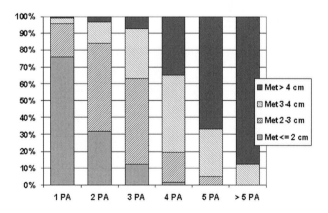

Fig. 25.5. The graph show the number of laser applicators which were inserted for the treatment of one single metastasis with respect to the size of the metastases. PA=power laser applicator

The approach to the lesion depends on the localization of the lesion (Fig. 25.6). Transpleural approaches are avoided in all cases. The most common approach to lesions located in liver segments 7 and 8 is the angulated lateral approach. The most common approach for lesions located in liver segments 2 and 3 is an approach from ventral. An approach is classified as dorsal, lateral or ventral if the angulation of the puncture direction is more than 15° from the scan plane. A transpleural approach is avoided in all cases, therefore the approach to most of the lesions in liver segments 7 or 8 is a lateral angulated approach (Fig. 25.7).

The mean energy for metastases with a diameter of 2 cm or smaller is 48 KJ, for metastases between 3 and 4 cm the mean energy is 140 KJ. The mean values of the applied energy are statistically significantly higher in liver metastases from colorectal carcinoma versus liver metastases from breast carcinoma and hepatocellular carcinoma (Fig. 25.8).

The volume of the induced coagulative necrosis 24 h after LITT treatment exceeds the volume of the initial tumor significantly ($p<0.001$). During follow-up examinations the volume of the induced necrosis is getting smaller again due to resorption and shrinking of the lesion. In the 3-month control the volume of the coagulative necrosis is already roughly half of the initial volume of the necrosis, but still larger than the initial tumor volume.

Evaluation of the MR thermometry data during MR-guided laser-induced thermotherapy demonstrates that metastatic tissue is very sensitive to heat,

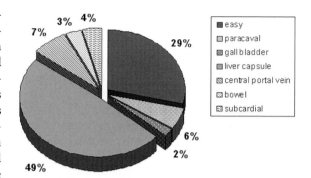

Fig. 25.7. The graph shows the distribution of the liver metastases with respect to the localization of the lesion. A localization was classified as easy if the lesion was sufficiently surrounded by normal liver parenchyma without relationship to any of the other listed structures. A lesion was classified as paracaval if there was a contact to the vena cava inferior. Other important relationships were the liver capsule, the gall bladder, the bowel and the central portal vein structures (including the central bile ducts). A lesion was classified as subcardial, if the lesion was located in liver segment II and the distance between the lesion and the pericardium was less than 8 mm

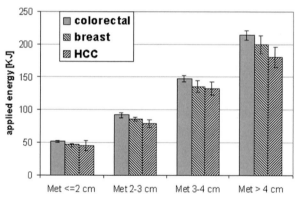

Fig. 25.8. The graph shows the applied energy per metastasis for colorectal cancer liver metastases, liver metastases from breast cancer and hepatocellular tumors for lesions 2 cm or less in diameter, lesions between 2 and 3 cm, lesions between 3 and 4 cm and lesions larger than 4 cm in diameter. Values are expressed as mean plus/minus standard error of mean, which is the measurement of how much the value of the mean may vary from sample to sample taken from the same distribution. It is the standard deviation of the distribution of all possible means, if samples of the same size are repeatedly taken

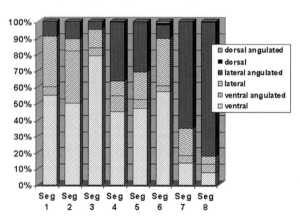

Fig. 25.6. The diagram presents the different approach to the lesion with respect to the different liver segments. An approach was classified as dorsal, lateral or ventral if the angulation of the puncture direction was more than 15° from the scan plane. A transpleural approach was avoided in all cases. Therefore the approach to most of the lesions in liver segments VII or VIII was a lateral angulated approach

showing earlier and more widespread temperature distribution of the delivered thermal energy than does surrounding liver parenchyma. Online MR-thermometric changes correlates exactly with the findings from contrast-enhanced T1-weighted sequences obtained after therapy. The mean volume of necrosis 24 h after LITT treatment is 60 ml (range: 3 ml to 460 ml). After 3 months the mean volume of necrosis is 40 ml (range: 2 to 230 ml) due to shrinking of the lesion. The number of treated metastases and laser applicators is shown in Table 25.2. Plain and contrast-enhanced MR is performed in all cases for verifying the obtained necrosis.

Table 25.2. Distribution of the metastases and laser applications in patients with colorectal liver metastases

	Mean	Median	Minimum	Maximum
Number of metastases	3.2	2.0	1	21
Number of laser applicators per metastasis	2.28	-	1	6
Number of laser applicators per patient	7.6	6	1	34
Treatment session per patient	2.7	2	1	13

25.3.1
Side Effects and Complications

All patients tolerated the intervention well under local anesthesia. Clinically relevant complications such as bleeding, infection, or pleural effusion were observed at the following rates (based on the number of treatment sessions): pleural effusion, 1.1%; intra-abdominal bleeding, 0.1%; liver abscess, 0.4%; 30-day mortality, 0.1%; pneumothorax, 0.1%; injury to bile duct, 0.1%; and bronchial-biliary fistula, 0.07%. The overall complication rate was 1.5%. However, except for the two patients who died within 30 days after the procedure, complications were not severe and could be treated either by drainage or puncture (pleural effusion, abscess) or percutaneous bile duct reconstruction by placing a stent. One patient died 4 weeks after treatment. This patient developed leakage in the jejunum following LITT of a liver metastasis in segment IVa. The patient underwent surgery but succumbed to peritonitis and acute respiratory distress syndrome. The death was considered possibly LITT-related, most likely due to stress ulceration of the jejunum. A second, 72-year-old patient died within 30 days after laser treatment, probably due to sepsis. Unfortunately this could not be proven as no autopsy was performed. One case of intra-abdominal bleeding was self-limiting and no treatment was necessary.

Imaging during LITT revealed a small, nonsymptomatic subcapsular hematoma in 1.9% of patients. Local infection at the puncture site was seen after treatment in two patients and treated with intravenous antibiotics. No seeding of metastases was found in our patients.

25.3.2
Local Tumor Control Rate and Survival Data

The local tumor control rate was determined using plain and contrast-enhanced MR images obtained 3 and 6 months after LITT treatment. Reflecting the development of the laser application systems and the increased experience of the physicians, the patients were divided into two groups for evaluation of the local tumor control rate. In group 1 (treated from June 1993 to September 1996, n=58 patients) the local tumor control rate was 70.4% in the 3-month follow-up. In group 2 (n=119), treated from October 1996 to September 1997 the local tumor control rate after 3 months was 79.4%. In group 3 (treated between October 1997 and May 2001, n=335) the local tumor control rate after 3 months was 97.6%. The contrast-enhanced MR control study 6 months after the laser treatment demonstrated a local tumor control rate of 45.1% in group 1, 64% in group 2 and 98.5% in group 3. This shows that MR-guided LITT results in definitive tumor destruction even in long-term follow-up. During the further follow-up period of up to 6 years after the laser treatment, plain and contrast-enhanced MR revealed no local recurrence later than 6 months after initial treatment. In the late follow-up period MR documented only scar tissue without any pathologic contrast enhancement.

Survival curves were evaluated using the Kaplan-Meier method (KAPLAN and MEIER 1958). The mean cumulative survival rate of patients with colorectal liver metastases was 3.8 years (95% confidence interval 3.4–4.1 years) (Fig. 25.9). The 1-year survival rate was 93%, the 2-year survival rate was 73%, the 3 year survival rate was 50%, and the 5-year survival was 28%. Maximum survival was 83.4 months. Patients with 1 or 2 initial metastases (mean survival 4.0 years, 95% confidence interval: 3.6–4.5 years) showed a superior survival than patients with 3 or 4 initial metastases (mean survival 2.8 years, 95% confidence interval: 2.6–3.3 years) (Fig. 25.10). However, the differences were not statistically significant when assessed with the log rank test, the Tarone-Ware test and the Breslow test for equality of survival distribution (log rank test p=0.13, Tarone-Ware p=0.14, Breslow test p=0.17). Patients with metachronous metastases showed superior survival compared with patients who had synchro-

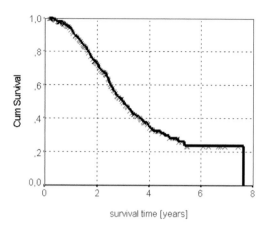

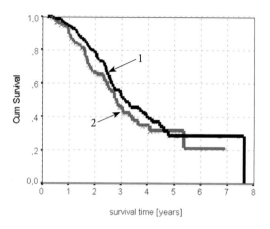

Fig. 25.9. Survival data of all patients (*n*=512) treated with LITT for colorectal liver metastases (*n*=1556)

Fig. 25.11. Comparison of survival of patients with respect to the initial staging of lymph nodes (*1, black line*, group 1: N0 and N1 stage; *2, grey line*, group 2: N2 or N3 stage)

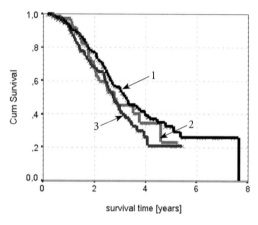

Fig. 25.10. Comparison of survival of patients with respect to the number of initial metastases (*1, black line*, group 1: 1 or 2 metastases; *3, dark grey line*, 3 or 4 metastases; *2, grey line*, group 2: more than 4 metastases)

nous metastases (metastases developed more than 6 months after detection of primary tumor) (*p*=0.11). In our patient collective we found a nearly equal distribution of synchronous and metachronous liver metastases. There were no statistically significant differences with regard to gender or size of treated metastases (*p*>0.05).

In the evaluation according to the primary lymph node stage it can be seen that patients with a N0 or N1 primary lymph node stages have superior survival compared to N2 and N3 patients. The mean survival in patients with N0 and N1 lymph node stage was 4.1 years (95% confidence interval: 3.6–4.6 years). The mean survival in patients with N2 and N3 lymph node stage was 3.5 years (95% confidence interval: 2.7–3.3 years) (Fig. 25.11).

25.4
Discussion

Liver metastases are the most common tumors in Europe and the United States and are twenty times more common in Africa, Japan and Eastern countries. The liver is the most common site of metastasis. Colorectal cancer is the third leading cause of death in Western communities, outnumbered only by lung and breast cancer. At the time of death, approximately two-thirds of patients with colorectal cancer have liver metastases (Stangl et al. 1994). Survival in metastatic liver disease depends on the extent of liver involvement and the presence of metastatic tumors. In several studies, liver metastases from colon carcinoma which were confined to one lobe and involved an area of less than 25% of the liver caused death in 6 months when untreated (Kemeny and Atiq 1999). When 25%–75% of the liver was involved, survival was 5.5 months; and when more than 75% of the liver was involved, death occurred in 3.4 months.

Therapeutic alternatives in the treatment of liver metastases include surgery, local ablation as LITT, radiofrequency (RF) ablation, cryotherapy (Charnley et al. 1989; Finlay et al. 2000; Hewitt et al. 1998; Seifert et al. 2000; Shapiro et al. 1998), microwave ablation and ethanol injection (Bartolozzi and Lencioni 1996; Amin et al. 1993; De Cobelli et al. 1994; Livraghi et al. 1990, 1993, 1995; Shiina et al. 1990; Sironi et al. 1991) or oncologic strategies such as systemic or locoregional chemotherapy (KEMENY 1995; GIACCHETTI et al. 1990; KAWAI et al. 1997; KEMENY et al. 1999; LORENZ et al. 2000). As a high number of tumors grow in damaged liver parenchyma with reduced hepatic functions, it is important for all methods which damage tumor cells to preserve functional reserve capacity, delaying terminal organ failure for as long as possible.

Therefore many local ablation techniques were developed in order to improve the survival of the patients (VOGL et al. 2004). Nowadays, the most common technique is RF ablation. Radiofrequency waves (RF waves) have been used since the 1960s for treating intracerebral tumors, controlled stereotactically. For some years RF treatment has also been used for treating soft tissue, focusing on the treatment of malignant liver tumors. As with LITT a coagulation necrosis is caused through a local temperature increase. Wavelengths between 300–500 kHz are introduced into the tissue through mono- or bipolar antennae systems resulting in the target area heating up to temperatures of 90°C, caused by high tissue resistance. In previous studies monopolar systems were used almost exclusively. The necessity for an external second electrode on patients makes an uncontrolled energy flow outside the required target zone possible in theory, as burns cannot be safely ruled out. Bipolar application systems integrate both poles in one applicator. Cooling the tip of the applicator in RF treatment was introduced to increase the size of the induced necrosis up to 5 cm in diameter.

Rossi et al. (1996) treated 11 patients with 13 metastases using mono- and bipolar systems and the multi-applicator technique. Despite the fact that the tumors were under 3.5 cm in size, one year after the operation only one patient was tumor-free and the relapse rate was around 55%. The findings for the 39 patients with HCC were better, as a relapse rate of only 10% and mean survival times of 44 months have been calculated (Rossi et al. 1996).

SOLBIATI et al. (1997) published a study of 29 patients with 44 liver metastases (size 1.3–5 cm) of colorectal, stomach, breast, and pancreatic carcinomas. Among them there were 20 patients with solitary lesions. The operation took place using cooled systems, and a complete tumor ablation was achieved in 91% of cases. At the 3- and 6-month check-up 66% of the treated lesions were still inactive. A survival rate of 100%, 94% and 86% after 6, 12, and 18 months was documented (SOLBIATI et al. 1997). LIVRAGHI et al. (1997) tried an approach using conventional systems and simultaneous irrigation with NaCl solution in 14 patients with 24 liver

metastases (1.2 to 4.5 cm in size) but only 52% of the lesions were inactive after 6 months.

LIVRAGHI et al. (1999) presented a direct comparison of RF therapy (42 patients, 52 lesions) with percutaneous alcohol injection (PAI) (44 patients with 60 tumors) in treating hepatocellular carcinomas (LIVRAGHI et al. 1999). This was the first direct comparison of these two different treatments in similarly structured patient populations. In all, 80% of tumors were removed completely using PAI and 90% using RF (no statistical significance). The main advantage of RF therapy proved to be the smaller number of treatment sessions (1.2 versus 4.8). On the other hand a higher complication rate (2% serious, 8% less serious complications versus 0% for PAI) was documented (DOUILLARD et al. 2000b). Side effects with regard to punctures are relevant here, i.e. pneumothorax or hemothorax (2%), injury of the bile ducts and the gall bladder, intraperitoneal bleeding (8%) and also pleural effusions. Depending on the procedure some cases had to be upgraded from local to general anesthesia due to severe pain during the energy application.

Our data in a large population of 891 patients with liver metastases from different primary tumors, mainly colorectal carcinomas show a very high local control rate (over 97% in 3- and 6-month control studies) and a very low local recurrence rate. LITT treatment can be performed easily under local anesthesia on an outpatient basis in metastases up to 5 cm in diameter with a 1 cm safety margin, which is very important for a low recurrence rate. Multiple applications can be performed simultaneously.

The wide range of the values of the energy which was applied to the metastases indicates that there is a high variance in heat distribution. Sometimes a couple of minutes are enough to treat a metastasis with a reliable safety margin and sometimes applications times of 30 min and more are necessary to get same necrosis in another metastasis of the same size. Therefore reliable nearly online monitoring of treatment is absolutely necessary in order to avoid over- or undertreatment of the metastases. Due to the fact that laser ablation is fully compatible with MR, which is the most reliable method for thermometry, MR is very well suited for monitoring thermal ablation like LITT.

The survival rates achieved, which represent the most relevant success criterion for a treatment, are slightly superior in patients with metastases from a colorectal carcinoma or a carcinoma of the breast to those in surgically resected patients. It must be considered, however, that a surgical resection was not or was no longer an option among most of the patients being treated due to metastatic relapse after surgical resection or a bilobate pattern of infestation. In spite of this it was possible to achieve survival rates comparable to surgical resection among these patients, who are actually in a group with a worse prognosis. Compared with the extensively published historic survival data after surgical metastatic resection, LITT offers a very good further treatment option (LORENZ and WALDEYER 1997; MARIETTE and FAGNIEZ 1992; HARRISON et al. 1997). Due to the survival data and local tumor control rates achieved so far, in our opinion randomized studies comparing LITT with chemotherapy solely in the case of patients who fulfill the inclusion criteria for LITT are no longer ethically tenable.

In the modern oncological concept of treatment the internationally defined terms of clinical benefit, performance status and quality of life are of the utmost importance. That applies predominantly to patients suffering from local and generally advanced tumors that are no longer curative. Above all, however, intensive chemotherapy, systemic or regional, with marked toxic side effects severely affects the quality of life in the majority of cases. Looking at it from this background all the more attention must be paid to the treatment concepts described here, because minimally invasive techniques are applied which adversely affect patients less and shorter-term.

Consequently the prerequisites are given to integrate these new procedures into oncological treatment programs which have been carried out up to now. LITT, which has been used for the past 8 years in the clinical routine, can play a great part in modern oncological treatment concepts.

At this time, liver resection is considered to represent the only potentially curative strategy in the treatment of colorectal liver metastases (CADY and STONE 1991; DODD et al. 2000; JENKINS et al. 1997). About 40% of the surgically treated patients survive for 3 years and 25% of them are alive at 5 years (BARTOLOZZI and LENCIONI 1996; ARDALAN et al. 1991; DOUILLARD et al. 2000a, 2000b; FINLAY et al. 2000). Repeated liver resections can be performed and can still achieve a 3-year survival rate of 30%. Clinical conditions, the presence of lesions in a central location, lesions in both hepatic lobes, or poor clinical status preclude surgical treatment. In an analysis of a population of 1568 patients with metastases confined to the liver which were surgically resected, there was a 5-year survival rate of 28% and a 5-year disease-free survival rate of 15%

(BARTOLOZZI and LENCIONI 1996). NORDLINGER et al. (1996) demonstrated that factors associated with increased risk of recurrence and death were related to the primary tumor, metastases, and the surgical procedure itself. By contrast there was no correlation with the location of the metastases or the extent of liver resection (DOCI et al. 1991; HOHENBERGER et al. 1988).

Liver resection can therefore be offered only to a small number of patients with a good chance of success. There is a demand for additional treatments to improve the success of resection and to diminish the incidence of recurrence after surgery, particularly in patients for whom surgery is not an option. Alternative methods include oncologic strategies, such as systemic or locoregional chemotherapy, and interventional techniques, including percutaneous alcohol injection, transarterial chemoembolization, microwave ablation, and percutaneous laser treatment (LIN et al. 1997).

Until now, most patients with unresectable liver metastases from colorectal carcinoma have received either systemic or locoregional chemotherapy. The reported mean and median survival rates in these patients are between 12.7 and 18.7 months (FONG and BLUMGART 1998). In contrast, for patients with unresectable liver metastases who fulfill the inclusion criteria mentioned above (maximum of five liver metastases, each one measuring less than 5 cm in diameter), MR-guided LITT offers a mean survival of 41.8 months, which is clearly superior to systemic and locoregional chemotherapy. The results of laser treatment of liver metastases support the surgical assumption that for improved survival liver metastases should be removed or destroyed whenever possible. This results are supported by a study performed on patients with initially unresectable liver metastases from colorectal cancer treated with a three-drug chemotherapy regimen followed by surgery of liver metastases whenever possible (LORENZ and MULLER 2000; FONG et al. 1997). Due to the strongly superior survival of patients who are candidates for LITT treatment compared to systemic or locoregional chemotherapy, we think that a randomized study of LITT versus chemotherapy alone is ethically unacceptable, as so far no study has been able to demonstrate a similar mean survival for patients with colorectal liver metastases who received chemotherapy alone even in a highly selected patient group.

The clinical success of MR-guided LITT depends on many factors. First, optimal positioning of one or more laser application systems in the lesion must be ensured, as determined in three dimensions. The real advantage of MR over CT and ultrasound lies in the heat-sensitivity of the MR sequence and the possibility of visualizing and quantifying the degree of induced necrosis of the malignant and surrounding parenchymal structures. It allows rapid acquisition of temperature maps, permitting nearly real-time documentation of LITT effects. Monitoring of these effects during ongoing therapy is advantageous for a number of reasons. The technique can be used to assure that the entire lesion has been treated, and if there is residual tissue within the lesion that has not been treated, the applicator can be re-positioned under MR guidance during the same treatment session. This technique allows safe destruction of metastases and well controlled coagulation of a safety margin surrounding the lesion.

Monitoring also minimizes destruction of healthy tissues, thus enhancing the safety of the procedure, particularly in the vicinity of vital structures such as large vessels or the central bile ducts in the liver. MR provides unparalleled topographic accuracy, due to its excellent soft-tissue contrast and high spatial resolution. This allows early detection of complications.

Several factors may influence the size and morphology of the areas of induced necrosis, including tumor geometry and adjacent structures such as arteries, portal and hepatic veins, and the biliary tree. The relationship of the tumor to the liver capsule is an essential factor in planning treatment of the lesion.

The major advantage of MR-guided LITT is that it can easily be performed under local anesthesia in outpatients with a low complication rate. Long-term studies yielded a local tumor control rate that depended largely on the technique used and the experience of the interventional group performing the procedure. In our series, the local tumor control rate after MR-guided laser-induced thermotherapy was 99.2%, including power laser and multiapplicator techniques. One imaging system serves in the planning, targeting, monitoring and control of the disease.

Additionally, the factor of a lower degree of therapeutically induced liver regeneration with a lower factor of possible tumor stimulation has to be discussed.

In summary, MR-guided LITT is a safe and effective treatment modality for oligonodal colorectal liver metastases. Our data show that MR-guided LITT allows a local tumor control rate of 97% and more after 3 months and 98% after 6 months, even in nonsurgical candidates. Although the intention of LITT was originally a palliative one, its favorable survival rates compared to those obtained with surgical resection of liver metastases, based on analyses of large surgical series with a clearly lower complication rate, are most encouraging (ADSON 1987; ADSON et al. 1984; AMIN et al. 1993; ARDALAN et al. 1991; BALLANTYNE and QUIN 1993; BARTOLOZZI and LENCIONI 1996; BISMUTH et al. 1993; BUTLER et al. 1986). These data form the basis for an extension of the indication to surgical candidates if there are no more than five metastases with a maximum diameter of 5 cm.

References

Adson MA (1987) Resection of liver metastases – when is it worthwhile? World J Surg 11:511–520

Adson MA, Heerden van J, Adson MH, et al (1984) Resection of hepatic metastases from colorectal cancer. Arch Surg 119:647–651

Amin Z, Lees WR, Bown SG (1993) Hepatocellular carcinoma: CT appearance after percutaneous ethanol ablation therapy. Radiology 188:882–883

Ardalan B, Sridhar KS, Benedetto P, et al (1991) A phase I, II study of high-dose 5-fluorouracil and high-dose leucovorin with low-dose phosphonacetyl-L-aspartic acid in patients with advanced malignancies. Cancer 68:1242–1246

Ballantyne GH, Quin J (1993) Surgical treatment of liver metastases in patients with colorectal cancer. Cancer 71:4252–4266

Bartolozzi C, Lencioni R (1996) Ethanol injection for the treatment of hepatic tumors. Eur Radiol 6:682–696

Bismuth H, Chiche L, Adam R, et al (1993) Liver resection versus transplantation for hepatocellular carcinoma in cirrhotic patients. Ann Surg 218:145–151

Butler J, Attiyeh FF, Daly JM (1986) Hepatic resection for metastases of the colon and rectum. Surg Gynecol Obstet 162:109–113

Cady B, Stone MD (1991) The role of surgical resection of liver metastases in colorectal carcinoma. Semin Oncol 18:399–406

Charnley RM, Doran J, Morris DL (1989) Cryotherapy for liver metastases: a new approach. Br J Surg 76:1040–1041

De Cobelli F, Castrucci M, Sironi S, et al (1994) Role of magnetic resonance in the follow-up of hepatocarcinoma treated with percutaneous ethanol injection (PEI) or transarterial chemoembolization (TACE). Radiol Med 88:806–817

Doci R, Gennai L, Bignami P, et al (1991) One hundred patients with hepatic metastases from colorectal cancer treated by resection: analysis of prognostics determinants. Br J Surg 78:797–801

Dodd GD, Soulen MC, Kane RA, et al (2000) Minimally invasive treatment of malignant hepatic tumors: at the threshold of a major breakthrough. Radiographics 20:9–27

Douillard JY, Bennouna J, Vavasseur F, et al (2000a) Phase

I trial of interleukin-2 and high-dose arginine butyrate in metastatic colorectal cancer. Cancer Immunol Immunother 49:56–61

Douillard JY, Cunningham D, Roth AD, et al (2000b) Irinotecan combined with fluorouracil compared with fluorouracil alone as first-line treatment for metastatic colorectal cancer: a multicentre randomised trial. Lancet 355:1041–1047

Finlay IG, Seifert JK, Stewart GJ, et al (2000) Resection with cryotherapy of colorectal hepatic metastases has the same survival as hepatic resection alone. Eur J Surg Oncol 26:199–202

Fong Y, Cohen AM, Fortner JG, et al (1997) Liver resection for colorectal metastases. J Clin Oncol 15:938–946

Fong Y, Blumgart LH (1998) Hepatic colorectal metastasis: current status of surgical therapy. Oncology 12:1489–1498; discussion 1498-1500, 1503

Giacchetti S, Itzhaki M, Gruia G, et al (1990) Long-term survival of patients with unresectable colorectal cancer liver metastases following infusional chemotherapy with 5-fluorouracil, leucovorin, oxaliplatin and surgery. Ann Oncol 10:663–669

Harrison LE, Brennan MF, Newman E, et al (1997) Hepatic resection for noncolorectal, nonneuroendocrine metastases: a fifteen-year experience with ninety-six patients. Surgery 121:625–632

Hewitt PM, Dwerryhouse SJ, Zhao J, et al (1998) Multiple bilobar liver metastases: cryotherapy for residual lesions after liver resection. J Surg Oncol 67:112–116

Hohenberger P, Schlag P, Schwarz V, et al (1988) Leberresektion bei Patienten mit Metastasen colorektaler Carcinome. Ergebnisse und prognostische Faktoren. Chirurg 59:410–417

Hughes KS, Simon R, Songhorabodi S, et al (1988) Resection of the liver for colorectal carcinoma metastases: A multi-institutional study of indications for resections. Surgery 103:278–288

Jenkins LT, Millikan KW, Bines SD, et al (1997) Hepatic resection for metastatic colorectal cancer. Am Surg 63:605–610

Kaplan EL, Meier P (1958) Nonparametric estimation from incomplete observation. J Am Stat Assoc 53:457–481

Kawai S, Tani M, Okumura J, et al (1997) Prospective and randomized clinical trial of Lipiodol-transcatheter arterial chemoembolization for treatment of hepatocellular carcinoma: a comparison of Epirubicin and Doxorubicin (Second Cooperative Study). Semin Oncol 24:38–45

Kemeny NE (1995) Regional chemotherapy of colorectal cancer. Eur J Cancer 31A:1271–1276

Kemeny NE, Atiq OT (1999) Non-surgical treatment for liver metastases. Baillieres Best Pract Res Clin Gastroenterol 13:593–610

Kemeny NE, Huang Y, Cohen AM, et al (1999) Hepatic arterial infusion of chemotherapy after resection of hepatic metastases from colorectal cancer. N Engl J Med 341:2039–2048

Lin DY, Lin SM, Liaw YF (1997) Non-surgical treatment of hepatocellular carcinoma. J Gastroenterol Hepatol 12: S319–328

Livraghi T, Lazzaroni S, Pellicano S, et al (1993) Percutaneous ethanol injection of hepatic tumors: single-session therapy with general anesthesia. AJR Am J Roentgenol 161:1065–1069

Livraghi T, Giorgio A, Marin G, et al (1995) Hepatocellular carcinoma and cirrhosis in 746 patients: long-term results of percutaneous ethanol injection. Radiology 197:101–108

Livraghi T, Goldberg SN, Monti F, et al (1997) Saline-enhanced radio-frequency tissue ablation in the treatment of liver metastases. Radiology 202:205–210

Livraghi T, Goldberg SN, Lazzaroni S, et al (1999) Small hepatocellular carcinoma: treatment with radio-frequency ablation versus ethanol injection. Radiology 210:655–661

Livraghi T, Lazzaroni S, Vettori C (1990) Percutaneous ethanol injection of small hepatocellular carcinoma. Rays 15:405–410

Lorenz M, Heinrich S, Staib-Sebler E, et al (2000) Relevance of locoregional chemotherapy in patients with liver metastases from colorectal primaries. Swiss Surg 6:11–22

Lorenz M, Waldeyer M (1997) The resection of the liver metastases of primary colorectal tumors. The development of a scoring system to determine the individual prognosis based on an assessment of 1568 patients. Strahlenther Onkol 173:118–119

Lorenz M, Muller HH (2000) Randomized multicenter trial of fluorouracil plus leucovorin administered either via hepatic arterial or intravenous infusion versus fluorodeoxyuridine administered via hepatic arterial infusion in patients with nonresectable liver metastases from colorectal carcinoma [see comments]. J Clin Oncol 18:243–254

Lorenz M, Waldeyer M, Muller HH (1996) Comparison of lipiodol-assisted chemoembolization versus only conservative therapy in patients with nonresectable hepatocellular carcinomas. Z Gastroenterol 34:205–206

Maksan SM, Lehnert T, Bastert G, et al (2000) Curative liver resection for metastatic breast cancer. Eur J Surg Oncol 26:209–212

Mariette D, Fagniez PL (1992) Hepatic metastasis of noncolorectal cancers. Results of surgical treatment. Rev Prat 42:1271–1275

Nordlinger B, Guiguet M, Vaillant JC, et al (1996) Surgical resection of colorectal carcinoma metastases to the liver. A prognostic scoring system to improve case selection, based on 1568 patients. Association Francaise de Chirurgie. Cancer 77:1254–1262

Petrelli NJ, Nambisan RN, Herrera L, et al (1985) Hepatic resection for isolated metastasis from colorectal carcinoma. Am J Surg 149:205–208

Ramsey WH, Wu GY (1995) Hepatocellular carcinoma: update on diagnosis and treatment. Dig Dis 13:81–91

Rossi S, Di Stasi M, Buscarini E, et al (1996) Percutaneous RF interstitial thermal ablation in the treatment of hepatic cancer. AJR Am J Roentgenol 167:759–768

Sato M, Watanabe Y, Tokui K, et al (2000) CT-guided treatment of ultrasonically invisible hepatocellular carcinoma. Am J Gastroenterol 95:2102-2106

Scheele J, Altendorf-Hofmann A, Stangl R, et al (1996) Surgical resection of colorectal liver metastases: gold standard for solitary and completely resectable lesions. Swiss Surg [Suppl 4]:4–17

Seifert JK, Achenbach T, Heintz A, et al (2000) Cryotherapy for liver metastases. Int J Colorectal Dis 15:161–166

Shapiro RS, Shafir M, Sung M, et al (1998) Cryotherapy of metastatic carcinoid tumors. Abdom Imaging 23:314–317

Shiina S, Tagawa K, Unama T, et al (1990) Percutaneous ethanol injection therapy of hepatocellular carcinoma: Analysis of 77 patients. AJR Am J Roentgenol 155:1221–1226

Sironi S, Livraghi T, Del Maschio A (1991) Small hepatocellular carcinoma treated with percutaneous ethanol injection: MR imaging findings. Radiology 180:333–336

Solbiati L, Goldberg SN, Ierace T, et al (1997) Hepatic
metastases: percutaneous radiofrequency ablation with
cooled-tip electrodes. Radiology 205:367–373

Stangl R, Altendorf Hofmann A, Charnley RM,et al (1994)
Factors influencing the natural history of colorectal
liver metastases. Lancet 343:1405–1410

Vogl TJ, Mack MG, Roggan A (2000a) Magnetresonanztomographisch gesteuerte laserinduzierte Thermotherapie von Lebermetastasen. Deutsches Ärzteblatt 37:
B2039–2044

Vogl TJ, Mack MG, Straub R (2000b) Perkutane interstitielle
Thermotherapie maligner Lebertumoren. Rofo Fortschr
Geb Rontgenstr Neuen Bildgeb Verfahr 172:12–22

Vogl TJ, Trapp M, Schroeder H (2000c) Transarterial chemoembolization for hepatocellular carcinoma: volumetric
and morphologic CT criteria for assessment of prognosis and therapeutic success-results from a liver transplantation center. Radiology 214:349–357

Vogl TJ, Straub R, Eichler K, et al (2002) Malignant
liver tumors treated with MR imaging-guided laser-
induced thermotherapy: experience with complications in 899 patients (2,520 lesions). Radiology
225:367–377

Vogl TJ, Mack MG, Balzer J, et al (2003) Liver metastases:
neoadjuvant downsizing with transarterial chemoembolization before laser-induced thermotherapy. Radiology 229:457–464

Vogl TJ, Straub R, Eichler K, et al (2004) Colorectal carcinoma metastases in liver: laser-induced interstitial thermotherapy – local tumor control rate and survival data.
Radiology 230:450–458

Wang SS, Vander Brink BA, Regan J, et al (2000) Microwave
radiometric thermometry and its potential applicability to ablative therapy. J Interv Card Electrophysiol
4:295–300

Weiss L (1994) Inefficiency of metastasis from colorectal
carcinomas. Relationship to local therapy for hepatic
metastasis. Cancer Treat Res 69:1–11

Weiss L, Grundmann E, Torhorst J, et al (1986) Haema-
togenous metastatic patterns in colonic carcinoma: an
analysis of 1541 necropsies. J Pathol 150:195–203

Yoon SS, Tanabe KK (1999) Surgical treatment and other
regional treatments for colorectal cancer liver metastases. Oncologist 4:197–208

26 Multimodality Treatment of Hepatic Metastases

Karl Heinrich Link, Volker Apell, Klaus Tischbirek, Matthias Holtappels, Karim Zayed, Tolga Atilla Sagban, Matthias Mörschel, Thomas Friedrich Weigel, Klaus Maria Josten, Ralf Thimm, and Ludger Staib

CONTENTS

K. H. Link, MD, PhD; V. Apell, MD; M. Holtappels, MD; K. Zayed, MD; T.A. Sagban, MD; M. Mörschel, MD; T. F. Weigel, MD
Surgical Center, Asklepios Paulinen Klinik (APK) and Asklepios Tumortreatment Center Rhein-Main (ATC), Geisenheimerstrasse 10D, 65197 Wiesbaden, Germany
K. Tischbirek, MD
Department Medical Oncology and Gastroenterology, Asklepios Paulinen Klinik (APK) and Asklepios Tumortreatment Center Rhein-Main (ATC) Geisenheimerstrasse 10D, 65197 Wiesbaden, Germany
K. M. Josten, MD
Interdisciplinary Outpatient Oncology, Asklepios Paulinen Klinik (APK) and Asklepios Tumortreatment Center Rhein-Main (ATC), Geisenheimerstrasse 10D, 65197 Wiesbaden, Germany
R. Thimm, MD
Department of Radiology, Asklepios Paulinen Klinik (APK) and Asklepios Tumortreatment Center Rhein-Main (ATC), Geisenheimerstrasse 10D, 65197 Wiesbaden, Germany
L. Staib, MD
Department of Surgery I and Ulm Cancer Center, University of Ulm, 89075 Ulm, Germany

26.1 Introduction

Treatment concepts for liver metastases are determined by the biology of the disease and, in the case of the disease being confined to the liver, by the number and topographic location of the metastases. Colorectal liver metastases are the most frequent indication for the use of regional treatment concepts for the liver. Liver metastases from other primary tumors, such as the breast, neuroendocrine tumors (carcinoids), ocular melanoma, renal cell cancer, and sarcoma, have also been removed by treatment approaches confined to the liver with curative intent.

The opinion that resection of liver metastases is not indicated, which unfortunately is still part of many medical and oncological approaches, should be seen as dated in the light of the results from both the established and new strategies, which using multimodal treatment offer long-term survival or cure even in advanced cases.

Based on single and multi-institutional reports in the literature, surgical resection has been the standard procedure recommended in the various national guidelines (Hermanek 2000; Baker et al. 1997). Recent developments in interventional radiology have shown that the local controlled destruction of liver metastases, mainly of colorectal origin, by radiofrequency (RF) or laser (LITT) induced thermal ablation, may yield results comparable to those for liver surgery (Lencioni et al. 1994; Vogl et al. 2000). Systemic or regional neoadjuvant chemotherapy and regional adjuvant chemotherapy seem to improve the surgical oncological long-term results (Adam 2003; Giacchetti et al. 1999; Kemeny et al. 2003; Link et al. 1999a). The benefit of adding these modalities to the thermal ablative procedures is currently being examined.

Surgery and interventional treatment approaches are competitive on the one hand, but could be additive and open up therapeutic perspectives on the other (Germer et al. 1999; Link et al. 2000a).

Therefore, each individual patient with metasta-ses confined to the liver should be considered and treated on an interdisciplinary basis. This report on the current concepts in the treatment of hepatic metastases from surgical and interdisciplinary on-cological viewpoints provides data to enable the optimal single or multiple treatment modality to be chosen for an individual patient with metastases to the liver.

26.2
Biology of Colorectal and Other Liver Metastases

More than 50% of patients with colon or rectal pri-mary tumors develop synchronous or metachro-nous metastases to the liver, in 25% of patients colorectal liver metastases are confined to the liver ("isolated") and roughly 25% of patients with iso-lated liver metastases are resectable using conven-tional criteria (BALLANTYNE and QUINN 1993). In the case of gastrointestinal cancers, liver metasta-ses develop via the portal pathway by tumor cell shedding via the hepatic-pulmonary-peripheral arterial cascade, which has a surprisingly low ef-ficiency, especially in cirrhotic patients (EDER and WEISS 1991; WEISS and WARD 1991; GERVAZ et al. 2003). Depending on interactions of the target organ and shed tumor cell(s), metastases might be confined to the liver, which is more likely in colorectal than other GI cancers (EDER and WEISS 1991). Solitary to multiple metastatic growth con-fined to the liver is also observable in ocular mela-noma, breast cancer, neuroendocrine tumors, renal cell cancers and sarcomas (LINK 1998; HUGHES and SUGARBAKER 1987; ELIAS et al. 2003a; LEYVRAZ et al. 1997). The biologically relevant confinement of metastases to the liver is indirectly proven by the fact that 5- and 10-year survival is possible af-ter resection of these metastases. Liver metastases usually expand locally in the liver segments, can metastasize within the liver, and might be the focus for extrahepatic hematogenous spread (EDER and WEISS 1991; SCHEELE 1989; SCHEELE 2001; WEISS et al. 1985). The doubling time (growth rate) of overt liver metastases in patients with colorectal cancer was estimated to be 155 ± 34 days, that of occult liver metastases 86 ± 12 days, and the correspond-ing ages calculated to be 3.7 ± 0.9 and 2.3 ± 0.4 years, respectively (FINLAY et al. 1988). In the sponta-neous course of colorectal liver metastases origi-nally confined to the liver, local expansion leads to hepatic dysfunction and death in 25% of patients presenting with hepatic disease (TAYLOR 1962). In the case of neuroendocrine tumors, not only local expansion but also severe endocrine dysfunctions (e.g. carcinoid syndrome or hypoglycemia) limit the quality and duration of patients' lives (ELIAS et al. 2003a; KOCKERLING et al. 1991). Thus, the spon-taneous course is determined by intrahepatic tu-mor load expansion and eventually by extrahepatic tumor spread to the lungs and other (rare) organ sites. Without specific treatment, the median sur-vival time of 104 (historical) patients with isolated colorectal liver metastases registered in Surgical Department I, University of Ulm, was 11.7 months (range 2 days–57 months), and the survival rates after 1, 2, and 3 years were 49%, 17%, and 5%, respectively (Table 26.1). In 47 patients who also had extrahepatic metastases, the median survival time was 6.6 months (VOGEL 2000). According to a number of reports in the literature, the median sur-vival times in the spontaneous course vary between 4.8 and 24 months and depend on the number and dissemination type of metastases (HUGHES and SUGARBAKER 1987). Most interesting is the data of historical patients, whose metastases would have been resectable; their median survival times were also limited to the range of 6–16 months, and 5-year survivors are extremely rare sporadic cases (HUGHES et al. 1988; SCHEELE et al. 1990). In a subset of the Ulm historical patients with isolated untreated liver metastases, the median time to extrahepatic disease progression was 3.5 months after diagnosis (VOGEL 2000). The various biologi-cal factors contributing to the spontaneous course and metastatic cascade have been the basis for the European, Japanese (JCCR 2003), and UICC (TNM 2003) classification systems (Table 26.2) (GENNARI et al. 1986a).

Knowledge about the biology and spontaneous course of colorectal and other liver metastases is the basis for various treatment strategies, which from our point of view should be stage adapted. The treatment modalities available are surgical resec-tion, thermoablation, radiotherapy, radionuclide therapy, systemic and regional intra-arterial infu-sion chemotherapy, and chemoembolization. The currently most effective and widely applied methods worldwide are surgery, systemic and, less frequently, regional chemotherapy; also of increasing impor-tance is thermal ablation. The methods and results of these modalities, used either alone or in combina-tion, are reported below.

Table 26.1. Colorectal liver metastases: treatment. Course of isolated colorectal liver metastases (1979–2002, Department of Surgery I, Ulm, Germany). FA, folinic acid; HAI, hepatic artery infusion; i.a., intra-arterial; i.v. intravenous (systemic); MFFM, mitoxantrone + 5-FU + FA + mitomycin C; n.d., no data; 5-FUDR, 5-fluorodeoxyuridine; 5-FU, 5-fluorouracil

	Patients	CR+PR[a]	Survival rates (%)					Median survival (months)
			1 y	2 y	3 y	4 y	5 y	
a) Spontaneous	104	-	49	17	5	-	<1	11.7
b) Resection and adjuvant therapy (all)	34	-	94	80				n.d.
5-FUDR i.a.+i.v.	14	-	100	86				60
5-FU+FA i.a.	20	-	90	75				>60
c) Palliative therapy								
5-FUDR i.a.+i.v	114	41–46%	-	-	-	-	-	21
FU+FA i.a.	24	45%	-	-	-	-	-	18
MFFM	63	54%	-	54	29	10	-	24
HAI in patients with:								
– Chemosensitivity	13	77%	-	-	-	-	-	32
– Chemoresistance	11	9%	-	-	-	-	-	17
d) HAI downstaging + Resection	12[b]	-	-	-	-	-		≤39

[a] CR+PR: response with complete or partial tumor remission (WHO criteria)

[b] 12/87 primarily nonresectable patients (14%) treated with protocols 5-FU+FA (24 patients) and MFFM (63 patients)

Table 26.2. Staging according to GENNARI et al. (1986b)

H1	Liver involvement	<25%
H2	Liver involvement	>25% ≤50%
H3	Liver involvement	>50%
S	Solitary metastasis	
M	Multiple metastases	
B	Bilateral metastases	
I	Infiltration of the surrounding tissue	
F	Liver dysfunction	

Stages:

I	H1s
II	H1m, b or H2s
III	H2m, b or H3s, m, b
IV	A. "Minimal" intra-abdominal extrahepatic metastases, first proven by laparotomy
	B. Extrahepatic metastases

26.3
Treatment of Resectable Isolated Liver Metastases

26.3.1
Surgical Resection: Indications, Methods and Results of Colorectal Liver Metastases and Other Primary Tumors

The indications for the different tumor types are given above, and are based on long-term survival and cures being possible by surgical removal of the liver metastases. The principles are the achievement of an R-O resection and the retention of sufficient function of the remaining liver parenchyma for the perioperative and postoperative course. The decision to resect is influenced by established disease-specific prognostic factors (e.g. the number and volume/diameter of metastases, their distribution within the liver segments, sectors, or lobes), the topographic location (distance to main branches of the bile duct, portal vein and hepatic vein systems), the prospective function of the remaining liver parenchyma, and the surgical technique/experience (SCHEELE 2001; GEOGHEGAN and SCHEELE 1999; HUGHES et al. 1988; NORDLINGER et al. 1992). Some limits may be overcome by downstaging metastasis, by adding thermal cryotherapeutic or RF ablation to surgery, by preoperative portal embolization to increase the remaining normal liver parenchyma, or even by split time resection (SEIFERT and JUNGINGER 1994; SEIFERT and MORRIS 1998; AZOULAY et al. 2001; BISMUTH et al. 1996; ELIAS et al. 2003b; GANSAUGE et al. 1993; LINK et al. 1999a; LINK et al. 2001). Age should not be a general contraindication, if there are, as in all patients planned for resection, no general risk factors for surgery and anesthesia (Fig. 26.1a–c).

The resection is performed after pre- (contrast enhanced MRT-, CT-, or PET-CT scans, X-rays or CT scans of the lungs) and intraoperative (ultrasound and bimanual palpation, extrahepatic disease?)

staging with the patient in the 30° elevated position, under low central venous and end expiratory pressures, and, if necessary, with intermittent clamping. Up to 75% of the normal liver may be resected, and determination of cholinesterase and the indocyanine excretion test (ICN) may help for estimation of the preoperative liver function. For dissection of the parenchyma, various devices, such as ultrasonic destruction (Cusa, Tyco), a water jet (Erbe), microsuction/thermal coagulation (PMOD, Prof. Ji, Nantong, China, personal communication), or an argon-plasma beamer (Erbe), are used. The destroyed liver tissue usually is sucked away during the dissection with the instruments. Alternatively, at defined locations, clamping and stapling (Tyco) may also be applied. In the case of major resections (lobectomy/sectorectomy), the main supplying artery/portal vein branch(es) and draining hepatic vein(s) should be ligated as the first step for resection. Total vascular clamping or ex situ resections are extremely specialized techniques increasing the technical possibilities of resection, but also the risk of no proven benefit (Geoghegan and Scheele 1999; Oldhafer et al. 2001). On the remaining cut surface, blood and bile fluid control is achieved by ligations and argon plasma coagulation or (more expensive) hemostyptic products (Fig. 26.1d–f).

Usually, the patient is extubated and monitored for 1–3 days at the intensive care unit. Using these techniques, the resection as a rule can be planned and performed anatomically, possibly normal liver parenchyma, and with minimized blood loss. Thus, liver resection today can be performed safely with low morbidity and mortality (Scheele 2001; Rau et al. 2001). Laparoscopic liver resection is evolving for selected indications (Gigot et al. 2002). Only in selected cases with functionally active metastases from biologically slowly growing endocrine tumors may there be an extraordinary indication for organ replacement. If liver resection is performed with strict indications and by teams with expertise, postoperative morbidity is lower than 35% and mortality below 5%. This treatment quality has been sustained for more than 2 decades (Tables 26.3, 26.4).

The 5-year survival rates after resection of isolated colorectal liver metastases have been 23–61%, and depend on selection, expertise, resectional status (R0 vs R1, 2), and, eventually the use of postoperative adjuvant (regional + systemic) chemotherapy, as alluded to later. Surgical cure is possible, since 89% of the patients tumor free at 5 years after resection remained disease free over the subsequent 5 years (Leslie et al.1995). Ten-year survival rates

of 16–21% are reported at median survival times of 18–34 months (Blumgart and Fong 1995). Cures by resection are not limited to solitary metastases, although the 5-year survival rates in solitary (36%) are higher than in multiple (26%) colorectal liver metastases (Ballantyne and Quinn 1993). Survival of 5 years and longer after resection is also possible in other types of liver metastases, but reports in the literature are less frequent and the percentage of long-term survivors is lower. The median hospital stay in modern series has been 14 days (Laurent et al. 2003).

Not all patients judged as resectable preoperatively will be resectable at the intraoperative examination. Prognostic factors accepted widely as contraindications are extrahepatic metastases, ≥4 metastases, and, most important, incomplete resectability (R1, 2) (Hughes et al. 1988; ISTO-Informationszentrum für Standards in der Onkologie 2004; Nordlinger et al. 1996). Positive factors influencing the decision for resection are sizes <8 cm and a possible safety margin >1 cm (Hughes et al. 1988; ISTO-Informationszentrum für Standards in der Onkologie 2004). These are guidelines for the pre- and intraoperative decision of whether to resect or not to resect. According to their independent risk factors for mortality/overall survival (age ≥60 years, primary tumor ≥T3, N-positive, liver metastases number ≥4, diameter ≥5 cm, margin <1 cm, interval ≥2 years; 1,568 resected patients analyzed), the French Association de Chirurgie defined, according to the presence of these factors, groups with low (0–2 positive factors, 2-year survival rate 79%), medium (three to four positive factors, 2 years 60%), and high risk (five to seven positive factors, 2 years 44%) (Nordlinger et al. 1996). Many other retrospective series have defined prognostic factors at liver resection, frequently with variations in results (Scheele 2001; Ercolani et al. 2002; Hughes et al. 1988; Kato et al. 2003; Mala et al. 2002; Nordlinger et al. 1996). A new aspect is the infiltrative morphology of liver metastases, which may be classified into various types in the preoperative CT scan; molecular prognostic factors relevant to the spontaneous course after resection have not yet been identified (Yamaguchi et al. 2002a; Yamaguchi et al. 2002b; Saw et al. 2002). A PET scan can contribute to a better preoperative patient selection for curative surgery in up to 40% of patients classified as resectable by conventional imaging (CT scan/ultrasound), and intraoperative ultrasound may change the surgical plans for 18% of patients (Conlon et al. 2003; Desai et al. 2003).

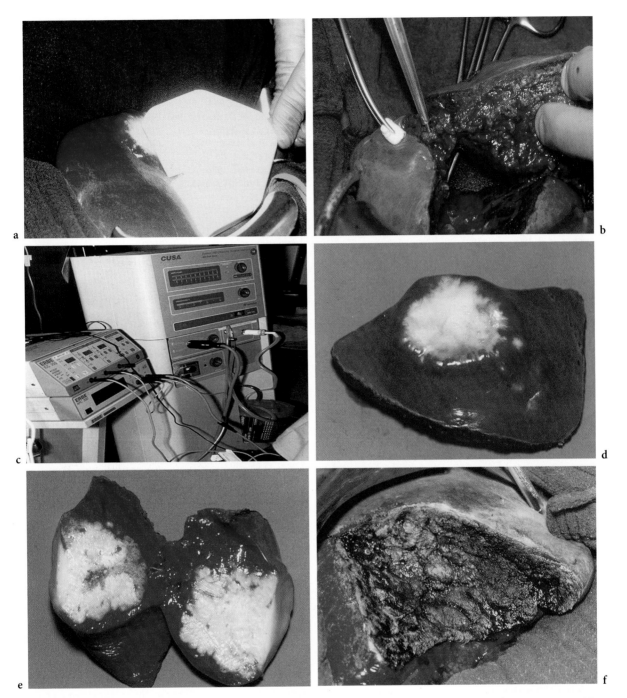

Fig. 26.1a–f. Surgical resection of a liver metastasis with satellite in segment VI using the Cusa technique. **a** Resectable liver metastasis. **b** Process of resection using the Cusa technique. **c** Cusa operating system. **d** Resected liver segment. **e** Intraoperative verification of safety margin. **f** After resection, coagulated liver tissue

In spite of the prognostic estimation, the decision to resect can also be made on an individual basis regarding the potentials of additive treatment possibilities such as intraoperative ablative therapy and postoperative modern "adjuvant" and palliative chemotherapy with reduced tumor load. The most important prognostic factor in various treatment strategies, surgery being the dominant procedure, is the histologically confirmed tumor free resection margin (R0) (SCHEELE 2001; GIACCHETTI et al. 1999; SCHEELE et al. 1996). In a single institution series, 34% of the 376 R0 resected patients lived disease free

Table 26.3. Colorectal liver metastases surgery: complication rates after resection

Author	Year	Patients	Morbidity	Mortality
FOSTER and LUNDY 1981	1981	231	-	6%
BENGMARK et al. 1982	1982	39	20%	5%
FORTNER et al. 1984	1984	65	27%	9%
CADY et al. 1985	1984	23	-	0%
AUGUST et al. 1985	1984	33	27%	0%
PETRELLI et al. 1985	1985	36	-	14%
GENNARI et al. 1986	1986	48	15%	2%
BUTLER et al. 1986	1986	62	26%	10%
1981–1986			**15–27%**	**0–14%**
STEELE et al. 1991	1991	69	13%	3%
VAN OIJEN et al. 1992	1992	118	35%	8%
DOCI et al. 1995	1995	208	35%	2%
SCHEELE et al. 1996	1996	1766	16%	5%
BILLINGSLAY	1998	400	26%	3%
JOURDAN et al. 1999	1999	70	37%	6%
HARMON et al. 1999	1999	110	34%	4%
1991–1999			**13–37%**	**2–8%**
BELGHITI et al. 2000	2000	747	-	4%
MALA et al. 2002	2002	137	27%	1.4%
LIU et al. 2002	2002	72	19%	4%
LAURENT et al. 2003	2003	311	30%	3%
2000–2003			**19–30%**	**1–4%**

Table 26.4. Colorectal liver metastases surgery: 5-year survival rates after resection

Author	Year	Patients	5-y survival
FOSTER and LUNDY 1981	1981	231	23%
FORTNER et al. 1984	1984	65	40%
CADY and MCDERMOTT 1985	1984	23	40%
AUGUST et al. 1985	1984	33	35%
ADSON et al. 1984	1984	141	25%
BUTLER et al. 1986	1986	62	34%
IWATSUKI et al. 1986	1986	60	45%
HUGHES and SUGARBAKER 1987	1987	859	33%
1981–1987			**23–45%**
DOCI et al. 1991	1991	100	30%
VAN OIJEN et al. 1992	1992	118	35%
NORDLINGER et al. 1992	1992	1818	26%
SUGIHARA et al. 1993	1993	109	48%
LEHNERT et al. 1995	1991	182	24%
SCHEELE et al. 1996	1996	1766	39%
WANG et al. 1996	1996	54	26%
NAKAMURA et al. 1997	1997	66	50%
OHLSSON et al. 1998	1998	111	25%
JOURDAN et al. 1999	1999	70	27%
HARMON et al.	1999	110	46%
KEMENY et al. 1999	1999	74	61%
1991–1999			**24–61%**
MALA et al. 2002	2002	137	25%
ERCOLANI et al. 2002	2002	245	34%
LIU et al. 2002	2002	72	32%
KATO et al. 2003	2003	585	39%
TOPAL et al. 2003	2003	105	37%
LAURENT	2003	311	36%
ELIAS et al. 2003b	2003	265	34%
ADAM et al. 2003	2003	615	41%
2000–2003			**25–41%**

after 5 years, while the longest survival time in the R1 and 2 resected group (65 patients) was 56 months. Moreover, the median survival time in this group was 14 months, and these findings were confirmed by a literature review (Table 26.5) (SCHEELE 2001).

The median survival times in R0 and R1,2 resected patients were 41 months vs 20 months, and the 5-year survival rates 34% vs 0.8%. The group reporting 5-year survivors in noncuratively resected patients, however, had a different definition for "curative" (tumor free margin >1 cm). The proportion of R1/2 resected patients was 14% (355/2,164). This proportion should be reduced, if possible, by a better preoperative evaluation, which is difficult. In one of the few prospective diagnostic/surgical studies involving 150 patients preoperatively judged as resectable (GITSG 6584), the Gastrointestinal Tumor Study Group found that 46% of these patients were R0 resected, with a median survival time of 35.5 months, 12% had an R2 resection with a median survival time of 20.8 months, and 42% were nonresectable with a median survival time of 16.5 months. Extrahepatic disease, a criterion for nonresectability, was found intraoperatively in 12% of the patients (BENOTTI and STEELE 1992). One of the extrahepatic tumor locations was the portal lymph nodes. The benefit of a routine portal lymph node dissection is under debate, and has been regarded as negative or positive in principle, negative in the case of macroscopic lymph node metastases, but potentially positive in the case of microscopic involvement. Patients with lymph node metastases near the hilum/along the pedicle may benefit, while patients with metastatic lymph nodes at the celiac trunk may not benefit, from LN dissection (JAECK 2003; BECKURTS et al. 1997; ELIAS et al. 1996; ERCOLANI et al. 2004; KATO et al. 2003).

As pointed out, R0 resection is the most important aim of resection. If a complete tumor removal is obtainable, the patients may benefit from a combination of hepatic and extrahepatic resections (SCHEELE 2001; BISMUTH et al. 1996; ELIAS et al. 2003b; SCHEELE et al.1996). This has been demonstrated by several authors in the case of simultaneous liver and lung metastases, with median survival

Table 26.5. Colorectal liver metastases surgery: re-resection of intrahepatic relapses

Author	Year	Patients	5-y survival	Median survival (months)
Nordlinger et al. 1992	1992	144	16%	-
Gouillat et al. 1993	1993	13	30%	17
Vaillant et al. 1993	1993	18	30%	-
Elias et al. 1993	1993	28	-	-
Scheele et al. 1994	1994	57	44%	44
Seifert and Junginger 1994	1994	20	-	38
Lamadé et al. 1994	1994	23	24%	24
Fernandez-T et al. 1995	1994	170	26%	30
Herfarth et al. 1995	1995	24	24%	32
Adam et al. 1997	1997	64	41%	-
1992–1997			**16–44%**	**17–44**

times ranging between 16 and 30 months and occasional cures (Bismuth et al. 1996; Elias et al. 2003b; Gough et al. 1994; Lehnert et al. 1999; Murata et al. 1998; Robinson et al. 1999). Compared to a group with isolated colorectal liver metastases, patients with additionally resected extrahepatic disease had a 5-year survival rate of 20% (111 patients) vs 34% (265 patients) (Elias et al. 2003b).

26.3.2
Patterns of Recurrence: Intrahepatic Relapses, Prevention and Re-resections

Patients may have intra- or extrahepatic micrometastases at the time of resection, and the surgical procedure could lead to hepatic venous tumor cell shedding (Vlems et al. 2003; Schimanski et al. 2003). The removal of a macroscopic tumor might also accelerate growth of any tumor tissue left in place after hepatectomy (Tanaka et al. 2003). The majority of the resected patients develop intrahepatic relapses and/or distant metastases.

The analysis of relapse patterns after resection of colorectal liver metastases showed that at the time of recurrence the liver is the relapse site in 21–35% of all resected patients in the case of relapse, and may be the only site in 28–29% of the relapsed patients (Blumgart and Fong 1995; Hughes et al. 1986; van Ooijen et al. 1992). In the long-term course, however, relapses have been confined to the liver in only 16% of relapsed patients (Hughes and Sugarbaker 1987). The intrahepatic recurrence rate in a large Japanese series of 585 resected patients was 41% (Kato et al. 2003). In a series of 105 patients, Topal et al. (2003) observed that at 2 years, the intra- and extrahepatic recurrence rates may be similar (58% vs 59%); after 2 years, the hepatic relapse rate re-

mains constant, while the extrahepatic progression continues to develop. These data provide the basis for the indication to re-resect, and to apply regional + systemic adjuvant chemotherapy. Re-resections may be indicated in 8–10% of resected patients, and the results of re-resection reported from experienced groups are similar to those of the first resection in terms of morbidity and oncological results (Table 26.4) (Rougier and Neoptolemos 1997). The 5-year survival rates range between 16% and 44% and median survival times between 17 and 44 months. Even three or more consecutive hepatectomies may be justified (Table 26.6) (Adam et al. 2003; Imamura et al. 2003).

Table 26.6. Relapse patterns after resection of isolated colorectal liver metastases

Overall relapse rates	Initial	Initial plus late
Liver isolated	28%	16%
Lung isolated	14%	7%
Others	20%	13%
Combined localization	8%	43%
Disease free	30%	30%

26.3.3
Resection of Noncolorectal Liver Metastases

Due to their biologic properties, a variety of other liver metastases may be resected with the prospect of the patient living 5 years or longer, and of being relieved of symptoms, i.e., due to hormonal secretion of neuroendocrine metastases. Selected isolated liver metastases from breast cancer, sarcoma, renal cell cancer and Wilms' tumors, melanoma, other GI cancers, melanoma, and, most frequently, endocrine tumors may benefit from resection. In well differentiated metastatic endocrine tumors, a maximal surgical reduction of the tumor load is indicated and beneficial even in palliative treatment concepts (Elias et al. 2003a). The reported 5-year survivors/survival rates are shown in Table 26.7. Overall the 5-year survival rates after resection of liver metastases not of colorectal origin (noncolorectal liver metastases) may approach 30% (Table 26.7) (Yedibela et al. 2004).

Table 26.7. Noncolorectal liver metastases surgery: 5-year survival rates after resection

Cancer location	Patients	5-year survival
Endocrine tumors[a]	203	70–73%
Breast[b]	105	9–19%
Stomach[c]	21	4 pts.
Wilms' tumor[a]	20	6 pts.
Leiomyosarcoma[a]	16	2 pts.
Melanoma[a]	13	1 pt.
Renal cell cancer[d]	11	3 pts.
Pancreas[a]	8	1 pt.
Adrenal cancer[a]	4	2 pts.
Esophagus[a]	3	1 pt.

[a]Elias et al. (2003a)
[b]Link (1998)
[c]Ochiai et al. (1994)
[d]Hughes and Sugarbaker (1987)

26.3.4
Adjuvant Therapy

Postoperative adjuvant chemotherapy may be effective according to phase III trials involving either regional intra-arterial or intra-arterial + systemic chemotherapy in resected colorectal liver metastases, although, due to conflicting results, this therapy has not yet been recommended for routine use (ISTO Informationszentrum für Standards in der Onkologie 2004) (Table 26.8). Patt et al. (1987) (MDA/Texas) were the first to report a larger series of patients with resected colorectal liver metastases and postoperative hepatic artery infusion with mitomycin C and 5-fluodeoxyuridine (FUDR). This protocol was effective in R0 and R1 resected patients, but of significant regional toxicity to the liver and duodenum (Patt et al. 1987). The most recent phase III trial of an interdisciplinary monoinstitutional expert group at the Memorial Sloan-Kettering Cancer Center significantly improved the intrahepatic relapse and 2-year survival rates using a combination of hepatic artery infusion with 5-FUDR + dexameth-asone (to effectively reduce regional toxicity) and systemic chemotherapy: a patient group with adjuvant intra-arterial 5-FUDR/dexa + systemic 5-FU + folinic acid was compared with a group receiving systemic 5-FU + folinic acid adjuvant chemotherapy only. The 2-year survival rates differed significantly, with 86% in the first and 72% in the second group, respectively ($p=0.03$), at high median survival times of 72 vs 59 months, and 5-year survival rates of 61% vs 49% (Kemeny et al. 1999). A Japanese group confirmed these results in principle (Tono et al. 2000). Both groups were able to reduce the intrahepatic relapse rates significantly from 40% to 10% and from 80% to 33% (Kemeny et al. 1999; Tono et al. 2000). In an intergroup trial intrahepatic adjuvant 5-FUDR increased intrahepatic and overall progression free survival vs surgical controls (Kemeny et al. 2002; Kemeny et al. 2003). None of these achievements was reached in a German ALM multicenter trial comparing resection only with a continuous intra-arterial infusion of 5-FU + folinic acid via hepatic arterial ports (5 days, 6 cycles, 6 months). This trial had several weak points, such as the fact that nearly 20% of the patients did not receive the allotted adjuvant treatment, and protocol treatment was completed in only 34/87 patients, mainly due to technical problems. In the subgroup "as treated" the median survival times were 44.8 months vs 39.7 months and intrahepatic progression free times 44.8 months vs 23.3 months (Lorenz et al. 1998). Although severe systemic toxicities occurred in 63% of the treated patients, it should be noted that with continuous infusion of 5-FU the hepatic extraction rate is high, resulting in less effective systemic drug levels (Table 26.1) (Wagner et al. 1986).

At the Department of Surgery I, University of Ulm, patients received either adjuvant hepatic arterial infusion with continuous i.a. + i.v. 5-FUDR (14 patients) or a subsequent approach with folinic acid (10-min infusion) followed by 5-FU (2-h infusion) days 1–5, 4-week intermission, six cycles (20 patients). The second approach had the theoretical advantage of providing a high regional and sufficient systemic concentration × time ($c×t$) interaction (Link et al. 1993). The 2-year survival rates were 86% in the first group, and 75% in the second group, and the survival curves divided after 3 years with an advantage for hepatic artery infusion (HAI) with 5-FU+FA (Table 26.1). The median survival time in the FUDR group was 60 months, and for the 5-FU+FA group it has not been reached. There was a significant disadvantage for 5-FUDR in terms of regional toxicity with sclerosing cholangitis in 24–26%

and duodenal ulcers (LINK et al. 1993). Adjuvant hepatic artery infusion with 5-FU alone had no survival benefit in a large case control series, although this treatment was effective in nonresected patients (KATO et al. 2003).

If adjuvant therapy is considered, HAI with 5-FU+FA according to the Ulm/ART protocol or HAI with 5-FUDR+5-FU/folinic acid or CPT 11 i.v. with strict adherence to the infusion times, dose modifications and supportive therapies could be treatment options (KEMENY et al. 2003; LINK et al. 1993). Due to the hepatotoxicity (sclerosing cholangitis) of HAI with 5-FUDR, this adjuvant treatment could reduce the patient's quality of life, induce life-threatening biliary cirrhosis, and increase the risk in (the rare) cases where (re-)resection is indicated (HODGSON 1986; HOHN et al. 1988; ONAITIS et al. 2003).

To date, there has not been a positive trial confirming the benefit of systemic adjuvant chemotherapy although this treatment has been applied by oncologists in more than 50% of cases (O'CONNELL and ADSON 1985; LANGER et al. 2002; PORTIER et al. 2002).

Adjuvant intraportal infusion after resection of colorectal liver metastases has not been effective, like palliative intraportal infusion (TSUJITANI and WATANABE 1991; SIGURDSON et al. 1987). Prophylactic intraportal infusion has been tested in several adjuvant trials after curative primary colon and rectal cancer resection. Although hepatic progression was reduced in some of the trials, this could not be translated into a definite survival benefit (LINK et al. 1986). In view of the proven benefit of systemic chemotherapy in reducing progression and improving survival, systemic adjuvant chemotherapy is the method of choice in reducing the frequency of hepatic and extrahepatic metastasis (LINK et al. 1996a). As a new approach, adjuvant hepatic arterial infusion with 5-FU might reduce hepatic progression and improve survival significantly

after curative resection of stage III colon cancer (SADAHIRO et al. 2004).

New adjuvant trials involving optimal regional + systemic treatment protocols are mandatory, and one of the improvements may be the combination of intra-arterial infusion of 5-FUDR + dexamethasone and systemic chemotherapy with CPT 11 (Table 26.8) (KEMENY et al. 2003).

26.3.5
Neoadjuvant Therapy

In view of the fact that modern systemic protocols like FOLFOX or FOLFIRI are able to downstage nonresectable liver metastases in a similar way to that reported with hepatic arterial infusion trials, the a priori pre-treatment of resectable metastases (neoadjuvant) has been the objective of recent phase II and III trials. Wein et al. treated 20 patients with resectable colorectal liver metastases within a monoinstitutional phase II trial at the University of Erlangen-Nuernberg with weekly systemic high-dose 5-FU + folinic acid and oxaliplatin (modified FOLFOX). All patients responded to therapy (CR 10%, PR 90%), and the curative resectability rate was 80%, the 2-year cancer related survival rate was 72% in all patients, and 80% in the 16 patients resected for cure (WEIN et al. 2003). An EORTC phase III trial comparing neoadjuvant FOLFOX to surgery only is still recruiting. In a retrospective study, neoadjuvant chemotherapy with FOLFOX, FOLFIRI or hepatic artery infusion with 5-FU+FA+CDDP compared to surgery only in advanced (≥5, bilobar) principally resectable colorectal liver metastases had an independent positive prognostic impact on survival and reduced the extent of surgery (TANAKA et al. 2003). Neoadjuvant chemotherapy seems to extinguish free disseminated tumor cells (VLEMS et al. 2003).

Table 26.8. Colorectal liver metastases surgery: adjuvant treatment after resection

Author	Year	Patients	Treatment	rHep	2-y survival	5-y survival	Median survival (months)
M. KEMENY (ECOG, SWOG)	2002	30	HAI+i.v. CT	50%c	~65%	~55%	64
		45	Observation	69%	~55%	~40%	49
N. KEMENY (MSKCC)	1999	74	HAI+i.v. CT	10%[a]	86%[b]	61%	72
		82	i.v. CT	40%	72%	49%	59
M. LORENZ (ALM)	1998	113	HAI	33%	~61%	?	35
		113	Observation	37%	~60%	?	41
K. H. LINK	2003	21	HAI 5-FU+FA	20%	75%	>60%?	Not reached

26.4
Treatment of Nonresectable Isolated Liver Metastases

26.4.1
Systemic Chemotherapy, Downstaging and Resection

The majority of patients with colorectal and other liver metastases are not candidates for resection due to extensive intrahepatic nonresectable disease or simultaneous extrahepatic spread. Palliative liver resection may be indicated in hormonally active endocrine liver metastases, but not in colorectal cancer, since R2 resection of colorectal liver metastases results in median survival times between 15 and 23 months (Benotti and Steele 1992; Steele et al. 1991). In these patients palliative chemotherapy is indicated, especially since the chemotherapeutic results have improved dramatically during the last decade (Table 26.9).

There is no doubt that chemotherapy improves survival time and quality compared to supportive treatment, which was frequent practice in the 5-FU i.v. monotherapy era (Allen-Mersh 1994; Jonker et al. 1999; Rougier et al. 1992; Scheithauer et al. 1993; The Nordic Gastrointestinal Tumor Adjuvant Therapy Group 1992). In the 1980s and early 1990s, 5-FU monotherapy in patients with hepatic and extrahepatic metastasis was improved by modulation with folinic acid to significantly higher response rates (22–23%), and, marginally, median survival times of 11–11.5 months (Advanced Colorectal Cancer Meta-Analysis Project 1992; Meta-analysis Group In Cancer 1998). In patients with nonresectable metastases confined to the liver, the median survival times of 11.3–12.7 months were similar to the whole group with metastatic colorectal cancer, and therefore definitely lower than 35–46 months in the patients with the option for surgical cure by resection, and 5-year

survival under systemic chemotherapy was sporadic (Scheele 2001; Thirion et al. 1999). The effectiveness of modern protocols combining the modulated fluoropyrimidine treatment with either oxaliplatin (e.g. FOLFOX) or CPT 11 (FOLFIRI) increased dramatically to response rates of 34–67% and median survival times of 15–19 months (Table 26.9). A major achievement of these modern protocols from a surgical oncological point of view is the fact that responding "downstaged" metastases could be resected with the option for cure (Bismuth et al. 1996; Giacchetti et al. 1999). Bismuth et al. (1996) were the first to report the possibility of resecting metastases responding to FOLFOX in 13% of a large group of patients who were considered primarily nonresectable with hepatic ± extrahepatic metastases, with a 5-year survival rate of 33%. Giacchetti et al. (1999) reanalyzed the subset of 151 nonresectable patients with isolated nonresectable liver metastases who were treated with a chronomodulated FOLFOX regime and, eventually, resected at Hôpital Paul Brousse, Villejuif, France. Of the 151 patients receiving palliative chronomodulated 5-FU+FA+oxaliplatin, 59% responded, the median survival time was 24 months, and the 5-year survival rate was 28%. More than 50% (77/151) of the patients were operated on, and 38% (58/151) had a complete resection of their liver metastases, resulting in a complete resection rate of 75% in the operated subgroup (58/77). The 5-year survival rates were 50% in the operated group (median survival time 48 months), 58% in the R0-resected patients, and <5% in the non-operated group (median survival time 15.5 months). Downstaging and secondary resection of primarily nonresectable disease is also possible with FOLFIRI (Adam 2003). These new developments in systemic chemotherapy underline the importance of treating patients with active protocols involving effective chemotherapy and aggressive surgery within interdisciplinary programs (Table 26.10) (Adam et al. 2001; Bismuth et al. 1996; Giacchetti et al. 1999).

Table 26.9. Systemic chemotherapy in metastasized colorectal cancer. 5-FU, 5-fluorouracil; FA, folinic acid; c.i., continuous infusion; Oxa, oxaliplatin; CPT11, irinotecan

Treatment protocol	Response rate	Median survival time (months)
5-FU (Advanced Colorectal Cancer Meta-analysis Project 1997)	11%	11
5-FU+FA (Advanced Colorectal Cancer Meta-analysis Project 1997)	23%	11.5
5-FU+FA c.i. (Meta-analysis Group In Cancer 1998)	22%	"Better"
5-FU+FA+Oxa (Giacchetti et al. 2000)	34–67%	15–19
5-FU+FA+CPT11 (Douillard et al. 2000; Saltz et al. 2000)	39–49%	15–17

Table 26.10. Colorectal liver metastases surgery: neoadjuvant treatment of nonresectable isolated liver metastases, downstaging and resection

	Resectable	Resection rate	Survival (months)
HAI			
Ulm 1997/1999 (FORMENTINI et al. 1997; LINK et al. 1999; LINK et al. 2001)	11/74	15%	<81
Ulm 2001 (FORMENTINI et al. 1997; LINK et al. 1999; LINK et al. 2001)	9/63	14%	39.2
Literature (HODGSON et al. 1986; HELIAS et al. 1995; MARNO et al. 1996; FUJITA et al. 1998; LORENZ et al. 1997; WADLER et al. 1989)	44/383	5–25%	14–60
i.v. CT			
Bismuth (BISMUTH et al. 1996)	53/330	16%	5-y survival 40%

26.4.2
Regional Chemotherapy, Downstaging and Resection

During the fluoropyrimidine monotherapy period, many surgical and medical oncologists have favored regional intra-arterial chemotherapy in patients with isolated nonresectable liver metastases, since response rates were significantly higher than in systemic chemotherapy (CHRISTOFORIDIS et al. 2002; LINK et al. 1999b; META-ANALYSIS GROUP IN CANCER 1996). Regional chemotherapeutic protocols traditionally have induced higher response rates, and a significant number of long-term survivors without surgical resection (FUJIMOTO et al. 1985; LINK et al. 1999b). In a meta-analysis of phase III trials comparing regional vs systemic fluoropyrimidine therapy, the response rates were 41% vs 14% ($p<10^{-10}$) and median survival times 15 months vs 10 months ($p<0.0009$). In view of the modern systemic combination protocols, regional chemotherapy seems to have lost importance, although phase III data comparing intra-arterial (+systemic) vs systemic chemotherapy are not available yet. Due to the high response rates, resection after downstaging has been reported longstanding by various groups using hepatic artery infusion protocols based on 5-FU.

Although expert teams at specialized centers can safely and effectively apply 5-FUDR, this hepatic arterial treatment via infusion pumps has shown no advantage in comparison to 5-FU + folinic acid i.a. or i.v. in a German multicenter trial in terms of survival, and may be associated with potentially lethal hepatotoxicity, which increases the risk for resection after downstaging (LORENZ and MULLER 2000; KEMENY et al. 1994; KEMENY et al. 1999; HOHN et al. 1988; HODGSON 1986; PATT et al. 1987). With regard to the 5-FUDR induced hepatotoxicity, we had stopped this treatment protocol in favor of 5-FU + folinic acid, and developed this new protocol by translational in vitro research on chemosensitivity of tumor cells from individual colorectal liver metastatic biopsies (Table 26.1) (LINK et al. 1993; LINK et al. 1998). The response rate to the Ulm protocol of mitoxantrone + 5-FU + folinic acid + mitomycin C (MFFM) was 54%, and the median survival time 24 months (LINK et al. 2001). If the Ulm chemotherapeutic protocol was tailored according to the individual cell culture and PCR test based chemosensitivity of a patient, the response rates and median survival times in the chemosensitive patients (CR+PR 77%, median survival 32 months) were significantly higher than in the potentially resistant group (CR+PR 9%, median survival 17 months). The predictability of response was improved by adding a test for quantitative expression of thymidylate synthase (TS) using a reverse transcriptase PCR, developed by P.V. and K. Danenberg, to the cell culture assay (LINK et al. 1986; LINK et al. 1994; LINK et al. 1996b; LINK et al. 2000b; KORNMANN et al. 1997). Testing for chemosensitivity, proven to be effective in regional chemotherapy, might increase the response (=downstaging) and thereupon the probability of receiving a potentially curative resection in combination with effective chemotherapy (Fig. 26.2).

In Fig. 26.2, a case with split time resection and sensitivity directed hepatic arterial chemotherapy during the interval between the two resections is shown. We were also able to downstage and resect patients with nonresectable liver metastases (LINK et al. 1999a). In the MFFM group, 9/63 patients (12%) could be resected after downstaging, and this subgroup had a median survival time of 39 months after the start of chemotherapy, and 22.8 months after resection. Even in patients with nonresectable primary tumors and disseminated nonresectable liver metastases, downstaging and resection of the rectal cancer by radiotherapy combined with systemic chemotherapy, and subsequent liver resection after response to hepatic artery infusion, may offer a chance for cure (KORNMANN and LINK 2002). The

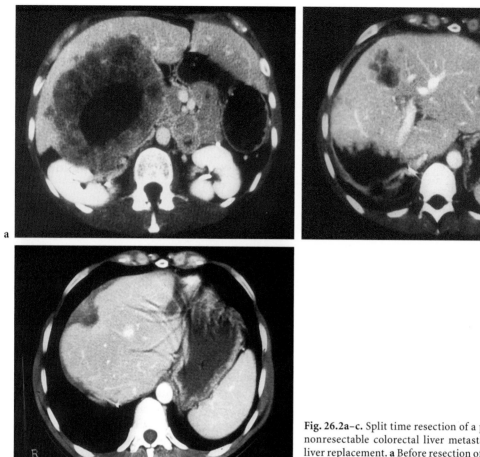

Fig. 26.2a–c. Split time resection of a patient with primarily nonresectable colorectal liver metastases, due to extended liver replacement. **a** Before resection of the right lobe. **b** After resection before HAI. **c** After second resection (left lobe resected)

modern Ulm protocols induced no sclerosing cholangitis (Table 26.1). Regional chemotherapeutic protocols can be improved by adding oxaliplatin or CPT 11 to a standard protocol or adding systemic (i.v.) drugs like CPT 11 to the intra-arterial (i.e., 5-FUDR) protocol; these strategies might increase intrahepatic response and the "adjuvant" effect against occult extrahepatic disease, preventing the imminent extrahepatic progression (KEMENY et al. 2001; KERN et al. 2001; KORNMANN et al. 2000; VAN RIEL et al. 2002). Systemic CPT-11 might be more effective than 5-FU+FA, since lung metastases have a different TS expression (KEMENY et al. 2003).

26.4.3
Thermoablation

Thermoablation is more effective than systemic or regional chemotherapy to achieve complete tumor destruction and long-term survival in selected non-

resectable patients. LENCIONI et al. (1998) was one of the first in Europe to report the feasibility and effectiveness of cooled-tip RF ablation of colorectal metastasis (LENCIONI et al. 1998).

If the limits of this procedure are respected (i.e., diameter ≤5 cm, number ≤5), high rates of complete destruction, 2-year survival rates of 70–80%, and median survival times of 27–37 months are obtainable with RF ablation or LITT (VOGL et al. 2000). These results were obtained in nonresectable liver metastases, intrahepatic relapses, and resectable metastases. The thermoablative treatment of resectable colorectal liver metastases (and metastases from other primary tumors) is not (yet) recommended in guidelines as standard, but is supposed to avoid unnecessary surgery in nearly 50% of patients who, e.g., are prone to developing extrahepatic progression, and it is claimed to be as effective as resection, with median survival times of 25 months in resected vs 27 months in RF-treated patient groups (LIVRAGHI et al. 2003; SHIBATA et al. 2000). Comparative studies in solitary colorectal liver metastases indicate, with median survival times/3-year survival rates of 41 months/55% (surgery) vs 37 months/53% (RF), that radiofrequency ablation is less invasive and the outcome comparable to resection at lower morbidity (Oshowo et al. 2003). If technically possible and indicated, interventional thermoablative treatment is indicated in nonresectable patients and patients with intrahepatic relapses (Lencioni et al. 1994; Vogl et al. 2000; Vogl et al. 2004). LITT or RF is also applied in resectable liver metastases, but data from phase III trials supporting this concept with a high level of evidence are pending (Livraghi et al. 2003; Oshowo et al. 2003; Shibata et al. 2000; Vogl et al. 2000; Vogl et al. 2004). At least in large, complex lesions, RF ablation should not replace resection as the primary treatment in resectable tumors (Bleicher et al. 2003). Regarding the limits of each procedure – surgery and RF ablation – both methods could be complementary with the aim of completely removing/destroying all viable tumor (Evrard et al. 2004).

26.4.4
Combination of Procedures

The benefit of combining chemotherapy with surgery has been demonstrated by reports from Hôpital Paul Brousse and others involving systemic chemotherapy, and numerous groups applying regional chemotherapy (Adam 2003; Maruo and Kosaka 1994; Adam et al. 2001; Bismuth et al. 1996; Elias et al. 1995; Fowler et al. 1992; Giacchetti et al. 1999; Kemeny et al. 1999; Link et al. 2000a; Patt et al. 1987). Physical principles might also be effectively added to resection. The intraoperative addition of cryotherapy to resection $\pm$ postoperative hepatic artery infusion or preoperative + postoperative chemotherapy in nonresectable liver metastases has been put forward by various groups (Link 2000; Rivoire et al. 2002; Shen et al. 2002; Yan et al. 2003). In the Australian report from the group of Morris, out of 172 patients with primarily unresectable liver metastases, 85% were tumor free after resection, and the 5-year survival rate was 15% (Yan et al. 2003). Additive cryotherapy to nonresectable metastases, split time resection, preoperative portal vein embolization and postoperative chemotherapy, in addition to preoperative chemotherapy, have been the oncologic tools used at Centre Hepato Biliare Paul Brousse, Paris, to achieve complete intrahepatic disease control in patients who could not be

cured by anatomical standard resection (Adam 2003). The combination of resection with intraoperative RF ablation is feasible and effective. The cure rate is higher than with either method alone, and the morbidity of resection is reduced (Evrard et al. 2004; Pawlik et al. 2003).

Portal vein embolization and split time resection increase the remnant liver volume and thus help to avoid postinterventional liver dysfunction (Fig. 26.3) (Azoulay et al. 2001; Hemming et al. 2003).

Most recent approaches add resection, intraoperative RF ablation, and postinterventional chemotherapy to the treatment of advanced or systemically pre-treated colorectal liver metastases with the aim of locally controlling the disease as long as possible with multimodal multiple interventions. Regional chemotherapy added to RF ablation, with or without resection, was studied as one of the various possible combinations. Extrahepatic progression and regional 5-FUD-related toxicity were the major problems of this procedure (Scaife et al. 2003). If 5-FU+FA (ART Protocol) or combinations with 5-FU+FA are used, regional toxicity compared to 5-FUDR according to our data is reduced, and 5-FU+FA has potentially active systemic levels (AUCs), so that this therapy can also be safely used for combination treatments (Fig. 26.3) (Link et al. 1993).

26.5
Stage Adapted Individualized Treatment Concept

Surgery, ablation, and chemotherapy of liver metastases and their combinations have evolved dramatically during recent years, offering the chance for unexpected cures in patients traditionally considered unresectable and thus prone to die of metastatic disease. The eminent new treatment perspectives and exciting results in stage adapted resection and multimodal therapy of colorectal and other liver metastases are highly stimulating and should definitely convince those hesitating to treat (isolated) colorectal liver metastases by observation or "soft" chemotherapy. Nowadays there is a multiplicity of treatment methods to offer patients with metastases confined to the liver the chance for cure or long-term survival. Most experience has been gained with colorectal liver metastases. In this indication either single or multimodal treatment approaches are possible on the one hand, but the multiplicity of treatment possibilities might confuse on the other.

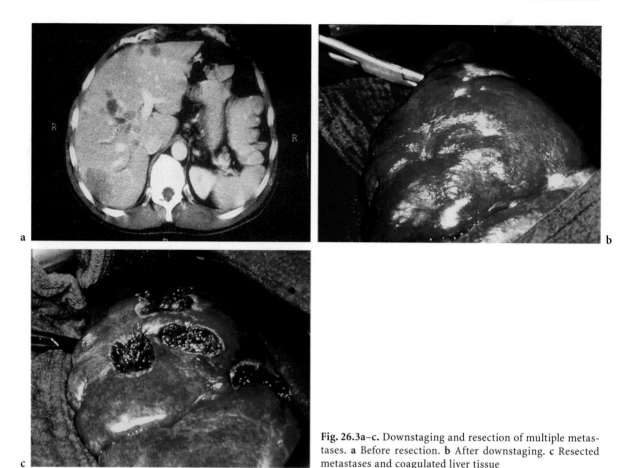

Fig. 26.3a–c. Downstaging and resection of multiple metastases. **a** Before resection. **b** After downstaging. **c** Resected metastases and coagulated liver tissue

The optimal procedure(s) can be offered by qualified expert teams on an individual basis. Treatment efforts should be stage and risk adapted, and of the therapeutic modalities a variety of combinations are possible. Regarding the potentials of these combinations, an algorithm could be designed for a clear treatment strategy which should offer patients the best perspective and convince referring colleagues, since skepticism against resection/ablation of liver metastases is still widespread. To provide a solid basis for algorithms or individual procedures, the methods available for the treatment of liver metastases have been outlined in this review.

26.5.1
Resection and Local Ablative Therapies

Surgery is the established method for cure and recent results have shown that the scope for resection has increased. Thermal ablation results during the rapid development of this method indicate that

RF/LITT, in limited indications, may come close to surgical resection.

Even in the 1990s skeptical opinions arguing against resection were published although many surgeons at this time had reported cures at low surgical morbidity/mortality, and it had become clear that surgery of liver metastases by far is superior to observation of the rapid spontaneous course or systemic chemotherapy (BALLANTYNE and QUINN 1993; BOZZETTI et al. 1993; FINLAY et al. 1988; HUGHES et al. 1988; HUNT et al. 1990). Long-term survivors with resectable metastases in the (nonresected) spontaneous course or under systemic chemotherapy are only sporadic, and only with regional chemotherapy applied as a single treatment modality has long-term survival been reported (HUGHES et al. 1988; FJIMOTO et al. 1985; LINK et al. 2001). Surgery is the established treatment offering cure, and thermoablation is evolving in specialized units as a treatment alternative but not as a substitute. The 5-year survival rates of surgical resection in patients with liver metastases of colorectal origin between 1981 and 1987 were 23–45%, and from 1991 to present 24–50%, and morbidity/mortality was 13–37%/0–14% (Table 26.3, 26.4). In the 1990s, radiofrequency (RF) and laser induced (LITT) thermoablative procedures were introduced in addition to the "old" cryo-therapy with potentials similar to surgery at a significantly lower morbidity/mortality of 7.6%/0.2% (VOGL et al. 2000). Optimistic authors from single institutions have proposed that the interventional (hyperthermic) procedures might be adequate or even superior to surgery, i.e., in patients with up to five metastases less than 5 cm in diameter (VOGL et al. 2000). These individual opinions are certainly stimulating the therapeutic revolution for the benefit of patients with resectable liver metastases, who, unfortunately, even today are recommended resection by their family practitioners in less than 50% of cases with clear indications. In general, regarding the excellent control rates of thermoablation with complete tumor destruction in, i.e., 60%, median survival times of 27–37 months, and 5-year survival rates of potentially 33%, this method is an excellent alternative for those who are not qualified for or refuse open surgery (Table 26.11) (LIVRAGHI et al. 2003).

The optimism that RF/LITT could fully replace surgery should be put into the perspective of the results obtained by open surgery (and adjuvant therapy) in patients who often have similar inclusion criteria set as limits for, i.e., LITT (≤5 metastases, ≤5 cm in diameter), or who are not qualified for RF/LITT. In addition, open surgery offers exact staging and controlled R0 resection for all intrahepatic, and, if indicated, extrahepatic disease. In patients deemed to have isolated resectable liver metastases by preoperative staging, only 46% at surgery were resectable for cure (median survival 35.5 months), 12% had extrahepatic disease, and, including these patients, 42% were nonresectable (median survival 16.5 months) (BENOTTI and STEELE 1992; STEELE et al. 1991). Interventional therapy thus has the risk of treating understaged patients who could have had more metastases removed by open surgery for cure (R0) or whose qualification for multimodal therapy would be defined by the open procedure. Although LITT or RF is applied in resectable liver metastases, this indication must be confirmed in phase III trials comparing resection vs thermoablation, trained on a broad base, and the indications/methods incorporated into up to date guidelines (LIVRAGHI et al. 2003; SHIBATA et al. 2000; VOGL et al. 2000). So

far the data for resection are superior with regard to long-term experience and survival data.

Complete (R0) resection (or destruction) at the initial treatment is of the utmost importance so that the chance of cure is not missed. The average 5-year survival rates and median survival times of more than 2,100 pathologically confirmed R0 resected patients reported in the literature from multiple institutions are 34% (range 30–48%) and 41 months (35–46 months), and the 5-, 10-, and 20-year survival rates in a single series involving 376 patients with nearly complete follow-up are 39%, 26%, and 21%, respectively (SCHEELE 2001; SCHEELE et al. 1996). Outstanding results were reported from the interdisciplinary team from the Hepatic Unit at MSKCC/New York with a median survival time of 72.2 months and 2/5-year survival rates of 86%/61% (KEMENY et al. 1999). Although potential candidates for thermoablation, re-resection in carefully selected patients offers results similar to the first resection, with median survival times ranging between 17 and 44 months (Table 26.5).

The fate of patients with noncurative resections (R1/2) is limited to sporadic 5-year survivors (0.8%), and an average median survival time of 20 months (15–23 months), which can also be obtained by systemic or regional chemotherapy or interventional treatment. Thus, the crucial point for selecting the patient for one or other of the single treatment modalities is the exact preoperative staging and determination of curative resectability and the desires/risk factors of the patient. The art is to select patients according to (individual) prognostic and risk factors, to resect completely (R0), at lowest morbidity and blood transfusion, as these factors, R1/2 and morbidity are independent negative prognostic factors in multivariate analysis, and may have a negative prognostic impact on the surgical oncological results (SCHEELE 2001; KOOBY et al. 2003; LAURENT et al. 2003).

The indication for surgical resection regarding prognostic factors of metastasis is given when all metastases are R0 resectable at margins ≥1 cm. Contraindications are positive nodes in the hepatoduodenal ligament or extrahepatic disease, except for resectable lung metastases or resectable local relapses (ISTO-INFORMATIONSZENTRUM FÜR STANDARDS IN DER ONKOLOGIE 2004). Resectable patients with colorectal liver metastases (and resectable intrahepatic isolated recurrences) should be resected, or, alternatively, receive RF/LITT therapy. However, new developments clearly show that both methods can be complementary for the benefit of increasing the perspective for cure (EVRARD et al. 2004). Patients with additional resectable lung metastases should also be resected, first in the liver, and then in the lungs, since at liver resection extrahepatic intra-abdominal disease precluding resection has been identified (ROUGIER and NEOPTOLEMOS 1997).

Additional indications for resection/ablation are isolated liver metastases of breast cancer, renal cell cancer and Wilms' tumors, sarcoma, melanoma (mostly of ocular origin), and, rarely, other GI cancers; neuroendocrine liver metastases are a frequent indication for curative resection or cytoreductive surgery in combination with the primary tumor location and extrahepatic metastases.

26.5.2
Chemotherapy and Combination of Therapies

Chemotherapy improves survival time and offers the chance for cure when combined with resection in downstaged patients.

While the limited success of systemic chemotherapy with 5-FU or its modulations, with median survival times of 11.3–12.7 months in patients with colorectal metastases confined to the liver and some benefit vs observation, did not seem to warrant suggesting this treatment to all qualified patients, the highly stimulating results of recent years have started a new era with encouraging perspectives for previously noncurable patients (THE NORDIC GASTROINTESTINAL TUMOR ADJUVANT THERAPY GROUP 1992; SCHEITHAUER et al. 1993; THIRION et al. 1999). The new combination protocols (developed in France with drugs designed in Japan) combining either oxaliplatin (i.e., "FOLFOX") or CPT 11 (i.e., "FOLFIRI") with 5-FU + folinic acid have led to consistently high remission rates of 34–67%, and median survival rates of 15–19 months, which were significantly better than with 5-FU+FA alone. Since the diameter of metastases or their topographic location with respect to vital intrahepatic structures is frequently a contraindication for curative resection, a response might lead to downstaging, turning the metastases resectable. As the doubling time of occult metastases is reported to be 86±12 days and lung metastases seem to show a different response to chemotherapy than liver metastases due to a different TS expression, the fact that during chemotherapy and the response in the liver there is no development of extrahepatic disease, which is most frequently expected in the lungs, facilitates

the decision to resect a previously nonresectable downstaged patient (KEMENY et al. 2001; KEMENY et al. 2003). This procedure has been successfully practiced by several groups who have used regional chemotherapy for treatment of isolated nonresectable liver metastases, since response rates to hepatic artery infusion have been significantly superior to i.v. chemotherapy, at least during the 5-FU+FA monotherapy era (MARUO and KOSAKA 1994; ELIAS et al. 1995, LINK et al. 1999a; LINK et al. 1999b; META-ANALYSIS GROUP IN CANCER 1996). Within an own phase II trial using MFFM, the response rate of isolated colorectal liver metastases to hepatic artery infusion was 54%, the median survival time 24 months, and in the 14% of downstaged and resected patients 39 months, respectively (LINK et al. 2001). The principle of resecting downstaged patients whose disease remains confined to the original tumor site(s) has gained widespread acceptance in the medical oncological community, since the groups at the "Centre de Chronotherapie" and "Centre Hepato-Biliaire" at Hôpital Paul Brousse, Villejuif, France, reported similar achievements with the new protocol of chronomodulated 5-FU + folinic acid combined with oxaliplatin (BISMUTH et al. 1996; GIACCHETTI et al. 1999). Previously nonresectable patients with colorectal metastases to the liver ± extrahepatic sites had a 5-year survival rate of 33% after successful downstaging and aggressive surgery (ADAM et al. 2001; BISMUTH et al. 1996). In these patients who had the disease confined to the liver, 51% could be operated on with a 5-year survival rate of 50% and a median survival time of 48 months; in the whole group of 151 patients the response rate was 59%, the median survival time 24 months, and the 5-year survival rate 28% (GIACCHETTI et al. 1999). With respect to the perspectives of the 5-FU+FA monotherapy era (response to i.v. therapy 21%, median survival times 11.3–12.7 months, hardly any 5-year survivors), these achievements are excellent and convincing. Currently the response rates to standard systemic or regional intra-arterial protocols at 34–67% and >50%, respectively, are comparable. The response to intra-arterial chemotherapy, according to our own experience, may be significantly increased to 77% if drugs active in vitro against the individual metastatic tumor cells were used for therapy (LINK et al. 2000b). This might increase the rate of downstaging and secondary resection. The effects of oxaliplatin and CPT 11 in hepatic arterial chemotherapy protocols are currently under evaluation. Patients with nonresectable colorectal liver metastases should receive systemic, or in selected cases, regional chemotherapy with the modern protocols that both might offer long-term survival, if resection is performed after downstaging. Therefore, the treatment indication and response evaluation are an interdisciplinary task that should involve oncologically experienced surgeons to discuss the possibility of secondary resection after successful downstaging.

The combination of treatment methods in the palliative and curative situation are feasible if complete removal or destruction of metastatic tumor tissue is achievable.

Surgical-oncological treatments must be individualized and flexible. The possibilities of treatment modality combinations provide potential for a variety of trials. As pointed out by various authors, resection/ablation of colorectal and other types of liver metastases can be completely achieved by applying various resection strategies, with the addition of intraoperative RF ablation or cryotherapy of metastases not amenable to resection or cryotherapy of nonsecure resection margins (ADAM et al. 2001; AZOULAY et al. 2001; EVRARD et al. 2004; LINK et al. 2000a; YAN et al. 2003). The techniques are complementary and depend on the size and topography of the lesions to be treated. To avoid hepatic failure split time resection or preoperative portal embolization of the liver lobe/sector to be resected are possible and effective. RF ablation, such as resection, may be combined with postinterventional "adjuvant" chemotherapy. Stereotactic irradiation, interstitial brachytherapy, and regional intra-arterial radionuclide therapy are evolving treatment techniques that might compete with the more established surgical and ablative techniques. Percutaneous radiotherapy has no proven benefit (WITTE et al. 2001).

The benefit of neoadjuvant chemotherapy in principle is not proven; modern adjuvant chemotherapy after resection (of colorectal liver metastases) may improve survival.

Although chemotherapy has been proven to downstage nonresectable metastases to secondary resectability, preoperative systemic chemotherapy in all resectable metastases has no evidence of level I proven benefit. In a single institution phase II neoadjuvant trial, WEIN et al. (2003) treated patients planned for resection with 2–3 cycles modified FOLFOX. As a result, all patients responded, and the resectability at 80% was relatively high. The 2-year survival rate ("cancer related") of 80% was similar to the 2-year survival rates achieved by regional + systemic chemotherapy in the trial of the MSKCC team (86% overall survival) or in our own observation trials (77–83%). While the benefit of adjuvant chemotherapy according to the trials with modern protocols (5-FUDR i.a. + 5-FU+FA i.v. or 5-FU+FA according to the ART protocol) is evident, but, according to other multicentric and historical control trials, concerning overall survival, not unanimously acceptable, the true benefit of neoadjuvant therapy in principle is open and being studied in an ongoing EORTC trial (LORENZ et al. 1998; ONAITIS et al. 2003). Since by far not all patients will be resectable, neoadjuvant therapy could be an overtreatment compared to adjuvant therapy, where only the resected patients receive therapy.

Regional chemotherapy combined with systemic chemotherapy reduces hepatic progression and may improve 2-year survival significantly according to phase III trials (KEMENY et al. 1999). Neoadjuvant chemotherapy may improve survival and extent of surgery according to phase II and historical control trials (TANAKA et al. 2003; WEIN et al. 2003).

The best "treatment" for colorectal liver metastases is their prevention by effective systemic adjuvant primary tumor therapy.

Based on the understanding of the pathogenesis of colorectal liver metastasis via portal dissemination, intraportal chemotherapy after primary tumor resection was tested in several phase III trials. Neither a reduction of hepatic progression nor a survival benefit could be unanimously observed, so

Table 26.11. Colorectal liver metastases surgery: thermoablative treatment

Author	Year	Patients	2-y survival	5-y survival	Median survival (months)
RF – radiofrequency ablation					
GILLAMS and LEES 2000	2000	69	-	-	27
SOLBIATI et al. 2001	2001	117	69%	-	36
SIPERSTEIN et al. 2002	2002	110	79%	-	-
LITT – laser induced thermotherapy					
VOGL	2000	360	~70%	~33%	37

that intraportal chemotherapy is not recommended for routine use (LINK et al. 1996a). Systemic effective adjuvant chemotherapy, however, has reduced systemic progression, including liver metastasis, and is recommended for routine use in UICC III colon, and UICC II+III rectal cancers. In the FOGT1 trial for adjuvant chemotherapy the hepatic progression rates in patients treated either with 5-FU + levamisole or 5-FU + folinic acid + levamisole in an initial evaluation were 15% vs 12% respectively (STAIB et al. 2001). Interestingly, hepatic arterial chemotherapy after primary colon cancer resection may reduce hepatic progression and improve survival, so that this modality deserves to be studied in large scale trials (Table 26.12) (SADAHIRO et al. 2004).

26.6
Stage Dependent Treatment Strategies

The principal aim is to remove all liver metastases with a safety margin >1 cm or, at least as a secure R0 resection. If possible this should be performed surgically, eventually with additional intraoperative thermal ablation, i.e., RF ablation. Positive lymph nodes, if located ventral to the hepatoduodenal ligament, are not a strict contraindication, but a location at the celiac trunk or the common hepatic artery. If the patient requests adjuvant therapy after resection of colorectal liver metastases, either hepatic artery infusion with 5-FUDR + additional systemic chemotherapy with 5-FU + folinic acid with strict adherence to the dose modification scheme according to the Kemeny protocol may be chosen (via pump) or, alternatively HAI with 5-FU+FA via a port according to the ART protocol with strict adherence to the infusion times may be the method of choice. In the case of an isolated intrahepatic relapse, re-resection or, alternatively, RF ablation are recommendable. Nonresectable liver metastases can be treated by thermal ablation if possible or by systemic chemotherapy. If the patient is explored for resection and turns out to be nonresectable, a hepatic artery port may be implanted and infusion chemotherapy conducted either according to the Ulm protocol

Table 26.12. Recommendations. 5-FU, 5-fluorouracil; FA, folinic acid; c.i., continuous infusion; Oxa, oxaliplatin; CPT11, irinotecan; RF, radiofrequency; LITT, laser-induced thermotherapy; CT, intravenous chemotherapy; HAI, hepatic artery infusion; MFFM, mitoxantrone + 5-FU + FA + mitomycin C; PVI, portal venous infusion

---

1. After primary tumor resection (UICC III)
   • Adjuvant systemic CT (5-FU+FA (e.g. FOGT1 arm b)
   • PVI or HAI experimental

2. Resectable "limited" disease
   • Resection
   • Additional or alternative RF/LITT ablation
   • "Adjuvant" HAI with 5-FU+FA
     (or 5-FUDR i.a. +5-FU+FA i.v.)

3. Nonresectable disease
   • Systemic CT (5-FU c.i.+FA+CPT11 or Oxa)
   • HAI MFFM or individualized
     (primary or second line treatment)
   • Split time resection

4. Response of nonresectable disease after i.v. CT/HAI
   • Resection
   • Additional or alternative RF/LITT
   • "Adjuvant" HAI with MFFM or individualized

5. Decision for therapy:• Multidisciplinary + patient's preference!

(MFFM, possibly modified according to individual chemosensitivity) or the MSKCC protocol (5-FUDR+Dexa, Kemeny). In case the patient responds and the metastases turn out to be resectable (with no extrahepatic disease), treatment as outlined under "resectable" should be performed. Resectable liver and lung metastases may be resected, first liver, then lung. Nonresectable hepatic and extrahepatic disease should receive primary systemic chemotherapy; in the case of a good response, combined resections may be considered individually and interdisciplinarily. The decisions and methods for treating colorectal liver metastases are multifarious and the new perspectives of the "aggressive" therapy are exciting. The best outcome for the patient can only be achieved by true interdisciplinary management, involving surgery, medical oncology, interventional radiology, radiotherapy, and pathology (Fig. 26.4).

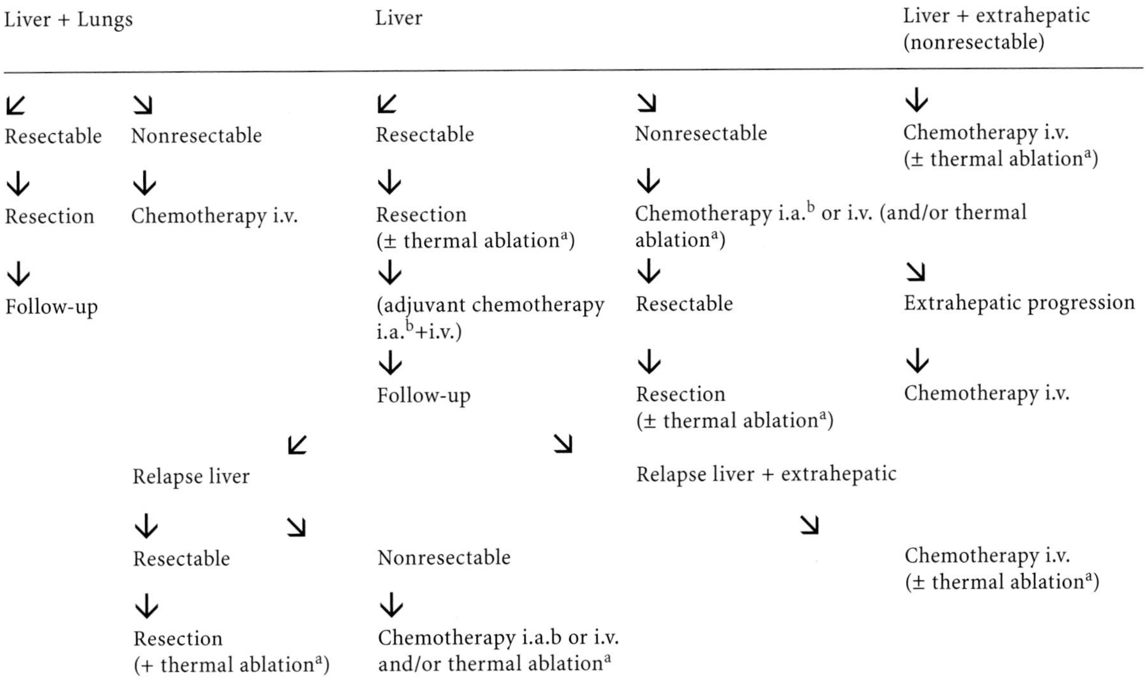

Liver + Lungs		Liver		Liver + extrahepatic (nonresectable)
↙	↘	↙	↘	↓
Resectable	Nonresectable	Resectable	Nonresectable	Chemotherapy i.v. (± thermal ablation[a])
↓	↓	↓	↓	
Resection	Chemotherapy i.v.	Resection (± thermal ablation[a])	Chemotherapy i.a.[b] or i.v. (and/or thermal ablation[a])	
↓		↓	↓	↘
Follow-up		(adjuvant chemotherapy i.a.[b]+i.v.)	Resectable	Extrahepatic progression
		↓	↓	↓
		Follow-up	Resection (± thermal ablation[a])	Chemotherapy i.v.
	↙ ↘			
Relapse liver		Relapse liver + extrahepatic		
↓	↘		↘	
Resectable	Nonresectable			Chemotherapy i.v. (± thermal ablation[a])
↓	↓			
Resection (+ thermal ablation[a])	Chemotherapy i.a.b or i.v. and/or thermal ablation[a]			

[a] Less than five metastases, diameter of metastases <5 cm, center of expertise, refusal of surgery at first place by patient/doctor involved in follow-up, intraoperative cryotherapy or thermal RF ablation in case of positive/narrow margin or nonresectable metastases <5 cm

[b] Intra-arterial chemotherapy in centers with expertise

Fig. 26.4. Flow chart for interdisciplinary treatment of colorectal liver metastases (resection-chemotherapy-thermal ablation)

References

Adam R (2003) Chemotherapy and surgery: new perspectives on the treatment of unresectable liver metastases. Ann Oncol 14:13–16

Adam R, Bismuth H, Castaing D, et al (1997) Repeat hepatectomy for colorectal liver metastases. Ann Surg 225:51–62

Adam R, Avisar E, Ariche A, et al (2001) Five-year survival following hepatic resection after neoadjuvant therapy for nonresectable colorectal. Ann Surg Oncol 8:347–353

Adam R, Pascal G, Azoulay D, et al (2003) Liver resection for colorectal metastases: the third hepatectomy. Ann Surg 238:871–884

Adson MA, van Heerden JA, Adson MH, et al (1984) Resection of hepatic metastases from colorectal cancer. Arch Surg 119:647–651

Advanced Colorectal Cancer Meta-Analysis Project (1992) Modulation of fluorouracil by leucovorin in patients with advanced colorectal cancer: evidence in terms of response rate. J Clin Oncol 10:896–903

Allen-Mersh TG, Earlam S, Fordy C, et al (1994) Quality of life and survival with continuous hepatic-artery floxuridine infusion for colorectal liver metastases. Lancet 344:1255–1260

August DA, Sugarbaker PH, Ottow RT (1985) Hepatic resection of colorectal metastases. Influence of clinical factors and adjuvant intraperitoneal 5-FU via Tenckhoff catheter on survival. Ann Surg 201:210–218

Azoulay D, Adam R, Castaing D, et al (2001) Multistage liver resections in colorectal liver metastases. The Paul Brousse concept. Chirurg 72:765–769

Baker J, Bleiberg H, Hutchison G, et al (1997) An international multidisciplinary approach to the management of advanced colorectal cancer. Eur J Surg Oncol 23:1–66

Ballantyne GH, Quin J (1993) Surgical treatment of liver metastases in patients with colorectal cancer. Cancer 71:4252–4256

Beckurts KT, Holscher AH, Thorban S, et al (1997) Significance of lymphnode involvement at the hepatic hilum in the resection of colorectal liver metastases. Br J Surg 84:1081–1084

Belghiti J, Hiramatsu K, Benoist S, et al (2000) Seven hundred forty-seven hepatectomies in the 1990s: an update to evaluate the actual risk of liver resection. J Am Coll Surg 191:38–46

Bengmark S, Hafstrom L, Jeppsson B (1982) Metastatic disease in the liver from colorectal cancer: An appraisal of liver surgery. World J Surg 6:61–65

Benotti P, Steele G (1992) Patterns of recurrent colorectal cancer and recovery surgery. Cancer 70:1409–1413

Bismuth H, Adam R, Levi F, et al (1996) Resection of nonresectable liver metastases from colorectal cancer after neoadjuvant chemotherapy. Ann Surg 224:509–522

Bleicher RJ, Allegra DP, Nora DT, et al (2003) Radiofrequency ablation in 447 complex unresectable liver tumors: lessons learned. Ann Surg Oncol 10:52–58

Blumgart LH, Fong Y (1995) Surgical options in the treatment of hepatic metastasis from colorectal cancer. Curr Probl Surg 32:333–421

Bozzetti F, Cozzaglio L, Boracchi P, et al (1993) Comparing surgical resection of limited hepatic metastases from colorectal cancer to non-operative treatment. Eur J Surg Oncol 19:162–167

Butler J, Attiyeh FF, Daly JM (1986) Hepatic resection for metastases of the colon and rectum. Surg Gynecol Obstet 162:109–113

Cady B, McDermott WV (1985) Major hepatic resection for metachronous metastases from colon cancer. Ann Surg 201:204–209

Christoforidis D, Martinet O, Lejeune FJ, et al (2002) Isolated liver perfusion for non-resectable liver tumours: a review. Eur J Surg Oncol 28:875–890

Conlon R, Jacobs M, Dasgupta D, et al (2003) The value of intraoperative ultrasound during hepatic resection compared with improved preoperative magnetic resonance imaging. Eur J Ultrasound 16:211–216

Desai DC, Zervos EE, Arnold MW, et al (2003) Positron emission tomography affects surgical management in recurrent colorectal cancer patients. Ann Surg Oncol 10:59–64

Doci R, Gennari L, Bignami P, et al (1991) One hundred patients with hepatic metastases from colorectal cancer treated by resection: analysis of prognostic determinants. Br J Surg 78:797–801

Doci R, Gennari L, Bignami P, et al (1995) Morbidity and mortality after hepatic resection of metastases from colorectal cancer. Br J Surg 82:377–381

Douillard JY, Cunningham D, Roth AD, et al (2000) Irinotecan combined with fluorouracil compared with fluorouracil alone as first-line treatment for metastatic colorectal cancer: a multicenter randomised trial. Lancet 355:1041–1047

Eder M, Weiss M (1991) Hämatogene Lebermetastasen – humanpathologische Grundlagen. Chirurg 62:705–709þ

Elias D, Lasser P, Hoang JM, et al (1993) Repeat hepatectomy for cancer. Br J Surg 80:1557–1562

Elias D, Lasser P, Rougier P, et al (1995) Frequency, technical aspects, results, and indications of major hepatectomy after prolonged intra-arterial hepatic chemotherapy for initially unresectable hepatic tumors. J Am Coll Surg 180:213–219

Elias D, Saric J, Jaeck D, et al (1996) Prospective study of microscopic lymph node involvement of the hepatic pedicle during curative hepatectomy for colorectal metastases. Br J Surg 83:942–945

Elias D, Lasser P, Ducreux M, et al (2003a) Liver resection (and associated extrahepatic resections) for metastatic well differentiated endocrine tumors: a 15-year single center prospective study. Surgery 133:375–382

Elias D, Ouellet JF, Bellon N, et al (2003b) Extrahepatic disease does not contraindicate hepatectomy for colorectal liver metastases. Br J Surg 90:567–574

Ercolani G, Grazi GL, Ravaioli M, et al (2002) Liver resection for multiple colorectal metastases: influence of parenchymal involvement and total tumor volume, vs number or location, on long-term survival. Arch Surg 137:1187–1192

Ercolani G, Grazi GL, Ravaioli M, et al (2004) The role of lymphadenectomy for liver tumors: further considerations on the appropriateness of treatment strategy. Ann Surg 239:202–209

Evrard S, Becouarn Y, Fonck M, et al (2004) Surgical treatment of liver metastases by radiofrequency ablation, resection, or in combination. Eur J Surg Oncol 30:399–406

Fernandez-Trigo V, Shamsa F, Sugarbaker PH (1995) Repeat liver resection from colorectal metastases. Repeat Hepatic Metastases Registry. Surgery 117:296–304

Finlay IG, Meek D, Brunton F, et al (1988) Growth rate of hepatic metastases in colorectal carcinoma. Br J Surg 75:641–644

Formentini A, Link KH, Pillasch J, et al (1997) Neoadjuvant regional chemotherapy for non-resectable pancreatic and hepatic tumors. Int J Oncol (S1)

Fortner JG, Silva JS, Golbey RB (1984) Multi-variate analysis of a personal series of 247 consecutive patients with liver metastases from colorectal cancer. I Treatment by hepatic resection. Ann Surg 199:306–316

Foster JH, Lundy J (1981) Liver metastases. Curr Probl Surg 18:157–202

Fowler WC, Eisenberg BL, Hoffman JP (1992) Hepatic resection following systemic chemotherapy for metastatic colorectal carcinoma. J Surg Oncol 51:122–125

Fujimoto S, Miyazaki M, Kitsukawa Y, et al (1985) Long-term survivors of colorectal cancer with unresectable hepatic metastases. Dis Colon Rectum 28:588–591

Fujita S, Miyake H, Akasu T, et al (1998) Hepatic arterial infusion (HAI) of 5-FU for unresectable liver metastases from colorectal cancer. J Jpn Soc Coloproctol 51:974

Gansauge F, Link KH, Büchler M, et al (1993) Split-time resection of 'unresectable' colorectal liver metastases supported by chemosensitivity directed hepatic artery infusion. International Conference on Regional Cancer Treatment (ICTCT 93). Wiesbaden, 12–14 July 1993

Gennari L, Doci R, Bozzetti F, et al (1986a) Surgical treatment of hepatic metastases from colorectal cancer. Ann Surg 203:49–54

Gennari L, Doci R, Bozzetti F, et al (1986b) Proposal for staging liver metastases. Recent Res Cancer Res 100:80–84

Geoghegan JG, Scheele J (1999) Treatment of colorectal liver metastases. Br J Surg 86:158–169

Germer CT, Isbert C, Albrecht D, et al (1999) Laser-induced thermotherapy combined with hepatic arterial embolization in the treatment of liver tumors in a rat tumor model. Ann Surg 230:55–62

Gervaz P, Pakart R, Nivatvongs S, et al (2003) Colorectal adenocarcinoma in cirrhotic patients. J Am Coll Surg 196:874–879

Giacchetti S, Itzhaki M, Gruia G, et al (1999) Long-term survival of patients with unresectable colorectal cancer liver metastases following infusional chemotherapy with 5-fluorouracil, leucovorin, oxaliplatin and surgery. Ann Oncol 10:663–669

Giacchetti S, Perpoint B, Zidani R, et al (2000) Phase III multicenter randomized trial of oxaliplatin added to chronomodulated fluorouracil-leucovorin as first-line treatment of metastatic colorectal cancer. J Clin Oncol 18:136–147

Gigot JF, Glineur D, Santiago AJ, et al (2002) Laparoscopic

liver resection for malignant liver tumors: preliminary results of a multicenter European study. Ann Surg 236:90–97

Gillams AR, Lees WR (2000) Survival after percutaneous, image-guided, thermal ablation of hepatic metastases from colorectal cancer. Dis Colon Rectum 43:656–661

Gough DB, Donohue JH, Trastek VA, et al (1994) Resection of hepatic and pulmonary metastases in patients with colorectal cancer. Br J Surg 81:94–96

Gouillat C, Ducerf C, Partensky C, et al (1993) Repeated hepatic resections for colorectal metastases. Eur J Surg Oncol 19:443–447

Harmon KE, Ryan JA Jr, Biehl TR, et al (1999) Benefits and safety of hepatic resection for colorectal metastases. Am J Surg 177:402–404

Hemming AW, Reed AI, Howard RJ, et al (2003) Preoperative portal vein embolization for extended hepatectomy. Ann Surg 237:686–693

Herfarth C, Heuschen UA, Lamade W, et al (1995). Rezidiv-Resektionen an der Leber bei primären und sekundären Lebermalignomen. Chirurg 66:949–958

Hermanek P (2000) Qualitätssicherung in der Onkologie: Kurzgefasste interdisziplinäre Leitlinien 2000. Zuckschwerdt Verlag, München, pp 182–188

Hodgson WJ, Friedland M, Ahmed T, et al (1986) Treatment of colorectal hepatic metastases by intrahepatic chemotherapy alone or as an adjuvant to complete or partial removal of metastatic disease. Ann Surg 203:420–425

Hohn DC, Shea WJ, Gemlo BT, et al (1988) Complications and toxicities of hepatic arterial chemotherapy. Contr Oncol 29:169–180

Hughes KS, Sugarbaker PH (1987) Resection of the liver for metastatic solid tumors. In: Rosenberg SA (ed) Surgical treatment of metastatic cancer. Lippincott, Philadelphia, pp 125–164

Hughes KS, Simon R, Songhorabodi S, et al (1986) Resection of the liver for colorectal carcinoma metastases: a multi-institutional study of indications for resection. Surgery 100:278–284

Hunt TM, Carty N, Johnson CD (1990) Resection of liver metastases from a colorectal carcinoma does not benefit the patient. Ann R Coll Surg Engl 72:199–205

Imamura H, Sano K, Harihara Y, et al (2003) Complete remission of disease for 5 years following initial and repeat resection of the liver for the removal of 22 metastases of colorectal origin. J Hepatobiliary Pancreat Surg 10:321–324

ISTO (2004) Informationszentrum für Standards in der Onkologie. Kurzgefasste Interdisziplinäre Leitlinien 2004. Deutsche Krebsgesellschaft e.V. 2004. Qualitätssicherung in der Onkologie, Diagnostik und Therapie maligner Erkrankugen. W. Zuckschwerdt Verlag, Munich

Iwatsuki S, Esquivel C, Gordon RD, et al (1986) Liver resection for metastatic colorectal cancer. Surgery 100:804–810

Jaeck D (2003) The significance of hepatic pedicle lymph node metastases in surgical management of colorectal liver metastases and of other liver malignancies. Ann Surg Oncol 10:1007–1011

Jonker D, Maroun J, Kocha W (2000) Survival benefit of chemotherapy in metastatic colorectal cancer: a meta-analysis of randomized controlled trials. Br J Cancer 82:1789–1794

Jourdan JL, Cannan R, Stubbs R (1999) Hepatic resection for metastases in colorectal carcinoma. N Z Med J 112:91–93

Kato T, Yasui K, Hirai T, et al (2003) Therapeutic results for hepatic metastasis of colorectal cancer with special reference to effectiveness of hepatectomy: analysis of prognostic factors for 763 cases recorded at 18 institutions. Dis Colon Rectum 46:S22–S31

Kemeny N, Conti JA, Cohen A, et al (1994) Phase II study of hepatic arterial floxuridine, leucovorin and dexamethasone for unresectable liver metastases from colorectal carcinoma. J Clin Oncol 12:2288–2295

Kemeny N, Huang Y, Cohen AM, et al (1999) Hepatic arterial infusion of chemotherapy after resection of hepatic metastases from colorectal cancer. N Engl J Med 341:2039–2048

Kemeny N, Gonen M, Sullivan D, et al (2001) Phase I study of hepatic arterial infusion of floxuridine and dexamethasone with systemic irinotecan for unresectable hepatic metastases from colorectal cancer. J Clin Oncol 19:2687–2695

Kemeny MM, Adak S, Gray B, et al (2002) Combined-modality treatment for resectable metastatic colorectal carcinoma to the liver: surgical resection of hepatic metastases in combination with continuous infusion of chemotherapy: an intergroup study. J Clin Oncol 20:1499–1505

Kemeny N, Jarnagin W, Gonen M, et al (2003) Phase I/II study of hepatic arterial therapy with floxuridine and dexamethasone in combination with intravenous irinotecan as adjuvant treatment after resection of hepatic metastases from colorectal cancer. J Clin Oncol 21:3303–3309

Kern W, Beckert B, Lang N, et al (2001) Phase I and pharmacokinetic study of hepatic arterial infusion with oxaliplatin in combination with folinic acid and 5-fluorouracil in patients with hepatic metastases from colorectal cancer. Ann Oncol 12:599–603

Köckerling F, Scheele J, Schneider C, et al (1991) Chirurgische Therapie von Lebermetastasen bei Karzinoidtumoren. In: Herfarth Ch, Schlag P (eds) Neue Entwicklungen in der Therapie von Lebermetastasen. Springer, Berlin, pp 345–352

Kooby DA, Stockman J, Ben-Porat L, et al (2003) Influence of transfusions on perioperative and long-term outcome in patients following hepatic resection for colorectal metastases. Ann Surg 237:860–869

Kornmann M, Link KH (2002) Conversion of locally inoperable primary rectal cancer with multiple liver metastases to an option for cure after local down-staging and hepatic arterial infusion chemotherapy. Langenbecks Arch Surg 387:90–93

Kornmann M, Link KH, Lenz HJ, et al (1997) Thymidylate synthase is a predictor for response and resistance in hepatic artery infusion chemotherapy. Cancer Lett 118:29–35

Kornmann M, Butzer U, Blatter J, et al (2000) Pre-clinical evaluation of the activity of gemcitabine as a basis for regional chemotherapy of pancreatic and colorectal cancer. Eur J Surg Oncol 26:583–587

Lamadé W, Hohenberger P, Hinz U, et al (1994) Hepatic reresection for recurrent liver metastases from colorectal cancer. Eur J Surg Oncol 20:317

Langer B, Bleiberg H, Labianca R, et al (2002) Fluorouracil (FU) + l-Feucovorin (l-LV) versus observation after potentially curative resection of liver metastases from colorectal cancer (CRC): Results of the ENG (EORTC/NCIC CTG/GIVIO) randomized trial. Proc Am Soc Oncol 21:A592

Laurent C, Sa Cunha A, Couderc P, et al (2003) Influence of postoperative morbidity on long-term survival following liver resection for colorectal metastases. Br J Surg 90:1131–1136

Lehnert T, Otto G, Herfarth C (1995) Therapeutic modalities and prognostic factors for primary and secondary liver tumors. World J Surg 19:252–263

Lehnert T, Knaebel HP, Dück M, et al (1999) Sequential hepatic and pulmonary resections for metastatic colorectal cancer. Br J Surg 86:241–243

Lencioni R, Vignali C, Caramella D, et al (1994) Transcatheter arterial embolization followed by percutaneous ethanol injection in the treatment of hepatocellular carcinoma. Cardiovasc Intervent Radiol 17:70–75

Lencioni R, Goletti O, Armillotta N, et al (1998) Radiofrequency thermal ablation of liver metastases with a cooled-tip electrode needle: results of a pilot clinical trial. Eur Radiol 8:1205–1211

Leslie KA, Rossi R, Hughes K, et al (1995) Survival expectancy of patients alive 5 years after hepatic resection for metastatic colon carcinoma: report from the registry of hepatic metastases. Proc Am Soc Oncol 14:200

Leyvraz S, Spataro V, Bauer J, et al (1997) Treatment of ocular melanoma metastatic to the liver by hepatic arterial chemotherapy. J Clin Oncol 15:2589–2595

Link KH (1998) Chirurgisch-onkologische Therapie von Mammakarzinom-Lebermetastasen. In: Kreienberg R, Möbus V, Alt D (eds) Management des Mammakarzinoms. Springer, Berlin, pp 274–287

Link KH (2000) Adjuvante Therapie bei Kolon- und Rektumkarzinomen: Zwischenergebnisse einer prospektiven, randomisierten Multicenterstudie (FOGT 1+2). 2/6-05-2000.117. Kongress der Deutschen Gesellschaft für Chirurgie, Berlin

Link KH, Aigner KR, Kuehn W, et al (1986) Prospective correlative chemosensitivity testing in high-dose intraarterial chemotherapy for liver metastases. Cancer Res 46:4837–4848

Link KH, Kreuser ED, Safi F, et al (1993) Die intraarterielle Chemotherapie mit 5-FU und Folinsäure (FA, Rescuvolin) im Therapiekonzept bei nicht resektablen kolorektalen Lebermetastasen. Tumordiagnostik Therapie 14:224–231

Link KH, Kornmann M, Safi F, et al (1994) Response prediction in hepatic artery infusion with Fluoropyrimidines using cell culture and polymerase chain reaction techniques. Eur J Surg Oncol 20:317–318

Link KH, Kornmann M, Leder GH, et al (1996) Regional chemotherapy directed by individual chemosensitivity testing in vitro: a prospective decision aiding trial. Clin Cancer Res 2:1469–1474

Link KH, Staib L, Kreuser ED, et al (1996) Adjuvant treatment of colon and rectal cancer: Impact of chemotherapy, radiotherapy and immunotherapy on routine postsurgical patient management. Recent Res Cancer Res 142:311–352

Link KH, Leder G, Pillasch J, et al (1998) In vitro concentration response studies and in vitro phase II tests as the experimental basis for regional chemotherapeutic protocols. Semin Surg Oncol 14:189–201

Link KH, Pillasch J, Formentini A, et al (1999a) Downstaging by regional chemotherapy of non-resectable isolated colorectal liver metastases. Eur J Surg Oncol 25:381–388

Link KH, Kornmann M, Formentini A, et al (1999b) Regional chemotherapy of non-resectable liver metastases from colorectal cancer – literature and institutional review. Langenbecks Arch Surg 384:344–353

Link KH, Germer CT, Seifert JK, et al (2000a) Neue Wirkprinzipien in der chirurgischen Onkologie. Onkologie 5:450–457

Link KH, Kornmann M, Butzer U, et al (2000b) Thymidylate synthase quantitation and in vitro chemosensitivity testing predicts responses and survival of patients with isolated nonresectable liver tumors receiving hepatic arterial infusion chemotherapy. Cancer 89:288–296

Link KH, Sunelaitis E, Kornmann M, et al (2001) Regional chemotherapy of nonresectable colorectal liver metastases with mitoxantrone, 5-fluorouracil, folinic acid, and mitomycin C may prolong survival. Cancer 92:2746–2753

Liu CL, Fan ST, Lo CM, et al (2002) Hepatic resection for colorectal liver metastases: prospective study. Hong Kong Med J 8:329–333

Livraghi T, Solbiati L, Meloni F, et al (2003) Percutaneous radiofrequency ablation of liver metastases in potential candidates for resection: the "test-of-time approach". Cancer 97:3027–3035

Lorenz M, Muller HH (2000) Randomized, multicenter trial of fluorouracil plus leucovorin administered either via hepatic arterial or intravenous infusion versus fluorodeoxyuridine administered via hepatic arterial infusion in patients with nonresectable liver metastases from colorectal carcinoma. J Clin Oncol 18:243–254

Lorenz M, Müller HH, Staib-Sebler E, et al (1997) Standard/studies for regional treatment of colorectal metastases (ALM study). Eighth International Conference of Regional Cancer Treatment. Reg Cancer Treat (S)72

Lorenz M, Muller HH, Schramm H, et al (1998) Randomized trial of surgery versus surgery followed by adjuvant hepatic arterial infusion with 5-fluorouracil and folinic acid for liver metastases of colorectal cancer. German Cooperative on Liver Metastases (Arbeitsgruppe Lebermetastasen). Ann Surg 228:756–762

Mala T, Bohler G, Mathisen O, et al (2002) Hepatic resection for colorectal metastases: can preoperative scoring predict patient outcome? World J Surg 26:1348–1353

Maruo H, Kosaka A (1994) Evaluation of cases of metastatic liver tumors resected following intra-arterial infusion chemotherapy. Gan To Kagaku Ryoho 21:2143–2146

Meta-analysis Group in Cancer (1996) Reappraisal of hepatic arterial infusion in the treatment of nonresectable liver metastases from colorectal cancer. J Natl Cancer Inst 88:252–258

Meta-analysis Group in Cancer (1998) Efficacy of intravenous continuous infusion of fluorouracil compared with bolus administration in advanced colorectal cancer. J Clin Oncol 16:301–318

Murata S, Morya Y, Akasu T, et al (1998) Resection of both hepatic and pulmonary metastases in patients with colorectal carcinoma. Cancer 83:1086–1093

Nakamura S, Suzuki S, Baba S (1997) Resection of liver metastases of colorectal carcinoma. World J Surg 21:741–747

Nordic Gastrointestinal Tumor Adjuvant Therapy Group (1992) Expectancy or primary chemotherapy in patients with advanced asymptomatic colorectal cancer: a randomized trial. J Clin Oncol 10:904–911

Nordlinger B, Jaeck D, Guiguet M, et al (1992) Surgical resection of hepatic metastases: multicentric retrospective study by the French Association of Surgery. In: Nordlinger B, Jaeck D (eds) Treatment of hepatic metastases of colorectal cancer. Springer, New York, pp 129–161

Nordlinger B, Guiguet M, Vaillant JC, et al (1996) Surgical resection of colorectal carcinoma metastases to the liver. A prognostic scoring system to improve case selection, based on 1568 patients. Association Francaise de Chirurgie. Cancer 77:1254–1262

Ochiai T, Sasako M, Mizuno S, et al (1994) Hepatic resection for metastatic tumours from gastric cancer: analysis of prognostic factors. Br J Surg 81:1175–1178

O'Connell MJ, Adson MA, Schutt AJ, et al (1985) Clinical trial adjuvant therapy after surgical resection of colorectal cancer metastatic to the liver. Mayo Clin Proc 60:517–520

Ohlsson B, Stenram U, Tranberg KG (1998) Resection of colorectal liver metastases: 25-year experience. World J Surg 22:268–277

Oldhafer KJ, Lang H, Malago M, et al (2001) Ex situ Resektion und Resektion an der in situ perfundierten Leber – Gibt es noch Indikationen? Chirurg 72:131–137

Onaitis M, Morse M, Hurwitz H, et al (2003) Adjuvant hepatic arterial chemotherapy following metastasectomy in patients with isolated liver metastases. Ann Surg 237:782–789

Oshowo A, Gillams A, Harrison E, et al (2003) Comparison of resection and radiofrequency ablation for treatment of solitary colorectal liver metastases. Br J Surg 90:1240–1243

Patt YZ, McBride CM, Ames FC, et al (1987) Adjuvant perioperative hepatic arterial mitomycin C and floxuridine combined with surgical resection of metastatic colorectal cancer in the liver. Cancer 59:867–873

Pawlik TM, Izzo F, Cohen DS, et al (2003) Combined resection and radiofrequency ablation for advanced hepatic malignancies: results in 172 patients. Ann Surg Oncol. 10:1059–1069

Petrelli NJ, Nambisan RN, Herrera L (1985) Hepatic resection for isolated metastasis from colorectal carcinoma. Am J Surg 149:205–209

Portier G, Rougier PJ, Milan C, et al (2002) Adjuvant systemic chemotherapy (CT) using 5-fluorouracil (FU) and folinic acid (AA) after resection of liver metastases (LM) from colorectal (CRC) origin. Results of an intergroup phase III study (Trial FFCD - ACHBT - AURC 9002). Proc Proc Am Soc Oncol 21:133a

Rau HG, Schauer R, Pickelmann S, et al (2001) Dissektionstechniken in der Leberchirurgie. Chirurg 72:105–112

Rivoire M, De Cian F, Meeus P, et al (2002) Combination of neoadjuvant chemotherapy with cryotherapy and surgical resection for the treatment of unresectable liver metastases from colorectal carcinoma. Cancer 95:2283–2292

Robinson BJ, Rice TW, Strong SA, et al (1999) Is resection of pulmonary and hepatic metastases warranted in patients with colorectal cancer? J Thorac Cardiovasc Surg 117:66–76

Rougier P, Neoptolemos JP (1997) The need for a multidisciplinary approach in the treatment of advanced colorectal cancer: a critical review from a medical oncologist and surgeon. Eur J Surg Oncol 23:385–396

Rougier P, Laplanche A, Huguier M, et al (1992) Hepatic arterial infusion of floxuridine in patients with liver metastases from colorectal carcinoma: long-term results of a prospective randomized trial. J Clin Oncol 10:1112–1118

Sadahiro S, Suzuki T, Ishikawa K, et al (2004) Prophylactic hepatic arterial infusion chemotherapy for the prevention of liver metastasis in patients with colon carcinoma: a randomized control trial. Cancer 100:590–597

Saltz LB, Locker PK, Pirotta N, et al (2000) Weekly irinotecan (CPT-11) leucovorin (LV), and fluorouracil (FU) is superior to daily ×5LV/FU in patients (pts) with previously untreated metastatic colorectal cancer (CRC). Proc Am Soc Clin Oncol 18:898 Abstract

Saw RP, Koorey D, Painter D, et al (2002) p53, DCC and thymidylate synthase as predictors of survival after resection of hepatic metastases from colorectal cancer. Br J Surg 89:1409–1415

Scaife CL, Curley SA, Izzo F, et al (2003) Feasibility of adjuvant hepatic arterial infusion of chemotherapy after radiofrequency ablation with or without resection in patients with hepatic metastases from colorectal cancer. Ann Surg Oncol 10:348–354

Scheele J (1989) Die segmentorientierte Leberresektion. Grundlagen – Technik – Stellenwert. Chirurg 60:251–265

Scheele J (2001) Anatomical and atypical liver resections. Chirurg 72:113–124

Scheele J, Stangl R, Altendorf-Hofmann A (1990) Hepatic metastases from colorectal carcinoma: impact of surgical resection on the natural history. Br J Surg 77:1241–1246

Scheele J, Stangl R, Altendorf-Hofmann A (1994) Repeated hepatic resection for colorectal liver metastases. Eur J Surg Oncol 20:315–316

Scheele J, Altendorf-Hofmann A, Stangl R, et al (1996) Chirurgische Resektion kolorektaler Lebermetastasen: Goldstandard für solitäre und radikal resektable Herde. Swiss Surg (S4):4–17

Scheithauer W, Rosen H, Kornek G, et al (1993) Randomised comparison of combination chemotherapy plus supportive care with supportive care alone in patients with metastatic colorectal cancer. BMJ 306:752–755

Schimanski CC, Linnemann U, Galle PR, et al (2003) Hepatic disseminated tumor cells in colorectal cancer UICC stage 4 patients: prognostic implications. Int J Oncol 23:791–796

Seifert JK, Morris DL (1998) Cryotherapy of the resection edge after liver resection for colorectal cancer metastases. Aust N Z J Surg 68:725–728

Seifert JK, Staupendahl D, Junginger T (1997) Repeat interventions in metastases. Chirurg 68:247–254

Shen P, Hoffman A, Howerton R, et al (2002) Cryosurgery of close or positive margins after hepatic resection for primary and metastatic hepatobiliary malignancies. Am Surg 68:695–703

Shibata T, Niinobu T, Ogata N, et al (2000) Microwave coagulation therapy for multiple hepatic metastases from colorectal carcinoma. Cancer 89:276–284

Sigurdson ER, Ridge JA, Kemeny N, et al (1987) Tumor and liver drug uptake following hepatic artery and portal vein infusion. J Clin Oncol 5:1836–1840

Siperstein AE, Rogers JS, Machi J, et al (2002) Long-term follow-up of patients undergoing radiofrequency thermal ablation of primary metastatic liver tumors: A multi-center study. ACS 88th Annual Clinical Congress, 9-10-2002, San Francisco, CA

Solbiati L, Livraghi T, Goldberg SN, et al (2001) Percutaneous radio-frequency ablation of hepatic metastases from colorectal cancer: long-term results in 117 patients. Radiology 221:159–166

Staib L, Link KH, Beger HG (2001) Toxicity and effects of adjuvant therapy in colon cancer: results of the German prospective controlled randomized multicenter trial FOGT 1. J Gastrointest Surg 5:275–281

Steele G, Bleday R, Mayer RJ, et al (1991) A prospective evaluation of hepatic resection for colorectal carcinoma metastases to the liver: Gastrointestinal Tumor Study Group Protocol 6584. J Clin Oncol 9:1105–1112

Sugihara K, Hojo K, Moriya Y, et al (1993) Pattern of recurrence after hepatic resection for colorectal metastases. Br J Surg 80:1032–1035

Tanaka K, Adam R, Shimada H, et al (2003) Role of neoadjuvant chemotherapy in the treatment of multiple colorectal metastases to the liver. Br J Surg 90:963–969

Taylor FW (1962) Cancer of the colon and rectum: a study of routes of metastases and death. Surgery 52:305–308

Thirion P, Wolmark N, Haddad E, et al (1999) Survival impact of chemotherapy in patients with colorectal metastases confined to the liver: a re-analysis of 1458 non-operable patients randomised in 22 trials and 4 meta-analyses. Meta-analysis Group In Cancer. Ann Oncol 10:1317–1320

Tono T, Hasuike Y, Ohzato H, et al (2000) Limited but definite efficacy of prophylactic hepatic arterial infusion chemotherapy after curative resection of colorectal liver metastases: a randomized study. Cancer 88:1549–1556

Topal B, Kaufman L, Aerts R, et al (2003) Patterns of failure following curative resection of colorectal liver metastases. Eur J Surg Oncol 29:248–253

Tsujitani S, Watanabe A, Kakeji Y, et al (1991) Hepatic recurrence not prevented with low-dosage long-term intraportal 5-FU infusion after resection of colorectal liver metastasis. Eur J Surg Oncol 17:526–529

Vaillant JC, Balladur P, Nordlinger B, et al (1993) Repeat liver resection for recurrent colorectal metastases. Br J Surg 80:340–344

van Ooijen B, Wiggers T, Meijer S, et al (1992) Hepatic resections for colorectal metastases in The Netherlands. A multi-institutional 10-year study. Cancer 70:28–34

van Riel JM, van Groeningen CJ, Kedde MA, et al (2002) Continuous administration of irinotecan by hepatic arterial infusion: a phase I and pharmacokinetic study. Clin Cancer Res 8:405–412

Vlems FA, Diepstra JH, Punt CJ, et al (2003) Detection of disseminated tumour cells in blood and bone marrow samples of patients undergoing hepatic resection for metastasis of colorectal cancer. Br J Surg 90:989–995

Vogel KM (2000) Der natürliche Verlauf von Lebermetastasen kolorektaler Karzinome in abhängigkeit von mehreren prognostischen Kriterien. Medizinische Fakultät der Unversität Ulm, Ulm, Germany

Vogl TJ, Mack MG, Roggan A (2000) Magnetresonanztomographisch gesteuerte laserinduzierte Theramographie von Lebermetastasen. Dtsch Ärztebl 37:2039–2044

Vogl TJ, Straub R, Eichler K, et al (2004) Colorectal carcinoma metastases in liver: laser-induced interstitial thermotherapy – local tumor control rate and survival data. Radiology 230:450–458

Wadler S, Schwartz EL, Goldman M, et al (1989) Fluorouracil and recombinant alpha-2a-interferon: An active regimen against advanced colorectal carcinoma. J Clin Oncol 7:1769–1775

Wagner JG, Gyves JW, Stetson P, et al (1986) Steady-state nonlinear pharmacokinetics of 5-fluorouracil during hepatic arterial and intravenous infusion in cancer patients. Cancer Res 46:1499–1506

Wang JY, Chiang JM, Jeng LB, et al (1996) Resection of liver metastases from colorectal cancer: are there any truly significant clinical prognosticators? Dis Colon Rectum 39:847–851

Wein A, Riedel C, Bruckl W, et al (2003) Neoadjuvant treatment with weekly high-dose 5-fluorouracil as 24-hour infusion, folinic acid and oxaliplatin in patients with primary resectable liver metastases of colorectal cancer. Oncology 64:131–138

Weiss SM, Skibber JM, Mohiuddin M, et al (1985) Rapid intra-abdominal spread of pancreatic cancer. Influence of multiple operative biopsy procedures. Arch Surg 120:415–416

Weiss L, Ward PM (1991) Metachronous and synchronous seeding of target-organs in the mouse, after paracecal injection of colon-26 cancer cells: Is it relevant to human metastatic colorectal cancer? Reg Cancer Treat 4:55–59

Witte RS, Cnaan A, Mansour EG, et al (2001) Comparison of 5-fluorouracil alone, 5-fluorouracil with levamisole, and 5-fluorouracil with hepatic irradiation in the treatment of patients with residual, nonmeasurable, intra-abdominal metastasis after undergoing resection for colorectal carcinoma. Cancer 91:1020–1028

Yamaguchi J, Komuta K, Matsuzaki S, et al (2002a) Mode of infiltrative growth of colorectal liver metastases is a useful predictor of recurrence after hepatic resection. World J Surg 26:1122–1125

Yamaguchi J, Sakamoto I, Fukuda T, et al (2002b) Computed tomographic findings of colorectal liver metastases can be predictive for recurrence after hepatic resection. Arch Surg 137:1294–1297

Yan DB, Clingan P, Morris DL (2003) Hepatic cryotherapy and regional chemotherapy with or without resection for liver metastases from colorectal carcinoma: how many are too many? Cancer 98:320–330

Yedibela S, Jawad MK, Graz V, et al (2004) Vergleich der Indikation und Ergebnisse nach Resektion nicht-kolorektaler Lebermetastasen an der Chrirugischen Universitätsklinik Erlangen-Nuernberg bei 162 Patienten zwischen 1972 und 2001. 121. Kongress der Deutschen Gesellschaft für Chirurgie, 27–30 April, ICC, Berlin

27 Tumor Ablation: Interventional Management of Complications

RONALD S. ARELLANO, DEBRA A. GERVAIS, and PETER R. MUELLER

CONTENTS

27.1
Introduction

After approximately 10 years of clinical experience, radiofrequency ablation has become an established therapeutic option for the treatment of primary or metastatic hepatic malignancies. Whether performed as an open surgical procedure or by percutaneous methods, radiofrequency ablation offers minimally invasive therapy of malignant tumors without the 15%–30% morbidity associated with open surgical resection (FONG et al. 1995; MOLMENTI et al. 1999; STEELE et al. 1991). Nevertheless, even minimally invasive therapies have associated risks and potential complications. In the case of radiofrequency ablation of the liver, potential complications derive from two broad categories: (a) direct physical injury as a result of placement of the electrode into the liver and (b) thermal-induced injury of the liver or related structures as a result of treatment (Fig. 27.1) (RHIM et al. 2003). In addition, preexisting conditions such as prior abdominal surgery or impaired liver function can also adversely affect the outcome of ablative therapy. However, other complications associated with thermal ablation of the liver require treatment and intervention beyond the skill of the interventional radiologist. Thermal injuries of the

skin, for example, can develop from improper placement or insufficient surface area of grounding pads and should be managed by a dermatologist or surgeon who specializes in burn injuries (GOLDBERG et al. 2000; STEINKE et al. 2003; YAMAGAMI et al. 2002). Metabolic derangement such as electrolyte imbalances, liver failure or hepatorenal syndrome can develop following treatment of primary or metastatic liver tumors (KELTNER et al. 2001; SHANKAR et al. 2002; VERHOEVEN et al. 2002).

Treatment of these conditions requires consultation from medical specialists in hepatology and nephrology.

In many cases, complications are minor and do not result in adverse sequelae or prolonged hospitalization. Major complications, on the other hand, can be life threatening and therefore often require additional, unplanned or prolonged therapy and hos-

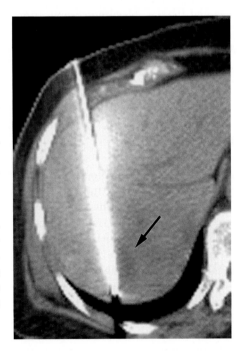

Fig. 27.1 Axial CT image of the liver demonstrating radiofrequency electrode within lesion in VII segment (*black arrow*)

R. ARELLANO, MD; D. A. GERVAIS, MD; P. R. MUELLER, MD
Department of Radiology, Massachusetts General Hospital, Division of Abdominal Imaging and Intervention, 55 Fruit Street, White 270, Boston, MA 02114, USA

pitalization (BURKE et al. 2003). The management of some radiofrequency induced major complications, such as hepatic failure or bowel perforation are beyond the expertise and skill of the interventional radiologist. However, several procedure-related major complications can be safely and effectively treated by percutaneous means. Therefore, recognition and experience with interventional management of radiofrequency related complications are essential in order to provide optimum patient care. This chapter will discuss the percutaneous management of complications associated with image-guided radiofrequency ablation of hepatic malignancies.

27.2
Complications

Major complication rates for image-guided percutaneous radiofrequency ablation range from 2.2-9.6% (BUSCARINI and BUSCARINI 2004; LIVRAGHI and MELONI 2002; DE BAERE et al. 2003; RHIM et al. 2003). While these rates compare favorably with to surgical resection, radiofrequency-induced complications can have a significant impact on patient care. Major complications that require additional interventional management include hepatic abscess, biliary-related complications such as bilomas, biliary strictures and fistulas, bleeding complications and complications involving the lung and the pleural space. Other complications such as skin burns, metabolic dysfunction and pain require medical management for resolution.

27.2.1
Hepatobiliary Complications

The liver and bile ducts are prone to procedure related complications due to direct injury by placement of the radiofrequency electrode and by the creation of devitalized hepatic tissue. Hepatic abscesses and bilomas derive from both mechanisms and must be suspected in any patient who develops significant pain or clinical signs of septicemia (i.e. tachycardia, fever, leukocytosis) beyond the first 2–4 weeks of the procedure. Adherence to strict sterile technique is essential in order to minimize the potentially life-threatening complication of overwhelming septicemia. Prophylactic intravenous antibiotics may further minimize the risk of post-procedure infections, though this practice remains controversial.

When an abscess is suspected, cross-sectional imaging with computed tomography imaging is necessary to localize and define the extent of disease.

Intralesional air that is generated within the lesion during treatment should resolve within 1 month of the treatment (LIM et al. 2001). Therefore, any fluid, air, or air-fluid levels within the treated lesion beyond the normal expectation should be regarded with clinical suspicion, especially accompanied by clinical signs and symptoms of infection (Fig. 27.2) (TITTON et al. 2003). Hepatic abscesses develop in up to 3% patients who undergo radiofrequency ablation for hepatic tumors (DE BAERE et al. 2000). Patients with preexisting biliary-enteric anastomoses may be more prone to develop postablation abscesses. Retrograde enteric flow into the biliary tree, altered lymphatic periportal drainage and vascular resection may all limit the effectiveness natural mechanisms to control spread of infectious organisms (SHIBATA et al. 2003). Patients with preexisting bile duct biliary stones or strictures may also be predisposed to hepatic abscess formation (ZAGORIA et al. 2002). Biliary strictures and obstruction have been described following radiofrequency treatment and centrally located lesions may result in clinically significant biliary complications (MULIER et al. 2002; RHIM et al. 2003). Treatment of hepatic abscesses or bilomas involves the combination of percutaneous drainage and intravenous antibiotics.

Drainage catheters of sufficient size (i.e. 8–14 F) to effectively drain purulent material can be placed using computed tomography, ultrasound or a combination ultrasound and fluoroscopic guidance (Fig. 27.3). Drainage catheters should be flushed on a daily basis

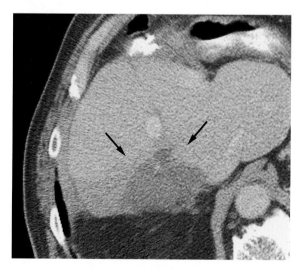

Fig. 27.2. Axial CT scan of the liver that demonstrates a low attenuation fluid collection 1 month following radiofrequency ablation (*black arrows*)

in order to ensure patency and to prevent encrustation of debris at the catheter tip. A sudden drop in the daily output may indication tube malposition, kinking or clogging, all of which require tube replacement or repositioning in order to restore drainage. Alternatively, persistently high output may be due to communication with the bile ducts in the setting of central obstruction (Figs. 27.4, 27.5) (TITTON et al. 2003). In such cases, a combination of percutaneous and endoscopic drainage may be necessary to achieve complete resolution (CURLEY et al. 2004; SHANKAR et al. 2003; SHIBATA et al. 2003; STIPPEL et al. 2003).

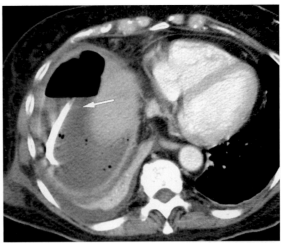

Fig. 27.5 Axial CT scan of the liver demonstrating drainage catheter within the biloma (*arrow*)

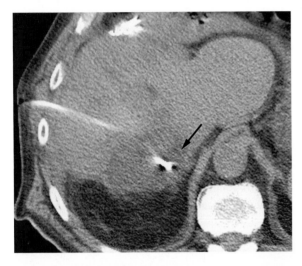

Fig. 27.3. Axial CT scan of the liver following percutaneous drainage of hepatic abscess, which developed following radiofrequency ablation (*arrow*)

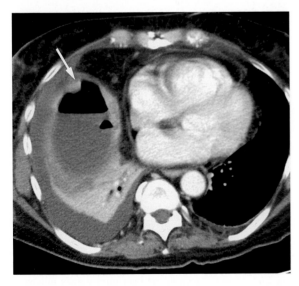

Fig. 27.4. Axial CT scan of the liver demonstrates large biloma, which developed following radiofrequency ablation for hepatocellular carcinoma (*arrow*)

27.2.2
Thoracic Complications

Thoracic complications can result from treatment of subcapsular lesions situated high in the hepatic dome. Treatment of hepatic dome lesions is technically challenging and potentially risky due to several factors, including the proximity of the diaphragm and lung, long trajectory from the skin to the lesion and difficulty in localizing lesions with imaging, especially when using ultrasound guidance. In order to overcome these limitations, several authors have described various techniques, which aid in detecting and isolating domes lesions in order to avoid potentially fatal complications (CURLEY et al. 2004; SHANKAR et al. 2003; SHIBATA et al. 2003; STIPPEL et al. 2003). Transpleural or transthoracic treatment of hepatic dome lesions can result in hemothorax, pleural effusions or pneumothorax (Fig. 27.6). Small, non-expanding pneumothoraces seldom lead to adverse clinical consequences and therefore can be treated conservatively. This is true as long as oxygenation is unaffected and the patient remains hemodynamically stable. On the other hand, patients who have severe or chronic underlying pulmonary disease often cannot tolerate even minor changes in respiratory dynamics. In this subgroup of patients, evacuation of the pleural air with needle aspiration or catheter drainage is necessary in order to restore normal respiration. Similarly, symptomatic pleural effusions and/or hemothoraces can be treated with thoracentesis using with small bore catheters or with thoracostomy.

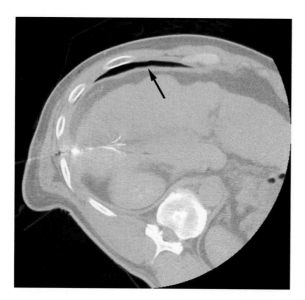

Fig. 27.6. Axial CT scan of the liver during radiofrequency ablation demonstrates a small pneumothorax that developed following placement of the radiofrequency electrode (*arrow*). The patient remained asymptomatic during the treatment and no treatment was necessary. In patients with underlying pulmonary disease, even small pneumothoraces can be symptomatic and may require thoracentesis or thoracostomy

27.2.3
Bleeding Complications

Bleeding complications arise as a result of needle puncture across the hepatic capsule (Fig. 27.7). Radiofrequency electrodes range in size from 14–15 gauge. Each puncture across the capsule creates the potential for bleeding. In addition, patients with hepatocellular carcinoma frequently have an underlying coagulopathy due to cirrhosis and compromised hepatic function. As a result, coagulation factors synthesized by the liver can be chronically low, causing prolongation of the prothrombin time and an increase in the international normalized ratio (INR). Added to this is the frequent finding in cirrhotic patients of hypersplenism and thrombocytopenia, which can lead to chronically low levels of circulating platelets. While no standardized algorithm exists for managing patients with coagulopathy, every effort should be made to correct a bleeding diathesis whenever possible. Intramuscular injections of vitamin K and infusions of fresh frozen plasma are indicated to correct a prolonged prothrombin time. A threshold platelet count of greater than 50,000/cm^3 is recommended prior to puncture across the hepatic capsule.

Procedure related bleeding can occur in several locations: (a) subcapsular, (b) intrahepatic, (c) intraperitoneal (BUSCARINI and BUSCARINI 2004; CURLEY et al. 2004; de BAERE et al. 2003; MULIER et al. 2002; RHIM et al. 2003; WOOD et al. 2000; ZAGORIA et al. 2002). Subcapsular and intrahepatic hematomas are usually self limiting and seldom require percutaneous intervention. Transfusions are indicated when sufficiently large subcapsular hematomas lower the hematocrit value to levels where the patient may experience hypotension. In the acute setting, drainage of large subcapsular hematomas may remove a natural tamponading mechanism that controls further bleeding and therefore drainage of fresh hematomas is not recommended. However, chronic hematomas cause pain due to capsular irritation or if they are suspected of becoming superinfected, and then image-guided percutaneous drainage is indicated. Drainage with a 10–14 F catheter is usually sufficient for complete evacuation of liquefied hematomas.

In contrast to subcapsular hematomas, intraperitoneal bleeding can rapidly evolve into an emergency situation; therefore, close hemodynamic monitoring by the anesthetist or the interventional nurse is essential to detect for signs of intraperitoneal hemorrhage. Clinically suspected acute hemorrhage can be confirmed by the detection of new high

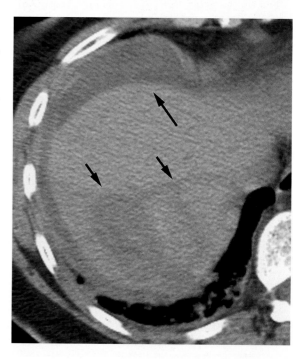

Fig. 27.7. Axial CT scan of the liver immediately following treatment, which demonstrates new fluid adjacent to the liver edge (*long black arrow*). The *small black arrows* point to the thermal lesion in the treated liver

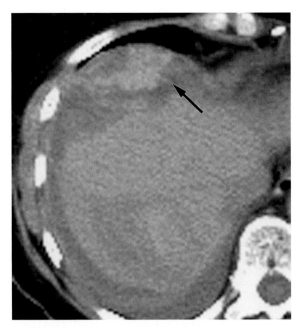

Fig. 27.8. Axial CT scan of the liver obtained 24 h after radiofrequency treatment. The *black arrow* points to new high density fluid adjacent to the liver, consistent with acute hemorrhage

density by computed tomography or by the development of complex fluid by ultrasound (Fig. 27.8). Immediately life-threatening intraperitoneal hemorrhage requires volume resuscitation and prompt control of the bleeding source. This subgroup of patients can be evaluated with angiography to identify and control the source of bleeding with embolization. Slower intraperitoneal bleeding can be managed more conservatively by following serial hematocrit levels, correcting any existing coagulopathies and by transfusions. Delayed bleeding complications from pseudoaneurysms of the hepatic arteries, have been described following treatment of colorectal metastases. These were successfully treated with coil embolization (BILCHIK et al. 2001). Transient thrombosis of the portal vein has been described as a consequence of radiofrequency ablation but this does not require interventional management (NG et al. 2003; ZHENG et al. 2003).

27.3
Conclusion

Of the potential complications associated with radiofrequency ablation of hepatic tumors, few require interventional management for resolution. As described above, these include hepatic abscesses, complications related to the biliary tree or collections, which develop in the pleura space. In almost all cases, resolution can be safely and effectively achieved with simple catheter drainage or other minimally invasive techniques.

References

Bilchik AJ, Wood TF, Allegra DP (2001) Radiofrequency ablation of unresectable hepatic malignancies: lessons learned. Oncologist 6:24–33

Burke DR, Lewis CA, Cardella JF, et al (2003). Quality improvement guidelines for percutaneous transhepatic cholangiography and biliary drainage. J Vasc Interv Radiol 14:S243–246

Buscarini E, Buscarini L (2004) Radiofrequency thermal ablation with expandable needle of focal liver malignancies: complication report. Eur Radiol 14:31–37

Curley SA, Marra P, Beaty K, et al (2004) Early and late complications after radiofrequency ablation of malignant liver tumors in 608 patients. Ann Surg 239:450–458

de Baere T, Elias D, Dromain C, et al (2000) Radiofrequency ablation of 100 hepatic metastases with a mean follow-up of more than 1 year. AJR Am J Roentgenol 175:1619–1625

de Baere T, Risse O, Kuoch V, et al (2003) Adverse events during radiofrequency treatment of 582 hepatic tumors. AJR Am J Roentgenol 18:695–700

Fong Y, Blumgart LH, Cohen AM (1995) Surgical treatment of colorectal metastases to the liver. CA Cancer J Clin 45:50–62

Goldberg SN, Solbiati L, Halpern EF, et al (2000) Variables affecting proper system grounding for radiofrequency ablation in an animal model. J Vasc Interv Radiol 11:1069–1075

Ishikawa T, Kohno T, Shibayama T, et al (2001) Thoracoscopic thermal ablation therapy for hepatocellular carcinoma located beneath the diaphragm. Endoscopy 33:697–702

Kapoor BS, Hunter DW (2003) Injection of subphrenic saline during radiofrequency ablation to minimize diaphragmatic injury. Cardiovasc Intervent Radiol 26:302–304

Keltner JR, Donegan E, Hynson JM, et al (2001) Acute renal failure after radiofrequency liver ablation of metastatic carcinoid tumor. Anesth Analg 93:587–589

Koda M, Ueki M, Maeda N, et al (2003) Diaphragmatic perforation and hernia after hepatic radiofrequency ablation. AJR Am J Roentgenol 180:1561–1562

Lim HK, Choi D, Lee WJ, et al (2001) Hepatocellular carcinoma treated with percutaneous radio-frequency ablation: evaluation with follow-up multiphase helical CT. Radiology 221:447–454

Livraghi T, Meloni F (2002) Treatment of hepatocellular carcinoma by percutaneous interventional methods. Hepatogastroenterology 49:62–71

Molmenti EP, Marsh JW, Dvorchik I, et al (1999) Hepatobiliary malignancies. Primary hepatic malignant neoplasms. Surg Clin North Am 79:43–57

Mulier S, Mulier P, Ni Y, et al (2002) Complications of radiofrequency coagulation of liver tumours. Br J Surg 89:1206–1222

Ng KK, Lam CM, Poon RT, et al (2003) Portal vein thrombosis after radiofrequency ablation for recurrent hepatocellular carcinoma. Asian J Surg 26:50–54

Rhim H, Yoon KH, Lee JM, et al (2003) Major complications after radio-frequency thermal ablation of hepatic tumors: spectrum of imaging findings. Radiographics 23:123–134

Schmidt-Mutter C, Breining T, Gangi A, et al (2003) Fatal bile pulmonary embolism after radiofrequency treatment of a hepatocellular carcinoma. Surg Endosc 17:2028–2031

Shankar S, Tuncali K, van Sonnenberg E, et al (2002) Myoglobinemia after CT-guided radiofrequency ablation of a hepatic metastasis. AJR Am J Roentgenol 178:359–361

Shankar S, van Sonnenberg E, Silverman SG, et al (2003) Diagnosis and treatment of intrahepatic biloma complicating radiofrequency ablation of hepatic metastases. AJR Am J Roentgenol 181:475–477

Shibata T, Iimuro Y, Ikai I, et al (2002) Percutaneous radiofrequency ablation therapy after intrathoracic saline solution infusion for liver tumor in the hepatic dome. J Vasc Interv Radiol 13:313–315

Shibata T, Yamamoto Y, Yamamoto N, et al (2003) Cholangitis and liver abscess after percutaneous ablation therapy for liver tumors: incidence and risk factors. J Vasc Interv Radiol 14:1535–1542

Steele G Jr, Bleday R, Mayer RJ, et al (1991) A prospective evaluation of hepatic resection for colorectal carcinoma metastases to the liver: gastrointestinal tumor study group protocol 6584. J Clin Oncol 9:1105–1112

Steinke K, Gananadha S, King J, et al (2003) Dispersive pad site burns with modern radiofrequency ablation equipment. Surg Laparosc Endosc Percutan Tech 13:366–371

Stippel DL, Tox U, Gossmann A, et al (2003) Successful treatment of radiofrequency-induced biliary lesions by interventional endoscopic retrograde cholangiography (ERC). Surg Endosc 17:1965–1970

Takeda Y, Hasuike Y, Ohmori S, et al (2002) Transdiaphragmatic radiofrequency ablation of malignant liver tumors. Gan To Kagaku Ryoho 29:2229–2233

Titton RL, Gryzenia PC, Gervais DA, et al (2003) Interventional radiology case conferences Massachusetts General Hospital. Continuous high-output drainage of hepatic abscess 3 months after radiofrequency ablation of hepatocellular carcinoma. AJR Am J Roentgenol 180:1079–1084

Verhoeven BH, Haagsma EB, Appeltans BM, et al (2002) Hyperkalaemia after radiofrequency ablation of hepatocellular carcinoma. Eur J Gastroenterol Hepatol 14:1023–1024

Wood TF, Rose DM, Chung M, et al (2000) Radiofrequency ablation of 231 unresectable hepatic tumors: indications, limitations, and complications. Ann Surg Oncol 7:593–600

Yamagami T, Nakamura T, Kato T, et al (2002) Skin injury after radiofrequency ablation for hepatic cancer. AJR Am J Roentgenol 178:905–907

Zagoria RJ, Chen MY, Shen P, et al (2002) Complications from radiofrequency ablation of liver metastases. Am Surg 68:204–209

Zheng RQ, Kudo M, Inui K, et al (2003) Transient portal vein thrombosis caused by radiofrequency ablation for hepatocellular carcinoma. J Gastroenterol 38:101–103

Subject Index

List of Contributors

ANDREAS ADAM, MB, BS, FRCP, FRCR, FRCS
Department of Radiology
St. Thomas' Hospital
Lambeth Palace Road
London SE1 7EH
UK

THOMAS ALBRECHT, MD
Department of Radiology and Nuclear Medicine
Campus Benjamin Franklin, Charité
Universitätsmedizin Berlin
Hindenburgdamm 30
12200 Berlin
Germany

VOLKER APELL, MD
Surgical Center
Asklepios Paulinen Klinik (APK) and
Asklepios Tumortreatment Center Rhein-Main (ATC)
Geisenheimerstrasse 10D
65197 Wiesbaden
Germany

RONALD S. ARELLANO, MD
Department of Radiology
Massachusetts General Hospital
Division of Abdominal Imaging and Intervention
55 Fruit St, White 270
Boston, MA 02114
USA

CARLO BARTOLOZZI, MD
Division of Diagnostic and Interventional Radiology
Department of Oncology, Transplants,
and Advanced Technologies in Medicine
University of Pisa
Via Roma 67
56126 Pisa
Italy

RAFFAELLA BASILICO, MD
Department of Radiology
Imaging Sciences Department
University G. D'Annunzio
Via dei Vestini
66013 Chieti
Italy

ELISA BATINI, MD
Division of Diagnostic and Interventional Radiology
Department of Oncology, Transplants,
and Advanced Technologies in Medicine
University of Pisa
Via Roma 67
56126 Pisa
Italy

MASSIMO BAZZOCCHI, MD
Institute of Radiology
University of Udine
Via Colugna 50
33100 Udine
Italy

CHRISTOPH D. BECKER, MD
Division of Diagnostic and Interventional Radiology
Geneva University Hospital
24, Rue Micheli du Crest
1211 Geneva 14
Switzerland

LUIGI BOLONDI, MD
Division of Internal Medicine
Department of Internal Medicine and Gastroenterology
University of Bologna
Via Albertoni 15
40138 Bologna
Italy

MARIA PIA BONDIONI, MD
Department of Radiology
University of Brescia
Spedali Civili di Brescia
Piazzale Spedali Civili 1
25023 Brescia
Italy

GIUSEPPE BRANCATELLI, MD
Department of Radiology
Policlinico Universitario
Via del Vespro 127
90127 Palermo
Italy

LORENZO BONOMO, MD
Department of Radiology
Imaging Sciences Department
Catholic University
Policlinico A. Gemelli
Largo A. Gemelli 8
00168 Rome
Italy

FILIPE CASEIRO-ALVES, MD, PhD
Department of Radiology
Faculdade de Medicina de Coimbra
Praceta Mota Pinto
3000 Coimbra
Portugal

MICHELA CELESTRE, MD
Department of Radiological Sciences
University of Rome "La Sapienza"
Policlinico Umberto I
Viale Regina Elena 324
00161 Rome
Italy

DANIA CIONI, MD
Division of Diagnostic and Interventional Radiology
Department of Oncology, Transplants,
and Advanced Technologies in Medicine
University of Pisa
Via Roma 67
56126 Pisa
Italy

MASSIMO COLOMBO, MD
Department of Gastroenterology and Endocrinology
IRCCS Maggiore Hospital
University of Milan
Via Pace 9
20122 Milano
Italy

ANDREA CONTI, MD
Division of Diagnostic and Interventional Radiology
Department of Oncology, Transplants,
and Advanced Technologies in Medicine
University of Pisa
Via Roma 67
56126 Pisa
Italy

DAVID O. COSGROVE, MD
Department of Imaging Sciences
Imperial College School of Medicine
Hammersmith Hospital
150, Du Cane Road
London W12 0HS
UK

LAURA CROCETTI, MD
Division of Diagnostic and Interventional Radiology
Department of Oncology, Transplants,
and Advanced Technologies in Medicine
University of Pisa
Via Roma 67
56126 Pisa
Italy

CHIARA DEL FRATE, MD
Institute of Radiology
University of Udine
Via Colugna 50
33100 Udine
Italy

CLOTILDE DELLA PINA, MD
Division of Diagnostic and Interventional Radiology
Department of Oncology, Transplants,
and Advanced Technologies in Medicine
University of Pisa
Via Roma 67
56126 Pisa
Italy

ANTONIA D'ERRICO, MD
Department of Pathology
Institute of Oncology F. Addarii
University of Bologna
Via Massarenti 9
40138 Bologna
Italy

FRANCESCA DI FABIO, MD
Department of Radiology
Imaging Sciences Department
University G. D'Annunzio
Via dei Vestini
66013 Chieti
Italy

KATHRIN EICHLER, MD
Department of Diagnostic and Interventional Radiology
University Hospital Frankfurt
Johann Wolfgang Goethe University
Theodor-Stern-Kai 7
60590 Frankfurt/Main
Germany

JEAN FASEL, MD
Department of Anatomy
University Hospitals of Geneva
24, Rue Micheli du Crest
1211 Geneva 14
Switzerland

MICHAEL P. FEDERLE, MD
Department of Radiology
Abdominal Imaging Offices
University of Pittsburgh Medical Center
Room 4660, CHP, MT,
200 Lothrop Street
Pittsburgh, PA 15213
USA

ANA FERREIRA, MD
Department of Radiology
Hospital Universitade de Coimbra
Praceta Mota Pinto
3000 Coimbra
Portugal

ANTONELLA FILIPPONE, MD
Department of Radiology
Imaging Sciences Department
University G. D'Annunzio
Via dei Vestini
66013 Chieti
Italy

DEBRA A. GERVAIS, MD
Department of Radiology
Massachusetts General Hospital
Division of Abdominal Imaging and Intervention
55 Fruit St, White 270
Boston, MA 02114
USA

ALICE R. GILLAMS, MD
Department of Medical Imaging
The Middlesex Hospital
Mortimer Street
London W1T 3AA
UK

J. ANTONY GOODE, MD
Department of Interventional Radiology
St Thomas' Hospital
Lambeth Palace Road
London SE1 7EH
UK

LUIGI GRAZIOLI, MD
Department of Radiology
University of Brescia
Spedali Civili di Brescia
Piazzale Spedali Civili 1
25023 Brescia
Italy

RENATE M. HAMMERSTINGL, MD
Department of Diagnostic and Interventional Radiology
J.W. Goethe University
University Hospital Frankfurt
Theodor-Stern-Kai 7
60590 Frankfurt/Main
Germany

THOMAS K. HELMBERGER, MD
Institute of Clinical Radiology
Klinikum Grosshadern
Ludwig Maximilians University
Marchioninistrasse 15
81377 Munich
Germany

MATTHIAS HOLTAPPELS, MD
Surgical Center
Asklepios Paulinen Klinik (APK) and
Asklepios Tumortreatment Center Rhein-Main (ATC)
Geisenheimerstrasse 10D
65197 Wiesbaden
Germany

KLAUS MARIA JOSTEN, MD
Interdisciplinary Outpatient Oncology
Asklepios Paulinen Klinik (APK) and
Asklepios Tumortreatment Center Rhein-Main (ATC)
Geisenheimerstrasse 10D
65197 Wiesbaden
Germany

CHRISTIANE KULINNA, MD
Department of Radiology
Medical University of Vienna
AKH Vienna
Waehringer Guertel 18-20
1090 Vienna
Austria

ROBERTO LAGALLA, MD
Department of Radiology
Policlinico Universitario
Via del Vespro 127
90127 Palermo
Italy

ANDREA LAGHI, MD
Department of Radiological Sciences
University of Rome "La Sapienza"
Policlinico Umberto I
Viale Regina Elena 324
00161 Rome
Italy

THOMAS LEHNERT, MD
Department of Diagnostic and Interventional Radiology
University Hospital Frankfurt
Johann Wolfgang Goethe University
Theodor-Stern-Kai 7
60590 Frankfurt/Main
Germany

RICCARDO LENCIONI, MD
Division of Diagnostic and Interventional Radiology
Department of Oncology, Transplants,
and Advanced Technologies in Medicine
University of Pisa
Via Roma 67
56126 Pisa
Italy

SIMONA LEONI, MD
Division of Internal Medicine
Department of Internal Medicine and Gastroenterology
University of Bologna
Via Albertoni 15
40138 Bologna
Italy

JACOPO LERA, MD
Division of Diagnostic and Interventional Radiology
Department of Oncology, Transplants,
and Advanced Technologies in Medicine
University of Pisa
Via Roma 67
56126 Pisa
Italy

KARL HEINRICH LINK, MD, PhD
Surgical Center
Asklepios Paulinen Klinik (APK) and
Asklepios Tumortreatment Center Rhein-Main (ATC)
Geisenheimerstrasse 10D
65197 Wiesbaden
Germany

PIERRE LOUBEYRE, MD
Department of Radiology
University Hospitals of Geneva
24, Rue Micheli du Crest
1211 Geneva 14
Switzerland

MARTIN MACK, MD
Department of Diagnostic and Interventional Radiology
University Hospital Frankfurt
Johann Wolfgang Goethe University
Theodor-Stern-Kai 7
60590 Frankfurt/Main
Germany

PIETRO MAJNO, MD
Departments of Surgery and Transplantation
University Hospitals of Geneva
24, Rue Micheli du Crest
1211 Geneva 14
Switzerland

DIDER MATHIEU, MD, PhD
Centre de Radiologie
Boulevard de la Republique 1
13100 Aix en Provence
France

GILLES MENTHA, MD
Departments of Surgery and Transplantation
University Hospitals of Geneva
24, Rue Micheli du Crest
1211 Geneva 14
Switzerland

MASSIMO MIDIRI, MD
Department of Radiology
Policlinico Universitario
Via del Vespro 127
90127 Palermo
Italy

MATTHIAS MÖRSCHEL, MD
Surgical Center
Asklepios Paulinen Klinik (APK) and
Asklepios Tumortreatment Center Rhein-Main (ATC)
Geisenheimerstrasse 10D
65197 Wiesbaden
Germany

SARA MONTAGNANI, MD
Division of Diagnostic and Interventional Radiology
Department of Oncology, Transplants,
and Advanced Technologies in Medicine
University of Pisa
Via Roma 67
56126 Pisa
Italy

PHILIPPE MOREL, MD
Departments of Surgery and Transplantation
University Hospitals of Geneva
24, Rue Micheli du Crest
1211 Geneva 14
Switzerland

KOENRAAD MORTELÈ, MD
Division of Abdominal Imaging and Intervention
Department of Radiology
Brigham and Women's Hospital
Francis Street 75
02115 Boston, MA
USA

PETER R. MUELLER, MD
Department of Radiology
Massachusetts General Hospital
Division of Abdominal Imaging and Intervention
55 Fruit St, White 270
Boston, MA 02114
USA

PASQUALE PAOLANTONIO, MD
Department of Radiological Sciences
University of Rome "La Sapienza"
Policlinico Umberto I
Viale Regina Elena 324
00161 Rome
Italy

ROBERTO PASSARIELLO, MD
Department of Radiological Sciences
University of Rome "La Sapienza"
Policlinico Umberto I
Viale Regina Elena 324
00161 Rome
Italy

FABIO PISCAGLIA, MD
Division of Internal Medicine
Department of Internal Medicine and Gastroenterology
University of Bologna
Via Albertoni 15
40138 Bologna
Italy

ROBERTO POZZI-MUCELLI, MD
Department of Radiology
University of Trieste
Cattinara's Hospital
Via Strada di Fiume 447
34149 Trieste
Italy

ERIKA ROCCHI, MD
Division of Diagnostic and Interventional Radiology
Department of Oncology, Transplants,
and Advanced Technologies in Medicine
University of Pisa
Via Roma 67
56126 Pisa
Italy

GUIDO RONCHI, MD
Department of Gastroenterology and Endocrinology
IRCCS Maggiore Hospital
University of Milan
Via Pace 9
20122 Milano
Italy

Tarun Sabharwal, MD
Department of Interventional Radiology
St Thomas' Hospital
Lambeth Palace Road
London SE1 7EH
UK

Tolga Atilla Sagban, MD
Surgical Center
Asklepios Paulinen Klinik (APK) and
Asklepios Tumortreatment Center Rhein-Main (ATC)
Geisenheimerstrasse 10D
65197 Wiesbaden
Germany

Ilaria Sansoni, MD
Department of Radiological Sciences
University of Rome "La Sapienza"
Policlinico Umberto I
Viale Regina Elena 324
00161 Rome
Italy

Wolfgang Schima, MD
Department of Radiology
Medical University of Vienna
AKH Vienna
Waehringer Guertel 18-20
1090 Vienna
Austria

Wolfram V. Schwarz, MD
Department of Diagnostic and Interventional Radiology
J.W. Goethe University
University Hospital Frankfurt
Theodor-Stern-Kai 7
60590 Frankfurt/Main
Germany

Ludger Staib, MD
Department of Surgery I and
Ulm Cancer Center
University of Ulm
89075 Ulm
Germany

Ralf Straub, MD
Department of Diagnostic and Interventional Radiology
University Hospital Frankfurt
Johann Wolfgang Goethe University
Theodor-Stern-Kai 7
60590 Frankfurt/Main
Germany

Sylvain Terraz, MD
Division of Diagnostic and Interventional Radiology
Geneva University Hospital
24, Rue Micheli du Crest
1211 Geneva 14
Switzerland

Ralf Thimm, MD
Department of Radiology
Asklepios Paulinen Klinik (APK) and
Asklepios Tumortreatment Center Rhein-Main (ATC)
Geisenheimerstrasse 10D
65197 Wiesbaden
Germany

Klaus Tischbirek, MD
Department Medical Oncology and Gastroenterology
Asklepios Paulinen Klinik (APK) and
Asklepios Tumortreatment Center Rhein-Main (ATC)
Geisenheimerstrasse 10D
65197 Wiesbaden
Germany

Annamaria Venturi, MD
Division of Internal Medicine
Department of Internal Medicine and Gastroenterology
University of Bologna
Via Albertoni 15
40138 Bologna
Italy

Valérie Vilgrain, MD
Department of Radiology
Hopital Beaujon
Avenue du General Leclerc 100
92118 Clichy Cedex
France

Thomas J. Vogl, MD
Department of Diagnostic and Interventional Radiology
University Hospital Frankfurt
Johann Wolfgang Goethe University
Theodor-Stern-Kai 7
60590 Frankfurt/Main
Germany

Thomas Friedrich Weigel, MD
Surgical Center
Asklepios Paulinen Klinik (APK) and
Asklepios Tumortreatment Center Rhein-Main (ATC)
Geisenheimerstrasse 10D
65197 Wiesbaden
Germany

Karim Zayed, MD
Surgical Center
Asklepios Paulinen Klinik (APK) and
Asklepios Tumortreatment Center Rhein-Main (ATC)
Geisenheimerstrasse 10D
65197 Wiesbaden
Germany

Chiara Zuiani, MD
Institute of Radiology
University of Udine
Via Colugna 50
33100 Udine
Italy

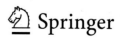

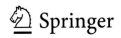 Springer

Printing and Binding: Stürtz GmbH, Würzburg